Most Commons in
Medicine

Most Commons in Medicine

■ **Edward F. Goljan, MD**
Professor and Chairman of Pathology
Oklahoma State University
College of Osteopathic Medicine
Tulsa, Oklahoma

W.B. SAUNDERS COMPANY
A Harcourt Health Sciences Company
Philadelphia ■ London ■ New York ■ Toronto ■ St. Louis ■ Sydney

W.B. SAUNDERS COMPANY
A Harcourt Health Sciences Company

The Curtis Center
Independence Square West
Philadelphia, Pennsylvania 19106

Library of Congress Cataloging-in-Publication Data

Most commons in medicine / Edward F. Goljan.

p.   cm.

ISBN 0–7216–8759–8

1. Clinical medicine—Handbooks, manuals, etc.   I. Title.
   [DNLM: 1. Clinical Medicine—Handbooks. WB 39 G626m 2000]

RC55.G565 2000 616—dc21

DNLM/DLC   99-048221

MOST COMMONS IN MEDICINE   ISBN 0–7216–8759–8

Printed in the United States of America.

Last digit is the print number: 9 8 7 6 5 4 3 2 1

This book is dedicated to my wife Joyce and our children—Keith, Lauren, and Renee—who epitomize the following quotes in the Psalms: *"Your wife shall be as a fruitful vine in your house and your children like olive plants around your table. Yes, children are a heritage of the Lord, and the fruit of the womb is His reward."* (Psalms 128:3, 127:3.)

■ PREFACE

Most Commons in Medicine is one of five books scheduled for the *Most Commons* series. The series includes *Most Commons in Pathology and Laboratory Medicine* (already available) and in Medicine, Surgery (in preparation), Pediatrics, and Obstetrics and Gynecology.

In the author's opinion, which is based on over 8 years of teaching USMLE step 1 and step 2 board reviews throughout the United States, there are very few concise review books that specifically target third and fourth year medical students who are fulfilling required clinical rotations through internal medicine. Major areas that are lacking in most of the available internal medicine review books and that are present in this *Most Commons in Medicine* include physical diagnosis, laboratory medicine, medical statistics (e.g., sensitivity, specificity), medical genetics, preventive medicine (e.g., immunizations, adult screening, nutrition), infectious disease arranged by systems, and USMLE steps 2 and 3 types of questions that focus on integration of the material.

In *Most Commons in Medicine,* the material is arranged in a tabular format with a Most Common column on the left and an Answer and Explanation column on the right. The most common cause of—e.g., sign/symptom of—in the left hand column is followed by a concise answer and explanation in the right hand column, with the leading cause/sign always in bold type and less common causes/signs in italics. Every aspect of a disease or topic is covered, including pathogenesis, signs and symptoms, complications, laboratory diagnosis, and management. A review question, answer, and discussion are at the end of every table. In most cases, the question has a multiple answer type format (e.g., SELECT 3 ANSWERS), similar to those currently used on the USMLE step 2 and step 3 examinations. An extensive index is provided at the end of the book that cross-references items that are present in different tables and chapters. The book is pocket-sized, which makes it available for quick reference.

Edward F. Goljan, M.D.

■ CONTENTS

CHAPTER

CLINICAL DECISION MAKING

CONTENTS

Table 1–1. LABORATORY TEST CHARACTERISTICS

Most Common...	Answer and Explanation
reasons for ordering lab tests	• *screen asymptomatic people*: e.g., * CH, * HDL, • *screen symptomatic people*: e.g., stress ECG for exertional angina • *confirm disease*: e.g., serum troponin-I in AMI, • *monitor disease or drug levels*: e.g., * glycosylated HbA_{1c} for glycemic control in DM, * digoxin levels
rationale for screening asymptomatic patients	• *disease has a high prevalence,* • *disease has a high morbidity/mortality,* • *effective therapy exists,* • *early detection is possible,* • *screening tests are inexpensive*
nomenclature for patient test results	• *true positive* (TP): patient with disease, • *false negative* (FN): normal test result in a patient with disease, • *true negative* (TN): person without disease, • *false positive* (FP): positive test result in a person without disease
use of a test with 100% sensitivity	*screen for disease*: e.g., serum ANA for SLE [Sensitivity = the chance a test is positive in a patient with disease: $$\frac{TP}{TP + FN} \times 100$$ A test with 100% sensitivity has no FNs. Negative test results exclude disease, while positive test results are either a TP or an FP ("includes and excludes disease"). No patient with disease is excluded when the test has 100% sensitivity.]

Table continued on following page

Table 1–1. LABORATORY TEST CHARACTERISTICS
Continued

Most Common...	Answer and Explanation
use of a test with 100% specificity	*confirming disease in a patient with a positive test result on a screening test* [Specificity = the chance a test will be negative in a person without the disease: $$= \frac{TN}{TN + FP} \times 100$$ A test with 100% specificity for a disease has no FPs. Therefore, a positive test must be a TP rather than an FP, hence its usefulness in confirming disease. However, a negative test does not distinguish a TN from an FN. For example, a positive VDRL test (screening test for non-treponemal antibodies in syphilis) is either a TP or an FP. The FTA-ABS, which detects treponemal antibodies, has a high specificity (very few FPs) for diagnosing syphilis. Hence, a positive FTA-ABS indicates that the positive VDRL is a TP rather than an FP, whereas a negative FTA-ABS indicates the VDRL result is an FP.]
cause of an FP test result	*low prevalence of disease* [Prevalence of a disease is the total number of people with disease in the total population under study: $$\text{Prevalence} = \frac{TP + FN}{TP + FN + TN + FP} \times 100$$ When disease prevalence is low, the predictive value of a positive test (PV⁺) result indicating disease is low, since there are more FPs than TPs. The formula for PV⁺ is as follows: $$PV^+ = \frac{TP}{TP + FP} \times 100$$ Tests with 100% specificity (no FPs) have a PV⁺ of 100%, hence their utility in confirming disease).]

Table 1–1. LABORATORY TEST CHARACTERISTICS
Continued

Most Common...	Answer and Explanation
cause of an FN test result	*low prevalence of disease* [When disease prevalence is low, the predictive value of a negative test result (PV⁻) is high, indicating that there are more TNs than FNs. The formula for PV⁻ is as follows: $$PV^- = \frac{TN}{TN + FN} \times 100$$ Tests with 100% sensitivity (no FNs) always have a PV⁻ of 100%, hence their utility in excluding disease.]
effect of altering the duration of a disease on the prevalence of the disease	• *decreasing disease duration decreases the prevalence of disease,* • *increasing duration increases the prevalence of disease* [Prevalence (P) = incidence (I) × duration (D). Incidence (I) is the number of newly discovered cases of disease within a certain time frame. Hence, (P) increases or decreases when (D) increases or decreases.]
statistical method for expressing the precision (reproducibility) of a test	*standard deviation (SD)* [Precision is a test's reproducibility after repetitive measurements on the same sample. A low SD indicates good precision and vice versa. Accuracy is how close the test results are to the true value.]
method for establishing the reference interval for a test	*2 SDs from the mean of the test in a normal population of people*: * 2 SDs include 95% of the normal population, * 5% (1:20) of normal people are outside the reference interval (FP test result), * example: mean of a test is 100 mg/dL, 1 SD = 2 mg/dL; reference interval = 96 − 104 mg/dL (2 SD = 4 mg/dL; 100 − 4 = 96 and 100 + 4 = 104.]
formula used to calculate percent chance of obtaining an FP test result per test	*% chance of an FP = $100 - (0.95^n \times 100)$, where n = the number of tests performed*: for example, if 12 tests are ordered: %FP = $100 - (0.95^{12} \times 100) = 46\%$.]

Table continued on following page

Table 1–1. LABORATORY TEST CHARACTERISTICS
Continued

Most Common...	Answer and Explanation
effect of raising the upper limit of a reference interval on the PV⁺ and PV⁻ of a test result	• *effect on PV⁺ test result:* * increases specificity, * increases PV⁺ test (less FPs), • *effect on PV⁻ test result*: decreases sensitivity of the test, * decreases the PV⁻ test result (more FNs) [For example, if the fasting glucose for diagnosing DM is raised from 115 mg/dL to 140 mg/dL, the PV⁺ of the test is increased (specificity increased), and PV⁻ test result is decreased (sensitivity decreased).]
effect of lowering the upper limit of a reference interval on the PV⁺ and PV⁻ of a test result	• *effect on PV⁺ test result*: * decreases specificity, * decreases PV⁺ test result (more FPs), • *effect on PV⁻ test result*: * increases sensitivity, * increases PV⁻ test result (less FNs) [For example, if the upper limit of a fasting glucose is lowered from 140 mg/dL to 126 mg/dL, this increases the PV⁻ test result (sensitivity increased) and decreases the PV⁺ test result (specificity decreased).]
effect on PV⁺ and PV⁻ when more than one test must be positive to confirm disease	• *effect on PV⁺:* * increases overall specificity, * increases PV⁺ test result, • *effect on PV⁻:* * decreases overall sensitivity, decreases PV⁻ test result [For example, if both CK-MB and troponin-1 are positive, an AMI is present.]
effects on PV⁺ and PV⁻ when only one of multiple tests must be positive to confirm disease	• *effect on PV⁻ test result:* * increases overall sensitivity, * increases PV⁻ test result, • *effect on PV⁺ test result*: * decreases overall specificity, * decreases PV⁺ test result [For example, if the criteria for an AMI are that either a CK-MB or a troponin-I must be positive, this increases the overall sensitivity of the tests and increases the PV⁻ test result. If both tests must be positive to confirm an AMI, this increases the overall specificity of the tests and increases the PV⁺ test result.]

Table 1–1. LABORATORY TEST CHARACTERISTICS
Continued

Question: Test X is positive in 90 out of 100 people with disease and normal in 60 out of 100 people without disease. Assuming a disease prevalence of 10%, what is the PV+ test result? **SELECT 1**

(A) 10%
(B) 20%
(C) 30%
(D) 40%
(E) 50%

Answer: (B): First the sensitivity and specificity of test X must be calculated. Since 90 out of 100 people with disease have a positive test, the TP rate is 90 and the FN rate is 10, hence the sensitivity is 90% (TP ÷ TP + FN = 90/90 + 10 = 90%). The test is normal in 60 out of 100 people without disease; therefore, the TN rate is 60 and the FP rate is 40. Hence, the specificity of test X is 60% (TN ÷ TN + FP = 60%). Assuming a population of 1000 people, a 10% prevalence of disease means that 100 have disease and 900 are normal. Since the test sensitivity is 90%, 90 out of 100 people with disease are TPs and 10 are FNs. Since the test specificity is 60%, 540 of the 900 normal people are TNs and 360 are FPs. The PV+ = 20% (TP/TP + FP = 90/90 + 360 = 20%). This indicates that there is an 80% chance that it is an FP test result (100 − 20 = 80%). The PV- = 98% (TN/TN + FN = 540/540 + 10 = 98%), which means that the FN rate is only 2%. This underscores the effect prevalence has on the PV+ and PV- test result.

AMI = acute myocardial infarction, ANA = antinuclear antibody, CH = cholesterol, CK-MB = creatine kinase MB, D = duration, DM = diabetes mellitus, ECG = electrocardiogram, FN = false negative, FP = false positive, FTA-ABS = fluorescent treponemal antibody absorption test, HbA_{1c} = glycosylated hemoglobin, HDL = high density lipoprotein, I = incidence, P = prevalence, PV- = predictive value of a negative test result, PV+ = predictive value of a positive test result, SD = standard deviation, SLE = systemic lupus erythematosus, TN = true negative, TP = true positive, VDRL = Venereal Disease Research Laboratories.

Table 1–2. SCREENING AND CONFIRMATORY TESTS (S/C)

Most Common...	Answer and Explanation
S/C for HIV	• *screen:* ELISA test, • *confirm:* Western blot assay
S/C for CAD	• *screen:* stress ECG, • *confirm:* coronary angiography
S/C for primary prevention of CAD (no previous history of CAD)	• *screen:* serum CH and HDL beginning at age 35 in men and 45 in women, • *confirm:* lipid profile (calculated LDL, measured TG, HDL, CH)

Table continued on following page

Table 1–2. SCREENING AND CONFIRMATORY TESTS (S/C) *Continued*

Most Common...	Answer and Explanation
S/C for typical pneumonia	• *screen:* chest x-ray, • *confirm:* sputum culture
S/C for ectopic pregnancy	• *screen:* β-hCG, • *confirm*: transvaginal ultrasonogram (laparoscopy, if non-diagnostic)
S/C for a UTI	• *screen*: complete urinalysis, • *confirm:* urine culture [A positive dipstick for nitrites and leukocyte esterase is highly predictive for a UTI.]
S/C for iron deficiency anemia	• *screen:* Hb and Hct, • *confirm*: serum ferritin [Early stages of iron deficiency may have abnormal iron study results before any anemia is present, hence Hb and Hct screening may have FNs. In most cases, only a ferritin is performed, since it has both a high sensitivity and specificity for diagnosing iron deficiency when it is decreased.]
S/C for DM	• *screen:* fasting glucose ≥126 mg/dL is presumptive evidence of DM, • *confirm:* fasting glucose ≥126 mg/dL on another day or a 2-hour glucose ≥200 mg/dL after a 75-g glucose challenge
S/C for GDM	• *screen:* * 50-g glucose challenge between 24–28 weeks' gestation, * glucose ≥140 mg/dL after 1 hour is presumptive evidence of GDM, • *confirm*: 100-g 3-hour glucose tolerance test
S/C for lead poisoning	*screen and confirm:* blood lead level
S/C for primary syphilis	• *screen*: RPR or VDRL, • *confirm:* FTA-ABS
S/C for suspected gonococcal urethritis	• *screen*: Gram stain of exudate, • *confirm:* culture or PCR test
S/C for Rh sensitization of a fetus	• *screen*: maternal serum antibody screen, • *confirm*: if anti-D is present, amniocentesis is performed to check for bilirubin pigment in the amniotic fluid indicating fetal RBC hemolysis
S/C for Down syndrome	• *screen:* * maternal serum β-hCG, AFP, and urine estriol, * positive screen if β-hCG is

Table 1–2. SCREENING AND CONFIRMATORY TESTS (S/C) *Continued*

Most Common...	Answer and Explanation
Continued	high, AFP low, and urine estriol low, • *confirm*: chromosome analysis of fetal cells
S/C for open neural tube defects in a fetus	• *screen*: maternal AFP, • *confirm*: ultrasonogram
S/C for sickle cell trait	• *screen:* sickle cell preparation (sodium metabisulfite), • *confirm:* Hb electrophoresis
S/C for Cushing's syndrome	• *screen:* * low dose dexamethasone test (cannot suppress cortisol in Cushing's), * 24-h urine for free estriol (increased in Cushing's), • *confirm:* high dose dexamethasone test (can suppress pituitary Cushing's but not adrenal or ectopic Cushing's syndrome)
S/C for multiple myeloma	• *screen:* serum protein electrophoresis (looking for a monoclonal spike), • *confirm:* bone marrow examination
S/C for breast cancer in a woman	• *screen:* annual mammography beginning at age 40, • *confirm:* if a mass is discovered, a fine needle aspiration is performed [Although controversial, most organizations recommend mammography every 1–2 years beginning at age 40, particularly those with a family history of breast cancer. All organizations agree that mammography should be performed annually on all women between 50 and 69 years of age.]
S/C for cervical cancer	• *screen:* cervical Papanicolaou smear following onset of sexual activity or at age 20 (whichever comes first) q every 3 years, • *confirm*: colposcopy with biopsy of suspicious areas
S/C for colorectal cancer	• *screen*: beginning at ≥50 years old, an annual stool for occult blood plus a flexible sigmoidoscopy q 3–5 years, • *confirm*: colonoscopy
S/C for prostate cancer	• *screen*: DRE and PSA beginning at ≥50 years old, • *confirm*: transrectal ultrasonogram with biopsy

Table continued on following page

Table 1–2. SCREENING AND CONFIRMATORY
TESTS (S/C) *Continued*

Question: Which of the following are generally considered screening rather than confirmatory tests? **SELECT 5**

(A) Bone marrow examination in a patient with anemia
(B) Hb and Hct
(C) Coronary angiogram in the work-up of angina
(D) PPD
(E) Western blot assay for HIV
(F) β-hCG
(G) Hb electrophoresis
(H) Chest radiograph in bacterial pneumonia
(I) FOBT
(J) Urine culture for a UTI

Answers: (B), (D), (F), (H), (I): Hb and Hct are screening tests (choice **B**) to rule out anemia, whereas a bone marrow examination (choice **A**) is often a confirmatory test for identifying the cause of certain anemias (e.g., aplastic anemia). A stress ECG is the screening test for angina, whereas coronary angiogram (choice **C is incorrect**) is the confirmatory test. A PPD (choice **D**) is a screening test for tuberculosis. The ELISA test is the screen for HIV and the Western blot (choice **E is incorrect**) the confirmatory test. A β-hCG (choice **F**) is a screening test for pregnancy. An Hb electrophoresis (choice **G is incorrect**) is the confirmatory test to document a hemoglobinopathy (e.g., sickle cell trait). A chest radiograph (choice **H**) is the screening test of choice for a bacterial pneumonia and culture is the confirmatory test. A FOBT (choice **I**) is a screen for colon cancer, whereas a colonoscopy with biopsy is the confirmatory test. A urine culture (choice **J is incorrect**) is a confirmatory test for a UTI, whereas a urinalysis is the initial screening test.

AFP = alpha-fetoprotein, β-hCG = human chorionic gonadotropin, CAD = coronary artery disease, CH = cholesterol, DM = diabetes mellitus, DRE = digital rectal examination, ECG = electrocardiogram, ELISA = enzyme-linked immunosorbent assay, FOBT = fecal occult blood test, FN = false negative, FTA-ABS = fluorescent treponemal antibody absorption test, GDM = gestational diabetes mellitus, Hb = hemoglobin, Hct = hematocrit, HDL = high density lipoprotein, HIV = human immunodeficiency virus, LDL = low density lipoprotein, PCR = polymerase chain reaction, PPD = purified protein derivative, PSA = prostate specific antigen, RBC = red blood cell, RPR = rapid plasma reagin, S/C = screen/confirm, TG = triglyceride, UTI = urinary tract infection, VDRL = Venereal Disease Research Laboratories.

Table 1–3. VARIABLES AFFECTING LABORATORY TEST RESULTS

Most Common...	Answer and Explanation
reasons to suspect an erroneous lab test result	• *test result does not make sense*: e.g., it is incompatible with life, • *test result is inconsistent with previous reports:* e.g., serum CK-MB at 12 hours post-chest pain is abnormal and at 24 hours it is normal, • *other tests are at odds with the test result*: e.g., patient has known polycythemia and the Hb is now 7 g/dL, • *test result differs from your clinical expectation*: e.g., you expected chronic respiratory acidosis and the ABG shows respiratory alkalosis
cause of an erroneous test result	*transcription error*
cause of a turbid blood sample	*increase in triglyceride (TG) in a patient who was not fasting prior to obtaining the sample*: * TG in a nonfasting state comes from saturated fats in the diet that are packaged into chylomicrons, * TG is also increased due to an increase in VLDL (liver synthesized TG)
tests requiring a fasting sample	• *lipid profile* (CH, TG, HDL, calculated LDL): fasting eliminates the effect of saturated fats in the diet on TG (not CH or HDL), which may falsely increase the measured TG concentration and spuriously lower the calculated LDL: (LDL = CH − HDL − ↑**TG/5**), • *fasting glucose:* a fasting glucose is one of three different ways of diagnosing DM (see Table 11–5).
lipids not affected by fasting	*CH and HDL:* * chylomicrons derived from the diet contain <3% CH (not enough to be significant), * HDL is measured as HDL bound to CH (also not significantly altered)
causes of an FP serum potassium	• **hemolysis of the blood sample:** called pseudohyperkalemia, • *collection tube with >100,000 WBCs/μL or >1,000,000 platelets/μL*: cells leak out potassium [Other analytes falsely increased due to RBC hemolysis are * LDH and * AST.]
cause of pseudoanemia in a CBC performed on an automated counter	*presence of cold agglutinins causing RBCs to agglutinate*

Table continued on following page

Table 1–3. VARIABLES AFFECTING LABORATORY
TEST RESULTS *Continued*

Most Common...	Answer and Explanation
causes of a falsely low platelet count performed on an automated counter	• **artifactual clumping of platelets in an EDTA collection tube**: draw the blood in a green top tube with heparin or a blue top tube with citrate for valid results, • *platelet satellitosis around WBCs*, • *finger-stick collections of blood causing platelets to clump*
effect of excess caffeine intake on lab results	*increases serum cortisol and catecholamines*: increases glycogenolysis and serum glucose
effect of increased TG >1000 mg/dL and total protein (>8 g/dL) on serum sodium	*pseudohyponatremia* [~93% of serum is water (aqueous phase) and 7% is composed of lipids and protein (nonaqueous phase). Sodium ions dissolve only in the aqueous phase of serum. Sodium concentration in a liter of normal saline is 154 mEq/L (no nonaqueous phase is present), but in serum, it is 0.93×154 mEq/L = 143 mEq/L owing to the nonaqueous phase displacing the aqueous phase. Increasing the nonaqueous phase (excess TG or protein) further displaces the aqueous phase and artifactually lowers serum sodium, since it is expressed in mEq/L. Instruments with ion-selective electrodes for sodium are not affected by lipids if the sample is *not diluted with water prior to measurement.* If the sample is diluted with water prior to measurement or a flame photometer is used in measuring the sodium, pseudohyponatremia will occur. When the TG concentration in mg/dL is multiplied by 0.002, it yields the artifactual reduction in sodium in mEq/L that must be added to the measured serum sodium. Similarly, if the protein concentration is increased, multiplying the protein concentration in g/dL by 0.25 yields the artifactual reduction in sodium in mEq/L that must be added to the measured serum sodium.]
cause of an elevated serum GGT and falsely low drug levels	*induction of the hepatic cytochrome P450 system by a drug*: * drugs like alcohol, barbiturates, and rifampin increase the synthesis of SER-located GGT, * induction enhances drug metabolism (e.g., theophylline)

Table 1–3. VARIABLES AFFECTING LABORATORY
TEST RESULTS *Continued*

Most Common...	Answer and Explanation
cause of an unexpected drug toxicity in a patient on an H_2 or proton blocker	*drugs block the hepatic cytochrome P450 system*: cimetidine, an H_2 blocker, and omeprazole, a proton blocker, block the cytochrome system and potentiate drug toxicity
vitamin toxicity associated with potentiation of oral anticoagulants	*vitamin E toxicity* [Vitamin E toxicity antagonizes vitamin K activity on γ-carboxylation of vitamin K-dependent coagulation factors II, VII, IX, and X (excess vitamin E acts like an anticoagulant) and the synthesis of the coagulation factors. This further prolongs the PT.]
cause of a falsely elevated serum creatinine in a patient with DKA	*ketoacids* [Ketoacids interfere with the Jaffe reaction, which is commonly used in assays for serum creatinine. Non-creatinine chromogens (e.g., ketoacids, acetone, glucose, cephalosporins) react with the picrate in the Jaffe test system, leading to a falsely elevated creatinine.]
effect of digoxin antibodies (Fab fragments) on the serum digoxin level after Rx for digoxin toxicity	*falsely elevated serum digoxin*: Fab fragments interfere with most immunoassay procedures since they bind to digoxin and are not differentiated from unbound digoxin
overall cause of hypocalcemia	*hypoalbuminemia* [Total calcium levels represent calcium bound to albumin (40%), other substrates (13%), and free, ionized calcium (47%, metabolically active). Hence, hypoalbuminemia automatically lowers the serum calcium without altering the ionized level (no tetany). Corrected serum calcium = (serum calcium − serum albumin) + 4.]
effect of alcohol excess on serum glucose	*possible fasting hypoglycemia* [The increase in NADH in alcohol metabolism causes the biochemical reaction involving LDH and NADH to favor conversion of pyruvate into lactate. This reduces the availability of pyruvate as a substrate for gluconeogenesis in the fasting state.]

Table continued on following page

**Table 1–3. VARIABLES AFFECTING LABORATORY
TEST RESULTS** *Continued*

Most Common...	Answer and Explanation
effect of alcohol excess on the anion gap (AG)	*increases the AG* [This is due to an increase in the production of lactate (see above) and β-hydroxybutyrate (β-OHB). Acetyl CoA, the end-product of alcohol metabolism, is increased in the blood and is converted in the liver into ketone bodies (AcAc and β-OHB). Excess amounts of NADH (see above) favor the conversion of AcAc into β-OHB. Owing to the increase in lactate and β-OHB anions, there is an increased AG metabolic acidosis in alcoholics. See Table 6–2.]
effect of alcohol on uric acid levels	*hyperuricemia* [The increase in lactate and β-OHB anions leads to hyperuricemia, since all acids compete for secretion in the same location in the proximal renal tubules. Hyperuricemia may precipitate acute gouty arthritis.]
effect of alcohol on TG levels	*hypertriglyceridemia* [The metabolic products of alcohol (NADH, acetate, acetyl CoA) are used by the liver to synthesize TG. The TG is packaged into VLDL (cause of a fatty liver) and released into the blood (type IV hyperlipoproteinemia).]
effect of cigarette smoking on ABGs	• **chronic respiratory acidosis,** • *hypoxemia;* an increase in $Paco_2$ always causes a decrease in Pao_2, • *increase in the A–a gradient:* refers to the oxygen gradient between the alveoli and arterial blood [Smoking also increases CO levels in the blood. See Table 6–2.]
effect of cigarette smoking on the WBC and RBC count	*increases total neutrophil and RBC count* [The neutrophil count is increased owing to the release of catecholamines, which interfere with the synthesis of adhesion molecules. This causes the marginating pool (normally 50% of the peripheral blood neutrophils) to enter the circulating pool of neutrophils. RBCs increase owing to a hypoxemic stimulus for erythropoietin release, which produces a secondary polycythemia.]

Table 1–3. VARIABLES AFFECTING LABORATORY TEST RESULTS *Continued*

Most Common...	Answer and Explanation
effect of volume depletion on serum BUN and albumin, Hb and Hct, and urine specific gravity	• *serum BUN, Hb, Hct, and albumin are all increased*: due to hemoconcentration of blood from a reduction in plasma volume, • *urine specific gravity is increased*: ADH is released in response to volume depletion, leading to the reabsorption of free water in the collecting tubule and concentration of urine
cause of an FP syphilis serology	*presence of anti-cardiolipin antibodies* [The test antigen in the RPR and VDRL is beef cardiolipin to which non-treponemal antibodies normally react in the test. Anti-cardiolipin antibodies in patients with SLE and other disorders cross-react with the cardiolipin in the test system, leading to an FP syphilis serology. The FTA-ABS is negative, since it measures specific treponemal antibodies.]
cause of neutropenia in African Americans	*normal increase in the marginating neutrophil pool* [Normally, the circulating and marginating (adherent to the endothelium) pool of neutrophils is equally distributed. An increase in the marginating pool in African Americans is a normal variation and does not hinder neutrophil response to infection.]
lab test alterations in children that differ from those in adults	• *increased serum alkaline phosphatase*: 3–5 times higher in children than in adults and due to increased osteoblast activity from active bone growth, • *increased serum phosphate*: phosphate is the driving force for depositing calcium in bone, • *lower Hb*: 11–12 g/dL
lab test results in women that significantly differ from those in men	*lower serum levels*: * serum iron, * percent transferrin saturation, * ferritin [The above differences are secondary to menses (~35–40 mL of blood loss per period), lower serum testosterone than men (less stimulation of erythropoiesis), and childbearing (lose 500 mg of iron per pregnancy if not on iron supplements).]

Table continued on following page

**Table 1-3. VARIABLES AFFECTING LABORATORY
TEST RESULTS** *Continued*

Most Common...	Answer and Explanation
lab test alterations in pregnancy that differ from those in non-pregnant women	• *two times greater increase in plasma volume than RBC mass:* this results in * decrease in Hb and Hct—dilutional effect, * increase in creatinine clearance—increased plasma volume, * low serum BUN—increased urine clearance, * low serum uric acid—increased urine clearance, * low serum creatinine—increased urine clearance, • *increased serum alkaline phosphatase:* * placental origin, * heat stable, • *respiratory alkalosis:* progesterone overstimulates the central respiratory center, • *increased total T$_4$ and cortisol:* estrogen increases synthesis of their binding proteins without altering the free hormone levels, • *mild glucose intolerance:* anti-insulin effect of hPL, • *glucosuria:* * lower renal threshold for glucose, * normal blood glucose
lab test alterations in the elderly	• *decreased creatinine clearance:* due to a * decrease in the GFR, * decrease in renal excretion of drugs (potential for nephrotoxicity), * decreased ability to concentrate urine, • *lower Hb concentration in men:* * drop in testosterone reduces erythropoiesis, * elderly men and women have the same Hb concentration, • *increase in serum autoantibodies:* decrease in CD$_8$ T suppressor cells allows CD$_4$ T helper cells to stimulate antibody production, • *decreased response to skin testing with common antigens:* * diminished DRH response, * cellular immunity slightly impaired, • *slight elevation in serum glucose:* due to down-regulation of insulin receptors as adipose increases, • *"obstructive" type of PFTs:* * lower PaO$_2$, * increased TLC and RV, * lower VC, TV, and FEV$_{1sec}$, • *slight increase in serum alkaline phosphatase:* due to osteophyte formation in osteoarthritis

Table 1–3. VARIABLES AFFECTING LABORATORY
TEST RESULTS *Continued*

Question: Which of the following clinical scenarios most likely represents FP test results? **SELECT 2**

- (A) Hyperkalemia in a patient with renal failure
- (B) Hyponatremia in a patient with type II hyperlipoproteinemia
- (C) $LDH_{1/2}$ flip in a hemolyzed blood sample
- (D) Low serum ferritin in a hemolyzed blood sample
- (E) Serum alkaline phosphatase elevation in an asymptomatic 4-year-old child
- (F) Elevated serum alkaline phosphatase in an elderly man with bone pain in the lower vertebral column
- (G) Elevated CK-MB 12 hours after severe chest pain in a 65-year-old man
- (H) Positive RPR and negative FTA-ABS in a patient with SLE

Answers: **(C)**, **(H):** The most common pathologic cause of hyperkalemia is renal failure **(choice A is a TP).** A type II hyperlipoproteinemia is associated with an increase in LDL (primary carrier of CH), which, unlike an increase in TG, does not produce serum turbidity and pseudohyponatremia **(choice B is a TP).** RBCs have a high concentration of the LDH_1 isoenzyme. Therefore, a hemolyzed sample produces an FP $LDH_{1/2}$ flip **(choice C is an FP).** A low serum ferritin in a hemolyzed sample is a TP for iron deficiency, since ferritin is not falsely elevated in hemolyzed RBCs **(choice D is a TP).** An elevated serum alkaline phosphatase in an asymptomatic child is normal for age **(choice E is a TP).** An elevated alkaline phosphatase in an elderly man with bone pain most likely represents osteoblastic metastasis from prostate cancer **(choice F is a TP).** An elevated CK-MB taken 12-h after chest pain is diagnostic of an AMI **(choice G is a TP).** A positive RPR and negative FTA-ABS is an FP syphilis serology **(choice H is an FP).** In a patient with SLE, the FP is most likely due to the presence of anti-cardiolipin antibodies.

A–a = alveolar/arterial gradient, ABG = arterial blood gas, AcAc = acetoacetate, ADH = antidiuretic hormone, AG = anion gap, AMI = acute myocardial infarction, AST = aspartate aminotransferase, β-OHB = β-hydroxybutyrate, BUN = blood urea nitrogen, CH = cholesterol, CK-MB = creatine kinase MB, CoA = coenzyme A, DKA = diabetic ketoacidosis, DM = diabetes mellitus, DRH = delayed hypersensitivity reaction, EDTA = ethylenediaminetetraacetic acid, FEV_{1sec} = forced expiratory volume in 1 second, FP = false positive, FTA-ABS = fluorescent treponemal antibody absorption test, GFR = glomerular filtration rate, GGT = γ-glutamyltransferase, H_2 = histamine, Hb = hemoglobin, Hct = hematocrit, HDL = high density lipoprotein, hPL = human placental lactogen, LDH = lactate dehydrogenase, LDL = low density lipoprotein, NADH = nicotinamide adenine dinucleotide (reduced form), $PaCO_2$ = partial pressure of arterial carbon dioxide, PaO_2 = partial pressure of arterial oxygen, PFTs = pulmonary function tests, PT = prothrombin time, RBC = red blood cell, RPR = rapid plasma reagin, RV = residual volume, Rx = treatment, SER = smooth endoplasmic reticulum, SLE =

systemic lupus erythematosus, T_4 = thyroxine, TG = triglyceride, TLC = total lung capacity, TN = true negative, TP = true positive, TV = tidal volume, VC = vital capacity, VDRL = Venereal Disease Research Laboratories, VLDL = very low density lipoprotein, WBC = white blood cell.

CHAPTER

2

PREVENTIVE MEDICINE AND PUBLIC HEALTH

CONTENTS

Table 2–1. RISK FACTORS ASSOCIATED WITH THE LEADING CAUSES OF DEATH IN THE UNITED STATES

Most Common...	Answer and Explanation
top five causes of death in the United States in descending order	• **heart disease**, • *cancer*, • *CVA*, • *COPD*, • *accidents*
top five risk factors leading to increased morbidity/mortality in the United States in descending order	• **cigarette smoking**, • *dietary factors and activity patterns:* * high saturated fat, * low-fiber diet, * lack of exercise, • *alcohol,* • *microbial agents,* • *toxic agents*
cause of accidental death from 1–24 years of age	*MVAs* [MVAs are most often associated with drunk driving. In white males, it is also the most common COD between 25 and 44 years of age. AIDS is the most common COD in African-American males and women between 25 and 44 years.]
COD in African-American males between 15 and 25 years of age	*homicide*
type of prevention used before the existence of disease in a patient	*primary prevention* [It removes/reduces risk factors before disease exists. Examples include * cessation of smoking, * health education, * air bags in cars, * bike helmets for

Table continued on following page

17

**Table 2–1. RISK FACTORS ASSOCIATED WITH THE
LEADING CAUSES OF DEATH IN THE UNITED STATES**
Continued

Most Common...	Answer and Explanation
Continued	children, * car seats for children, * immunizations, * blood pressure checks, * sex education
type of prevention that detects disease before it becomes symptomatic	*secondary prevention* [It refers to early detection and Rx of disease in a presymptomatic or preclinical stage with screening tests. Examples include * cervical Pap smear (detects cervical dysplasia, in situ cancer) * mammography (detects non-palpable masses).]
type of prevention that prevents future adverse health effects in a disease that already exists	*tertiary prevention* [It seeks measures to reduce future morbidity/mortality due to a disease that has already been diagnosed. Examples include * colon resection in colorectal cancer, * aspirin/β-blockers after an AMI, * tamoxifen Rx after recurrence of breast cancer, * physical rehabilitation in rheumatoid arthritis.]
risk factors for heart disease	• **age of the patient**: * ≥45 in a man, * ≥55 in a woman, • *family Hx of heart disease/ stroke,* • *smoking,* • *DM,* • *HTN,* • *HDL ≤35 mg/dL,* • *LDL ≥160 mg/dL*
primary prevention measures to reduce the incidence of CAD	• **normalize blood pressure**: weight reduction, • *diet high in fiber and low in saturated fats,* • *exercise,* • *stop smoking,* • *moderation with alcohol ingestion*
secondary prevention measures to reduce the incidence of CAD	• *CH and HDL measurement*: men aged 35–64, women aged 45–64, • *blood pressure:* periodic screening of BP in all persons ≥20 years of age, • *ECG:* for men >40 years old with more than two risk factors (see above) or sedentary person planning a vigorous exercise program, • *aspirin*: prevents coronary artery thrombosis (use ticlopidine if the patient is allergic to aspirin)
risk factors for lung cancer	• **cigarette smoking**, • *increasing age,* • *male sex* (2:1 male:female ratio), • *radon gas,* • *asbestos,* • *chromium,* • *nickel,* • *arsenic,* • *cadmium*
primary prevention measure to reduce the incidence of lung cancer	*stop smoking* [Screening with a chest radiograph or pulmonary cytology is not cost-effective.]

**Table 2–1. RISK FACTORS ASSOCIATED WITH THE
LEADING CAUSES OF DEATH IN THE UNITED STATES**
Continued

Most Common...	Answer and Explanation
risk factors for breast cancer in women	• **≥50 years of age,** • *other high-risk factors*: * personal Hx of breast cancer, * premenopausal family member with bilateral breast cancer, * Hx of family cancer syndrome, * Bx with atypical proliferative breast disease, • *moderate risk*: * breast cancer in mother and/or sister, * previous Hx of endometrial or ovarian cancer, * age at first pregnancy >30-y, * nulliparous, * obesity in postmenopausal woman, * upper socioeconomic class, • *low risk*: * early menarche (<12-y-old), * late menopause (>55-y-old), * moderate alcohol intake, * breast radiation from screening, * *smoking*
secondary prevention measure to reduce the incidence of breast cancer	• **annual screening mammography for women aged 40–69**: reduces mortality by 20–30%, • *yearly clinical breast exam ≥40-y-old* [Controversy exists over whether screening should begin at age 40. Most recommend mammography every 1–2 years and then annually from age 50–69. Clinical exam sensitivity 50–70%, specificity >90%. Mammography sensitivity 80–95% for women ≥50 y old and 60–80% <50 y old, specificity 95–99%. 10% of breast cancers detected clinically are not detected by mammography (less sensitive and more specific).]
STD cancer	*cervical cancer*
risk factors for cervical cancer	• **early onset of sexual activity**, • *multiple sexual partners*, • *smoking*, • *oral contraceptives*, • *drug immunosuppression*, • *Hx of STD* [HPV types 16, 18, and 31 are implicated in cervical cancer.]
secondary prevention of cervical cancer	*cervical Pap smear* [Cervical Pap smear sensitivity is 55–80% and specificity 90–99%. Screen at onset of sexual activity annually for 2 consecutive years and, if negative, every 1–3 y until age 65. Dysplastic cervical Pap is followed up with colposcopy. Cervical cancer is the least common gynecologic cancer owing to early detection and Rx of cervical dysplasia, the precursor lesion for squamous cancer and carcinoma in situ. Incidence and

Table continued on following page

Table 2–1. RISK FACTORS ASSOCIATED WITH THE LEADING CAUSES OF DEATH IN THE UNITED STATES
Continued

Most Common...	Answer and Explanation
Continued	mortality from cervical cancer have decreased 30–40% in recent decades owing to Pap smears.]
risk factors for ovarian cancer	• **age >50**, • *high-fat/low-fiber diet*, • *personal Hx of breast and/or endometrial cancer*, • *first-degree relative with Hx of ovarian cancer*, • *early menarche/late menopause:* increased number of ovulation years, • *Turner's syndrome*, • *nulliparity:* * the more times a woman ovulates the greater the risk, * patients on birth control pills have a decreased risk, • *late menopause* [Ovarian cancer is the most common COD due to a gynecologic cancer. Screening for ovarian cancer as a secondary prevention with CA-125, ultrasonography, or bimanual exam is not cost-effective.]
risk factors for endometrial cancer	• **unopposed estrogen**: unopposed estrogen stimulation may be due to * a woman taking estrogen without progesterone, * early menarche/late menopause, * obesity, * DM, * POS, * tamoxifen, * nulliparity, • *Hx of previous breast cancer*, • *HTN* [Endometrial cancer is the most common gynecologic cancer and the one with the best prognosis. Cervical Pap smears are not effective in detecting endometrial cancer.]
risk factors for skin cancer	• **exposure to UVB light**, • *dysplastic nevus syndrome* (risk for malignant melanoma), • *xeroderma pigmentosum:* AR disease with absent DNA repair enzymes, • *immunosuppression:* particularly squamous cell cancer [UVB-related skin cancers include * basal cell carcinoma (**most common**), * squamous cell carcinoma, and * malignant melanoma.]
primary prevention for skin cancer	• **use sunscreen with a sun protective factor of at least 15**, • *avoid sunlight between 11:00 AM and 2:30 PM*
secondary prevention for skin cancer	*patients with the dysplastic nevus syndrome should be evaluated by a dermatologist on an annual basis*

Table 2–1. RISK FACTORS ASSOCIATED WITH THE
LEADING CAUSES OF DEATH IN THE UNITED STATES
Continued

Most Common...	Answer and Explanation
risk factors for colorectal cancer	• **age >50 years old:** risk doubles every 7-y after 50, • *first-degree relative with colorectal cancer,* • *dietary factors:* * low fiber/high saturated fat diet, * fiber has come under attack recently as a factor, • *Hx of a polyposis syndrome:* 100% risk by 40 y of age), • *previous adenomatous polyps:* * size and percent villous component are most important, * requires 7–10 y for a polyp to become cancer, • *previous personal Hx of endometrial, ovarian, or breast cancer,* • *personal Hx of ulcerative colitis:* 50% risk with a 30–y Hx of the disease, • *smoking* [Colorectal cancer is the second most common cancer and cancer killer in men and women. Over 90% of colorectal cancers occur after 50–y of age. Smoking is not a risk factor. Aspirin helps prevent colorectal cancer.]
secondary prevention measure to reduce the incidence of colorectal cancer	*annual FOBT and flexible sigmoidoscopy every 3–5 years for all persons aged 50 and older* [The above screening regimen has reduced the cumulative mortality of colorectal cancer by 33%. FOBT sensitivity is 20–30% (not good for detecting polyps). Proctoscopy sensitivity is >90% (detects only 30% of cancers). Flexible sigmoidoscopy sensitivity is >90% (detects 60% of cancers). Barium enema and colonoscopy (gold standard) sensitivity is 85–95%.]
risk factors for prostate cancer	• **age** (prostate cancer is age-dependent), • *Hx of prostate cancer in first-degree relatives,* • *African American,* • *cadmium exposure* [Prostate cancer is the most common cancer in men and second most common cancer killer. It requires 10–15 y to grow from a tiny nidus to a clinically significant cancer.]
secondary prevention measure to reduce the incidence of prostate cancer	*annual DRE and PSA screening beginning at age 50* (age 40 if the patient is African American or has a family Hx of prostate cancer) [The argument against the above screening regimen is that screening has not reduced the morbidity/mortality of prostate cancer.]

Table continued on following page

**Table 2–1. RISK FACTORS ASSOCIATED WITH THE
LEADING CAUSES OF DEATH IN THE UNITED STATES**
Continued

Most Common...	Answer and Explanation
risk factors for a CVA	• **HTN**, • *old age*, • *smoking*, • *DM*, • *heart disease*, • *atrial fibrillation*: increased risk of embolization to middle cerebral artery, • *oral contraceptives in women who smoke*
secondary prevention measures to reduce the incidence of CVA	• **control the blood pressure**, • *aspirin*: ticlopidine should be used if the patient is allergic to aspirin
risk factors for COPD	• **smoking**, • *textile workers*, • *occupational exposure to coal dust, copper, tin*, • *passive smoke*
primary prevention measure to reduce the incidence of COPD	*stop smoking* (see Table 2–3)
risk factors for TB	• **HIV positive**, • *ethnicity*: foreign-born with recent immigration, • *nursing home resident*, • *prisoners*, • *living with a patient who has active TB* [TB is the most common infectious disease COD in the world.]
primary prevention of TB	*BCG vaccination* [Vaccination is 80% effective. It is primarily used in high-risk areas. It is not recommended in the United States. A positive PPD skin test in a patient with a BCG vaccination is considered active TB.]
screening test for TB	*PPD* (Mantoux) *intradermal skin test* (5-tuberculin units) [See Table 1–2 for discussion]
method of screening for TB in the elderly	*two-step PPD testing:* owing to relative anergy to skin testing in the elderly, a two-step procedure is used to enhance the reaction
work-up when a PPD is positive	• *chest radiograph*, • *clinical evaluation for active TB*
secondary prevention of TB when PPD is positive	*INH therapy:* 6–12 months of Rx is recommended for recent converters of * <2-y, * contacts of people with active TB with PPD >5 mm, * inadequately treated TB in the past, * patient <35-y old with positive PPD and no clinical evidence of active TB, * positive

Table 2–1. RISK FACTORS ASSOCIATED WITH THE
LEADING CAUSES OF DEATH IN THE UNITED STATES
Continued

Most Common...	Answer and Explanation
Continued	PPD with abnormal but stable chest radiograph. Liver enzymes should be evaluated every month in the elderly owing to increased risk of liver toxicity
risk factors for cirrhosis	• **excess alcohol intake**: * ~25% of alcoholics develop cirrhosis, * risk factors include— ♦ duration and magnitude of alcohol ingestion, ♦ sex of the patient (women have a greater risk even with less alcohol intake than men), ♦ presence of coexisting HCV, ♦ nutritional status, ♦ genetic factors, • *chronic HBV and HCV*, • *hemochromatosis*, • *Wilson's disease*, • *primary biliary cirrhosis*
risk factors for primary DM	• *HLA DR3/DR4*: type I DM, • *family Hx*: type II DM, • *obesity:* type II DM, • *gestational DM*, • *hemochromatosis*, • *chronic pancreatitis*, • *pentamidine*, • *endocrine disorders:* * Cushing's syndrome, * acromegaly, pheochromocytoma
risk factors for suicide	• *sex:* males more likely than females, • *divorced men*, • *adolescents of divorced parents*, • *occupational factors:* * psychiatrists, * lawyers, * women physicians, • *drug abuse, serious medical illness*

Question: High-fat and low-fiber diets, obesity, DM, hypertension, hypercholesterolemia, sedentary lifestyle, and smoking are the greatest overall group of risk factors for which of the following leading causes of death in the United States? **SELECT 1**
- (A) Heart disease
- (B) Cancer
- (C) Stroke
- (D) Atherosclerosis
- (E) COPD

Answer: (A): A high-fat/low-fiber diet is a risk factor for heart disease, cancer, stroke, DM, and atherosclerosis. Obesity is a risk factor for heart disease, cancer, stroke, and DM. HTN is a risk factor for heart disease, stroke, and DM. DM is a risk factor for heart disease and atherosclerosis. Hypercholesterolemia is a risk factor for heart disease, stroke, and atherosclerosis. A sedentary lifestyle is a risk factor for heart disease, cancer, DM, and atherosclerosis. Smoking is a risk factor for all of the choices including accidents, COPD, and pneumonia.

AIDS = acquired immunodeficiency syndrome; AMI = acute myocardial infarction, AR = autosomal recessive, BCG = bacille Calmette-Guérin, BP = blood pressure, Bx = biopsy, CAD = coronary artery disease, CH = cholesterol, COD = cause of death, COPD = chronic obstructive pulmonary disease, CVA = cerebrovascular accident, DM = diabetes mellitus, DRE = digital rectal examination, ECG = electrocardiogram, FOBT = fecal occult blood testing, HBV = hepatitis B virus, HCV = hepatitis C virus, HDL = high density lipoprotein, HIV = human immunodeficiency virus, HLA = human leukocyte antigen, HPV = human papillomavirus, HTN = hypertension, Hx = history, INH = isoniazid, LDL = low density lipoprotein, MVA = motor vehicle accident, POS = polycystic ovarian syndrome, PPD = purified protein derivative, PSA = prostate specific antigen, Rx = treatment, STD = sexually transmitted disease, TB = tuberculosis, UV = ultraviolet.

Table 2–2. ADULT IMMUNIZATION

Most Common...	Answer and Explanation
types of immunization	• *active immunization:* * patient develops antibodies, * antibodies usually last a lifetime, • *passive immunization:* * preformed antibodies, * immunity lasts up to 3 months
recommendations for influenza vaccination	• *yearly vaccination for all persons aged 65 and older,* • *vaccination for high-risk patients:* * chronic cardiopulmonary disease, * DM, * HbSS, * chronic liver disease, * patients who are immunocompromised [The killed-virus vaccine is 70–80% effective in preventing or reducing the severity of influenza (type A the most common type) in patients under 65 years of age. Vaccine contains 2 A-type viruses and 1 B-type virus. Chemoprophylaxis is with amantadine or rimantadine (70–90% effective in preventing illness due to influenza A, fever and some symptoms improved if given within 48 hours of contracting the virus).]
recommendations for pneumococcal vaccination	• *vaccination for all immunocompetent individuals who are aged 65 years or older,* • *vaccination for high-risk patients:* * chronic cardiopulmonary disease, * HbSS, * asplenic, * DM [It is a polysaccharide vaccine derived from 23 of the most common strains. The highest case-fatality rates occur in elderly patients (e.g., pneumonia, meningitis, sepsis). Titers of the vaccine persist for ~5 years. Revaccination every 6 years is recommended only for those at increased risk.]

Table 2–2. ADULT IMMUNIZATION *Continued*

Most Common...	Answer and Explanation
recommendation for tetanus and diphtheria (Td) immunization	*Td vaccine series* [Td is a toxoid vaccine. The Td series should be completed in adults who have not had the primary series at 0, 2, and 8–14 months and periodic boosters at least once every 10 years. Adults should receive two doses of Td 1–2 months apart followed by a booster dose 6–12 months later. Td is given to patients ≥7 years of age, whole DTP is for children <7 years of age.]
recommendation for a clean wound in immunized and nonimmunized patients	• *immunized*: * clean the wound, * no booster if last booster within 10 y, • *nonimmunized*: * clean wound, * give Td [Quaternary ammonium compounds are recommended for cleaning wounds.]
recommendation for dirty wounds in immunized and nonimmunized patients	• *immunized*: * clean wound, * if last booster within 5 y, no Td booster necessary, * if last booster >5 y, give Td booster, • *nonimmunized*: * clean wound, * ½ dose of immune globulin injected into the wound and ½ in another site, * give Td as well
recommendation for Td in pregnancy	*best to wait until second trimester:* Maternal antibodies confer immunity in newborn for a few months
recommendation for MMR vaccination	*administer (single dose) to all persons born after 1956 who lack serologic evidence of immunity to measles* [MMR is a live-attenuated virus vaccine. It is not recommended during pregnancy. MMR may be given to HIV+ patients; however, this recommendation does not extend to other immunocompromised patients. Revaccination is recommended before entering college or the health care profession. Vaccination is protective within 72 h of exposure to a patient with active disease. A single dose is 95% effective in producing long-term immunity. Risk for encephalitis in an adult with measles is 1:1000. In nonimmune adults, two doses of MMR are given at least 1 month apart
danger of rubella contracted during the first trimester by a nonimmunized woman	*congenital rubella syndrome:* up to 85% chance [Vaccination cannot be given during pregnancy. It may be given 3 months after delivery. Vaccination does not transmit the virus to other members. Arthralgias may occur 1–3 weeks after the vaccination.]

Table continued on following page

Table 2–2. ADULT IMMUNIZATION *Continued*

Most Common...	Answer and Explanation
recommendations for hepatitis B vaccination	• *vaccination for all young adults not previously immunized,* • *vaccination for susceptible adults in high-risk groups:* e.g., * homosexuals, * health care workers, * travelers to high-risk countries, * household contacts of HBV carriers [HBV vaccine is a recombinant vaccine that is given intramuscularly into the deltoid (not the gluteal muscles). Vaccine is given at 0, 1 month, and 6 months. Immunity lasts ~≥7 years (currently, revaccination is not recommended). Non-responders to vaccination (do not develop anti-HBs antibodies) may receive up to three additional doses at 1- to 2-month intervals with serologic testing after each dose.]
recommendation for immunization if nonimmune person is exposed to active HBV	*vaccine* (active immunization) *and immune globulin* (passive immunization)
recommendation for HBV vaccination during pregnancy	*advisable if the woman is at risk for HBV infection*
recommendation for hepatitis A vaccination	*vaccination for those 2 years of age or older who are at increased risk for developing HAV:* e.g., * military personnel, * travelers to endemic areas, * homosexuals, * institutionalized persons [HAV vaccine is an inactivated virus vaccine that provides permanent protection against HAV hepatitis. IM injection of immune globulin only provides temporary protection against patients exposed to HAV.]
recommendation for varicella vaccination	*vaccination for healthy adults with no Hx of varicella infection or previous immunization vaccination for high-risk groups:* e.g., * health care workers, * day care center workers, * non-pregnant women of childbearing age [Varicella vaccine is a live-attenuated vaccine that should not be given to any immunocompromised patient.]
recommendations for oral polio vaccine [OPV] and inactivated enhanced potency vaccine [IPV]	• *OPV vaccination is not recommended for primary vaccination of adults:* due to the risk for vaccine-associated paralytic poliomyelitis * OPV is a live-attenuated vaccine 1:1,000,000 risk after first dose and 1:2,000,000

Table 2-2. ADULT IMMUNIZATION *Continued*

Most Common...	Answer and Explanation
Continued	risk for susceptible household contact), • *IPV vaccination for nonimmunized adults traveling to developing countries:* only IPV is used to immunize susceptible adults
recommendations for nonimmunized adults who have children about to receive OPV	*IPV should be administered prior to the children receiving OPV owing to a potential risk for developing paralytic poliomyelitis* [There is no risk to nonimmunized adults exposed to children who have received MMR, which is also a live vaccine.]
recommendation for immunization in pregnant women	*routine immunization is best avoided during pregnancy* [If vaccination is indicated, inactivated viral vaccines such as * HBV, * influenza, and * pneumococcal vaccines may be administered. If the risk to the patient is great, the only live viral vaccines that may be used are OPV and yellow fever vaccines (MMR and varicella vaccines are contraindicated).]
recommendation for immunizations in women who are breast-feeding	*immunization poses no danger either to the lactating mother or infant with any live or killed vaccine*
polysaccharide vaccines	• *pneumococcus,* • *Hib*
toxoid vaccine	*Td*
recombinant viral vaccine	*HBV*
live viral vaccines	• *OPV,* • *MMR,* • *varicella,* • *yellow fever* [Except for OPV and yellow fever, live viral vaccines should not be given for at least 3 months after receiving immune globulin.]
killed viral vaccines	• *influenza,* • *IPV,* • *HAV,* • *rabies (human diploid)*
live bacterial vaccine	*BCG*
inactivated bacterial vaccines	• *cholera,* • *plague,* • *typhoid,* • *anthrax,* • *Hib,* • *meningococcal,* • *pneumococcal*
polysaccharide bacterial vaccines	• *Hib,* • *meningococcal,* • *pneumococcal*

Table continued on following page

Table 2–2. **ADULT IMMUNIZATION** *Continued*

Most Common...	Answer and Explanation
antitoxins	• *botulism*, • *diphtheria*, • *Crotalus antitoxin*: the antitoxin is against the venom of rattlesnakes [Antitoxins are a solution of antibodies derived from the serum of animals immunized with specific antigens.]
specific immune globulin preparations	• *HBV*, • *tetanus*, • *varicella/zoster*, • *rabies*
vaccines contraindicated in patients with egg allergy	• *MMR*, • *yellow fever*, • *influenza*
vaccines contraindicated in patients with reactions against neomycin	• *MMR*, • *OPV*, • *varicella*
vaccines contraindicated in patients with reactions against streptomycin	• *OPV*, • *IPV*
recommendation for nonimmunized travelers to countries with a high incidence of HBV	*active immunization with recombinant HBV vaccine at least 6 months prior to leaving the United States* [All travelers to foreign countries should have up-to-date immunization for tetanus, pertussis, polio, MMR, and HBV.]
recommendations for nonimmunized adults	• *Td*: see above, • *pneumococcal vaccine if 65 or older or have risk factors*, • *annual influenza vaccine ≥65 y*, • *HBV, if risk factors present*, • *MMR* (1–2 doses if born after 1956), • *varicella vaccination*
causes of rabies in the United States	• **skunk bite**, • *raccoons:* common cause in Northeast, • *fox*, • *bats:* bites or aerosolization, • *coyotes:* Texas, • *woodchucks:* only rodent. [In third world countries, rabid dogs are the most common cause of rabies.]
recommendation for a dog bite	*quarantine the dog for 10 d:* * no sign of rabies, no immunization necessary, * signs of rabies, decapitate dog and send head to state health department to check for rabies

Table 2–2. ADULT IMMUNIZATION *Continued*

Most Common...	Answer and Explanation
recommendation for bites by a bat, skunk, fox, coyote, or woodchuck	*active and passive immunization* [After cleaning the wound with quaternary ammonium soap, ½ of the Ig is injected into the wound and the other ½ is injected in another site. Active immunization is with human diploid vaccine.]

Question: Which of the following vaccines are recommended in all normal adult patients who have not been previously immunized? **SELECT 5**

- (A) Hib
- (B) Td
- (C) OPV
- (D) MMR
- (E) Varicella
- (F) IPV
- (G) Pneumococcal (≥65 y old)
- (H) aP
- (I) Influenza (≥65 y old)

Answers: (B), (D), (E), (G), (I): Hib (choice A) is a childhood immunization. Td (choice B) is recommended with a booster every 10 years. OPV (choice C) is not recommended in adults ≥18 years of age. IPV (choice F) is only recommended in high-risk patients (e.g., child in the home is going to receive OPV) who have not been immunized or in those who are traveling to countries where polio is endemic. MMR (choice D) and varicella immunizations (choice E) are recommended. Pneumococcal vaccine (choice G) is recommended if the patient is high risk or ≥65 years old. Acellular pertussis vaccine (aP, choice H) is recommended only for children. Influenza vaccine (choice I) is recommended annually for patients ≥65 years old.

anti-HBs = surface antibodies against hepatitis B surface antigen, aP = acellular pertussis vaccine, BCG = bacille Calmette-Guérin vaccine, DM = diabetes mellitus, DTP = diphtheria/tetanus/pertussis, HAV = hepatitis A virus, HbSS = sickle cell disease, HBV = hepatitis B virus, Hib = *Haemophilus influenzae* type b vaccine, HIV = human immunodeficiency virus, Ig = immune globulin, IM = intramuscular, IPV = inactivated enhanced potency polio vaccine, MMR = measles/mumps/rubella, OPV = oral polio vaccine, Td = tetanus/diphtheria.

Table 2–3. SMOKING RISKS

Most Common...	Answer and Explanation
cause of premature death in the United States	*cigarette smoking* [Smoking accounts for 20% of all deaths in the United States.]

Table continued on following page

Table 2–3. SMOKING RISKS *Continued*

Most Common...	Answer and Explanation
test used to document nicotine intake	*plasma or urine level of continine* [Nicotine is absorbed rapidly into the pulmonary circulation. It moves quickly into the brain where it attaches to nicotinic cholinergic receptors to produce its gratifying effects. Continine is only derived from the metabolism of nicotine.]
complication of smoking	*COPD:* * chronic bronchitis, * emphysema
single preventable cause of cancer	*smoking*
cancers in which smoking is the leading cause	• **lung cancer:** * squamous, * small cell, * adenocarcinoma to a lesser extent, • *oral squamous cancer,* • *pancreatic adenocarcinoma,* • *esophagus:* squamous, • *larynx:* squamous, • *transitional cell carcinoma of the bladder,* • *renal adenocarcinoma*
cancers in which smoking has been implicated but is not the most common risk factor	• *cervical cancer:* * squamous, * carcinogens have been found in cervical secretions, • *stomach adenocarcinoma,* • *breast adenocarcinoma:* in women who are slow acetylators of *N*-acetyltransferase 2 enzymes, • *prostate adenocarcinoma,* • *colon adenocarcinoma,* • *leukemia:* increased risk of both lymphoid and myeloid leukemias
cocarcinogen that enhances the risk of oropharyngeal, esophageal, and laryngeal cancers	*alcohol:* alcohol alone is a risk factor for oropharyngeal, esophageal, and laryngeal cancers, * alcohol + smoking further enhances the cancer risk.
cocarcinogen that enhances the risk for lung cancer	*asbestos* [Smoking + exposure to asbestos markedly increases the risk for primary lung cancer, but not mesothelioma, which has no association with smoking. However, whether the patient is a smoker or not, lung cancer is the most common cancer associated with asbestos exposure.]
genetic change associated with smoking-related cancer	*inactivation of the p53 suppressor gene by a point mutation on chromosome 17*

Table 2–3. **SMOKING RISKS** *Continued*

Most Common...	Answer and Explanation
cardiovascular effects of smoking	• **increased risk for AMI**: increased risk for recurrent AMI as well, • *sudden cardiac death,* • *peripheral vascular disease* [Smoking is responsible for ~20% of cardiovascular deaths. Contributing factors include * enhanced atherosclerosis, * nicotine effect on blood pressure and heart rate, * atherogenic lipid profile, * tissue hypoxia secondary to excess CO, and * hypercoagulability.]
pulmonary effects of smoking	• **COPD:** ~80%, • *recurrent infections:* * pneumonia, * URIs, • *exacerbates bronchial asthma,* • *cancer:* see above
GI effects	• **GERD,** • *delays the rate of ulcer healing,* • *increased risk for cancer:* see above
effects of smokeless tobacco (snuff, chewing tobacco)	• **nicotine addiction,** • *leukoplakia and cancer inside the lip, under the tongue or cheek:* verrucous squamous cancer, • *nasal cancer:* snuff users, • *aggravation of cardiovascular disease:* nicotine effect
effect of smoking on bone	*increases the risk for osteoporosis* [Smoking antagonizes the protective effect of estrogen in women and testosterone in men on the breakdown of bone.]
effects of smoking during pregnancy	• **increases the risk of having a low birthweight baby:** fetal tobacco syndrome, • *increases premature births,* • *increases the risk for spontaneous abortions, abruptio placentae, and PROM,* • *increases perinatal mortality,* • *reduces fertility* [The vasoconstrictive effects of nicotine produce placental ischemia. Endothelial damage due to smoke is also associated with an increased risk for thrombosis in placental vessels.]
effects of passive smoke on children	• *increases the incidence of SIDS,* • *increases risk for lung cancer,* • *exacerbates asthma,* • *increases risk for otitis media,* • *increases risk for recurrent upper and lower respiratory infections* [~75% of the total combustion product in a cigarette is exhaled, hence the risk of passive smoke on children as well as adults.]

Table continued on following page

Table 2–3. SMOKING RISKS *Continued*

Most Common...	Answer and Explanation
CNS effect of smoking	*increases risk for CVA*
renal effect of smoking in DM	*increases risk for developing proteinuria*
effect of smoking on the incidence of residential fires	*directly responsible for ~25% of residential fires*
beneficial effects of quitting smoking	• *longevity:* smokers who quit before 50 years of age have half the risk of dying over the next 15 years that a smoker has, • *lung cancer:* in 10 years, there is a 50% reduction in lung cancer when compared to a smoker and after 15 years, a 16% risk for lung cancer when compared to a smoker, • *AMI: AMI risk approaches that of a nonsmoker after 1 year of abstinence,* • *pregnancy:* pregnant women who stop smoking in the first trimester reduce the risk of a low birthweight baby to that of a nonsmoker, • *FEV$_{1sec}$: it is not improved by cessation of smoking, but the rate of decline is similar to that of a nonsmoker* [Smoking has declined in the United States. It is still more common in men than women; however, the incidence is increasing in women and decreasing in men.]

Question: Smoking is a risk factor for which of the following conditions? **SELECT 4**
- (A) Obesity
- (B) Hypothyroidism
- (C) Cervical cancer
- (D) Rheumatoid arthritis
- (E) Alzheimer's disease
- (F) Bladder cancer
- (G) Basal cell carcinoma
- (H) Abruptio placentae
- (I) Colorectal cancer

Answers: (C), (F), (H), (I): Currently, there is no relationship of smoking with obesity (**choice A is incorrect**), hypothyroidism (**choice B is incorrect**), rheumatoid arthritis (**choice D is incorrect**), Alzheimer's disease (**choice E is incorrect**), or basal cell carcinoma (**choice G is incorrect**). Cervical cancer (**choice C**), squamous carcinoma, transitional cell carcinoma of the bladder (**choice F**), abruptio placentae (**choice H**, vasoconstrictive effects of nicotine) and colorectal cancer (**choice I**) are all increased in patients who smoke.

AMI = acute myocardial infarction, CNS = central nervous system,

COPD = chronic obstructive pulmonary disease, CVA = cerebrovascular accident, DM = diabetes mellitus, FEV_{1sec} = forced expiratory volume in 1 second, GERD = gastroesophageal reflux disease, GI = gastrointestinal, PROM = premature rupture of membranes, SIDS = sudden infant death syndrome, URIs = upper respiratory infections.

Table 2–4. ALCOHOL ABUSE

Most Common...	Answer and Explanation
sites of alcohol reabsorption	• **small intestine:** 75%, • *stomach: 25%* [It is partially metabolized in the stomach by alcohol dehydrogenase.]
site of alcohol metabolism	*liver* [The breakdown is as follows: $$\text{alcohol} \xrightarrow{\text{alcohol dehydrogenase}} \text{acetaldehyde} + \text{NADH} \xrightarrow{\text{aldehyde dehydrogenase}} \text{acetate} + \text{NADH} \rightarrow \text{acetyl CoA}.$$
pharmacologic action of alcohol	*CNS depressant* [In descending order, its depressant effect is on the * cerebral cortex, * limbic system, * cerebellum, and * lower brain stem. It potentiates the action of inhibitory neurotransmitters like γ-aminobutyric acid.]
genetic defect affecting alcohol metabolism	*aldehyde dehydrogenase deficiency* [~40% of Asians are deficient in this enzyme. Alcohol intake leads to a build-up of acetaldehyde and GI upset.]
S/S at 50, 100, 125–150, 200–250, 300–350, >500 mg/dL	• *50 mg/dL:* * euphoria, * gregarious, * talkative, • *100 mg/dL:* * legally drunk, * slurred speech, * uncoordinated, • *125–150 mg/dL:* * combativeness, * unrestrained behavior, • *200–250 mg/dL:* lethargic, • *300–350 mg/dL:* stupor or coma, • >500 mg/dL: death
blood level accepted in most states as legal drunkenness	*≥100 mg/dL* [Some states have limits as low as 80 mg/dL or as high as 150 mg/dL. 50% of all drug fatalities and 25% of all suicides are associated with alcohol abuse.]
clinical findings in alcoholic blackouts	*amnesia lasting for several hours or more after a bout of heavy drinking:* Sign of impending or already existing alcohol addiction.

Table continued on following page

Table 2–4. ALCOHOL ABUSE *Continued*

Most Common...	Answer and Explanation
withdrawal states	• **tremulousness:** accompanied by insomnia and agitation • *rum fits* • *DTs*
S/S of rum fits	*generalized seizures* [These emerge when blood alcohol levels begin dropping. They may occur while drinking or a few hours after drinking. In one-third of cases, they are followed by DTs.]
Rx of rum fits	*IV diazepam*
S/S of DTs	• *tremulousness*, • disorientation, • *visual hallucinations*, • *agitation*, • β-*adrenergic signs:* * tachycardia, * sweating, * fear, * tachypnea, * HTN, • *incontinence* [The above emerge 3–5 days after complete withdrawal. They may occur while hospitalized for some other ailment.]
Rx of DTs	• **IV diazepam**, • *IV thiamine:* prevent or Rx Wernicke's syndrome
diseases in which alcohol is the leading cause	• *thiamine deficiency*: * Wernicke's syndrome, * Korsakoff's psychosis, * congestive cardiomyopathy, • *macrocytic anemia*: folate deficiency, • *acquired sideroblastic anemia,* • *Mallory-Weiss syndrome:* tear of the distal esophagus/proximal stomach from retching, • *Boerhaave's syndrome:* rupture of the distal esophagus/proximal stomach from retching, • *cirrhosis*, • *esophageal varices:* indirect effect of PH from alcoholic cirrhosis, • *fatty change in the liver*, • *alcoholic hepatitis*, • *chronic pancreatitis*, • *acute pancreatitis*: shares the lead with biliary tract disease
cancer risks associated with alcohol	• **squamous carcinoma**: * head and neck, * esophagus, * larynx—cocarcinogen with smoking, • *adenocarcinoma:* * stomach, * pancreas, * breast, * liver
nutritional effects of alcohol	• **protein-energy malnutrition**, • *thiamine deficiency* [Alcohol provides 7 calories per gram. These are empty calories and provide negligible amounts of vitamins, trace minerals, and protein.]

Table 2–4. **ALCOHOL ABUSE** *Continued*

Most Common...	Answer and Explanation
effects of alcohol on the CNS/PNS	• *Wernicke's syndrome,* • *Korsakoff's psychosis,* • *cerebellar degeneration:* Hu and Yo antibodies noted in spinal fluid, • *dementia,* • *DTs:* see above, • *distal peripheral neuropathy,* • *optic atrophy,* • *central pontine myelinolysis*
effects on the hematologic system	• *macrocytic anemia:* most commonly folate deficiency—nutritional basis, • *thrombocytopenia:* * direct toxic effect on megakaryocytes, * hypersplenism, • *leukopenia:* hypersplenism, • *sideroblastic anemia:* * most common cause, * ringed sideroblasts in the BM, • *iron deficiency:* bleeding from esophagitis, gastritis, esophageal varices, • *decreases platelet aggregation:* prolongs the bleeding time, • *prolonged PT:* coagulation factor deficiencies
effects of alcohol on the GI system	• *esophageal varices:* * most common cause, * related to PH, • *esophagitis,* • *GERD,* • *acute gastritis,* • *Mallory-Weiss/Boerhaave's syndrome*
effects of alcohol on the HB/pancreas system	• **fatty liver:** most common cause, • *alcoholic hepatitis,* • *cirrhosis:* most common cause, • *hemosiderosis:* acquired iron overload, • *gallstones,* • *acute/chronic pancreatitis:* most common cause
effects of alcohol on the CV system	• *congestive cardiomyopathy:* * direct toxic effect on myocardial tissue, * thiamine deficiency, • *cardiac arrhythmias:* * paroxysmal tachycardia, * hyperlipidemia—type IV hypertriglyceridemia
effects of alcohol on the GU system	• *impotence:* * decreases erectile capacity, * reduces testosterone levels by a direct toxic effect on Leydig cells, * inhibits gonadotropin release, * increases SHBG—increases binding of free testosterone, • *fetal alcohol syndrome:* * most common teratogen, * mental retardation, * facial and cardiac defects, • *secondary amenorrhea:* decreases gonadotropins

Table continued on following page

Table 2–4. **ALCOHOL ABUSE** Continued

Most Common...	Answer and Explanation
effects of alcohol on the respiratory system	• *lung abscesses*: aspiration of infected oropharyngeal secretions, • *Klebsiella pneumoniae pneumonia*, • *TB*, • *laryngeal cancer*
effects of alcohol on immune system	• *increased susceptibility to infection*, • *impaired healing*
effect of alcohol on the musculoskeletal system	• **myopathy**, • *rhabdomyolysis* [Painful myopathy may occur with an increase in serum CK. Rhabdomyolysis may occur abruptly particularly after a rum fit with all the seizure activity.]
lab findings in alcohol abuse	• *macrocytic anemia*: folate deficiency—most common cause, • *fasting hypoglycemia:* see Table 1–3, • *lactic and β-OHB acidosis*: Table 1–3, • *iron deficiency*: decreased iron, percent saturation, and ferritin, increased TIBC, • sideroblastic anemia: increased iron, percent saturation, ferritin, decreased TIBC, • *increased GGT*: * see Table 1–3, * levels >30 units/IU indicate heavy drinking, • *serum AST > ALT*: * AST is primarily in hepatocyte mitochondria, * alcohol is a mitochondrial poison causing preferential release of AST, • *hyperuricemia*: see Table 1–3, • *increased TG*: see Table 1–3, • *hypomagnesemia*: * nutritional deficiency, * diarrhea, • *hypokalemia*: * dietary deficiency, * vomiting, * secondary aldosteronism from cirrhosis, • *hypophosphatemia*: * dietary deficiency, * may lead to respiratory failure, especially if the patient is given fructose, a phosphate trapper, • *chronic respiratory alkalosis*: toxic metabolites in cirrhotic patients overstimulate the central respiratory center

Table 2–4. ALCOHOL ABUSE *Continued*

Question: Alcohol is causally related to which of the following conditions? **SELECT 4**
  (A) Metabolic acidosis
  (B) B_{12} deficiency
  (C) Chronic pancreatitis
  (D) Hemochromatosis
  (E) Hypertrophic cardiomyopathy
  (F) Rhabdomyolysis
  (G) Macrocytic anemia
  (H) Acute leukemia
  (I) Colorectal cancer

Answers: (A), (C), (F), (G): Metabolic acidosis **(choice A)** is secondary to increased production of both lactic and β-OHB. Folate deficiency as a cause of macrocytic anemia is far more common than B_{12} deficiency **(choice B is incorrect)**, since the liver stores last for only 3–4 months. Chronic pancreatitis **(choice C)** is most commonly associated with alcohol excess. Hemosiderosis is an acquired iron overload disease, which may be associated with alcohol excess. However, hemochromatosis **(choice D is incorrect)** is a genetic iron overload disease. Congestive rather than hypertrophic cardiomyopathy **(choice E is incorrect)** is seen in alcoholics. Rhabdomyolysis **(choice F)** may occur in alcoholics secondary to myopathy or hypophosphatemia. Currently, there is no association of alcohol with leukemia **(choice H is incorrect)** or colon cancer **(choice I is incorrect).**

ALT = alanine aminotransferase, AST = aspartate aminotransferase, BM = bone marrow, β-OHB = β-hydroxybutyric acid, CK = creatine kinase, CNS = central nervous system, CoA = coenzyme A, CV = cardiovascular, CVA = cerebrovascular accident, DTs = delirium tremens, GGT = γ-glutamyltransferase, GERD = gastroesophageal reflux disease, GI = gastrointestinal, GU = genitourinary, HB = hepatobiliary, HTN = hypertension, IV = intravenous, NADH = nicotinamide adenine dinucleotide (reduced form), PH = portal hypertension, PNS = peripheral nervous system, PT = prothrombin time, Rx = treatment, SHBG = sex hormone binding globulin, S/S = signs and symptoms, TB = tuberculosis, TG = triglyceride, TIBC = total iron binding capacity.

Table 2–5. DRUGS OF ABUSE (DOA)

Most Common...	Answer and Explanation
types of DOA	• *sedatives:* e.g., barbiturates, alcohol, • *stimulants:* e.g., cocaine, • *hallucinogens:* e.g., lysergic acid diethylamide [There is some overlap among the drugs in these groups.]
patient criteria for compulsive drug use	• *psychologic dependence*: craving and motivation for procuring the drug, • *physiologic*

Table continued on following page

Table 2–5. **DRUGS OF ABUSE (DOA)** *Continued*

Most Common...	Answer and Explanation
Continued	dependence: withdrawal symptoms occur when D/C the drug, • *tolerance*: dose of the drug must be increased to produce the same desired effects [Drug abuse is most common in the 18- to 25-year-old age group and is three times more common in males than females.]
CNS effects of long-term drug abuse	*damage to neurotransmitter receptor sites* [This may lead to psychiatric illness in the patient as well as poor job performance. Cerebral atrophy may occur with certain drugs, e.g., alcohol.]
groups of drugs that are water soluble	• *alcohol*, • *opioids*, • *stimulants* [Since they are water soluble, they are cleared more rapidly by the kidneys (often within 24 h), hence making their detection more difficult.]
groups of drugs that are lipophilic	• *THC*, • *barbiturates* [Lipophilic drugs take longer to clear out through the kidneys (days to months), since they must be rendered water soluble by the liver cytochrome system.]
factors affecting drug reabsorption in the GI tract	• *water or lipid solubility*, • *pKa of the drug*, • *pH of the drug*, • *gastric emptying time*, • *gastric pH*, • *intestinal motility*, • *presence of other drugs*, • *food interference* [Most weakly acidic drugs are in the nonionized state and are rapidly reabsorbed in the acid environment of the stomach. Highly ionized basic drugs are not absorbed in these conditions.]
factors affecting the distribution of a drug to its site of action	• *plasma protein concentration*, • *protein binding of the drug*, • *underlying disease conditions*, • *body composition*, • *degree of tissue perfusion* [Only the free drug can cross cell membranes. Acidic drugs (e.g., LSD) most often bind to albumin, while basic drugs (e.g., opioids, barbiturates) bind to α_1-acid glycoproteins. Drugs may be displaced from binding proteins, hence increasing their free concentration. The volume of distribution of a drug is dependent on body composition (lipophilic drugs distribute to adipose, while water-soluble drugs concentrate in the serum).]
site for drug metabolism	*hepatic microsomal* (cytochrome) *system* [The microsomal system renders drugs more water soluble. Microsomal enzyme systems act on classes of compounds with similar

Table 2–5. DRUGS OF ABUSE (DOA) *Continued*

Most Common...	Answer and Explanation
opiate DOA	• **heroin** (diacetylmorphine), • *morphine*, • *meperidine*, • *methadone*, • *codeine* [Opiates are depressant drugs. Heroin (morphine is a derivative of heroin) and codeine derive from the poppy plant, while methadone is a synthetic opioid. Both withdrawal symptoms and tolerance are associated with these drugs.]
methods of taking heroin	• **IV or SC**, • *snorting*, • *smoking* [Heroin is usually "cut" with some agent (e.g., quinine, talc), to which granulomatous reactions occur in the skin and lungs.]
opiate DOA among health professionals	*meperidine*
localized infection in IVDA	*skin abscesses, due to Staphylococcus aureus*
systemic infections in IVDA	• **HBV**, • *HIV:* IVDA accounts for 22% of all cases of HIV, • *infective endocarditis:* * right-sided (TV) and left-sided (AV) valvular disease, * *S. aureus* most common cause, • *brain abscesses*, • *osteomyelitis*, • *tetanus:* from "skin popping"
S/S of heroin overdose	• **respiratory depression**, • *miotic pupils:* they are mydriatic in the presence of acidosis, • *non-cardiogenic pulmonary edema:* frothing from the mouth is common
serious renal complication in IV heroin abuse	*focal segmental glomerulosclerosis:* FSG presents with HTN and the nephrotic syndrome
Rx for heroin overdose	*naloxone:* morphine derivative that has a high affinity for opioid binding sites of the mu receptor type
withdrawal symptoms of opioid abuse	• **adrenergic symptoms:** * anxiety, * sweating, * piloerection, • *fever*, • *rhinorrhea*, • *N/V*, • *cramping in the stomach* [Clonidine prevents the adrenergic symptoms.]

Table 2–5. DRUGS OF ABUSE (DOA) Continued

Most Common...	Answer and Explanation
Continued	structures, hence the possibility of drug competition for metabolism. In general, drugs are metabolized from an active to an inactive form. Some DOA enhance the microsomal system (e.g., alcohol), which increases the drug's metabolism, hence requiring a greater amount of the drug to produce the same effect (tolerance).]
site for drug excretion	*kidneys*
method used for drug screening	*immunoassays and/or chromatographic techniques* [Urine is the best screening medium for DOA; however, blood is also used in drug assays. Positive screens are confirmed with gas-liquid mass spectrophotometry, since many over-the-counter drugs cross-react with drugs of abuse (e.g., chlorpromazine with opioids).]
toxic syndromes associated with DOA	• *sympathomimetic*: e.g., * amphetamines, * cocaine, • *opiate/sedative*: e.g., * heroin, * benzodiazepines, * barbiturates, • *anticholinergic*: e.g., antidepressants, • *psychedelic/hallucinogenic*: e.g., * PCP, * LSD
S/S of sympathomimetic toxicity	• *tachycardia*, • *mydriasis*: pupillary dilatation, • *psychosis*, • *piloerection*, • *HTN*, • *hyperthermia*, • *sweating*, • *seizures*
S/S of opiate/ sedative toxicity	• *respiratory depression*, • *stupor/coma*, • *seizures*, • *miotic pupils*: * pinpoint pupils, * mydriasis occurs if acidosis is present, • *absent DTRs*, • *hypotension*
S/S of anticholinergic toxic syndromes	• *mydriasis*, • *fever elevation often into hyperthermic ranges*, • *dry skin*, • *dementia*, • *tachycardia*, • *myoclonic jerks*, • *seizures*
types of drug toxicities with anticholinergic S/S	• *antidepressants*, • *antihistamines*, • *antiparkinson-type medications*, • *atropine*, • *muscle relaxants*
antidotes used in unconscious patients	• *dextrose*: * R/O possible hypoglycemia from insulin overdose, * draw serum for glucose before giving dextrose, • *naloxone*: possible opiate overdose, • *intravenous thiamine*: * possible alcohol effect, * glucose may precipitate Wernicke's encephalopathy

Table continued on following page

Table 2–5. **DRUGS OF ABUSE (DOA)** *Continued*

Most Common...	**Answer and Explanation**
use of methadone	*detoxification of opiate abusers* [Methadone is a legal, synthetic opioid that is taken orally. A long-acting drug, it saturates the CNS opiate receptors and prevents the sudden euphoric action usually associated with heroin. It causes physical dependence and tolerance. Naloxone must be used for a longer time in drug overdose.]
symptoms of benzodiazepine toxicity	• *drowsiness*, • *dysarthria*, • *ataxia* [Benzodiazepines enhance the *frequency* of opening up of the $GABA_A$ receptor-chloride ion channels, which increases chloride ion conductance. GABA is an inhibitory neurotransmitter. In general, benzodiazepines depress mental and respiratory function, but to a lesser degree than barbiturates. Both withdrawal symptoms and tolerance are associated with the drugs. Their effect is enhanced in the presence of alcohol. They are used as tranquilizers, sedatives, muscle relaxants, anticonvulsants, and anesthetics and are the drug of choice for Rx of patients with the alcohol withdrawal syndrome.]
drug Rx of benzodiazepine toxicity	*flumazenil* [Flumazenil is an antagonist of benzodiazepine. It does not block barbiturates or other depressants, hence it does not work effectively if mixed overdoses with antidepressants are present.]
S/S of barbiturate overdose	• *respiratory and mental status depression*, • *coma*, • *loss of DTRs*, • *bullae over pressure points:* erythema multiforme, • *hypothermia*, • *hypotension* [Barbiturates enhance the *duration* of opening up of the $GABA_A$ receptor-chloride ion channels, which increases chloride ion conductance. They depress neuronal activity in the reticular activating system, which also inhibits the inhibitory effects of GABA and glycine (an amino acid inhibitory neurotransmitter). Both withdrawal symptoms and tolerance are associated with the drugs. They have a similar range of clinical uses noted above for benzodiazepines.]

Table continued on following page

Table 2–5. DRUGS OF ABUSE (DOA) *Continued*

Most Common...	Answer and Explanation
Rx of barbiturate overdose	• *maintain the airway and blood pressure,* • *gastric lavage with activated charcoal,* • *increase excretion of the drug in the urine with forced alkaline diuresis using sodium bicarbonate*
COD from an illicit drug in the United States	*cocaine overdose* [Cocaine blocks the uptake of neurotransmitters dopamine and NOR by the presynaptic axon. It is a sympathomimetic drug (e.g., produces mydriasis; *d* = dilate). It predisposes to * sudden death, * AMI, * pulmonary edema, * ventricular arrhythmias, * CVA, and * myocarditis. Both withdrawal symptoms and tolerance are associated with the drug.]
effects of maternal cocaine use on the newborn	• **microcephaly**: most common CNS effect, • *hyperactivity,* • *growth retardation,* • *interruption of blood flow leading to CNS, bowel, and limbs*—infarcts with missing digits
effects of cocaine abuse during pregnancy	• *stillbirths,* • *premature birth,* • *abruptio placentae,* • *SGA newborn*
S/S of cocaine overdose	• *HTN,* • *psychosis,* • *seizure activity,* • *perforated/ulcerated nasal septum,* • *mydriasis,* • *sinus tachycardia*
Rx of cocaine overdose	• *benzodiazepines control seizure activity,* • *lidocaine for ventricular arrhythmias,* • *labetalol for adrenergic symptoms*
S/S of amphetamine overdose	• *cardiovascular abnormalities:* * arrhythmias, * HTN, * tachycardia, * AMI, * circulatory collapse, • *extreme hyperexcitability,* • *hallucinations,* • *flushing,* • *rhabdomyolysis with myoglobinuria,* • *mydriasis,* • *hyperthermia* [Amphetamines release catecholamines from presynaptic terminals. Stimulant drugs listed as amphetamines include dextroamphetamine (used in treating obesity), methylphenidate (used in treating ADHD, narcolepsy), methamphetamine ("ice" is a street form of the drug). Both withdrawal symptoms and tolerance are associated with the drugs. Overdose S/S resemble those of schizophrenia.]

Table 2–5. **DRUGS OF ABUSE (DOA)** *Continued*

Most Common...	Answer and Explanation
drug Rx of amphetamine overdose	• *activated charcoal,* • *benzodiazepines for seizures and agitation,* • *haloperidol for hallucinations,* • *propranolol or lidocaine for arrhythmias*
illegal DOA used in the United States	*marijuana* [Marijuana contains the psychoactive stimulant Δ^9-tetrahydrocannabinol (THC), which derives from the leaves and flowering tops of hemp plants (*Cannabis sativa*). *Hashish* is the extracted resin of marijuana that has 5–10 times the potency of the parent compound. THC binds to receptors in the substantia nigra, globus pallidus, hippocampus, and cerebellum. Owing to its high lipid solubility, THC in the urine is present for more than a week.]
S/S of marijuana use	• *tachycardia,* • *reddening of the conjunctiva,* • *orthostatic hypotension,* • *euphoria,* • *uncontrollable laughter,* • *delayed reaction time,* • *inability to judge speed and distance,* • *gynecomastia,* • *lung disease:* * COPD, * cancer [No teratogenic effect has been documented. Withdrawal symptoms are occasionally observed, but there is no tolerance to the drug.]
clinical uses of marijuana	• *decrease N/V in cancer patients,* • *lower intraocular pressure in glaucoma,* • *analgesic*
S/S of LSD toxicity	• **hallucinations,** • *diaphoresis,* • *mydriasis,* • *HTN,* • *flashbacks* [LSD is an ergot alkaloid that binds to the D_2 dopamine receptor in the brain (it also blocks the 5-HT_2 serotonin receptor in peripheral tissue). It is not associated with withdrawal symptoms but tolerance has been observed. There is controversy over whether it predisposes to chromosomal breakage leading to congenital defects.]
S/S of PCP toxicity	• **agitation,** *hallucinations:* auditory and visual, • *violent behavior,* • *impervious to pain,* • *HTN,* • *coma with the eyes open,* • *hyperacusis,* • *myotonic jerks,* • *horizontal and vertical nystagmus,* • *hyperthermia* [PCP (angel dust) is the most dangerous of the hallucinogenic drugs. It was initially introduced as a dissociative anesthetic, in that it separated bodily functions from the mind without a loss

Table continued on following page

Table 2–5. DRUGS OF ABUSE (DOA) *Continued*

Most Common...	Answer and Explanation
Continued	of consciousness. It reacts with opioid-like sigma receptors and subtypes of glutamate receptors (antagonist)].
Rx of PCP toxicity	• *benzodiazepine for agitation,* • *propranolol for adrenergic symptoms,* • *diphenhydramine for myoclonic activity* [There is no withdrawal or drug tolerance. Acidification of the urine is no longer recommended.]
DOA in adolescents	• **marijuana**, • *alcohol*

Question: Which of the following drugs is characteristically associated with tachycardia and redness of the conjunctiva? **SELECT 1**
- (A) Cocaine
- (B) PCP
- (C) Amphetamines
- (D) LSD
- (E) Marijuana

Answer: (E): Marijuana (**choice E**) characteristically is associated with tachycardia, conjunctival irritation, and orthostatic hypotension. Cocaine toxicity (**choice A is incorrect**) is similar to amphetamine toxicity but is more likely to have perforation of the nasal septum. PCP (**choice B is incorrect**) is associated with violent behavior and toxicity (**choice C is incorrect**). Amphetamine toxicity (**choice C is incorrect**) is most often confused with schizophrenia. LSD (**choice D is incorrect**) is associated with hallucinations, diaphoresis, mydriasis, hypertension, and flashbacks.

ADHD = attention deficit and hyperactivity disorder, AMI = acute myocardial infarction, AV = aortic valve, CNS = central nervous system, COD = cause of death, CVA = cardiovascular accident, DOA = drug of abuse, D/C = discontinue, DTRs = deep tendon reflexes, FSG = focal segmental glomerulosclerosis, GABA = γ-aminobutyric acid, GI = gastrointestinal, HBV = hepatitis B, HIV = human immunodeficiency virus, HTN = hypertension, IV = intravenous, IVDA = intravenous drug abuse, LSD = lysergic acid diethylamide, NOR = norepinephrine, N/V = nausea/vomiting, PCP = phencyclidine, pka = ionization constant, R/O = rule out, Rx = treatment, SC = subcutaneous, SGA = small for gestational age, S/S = signs and symptoms, THC = tetrahydrocannabinol, TV = tricuspid valve.

CHAPTER

HUMAN GENETICS AND AGING

CONTENTS

Table 3–1. DIAGNOSTIC TECHNIQUES, MUTATIONS, CHROMOSOME DISORDERS

Most Common...	Answer and Explanation
diagnostic techniques used in genetics	• *history:* e.g., * family history, * ethnicity, • *pedigree analysis:* maps out the distribution of an inherited disease, • *physical exam,* • *prenatal testing:* e.g., * amniocentesis—16 weeks, * chorionic villous sampling—9–12 weeks, * fetal blood sampling, • *ultrasonogram:* e.g., R/O open tube defects, • *maternal screening:* e.g., serum AFP, • *recombinant DNA technology:* e.g., * nucleic acid probes, * RFLP
DNA technique used to locate gene abnormalities	*nucleic acid probes* [Probes contain specific amino acid sequences of portions of DNA. They are spliced into DNA strands and are allowed to hybridize with a corresponding segment of DNA from a patient sample.]
use of PCR in genetics	*amplifies DNA fragments that harbor abnormal gene loci*
gene technique used when the exact site of an abnormal gene is unknown	*restriction fragment length polymorphism (RFLP)* [Abnormal genetic sites must be linked to a harmless marker gene on the same chromosome. DNA fragments on the abnormal chromosome (DNA is cleaved by restriction endonucleases) from both normal family members and those with the disease are studied for variations in fragment lengths to de-

Table continued on following page

Table 3–1. DIAGNOSTIC TECHNIQUES, MUTATIONS, CHROMOSOME DISORDERS *Continued*

Most Common...	Answer and Explanation
Continued	tect abnormal genetic sites. Future children in that family can then be studied and compared with normal and affected family members.]
routine maternal screening tests for genetic disorders	• *AFP,* • β-*hCG,* • *urine for unconjugated estriol* [A low AFP and unconjugated estriol plus a high β-hCG occurs in Down syndrome in 60% of cases.]
screening test abnormality in open neural tube defects	*increased AFP* [AFP is fetal albumin. It must be correlated with the gestational age. Open neural tube defects have been causally related to folate deficiency.]
types of mutations	• **gene mutations**: * mendelian disorders secondary to deletion or insertions of nucleotide bases, * e.g., cystic fibrosis, • *genomic mutation*: * loss or gain of a whole chromosome, * e.g., trisomy 21, • *chromosome mutation:* * 1:180 births, * e.g., Down syndrome with 46 chromosomes [A mutation is a stable inheritable change in the DNA.]
cause of a genomic mutation	*nondisjunction* [In nondisjunction, there is a failure of one set of homologous chromosomes to separate during the first phase of meiosis. The gamete contains either 22 or 24 chromosomes (normal haploid number is 23). One-third of chromosome abnormalities involve *aneuploidy*, or an abnormal number of chromosomes.]
cause of a chromosome mutation	*translocations* [~34% of chromosome abnormalities involve translocations, deletions, duplications, or inversions. A translocation is where one part of a chromosome is transferred to a nonhomologous chromosome. It is a *balanced translocation* if the translocated fragment is still functional. A *Robertsonian translocation* is a type of balanced translocation in which there is a reciprocal translocation between the same two acrocentric chromosomes (e.g., chromosome 21) with the formation of one long chromosome. A parent has 45 chromosomes but is normal, while the patient has 46 chromosomes with 3 functional chromosomes 21s.]

Table 3–1. DIAGNOSTIC TECHNIQUES, MUTATIONS, CHROMOSOME DISORDERS *Continued*

Most Common...	Answer and Explanation
technique used to identify translocations, deletions, and other rearrangements	*chromosome analysis using banding and/or high-resolution techniques* [High-resolution techniques have identified microdeletion syndromes.]
examples of a microdeletion syndrome	• *Prader-Willi syndrome,* • *Angelman syndrome* [Both syndromes have a microdeletion at the same location on chromosome 15. In Prader-Willi syndrome, chromosome 15 is of paternal origin. In Angelman syndrome, chromosome 15 is of maternal origin. This is an example of *genomic imprinting*.]
cause of mosaicism	*mitotic nondisjunction:* unequal separation of chromosomes in mitotic division in the early embryonic period [Mosaicism is where two chromosomally different cell lines are derived from a single fertilized egg. Most cases involve the sex chromosomes (e.g., gonadal dysgenesis with XO/XX, XO/XY).]
types of gene mutations	• **point mutation with deletion of a single nucleotide**: e.g., * HbSS, * adenine replaces thymidine (valine replaces glutamic acid) in the sixth position of the β-globin chain, • *point mutation resulting in a stop codon*: e.g., * severe β-thalassemia, * the stop codon terminates β-globin chain synthesis, • *insertion of nucleotide bases leading to a frameshift mutation*: e.g., * Tay-Sachs disease, * a four-base insertion results in a defective hexosaminidase A, • *deletion of nucleotide bases*: e.g., * cystic fibrosis, * a three nucleotide base deletion coding for phenylalanine produces a defective transmembrane regulator protein for chloride ions, • *multifactorial (polygenic, complex) inheritance*: * multiple gene effects at independent sites along with certain environmental factors interact to produce a cumulative effect, * e.g., ♦ essential HTN, ♦ schizophrenia, ♦ CAD, ♦ gout, ♦ type II DM, ♦ cleft lip
type of mutation with the greatest risk of recurrence	*Mendelian disorders* [For example, AR diseases have a 25% rate of recurrence. A chromosomal disorder like trisomy 21 has only a

Table continued on following page

**Table 3–1. DIAGNOSTIC TECHNIQUES, MUTATIONS,
CHROMOSOME DISORDERS** *Continued*

Most Common...	Answer and Explanation
Continued	1% recurrence, and diseases exhibiting multi-factorial inheritance, have a 2–10% recurrence rate.]
genetic disorders in people of African origin	• **sickle cell trait/disease**: 8–10% prevalence, • *α- and β-thalassemia*, • *G6PD deficiency*, • *hereditary persistence of HbF*
genetic disorders in Ashkenazi Jews	• **factor XII deficiency**, • *Gaucher's disease*, • *Tay-Sachs disease*
genetic disorder in Northern Europeans	*cystic fibrosis* [CF is also the most common genetic disease interfering with the patient's ability to reproduce owing to early death or problems with fertility (e.g., absent vas deferens in male, thick cervical mucus in females).]
genetic disorder in Native Americans	*lactase deficiency*
genetic disorders in Mediterranean peoples	• **glucose 6-phosphate dehydrogenase deficiency**, • *sickle cell trait/disease*, • β-*thalassemia* [All of the above protect the patient from *Plasmodium falciparum* infections.]
Inuiet people	*21-hydroxylase deficiency*
genetic disorder in Southeast Asians	α-*thalassemia*
genetic syndrome associated with advanced maternal age	*trisomy 21 (Down syndrome)*
genetic syndromes associated with advanced paternal age	• **Marfan's syndrome**: prevalence 1:20,000, • *achondroplasia*: prevalence 1:26,000 [Increased paternal age leads to a greater number of cell divisions in germ cells, hence the greater risk for new mutations. Most of these produce an AD disease.]
genetic cause of mental retardation	*Down syndrome:* Increasing maternal age increases the risk for nondisjunction
clinical findings in Down syndrome	• **mental retardation**: ~50 IQ, • *CHD*: * 40%, * endocardial cushion defect, • *Alzheimer's disease*: occurs at an earlier age than usual, • *acute leukemia*, • *thyroid disease*, • *sterility in males*: females are fertile, • *duodenal atre-*

**Table 3–1. DIAGNOSTIC TECHNIQUES, MUTATIONS,
CHROMOSOME DISORDERS** *Continued*

Most Common...	Answer and Explanation
Continued	sia at birth: * vomiting of bile-stained fluid, * double bubble sign on abdominal x-ray, • *Hirschsprung's disease*, • *simian crease*
factor affecting longevity in adult Down syndrome patients	*Alzheimer's disease* [Chromosome 21 codes for β-amyloid protein, which is converted into amyloid that is toxic to neurons. Endocardial cushion defects is the most significant risk factor for *children* with Down syndrome.]
risk factors for having a child with Down syndrome	• **maternal age**: any women >35 years of age is at increased risk (1:385), • *risk of another affected child with trisomy 21 of 1–2%*, • *5–15% risk for parent with a balanced translocation of having another affected child*, • *female Down patient has a very high risk for having affected children* [The karyotype of the affected child should always be determined to determine the risk for siblings to have affected children.]
sex-chromosome disease recognizable at birth	*Turner's syndrome*
clinical findings in Turner's syndrome at birth	• **lymphedema of the hands and feet**, • *webbed neck*: redundant skin overlying dilated lymphatic channels, • *short fourth metacarpal*, • *preductal coarctation*: 30% with bicuspid aortic valve leading to heart failure
genetic cause of primary amenorrhea	*Turner's syndrome* [Oocytes are absent by 2 years of age, hence these patients have decreased estradiol levels with a subsequent lack of secondary sex characteristics and menses. There is no parental risk for having another affected child.]
cause of Turner's syndrome	*nondisjunction leading to a 45 XO genotype*: ~50–60% [Mosaics may also occur (XO/XY, XO/XX). Since one of the two X chromosomes is randomly inactivated to become a nuclear appendage called a Barr body, Turner's syndrome patients do not have any Barr bodies (a normal woman has one Barr body). Recall that ~50% of X-chromosomes are maternal and ~50% are paternal.

Table continued on following page

Table 3–1. DIAGNOSTIC TECHNIQUES, MUTATIONS, CHROMOSOME DISORDERS *Continued*

Most Common...	Answer and Explanation
study used to identify Barr bodies	*smear of the buccal mucosa squamous cells and identification of nuclear appendages representing Barr bodies*
ovarian tumors associated with Turner's syndrome	• **dysgerminoma**: germ cell tumor, • *gonadoblastoma:* mixed germ cell and sex cord/ stromal tumor [Presence of a Y chromosome confers an increased risk for ovarian cancer, hence the necessity of surgically removing the gonads.]
lab findings in Turner's syndrome	• *decreased estradiol and progesterone,* • *increased FSH and LH* [Decreased estradiol causes an increase in FSH and decreased progesterone, an increase in LH owing to negative feedback. Hypogonadism with an increase in FSH is called hypergonadotropic hypogonadism).]
cause of Klinefelter's syndrome	*nondisjunction resulting in an XXY genotype* [Normal males have no Barr bodies, while those with Klinefelter's syndrome have one Barr body.]
S/S of Klinefelter's disease	• *normal appearance before puberty,* • *arms and legs are disproportionately long,* • *hypogonadism,* • *female secondary sex characteristics*: * female hair distribution, * gynecomastia, • *learning disabilities,* • *atrophic testicles*: * atrophy/fibrosis of seminiferous tubules, * hyperplasia of Leydig cells, • *increased incidence of*: * DM, * autoimmune disease, * COPD, * malignant lymphoma, * breast cancer
cause of hyperestrinism in Klinefelter's syndrome	*aromatization of testosterone into estradiol in the Leydig cells* [Sertoli cells in the seminiferous tubules normally synthesize inhibin, which has a negative feedback with FSH. Absence of inhibin increases FSH, which increases Leydig cell synthesis of aromatase.]
lab findings in Klinefelter's syndrome	• *low testosterone,* • *azoospermia:* no sperm, • *high FSH*: low inhibin, • *high LH:* low testosterone, • *high serum estradiol* [This syndrome is an example of hypergonadotropic hypogonadism.]

Table 3–1. DIAGNOSTIC TECHNIQUES, MUTATIONS, CHROMOSOME DISORDERS *Continued*

Question: Which of the following ethnic groups has the greatest number of genetic disorders? **SELECT 1**

(A) Ashkenazi Jews
(B) Mediterranean peoples
(C) Southeast Asians
(D) African Americans
(E) Native Americans

Answer: (D): African Americans (**choice D**) have the greatest array of genetic disorders, including sickle cell trait/disease, G6PD deficiency, lactase deficiency, α and β-thalassemia, and hereditary persistence of HbF. Ashkenazi Jews (**choice A**) have an increase in Tay-Sachs, factor XII deficiency, and Gaucher's disease. Mediterranean peoples (**choice B**) have an increase in G6PD deficiency, HbSS, and β-thalassemia. Southeast Asians (**choice C**) have an increase in α-thalassemia and HbE disease. Native Americans (**choice E**) have an increase in 21-hydroxylase deficiency.

AD = autosomal dominant, AFP = alpha-fetoprotein, AR = autosomal recessive, β-hCG = human chorionic gonadotropin, CAD = coronary artery disease, CF = cystic fibrosis, COPD = chronic obstructive pulmonary disease, DM = diabetes mellitus, FSH = follicle-stimulating hormone, G6PD = glucose 6-phosphate dehydrogenase, HbF = fetal hemaglobin, HbSS = sickle cell disease, HTN = hypertension, LH = luteinizing hormone, PCR = polymerase chain reaction, RFLP = restriction fragment length polymorphism, R/O = rule out, S/S = signs and symptoms.

Table 3–2. MENDELIAN, MULTIFACTORIAL INHERITANCE, AND MITOCHONDRIAL DNA DISORDERS

Most Common...	Answer and Explanation
types of mendelian disorder in descending order of frequency	• **autosomal dominant** (AD), • *autosomal recessive* (AR), • *sex-linked recessive* (SXR), • *sex-linked dominant* (SXD)
clinical features of AD disorders	• *gene is strong enough to express itself in a heterozygous state*: * one normal allele (alternative form of the same gene) and one abnormal allele is enough to express the disease, * homozygosity is incompatible with life, • *50% of the siblings are affected and 50% are normal when one parent is affected* A a male with disease normal A AA A̲a (a̲ is the abnormal gene) female A AA Aa̲

Table continued on following page

**Table 3–2. MENDELIAN, MULTIFACTORIAL
INHERITANCE, AND MITOCHONDRIAL DNA DISORDERS**
Continued

Most Common...	Answer and Explanation
Continued	• *associated with structural defects in proteins and receptors*: enzyme deficiencies are uncommon (exceptions: AIP, C1 esterase inhibitor deficiency), • *late manifestations of disease*: e.g., in HD, chorea and dementia occur later in life, • *exhibits incomplete penetrance*: affected persons may never express the disease but can still transmit the gene to their children, • *exhibits variable expressivity*: affected people may have different levels of severity of the disease (e.g., mild, severe)
mechanisms of AD disease without a family Hx	• **incomplete penetrance**, • *new mutation*, • *somatic mosaicism:* gene defect in only some cells, including reproductive cells, • *incorrect assignment of paternity*
AD diseases	• **VWD**:1:125, • *familial hypercholesterolemia:* 1:500, • *APKD*: 1:1250, • *IHSS*: 1:1500, • *HD*: 1:2500, • *NF*: 1:3000, • *congenital spherocytosis*: 1:5000, • *familial polyposis*: 1:8000, • *AIP*: 1:10,000, • *osteogenesis imperfecta:* 1:15,000, • *Marfan's syndrome*: 1:20,000
genetic disease with the greatest overall mutational rate in gametes	*NF* (AD)
genetic defect causing NF	• **point mutation involving the NF-1 suppressor gene on chromosome 17**: * type I NF, * 85–90%, * ~50% arise from a new mutation, • *point mutation of NF-2 suppressor gene on chromosome 22:* type II NF
clinical findings in type I NF in adults	• **≥6 or more cafe-au-lait macules ≥1.5 cm**: * coffee-colored flat lesions, * long axes parallel underlying cutaneous nerve, • *axillary or inguinal freckling*, • *Lisch nodules*: hamartoma in iris, • *pigmented neurofibromas*: * benign tumors that involve all elements of the peripheral nerve, * first appear during puberty, • *plexiform neurofibromas*: grotesque overgrowth of soft tissue, • *CNS gliomas*: **optic nerve glioma most common CNS tumor associated with NF**, • *meningiomas*, • *skeletal deformities*: * **macrocephaly**, * short stature, * *kyphoscoliosis*, • *pheochromocytoma*:

Table 3–2. MENDELIAN, MULTIFACTORIAL
INHERITANCE, AND MITOCHONDRIAL DNA DISORDERS
Continued

Most Common...	Answer and Explanation
Continued	cause of HTN in NF, • *neurofibrosarcoma*: * <10%, * usually involve large nerve trunks, • *Wilms' tumor*
clinical findings in type II NF	• **bilateral acoustic neuromas**: * >90%, * benign tumor arising from Schwann cells, * involves the eighth cranial nerve, • *cafe-au-lait macules:* less common than in type I, • *CNS gliomas*, • *meningiomas*, • *subcapsular posterior cataracts*: not present in type I, • *absence of Lisch nodules and optic gliomas*
defect in Marfan's syndrome (AD)	*defect in fibrillin:* * fibrillin is a component of elastin in elastic tissue, * gene defect located on chromosome 15, * ~20% arise by a new mutation
skeletal defects in Marfan's syndrome	• *eunuchoid proportions:* * lower body length > upper body length, * arm span > height, * growth hormone is normal—reason for eunuchoidism, • *arachnodactyly*: spider hands, • *dolichocephaly*: narrow head, • *scoliosis:* * lateral curvature of the spine, * orthopedic surveillance recommended
CV abnormalities in Marfan's syndrome	• **dilatation of ascending aorta**: * progressive dilatation, * dilatation may lead to aortic dissection, • *mitral valve prolapse:* * 85%, * common cause of sudden death, * progressive disease, * mitral regurgitation may occur, * antibiotic prophylaxis recommended, • *aortic rupture*: * may occur from trauma, * no contact sports or strenuous exercise, * most common COD, * aortic regurgitation [Patients with Marfan's syndrome, regardless of age, should have annual echocardiograms to R/O aortic widening and MVP. Pregnancy is dangerous owing to increased plasma volume and increased risk for aortic dissection.]
eye and lung defects in Marfan's syndrome	• *dislocated lens:* * 50–80%, * defective suspensory ligament, * ophthalmologic surveillance recommended at an early age to correct visual acuity and potential for ♦ amblyopia, ♦ glaucoma, ♦ retinal detachment, • *spontaneous pneumothorax*

Table continued on following page

**Table 3–2. MENDELIAN, MULTIFACTORIAL
INHERITANCE, AND MITOCHONDRIAL DNA DISORDERS**
Continued

Most Common...	Answer and Explanation
genetic disease that has features very similar to Marfan's syndrome	*homocystinuria* [AR disease due to deficiency of cystathionine synthetase, which converts homocysteine (derived from methionine) into cystathione. Both homocysteine and methionine increase in serum. This is an example of *genetic heterogeneity.*]
clinical findings in homocystinuria	• *features resembling Marfan's syndrome*: * dislocated lens, * arachnodactyly, * eunuchoid, • *distinctive features*: * increase in plasma homocysteine levels leads to vessel damage and thrombosis, * mental retardation, * osteoporosis ("codfish" shaped, collapsed vertebra)
lab findings in homocystinuria	• *increased urine homocysteine*: positive nitroprusside reaction, • *increased serum/urine methionine* [Prenatal detection of the enzyme deficiency is available.]

clinical features of AR disease	• *abnormal gene must be present on both chromosomes to express the disease:* homozygous state, • *both parents must carry the abnormal gene*, • *heterozygotes are asymptomatic carriers*, • two asymptomatic carriers have a * 25% chance of having a child with the disease, * 50% chance of a child who is an asymptomatic carrier, and * 25% chance of a normal child
	          A a asymptomatic male
	                      carrier
	asymptomatic A AA Aa (a abnormal gene) carrier female a Aa aa (aa has the disease)
	• most AR diseases are enzyme deficiencies: * inborn errors of metabolism, * not enzyme deficiencies: ♦ CF, ♦ HbSS, ♦ hemochromatosis

AR diseases	• **non-classic 21-OHase deficiency**: see below, • *hemochromatosis:* 1:200, • *HbSS*: 1:625 blacks, • *CF*: 1:2500, • *AAT deficiency*: 1:4000, • *PKU*: 1:10,000, • *classic 21-OHase deficiency*: 1:14,000, • *Wilson's disease:* 1:100,000
enzyme deficiency in alkaptonuria	*homogentisate oxidase*: * AR disease, * converts homogentisate into maleylacetoacetate, * increase in homogentisic acid

**Table 3–2. MENDELIAN, MULTIFACTORIAL
INHERITANCE, AND MITOCHONDRIAL DNA DISORDERS**
Continued

Most Common...	Answer and Explanation
S/S of alkaptonuria	*severe joint and intervertebral disk disease* [Homogentisic acid is oxidized into a black pigment, which binds to collagen, leading to severe joint and intervertebral disk disease. It produces black urine on exposure to light.]
enzyme deficiency in McArdle's disease	*muscle phosphorylase*: * muscle glycogen cannot be catabolized into glucose for energy, * AR disease
clinical findings in McArdle's disease	• **fatigue easily**, • *rhabdomyolysis*: muscle necrosis with exercise, • *lab finding*: lactic acid does not accumulate after exercise, since anaerobic glycolysis cannot occur without glucose
clinical findings in SXR disorders	• **male dominant disorder**, • *affected male transmits the gene to all of his daughters and none of his sons*, • *all daughters are asymptomatic carriers*, • *carrier daughters transmit the gene to 50% of their sons (symptomatic) and to 50% of their daughters* X̲ Y symptomatic male normal X XX̲ XY XX is a asymptomatic carrier female X XX̲ XY X Y normal male carrier X̲ XX XY 50% males with disease female X̲ XX X̲Y
SXR diseases	• **fragile X syndrome**: 1:1000, • *G6PD deficiency*: 13% of African Americans, • *DMD*: 1:7000 males, • *hemophilia A and B*: 1:10,000 males, • *SCID*: * >1:100,000 males, * SCR variant is the most common type in the United States, * combined B and T cell ID, • *Wiskott-Aldrich syndrome*: * >1:100,000 males, * triad of ♦ B and T cell ID, ♦ eczema, ♦ thrombocytopenia, • *testicular feminization*, • *color blindness*, • *CHD of childhood*, • *Bruton's agammaglobulinemia*
cause of fragile X syndrome	*triplet repeats of 3 nucleotides* (CGG) [FXS is the * second most common genetic cause of mental retardation, the * most common cause of mental retardation in males, and the * most common mendelian disorder associated with mental retardation.]

Table continued on following page

Table 3–2. MENDELIAN, MULTIFACTORIAL
INHERITANCE, AND MITOCHONDRIAL DNA DISORDERS
Continued

Most Common...	Answer and Explanation
clinical findings in fragile X syndrome	• **mental retardation**, • *macroorchidism appearing at puberty*, • *increased incidence of MVP*, • *narrow face with large ears*, • *hyperactivity during childhood*, • mild general overgrowth [Unlike most SXR diseases, ~30% of female carriers are mentally retarded or have impaired learning. A special chromosome study is performed to identify the fragile X chromosome.]
method for detecting female carriers of fragile X syndrome	*DNA analysis:* Identification of the CGG triplet repeat is better than a fragile X study for confirming the disease
problem associated with future generation in patients with a triplet repeat mutation	*anticipation* [Size of the triplet repeat expands when transmitted from one generation to the next. Increased size of the triplet repeats increases severity of the disease.]
examples of triplet repeat disorders	• **fragile X syndrome** (SXR), • *HD* (AD), • *myotonic dystrophy* (AD), • *Friedreich's ataxia* (AR)
clinical findings in SXD disease	• *percentages of children with the abnormal gene are the same as those in SXR disorders*, • *dominant gene causes disease in both males and females*, • *affected woman transmits symptomatic disease to 50% of her daughters and 50% of her sons*, • *affected males transmit disease to all of their daughters and none of their sons*
examples of SXD disorders	• *familial hypophosphatemia*: * vitamin D–resistant rickets, * defect in the proximal reabsorption of phosphate and conversion of 25(OH)D to 1,25 (OH)$_2$D, • *Alport syndrome*: hereditary GN associated with nerve deafness
clinical findings in mitochondrial DNA disorders	• *mtDNA primarily codes for enzymes involved in mitochondrial oxidative phosphorylation reactions*, • *ova contain mitochondria, hence affected women transmit the disease to all their children*, • *sperm lose their mitochondria during fertilization, hence affected males do not transmit the disease to their children*

Table 3–2. MENDELIAN, MULTIFACTORIAL
INHERITANCE, AND MITOCHONDRIAL DNA DISORDERS
Continued

Most Common...	Answer and Explanation
examples of mtDNA disease	• *Leber's hereditary optic neuropathy,* • *myoclonic epilepsy,* • *lactic acid with stroke*
clinical findings in multifactorial inheritance	• *should be suspected when there is an increased prevalence of disease among the relatives of affected individuals,* • *parents and offspring have 50% of their genes in common,* • *second-degree relatives have an average of one-fourth of their genes in common,* • *third-degree relatives have one-eighth of their genes in common,* • *genes become diluted out in more distant relatives,* • *risk of an affected individual passing the disorder on to their offspring is conditioned by the number of mutant genes involved and the male-to-female prevalence of the disease*

Question: Which of the following are recessive diseases with an enzyme deficiency? **SELECT 3**
- (A) Testicular feminization
- (B) Sickle cell disease
- (C) Neurofibromatosis
- (D) AIP
- (E) Alcaptonuria
- (F) G6PD deficiency
- (G) Hemochromatosis
- (H) Congenital spherocytosis
- (I) Huntington's disease
- (J) 21-Hydroxylase deficiency
- (K) Fragile X syndrome

Answers: (E), (F), (J): Testicular feminization is SXR with an absent androgen receptor (**choice a is incorrect**). Sickle cell disease is AR and due to a point mutation (**choice B is incorrect**). Neurofibromatosis is AD with a point mutation of a suppressor gene (**choice C is incorrect**). AIP is an AD disease with a missing enzyme (uroporphyrinogen synthase, **choice D is incorrect**). Alcaptonuria is an AR disease with a missing enzyme (homogentisate oxidase, (**choice E is correct**). G6PD deficiency is an SXR disease with a missing enzyme (**choice F is correct**). Hemochromatosis is an AR disease with excessive reabsorption of iron from the small bowel (**choice G is incorrect**). Congenital spherocytosis is an AD disease with a defect in spectrin (**choice H is incorrect**). Huntington's disease is an AD disease with a triplet repeat defect (**choice I is incorrect**). 21-Hydroxylase deficiency is an AR disease with a missing enzyme (**choice J is correct**). Fragile X syndrome is SXR with a triplet repeat defect (**choice K is incorrect**).

AAT = α-1 antitrypsin, AD = autosomal dominant, AIP = acute intermittent porphyria, APKD = adult polycystic kidney disease, AR = autosomal recessive, CF = cystic fibrosis, CHD = chronic granulomatous disease, CNS = central nervous system, COD = cause of death, CV = cardiovascular disease, DMD = Duchenne's muscular dystrophy, G6PD = glucose 6-phosphate dehydrogenase, HbSS = sickle cell hemoglobin, HD = Huntington's disease, HTN = hypertension, Hx = history, ID = immunodeficiency, IHSS = idiopathic hypertrophic subaortic stenosis, mtDNA = mitochondrial DNA, MVP = mitral valve prolapse, NF = neurofibromatosis, OHase = hydroxylase, PKU = phenylketonuria, R/O = rule out, SCID = severe combined immunodeficiency, S/S = signs and symptoms, SXD = sex-linked dominant, SXR = sex-linked recessive, VWD = von Willebrand's disease.

Table 3–3. SEX DIFFERENTIATION DISORDERS, AGE-DEPENDENT AND RELATED DISORDERS

Most Common...	Answer and Explanation
determinant of genetic sex	*Y chromosome* [Absence of the Y chromosome results in differentiation of the germinal tissue into ovaries and apoptosis (individual cell death) of wolffian duct structures. Presence of the Y chromosome causes the germinal tissue to differentiate into testes. Müllerian inhibitory factor is responsible for apoptosis of müllerian tissue in the male fetus.]
functions of fetal testosterone and DHT	• *testosterone:* development of the * epididymis, * seminal vesicles, * vas deferens, • *DHT:* development of the * prostate, * external male genitalia by fusion of the labia to form the scrotum and extension of the clitoris to form a penis
function of 5-α-reductase	*converts testosterone into DHT*
clinical findings 5-α-reductase deficiency	• **ambiguous male genitalia**: * male pseudohermaphroditism, * due to absence of DHT effect on fetal external genitalia, • *testes located in the inguinal canals,* • *absence of the prostate gland:* DHT cannot be produced, • *presence of the epididymis, seminal vesicles, and vas deferens:* testosterone is present
cause of male pseudohermaphroditism	*testicular feminization* (SXR) [A male pseudohermaphrodite is a genotypic male (XY) who has the phenotypic appearance of a female that is usually manifested by the presence of ambiguous genitalia.]

Table 3–3. SEX DIFFERENTIATION DISORDERS, AGE-DEPENDENT AND RELATED DISORDERS *Continued*

Most Common...	Answer and Explanation
cause of testicular feminization	*deficiency of androgen receptors*
clinical findings in testicular feminization	• **neither the male accessory structures nor external genitalia develop**: * testosterone and DHT are present but no receptor, * external genitalia remain female, • *testicles located in the inguinal canal*: they are removed owing to a risk for seminoma, • *vagina ends as a blind pouch:* * upper part of vagina is of müllerian origin; therefore, it is absent, * lower part of the vagina represents urogenital sinus, which is the blind pouch, • *estrogen unopposed*: secondary female characteristics develop, • *patient is reared as a female*
lab findings in testicular feminization	• *normal testosterone*, • *increased LH*: LH does not respond to the negative feedback of testosterone
cause of Reifenstein syndrome (SXR)	*end-organ refractoriness* (complete or partial) *to the effect of testosterone and DHT*
cause of female pseudohermaphroditism	*adrenogenital syndrome* (AR) [A female pseudohermaphrodite is a genotypic female (XX) with a male phenotype. Adrenogenital syndrome is caused by enzyme deficiencies in steroid synthesis.]
enzyme deficiency in the adrenogenital syndrome	*21-hydroxylase (OHase) deficiency* [21-OHase converts 17-OHP into 11-deoxycortisol, which is further converted by 11-OHase into cortisol. The latter two compounds and their metabolites are measured as *17-OHCS* in the urine. 21-OHase also converts progesterone into 11-deoxycorticosterone, which is further converted by 11-OHase into corticosterone. 18-OHase in the zona glomerulosa (only location for this enzyme) converts corticosterone into aldosterone, the most powerful mineralocorticoid. Proximal to the 21- and 11-OHase reactions, the enzyme 17-OHase converts pregnenolone into DHEA and progesterone into androstenedione, which are weak androgens. DHEA and androstenedione are measured as *17-KS* in the urine. Androstenedione is further converted into testosterone by an oxidoreductase reaction.]

Table continued on following page

Table 3–3. SEX DIFFERENTIATION DISORDERS, AGE-DEPENDENT AND RELATED DISORDERS *Continued*

Most Common...	Answer and Explanation
S/S of classic 21-OHase deficiency	• **weakness and hypovolemia:** due to reduced synthesis of 11-deoxycorticosterone and renal loss of sodium, • *female pseudohermaphroditism:* due to accumulation of 17-ketosteroids proximal to the block that render the external genitalia ambiguous, • *precocious puberty in males:* due to an increase in the 17-KS, • *diffuse skin hyperpigmentation:* low cortisol increases ACTH, which stimulates melanin pigmentation
lab findings in classic 21-OHase deficiency	• **increased serum 17-OH-progesterone:** * proximal to the block, * excellent screen for 21- and 11-OHase deficiencies, • *increased urine pregnanetriol:* * urine metabolite of 17-OH-progesterone, * excellent screen for 21- and 11-OHase deficiencies, • *hyponatremia, hyperkalemia,* and *metabolic acidosis:* due to deficiency of the weak mineralocorticoids, • *increased 17-KS:* DHEA and androstenedione are proximal to the block, • *decreased 17-OHCS:* 11-deoxycortisol and cortisol are distal to the block, • *hypocortisolism:* cortisol is distal to the block, • *increased ACTH:* no cortisol feedback, • *increased urine sodium and low urine potassium:* due to weak mineralocorticoid deficiency [Prenatal testing is available for the enzyme defect.]
S/S of non-classic 21-OHase deficiency in adults	• **hirsutism in females:** * increased hair in hair-bearing areas, * virilization—development of male secondary sex characteristics does not occur as it does with the classic form of the disease, • *no signs of salt loss:* classic type has salt loss with hypovolemia, • *cystic acne in females,* • *secondary amenorrhea,* • *pseudoprecocious puberty in boys* [This variant occurs in 1:100 births, which makes it the most frequent AR disease and genetic disease in the United States.]
lab diagnosis for non-classic 21-OHase deficiency in children/adults	*screen for an increase in 17-OHP in blood* [This test is performed as a newborn screen in many states. If increased, an ACTH stimulation test is performed, which results in a further increase in 17-OHP if the enzyme defect is present.]

Table 3–3. SEX DIFFERENTIATION DISORDERS, AGE-DEPENDENT AND RELATED DISORDERS *Continued*

Most Common...	Answer and Explanation
S/S of classic 11-OHase deficiency	• **salt retention with hypertension**: increased 11-deoxycorticosterone proximal to the block, • *female pseudohermaphroditism*: accumulation of 17-KS proximal to the block, • *precocious puberty in males*: accumulation of 17-KS proximal to the block, • *diffuse skin hyperpigmentation*: decreased cortisol leaves ACTH uninhibited
lab findings in 11-OHase deficiency	• *increased 17-OH-progesterone and urine pregnanetriol*: * these are proximal to the block, * pregnanetriol is the metabolite of 17-OHP and is an excellent screening test, • *increased 17-KS*: proximal to the block, • *increased 17-OHCS*: increase in 11-deoxycortisol proximal to the block, • *hypocortisolism*: distal to the block, • *increased ACTH*: no cortisol negative feedback [There is a nonclassic type of 11-OHase deficiency, but it is uncommon.]
theories of aging	• *stochastic*: * cumulative injury to cells due to free radical injury, * increased cross-linking of proteins, * cumulative DNA damage from FRs, * accumulation of errors in protein synthesis adversely affects cellular function, • *programmed*: apoptosis genes are programmed to kill cells at a set time
age-dependent (inevitable) changes in body fat, lean body mass, TBW	• *increased body fat*: * increases the volume of distribution of fat-soluble drugs, * decreases the number of insulin receptors leading to glucose intolerance, • *decreased lean body mass/TBW*: reduces the volume of distribution of water-soluble drugs
age-dependent findings in the lungs with aging	• *obstructive type of pattern in PFTs*: so-called "senile emphysema" with decreased elasticity—reduced recoil on expiration, • *decreased FEV_{1sec} and FVC*, • *increased TLC and RV*, • *mild hypoxemia*
age-dependent changes in the aorta	• *loss of elasticity*: predisposes the patient to systolic hypertension—systolic pressure >160 mm Hg/diastolic <90 mm Hg, • *decreased baroreceptor sensitivity*: * increased risk for orthostatic hypotension, * impaired response to hypovolemia, • *decreased β-adrenergic responsiveness*: * decreased CO and heart rate

Table continued on following page

Table 3–3. SEX DIFFERENTIATION DISORDERS, AGE-DEPENDENT AND RELATED DISORDERS *Continued*

Most Common...	Answer and Explanation
Continued	in response to stress, * at rest, the CO is unchanged
age-dependent type of arthritis	*osteoarthritis in weight-bearing joints* [OA is the most common cause of pain in the elderly and disability from rheumatologic disease.]
age-dependent changes in the CNS	• *cerebral atrophy:* mild forgetfulness, • *impaired sleep patterns:* * insomnia, * early wakening, • *decreased dopaminergic synthesis*: parkinsonian-like gait
age-dependent disorders in the eyes	• **cataracts**: visual impairment increases the risk for falls, which is the most common cause of fractures in patients >65 years of age, • *arcus senilis*: ring of cholesterol around the cornea, • *presbyopia*: inability to focus on near objects
age-dependent disorders in the ears	• *presbycusis*: * sensorineural hearing loss, particularly at high frequency, * problems with discriminating speech, • *otosclerosis*: fusion of the ear ossicles producing conductive hearing loss
age-dependent changes in the immune system	*decreased T cell function* [This leads to an * increase in FP serum ANAs and RF, * decrease in skin reactions to antigens (e.g., ◆ PPD, ◆ common antigens in testing for cellular immunity).]
age-dependent changes in the skin	• *loss of skin elasticity*: increased cross-bridging of collagen, • *increase in body fat*, • *increase in vessel instability*: senile purpura over the dorsum of the hands and lower legs, which are areas subject to normal trauma • *decreased sweating*: * eccrine glands fibrosed, * danger of heat stroke
age-dependent changes in the GI tract	• *decreased gastric acidity:* * increase in serum gastrin, * predisposes to *Helicobacter pylori* infection, • *decreased colonic motility*: constipation, • *decreased activity of the hepatic microsomal enzyme system*: delayed metabolism of some drugs
age-dependent disorders in the reproductive tract in men	• **prostate hyperplasia**: * increased urine residual volume with subsequent increase in UTIs, * septic shock, • *prostate cancer*, • *decreased testosterone*: impotence

Table 3–3. SEX DIFFERENTIATION DISORDERS, AGE-DEPENDENT AND RELATED DISORDERS *Continued*

Most Common...	Answer and Explanation
age-dependent disorders in the reproductive tract in women	• *breast and vulvar atrophy*, • *decreased estrogen*, • *increased gonadotropins*: FSH and LH, owing to a decrease in estrogen and progesterone, respectively
age-dependent changes in the endocrine system	• *increased glucose intolerance*: increase in body fat leads to a decrease in insulin receptor synthesis, • *decreased PRA and aldosterone*: unknown mechanism, • *increased ADH*: tendency for hyponatremia, • *increased ANP*: tendency for hyponatremia, • *decreased absorption of vitamin D*: osteomalacia (decreased bone mineralization) with risk for fracture
age-dependent changes in the renal system	• *decreased GFR with concomitant reduction in the creatinine clearance*: risk of drug toxicity due to slow clearance, • *decreased ability to concentrate and dilute urine*: problem with excess water load and salt load, • *increased incidence of bacteriuria*
age-dependent changes affecting pharmacokinetics	• *increased α-1 glycoprotein*, • *increased body fat*, • *decreased renal function*, • *decreased hepatic blood flow*, • *decreased lean body mass*, • *decreased body water*
age-related (more common but not inevitable with aging) disorders in the CV system	• **atherosclerosis**, • *CAD*, • *temporal arteritis*, • *aortic stenosis*, • *diastolic dysfunction*: decreased compliance of the heart during diastole leading to a back-up of blood into the lungs and heart failure, • *aortic sclerosis*: hardening and fibrosis of the aortic cusps that is not hemodynamically significant but can cause benign murmurs, • *systolic HTN*
age-related disorders in the MS system	• *osteoporosis:* particularly the vertebral column in females, • *Paget's disease of bone*, • *RA*, • *Sjögren's syndrome*: * dry eyes, * dry mouth, * RA
age-related disorders in the respiratory system	• *pneumonia*: * usually *Streptococcus pneumoniae*, * diminished cough effectiveness, * decreased mucociliary clearing, • *primary lung cancer*
age-related disorders in the CNS	• *Alzheimer's disease*, • *Parkinson's disease*, • *strokes*, • *subdural hematomas*

Table continued on following page

64 MOST COMMONS IN MEDICINE

Table 3–3. SEX DIFFERENTIATION DISORDERS, AGE-DEPENDENT AND RELATED DISORDERS *Continued*

Most Common...	Answer and Explanation
age-related disorders in the eyes	• **macular degeneration**, • *limitation in upward gaze*
age-related disorders in the immune system	• *monoclonal gammopathies of undetermined significance*: most common cause of monoclonal gammopathy, • *multiple myeloma*
age-related disorders in the skin	• *BCC, squamous cell carcinoma, malignant melanoma:* all have a relation to excess exposure to UVB light, • *pressure sores:* * pressure on capillaries is the most important factor, * other factors include ♦ friction, ♦ shearing forces, ♦ maceration, * should check for underlying osteomyelitis with radionuclide scan
age-related disorders in the reproductive tract	• *women:* cancers of the * breast, * endometrium, * ovary, • *men:* malignant lymphoma of the testicle
age-related disorders in the kidneys	• *renovascular hypertension secondary to atherosclerosis*, * *renal adenocarcinoma*, • *urinary incontinence*: see Table 10–5
age-related disorder in the endocrine system	*type II DM*

Question: Which of the following are more likely to be age-dependent rather than age-related changes? **SELECT 6**
- (A) CAD
- (B) Otosclerosis
- (C) Decreased creatinine clearance
- (D) Breast cancer
- (E) Prostatic hyperplasia
- (F) Presbycusis
- (G) Senile purpura
- (H) Alzheimer's disease
- (I) Osteoarthritis

Answers: (B), (C), (E), (F), (G), (I): Otosclerosis (choice B), decreased creatinine clearance (choice C), prostatic hyperplasia (choice E), presbycusis (choice F), senile purpura (choice G), and osteoarthritis (choice I) are all age-dependent. CAD (choice A is incorrect), breast cancer (choice D is incorrect), and Alzheimer's disease (choice H is incorrect) are age-related disorders.

ACTH = adrenocorticotropic hormone, ADH = antidiuretic hormone, ANA = antinuclear antibody, ANP = atrial natriuretic peptide, AR = autosomal recessive, BCC = basal cell carcinoma, CAD = coronary artery disease, CNS = central nervous system, CV = cardiovascular, DHEA =

dehydroepiandrosterone, DM = diabetes mellitus, DHT = dihydrotestosterone, FEV_{1sec} = forced expiratory volume in 1 second, FP = false positive, FR = free radical, FSH = follicle stimulating hormone, FVC = forced vital capacity, GI = gastrointestinal, GFR = glomerular filtration rate, HTN = hypertension, KS = ketosteroids, LH = luteinizing hormone, MS = musculoskeletal, OA = osteoarthritis, OHase = hydroxylase, OHCS = hydroxycorticoids, OHP = hydroxyprogesterone, PFT = pulmonary function test, PPD = purified protein derivative, PRA = plasma renin activity, RA = rheumatoid arthritis, RF = rheumatoid factor, RV = residual volume, S/S = signs and symptoms, SXR = sex-linked recessive, TLC = total lung capacity, TBW = total body water, UTI = urinary tract infection, UV = ultraviolet.

CHAPTER

4

CLINICAL ONCOLOGY

CONTENTS

Table 4–1. OVERVIEW OF NEOPLASIA

Most Common...	Answer and Explanation
contributory factor responsible for cancer in the United States	*cigarette smoking* [Cancer is the second most common COD in the United States.]
primary prevention modalities in cancer	• *lifestyle modification*: * stop smoking, * increase fiber/decrease saturated fat in the diet, * reduce alcohol intake, * reduce weight • *aspirin*: decreases the incidence of * esophageal, * stomach, * colon, and * rectal cancers, • *isotretinoin*: decreases leukoplakia in the lungs and GI tract, • *tamoxifen*: * reduces risk for a second primary malignancy in the remaining breast in a woman with previous breast cancer, * may reduce the incidence of a primary malignancy in women who have a strong family Hx of breast cancer
secondary preventation modalities in cancer	*screening*: see Tables 1–2 and 2–1
name applied to malignant tumors derived from epithelium	*carcinomas* [Carcinomas are designated * squamous (e.g., SCC of the lungs), adenocarcinoma (form glands, e.g., prostate adenocarcinoma), or * transitional epithelium (e.g., bladder cancer).]
name applied to malignant tumors derived from connective tissue	*sarcomas*: e.g., * adipose—liposarcoma, * bone—osteogenic sarcoma

Table continued on following page

Table 4–1. OVERVIEW OF NEOPLASIA *Continued*

Most Common...	Answer and Explanation
sarcoma in adults	*malignant fibrous histiocytoma:* liposarcoma is a close second
cancer derived from the BM	*leukemia:* * derived from hematopoietic stem cells, * CLL is the most common adult leukemia
cancer derived from the lymph nodes	*malignant lymphoma*: NHL is more common than Hodgkin's lymphoma
extranodal site for malignant lymphoma	• **stomach**, • *terminal ileum*
feature that differentiates a benign from a malignant tumor	*tumor's capacity to metastasize to another site* [A benign tumor that metastasizes is an invasive mole. A malignant tumor that does not metastasize is a BCC.]
carcinomas that invade blood vessels	• **renal adenocarcinoma**, • *follicular carcinoma of the thyroid*, • *HCC* [Carcinomas most commonly spread first to the regional lymph nodes and from there into the blood stream.]
sarcomas that invade lymphatics	*rhabdomyosarcoma* [Sarcomas usually by-pass the lymphatics and spread directly via the blood stream, hence their proclivity for lung (most common) and bone metastasis.]
cell cycle characteristics of malignant tumors	*longer cell cycle than the parent tissue* [The G1 phase is usually longer in a malignant tumor than in its normal counterpart. In addition, more malignant cells stay in the cell cycle than normal cells, hence they accumulate. This is due to inactivation of the p53 suppressor gene, which codes for factors that modulate the kinases that control the movement from one phase of the cycle to the next.]
number of doubling times before tumors are clinically detectable	*30 doubling times:* equivalent to * 10^{-9} cells, * 1 g of tissue, * volume of 1 mL
DNA lab findings in highly aggressive malignancies	• *aneuploidy*: uneven multiple of 23 chromosomes, • *S phase fraction >5%*: measure of the number of malignant cells in the proliferating pool

Table 4-1. OVERVIEW OF NEOPLASIA *Continued*

Most Common...	Answer and Explanation
types of metastasis	• **lymphatic**, • *hematogenous*, • *seeding*: * spreading of tumor within body cavities, * e.g., peritoneal cavity
sites for seeding	• **peritoneal cavity: ovarian**, GI, or pancreatic cancers, • *pleural cavity*: primary or metastatic lung cancer, • **subarachnoid space**: * GBM, * medulloblastoma
bone sites for metastasis	• **vertebral column**, • *proximal femur* [The Batson vertebral venous plexus extends along the vertebral column from the cranial plexus to the pelvis. Tributaries penetrate the vertebra and surround the spinal cord. The plexus also connects with the vena cava, hence the movement of tumor emboli from the IVC into the Batson plexus and into the vertebral column.]
symptom of bone metastasis	*pain* [Pain is best relieved by local radiation therapy. Bisphosphonates may relieve pain by inhibiting bone resorption. ERA positive tumors of the breast respond well to tamoxifen, while anti-androgen drugs work best for prostate cancers.]
radiographic techniques to identify bone metastases	• **radionuclide bone scan**, • *plain x-rays*: 30–50% of cortical bone must be involved to be visualized, • *CT scan*: most useful in vertebral metastasis
cancer with osteoblastic metastasis	*prostate cancer*: radiodense loci are noted on plain films
enzyme elevated in osteoblastic metastases	*alkaline phosphatase*: indicates increased mineralization of bone by osteoblasts activated by cytokines in the tumor .
malignancies that produce purely osteolytic metastases	• **lung**, • *kidney* [lytic metastases produce lucencies in bone on plain films.]
factors released by tumors leading to activation of osteoclasts	• *PTH-like peptide*: * primary SCC of lung, * renal adenocarcinoma, • *vitamin D-like steroids*, • *prostaglandins*, • *cytokines*, • *osteoclast-activating factor*: IL-1 [Pathologic fractures commonly occur.]

Table continued on following page

Table 4–1. OVERVIEW OF NEOPLASIA *Continued*

Most Common...	Answer and Explanation
immunohistologic stain used to identify leukocyte malignancies	*CD45*
immunohistologic stain used to identify a neuroendocrine tumor	*S100 antigen* [It is positive in tumors of neural crest origin, such as malignant melanoma, small cell carcinoma of the lung, carcinoid tumors, and neuroblastoma.]
immunohistologic stains used to identify a malignant melanoma	• *S100 antigen*, • *HB45*
immunohistologic stains used to identify carcinomas	• *cytokeratin intermediate filaments*, • *CEA*, • *epithelial membrane antigen*
immunohistologic stain used to identify sarcomas	*desmin:* specific for muscle-derived sarcomas
organ metastasized to	*lymph nodes*
malignancy of lymph nodes	*metastasis*: * breast, * lung
primary malignancy of lymph nodes	*NHL*
malignancy of the lungs	*metastasis*: breast most common primary site
primary malignancy of the lung	*adenocarcinoma*
malignancy of the brain	*metastasis*: lung most common primary site
malignancy of the liver	*metastasis*: lung most common primary site
primary cancer of the liver	*HCC*: secondary to HBV postnecrotic cirrhosis
malignancy of bone	*metastasis:* breast most common primary site
primary malignancy of bone	*multiple myeloma*

Table 4–1. OVERVIEW OF NEOPLASIA *Continued*

Most Common...	Answer and Explanation
malignancy of the adrenal glands	*metastasis:* lung most common primary site
cancer metastatic to Virchow's node	*stomach adenocarcinoma*: left supraclavicular lymph node, or Virchow's node, drains the abdominal cavity
metastatic sites for breast cancer in descending order	• **lung**, • *bone*, • *liver*, • *adrenal*, • *brain*
metastatic sites for colorectal cancer in descending order	• **liver**, • *adrenal*, • *bone*, • *lung*
metastatic site for renal adenocarcinoma	*lungs*
metastatic site for TCC of the bladder	*adrenals*
metastatic sites for lung cancer in descending order	• **liver**, • *bone*, • *brain-adrenal*: same
metastatic sites for melanoma in descending order	• **liver-lung**: same, • *adrenal-brain-bone-skin*: approximately the same
metastatic sites for ovarian cancer in descending order	• **liver**, • *lung*, • *adrenal*
metastatic sites for prostate cancer in descending order	• **bone**, • *lung*, • *liver*
Rx for a woman with metastasis to axillary lymph nodes but no primary site	*Rx as a primary breast cancer* [~5–10% of all metastatic carcinomas have an unknown primary. The majority are undifferentiated adenocarcinomas.]
Rx for peritoneal carcinomatosis in a woman with no obvious primary site	• *exploratory laparotomy*, • *surgical cytoreduction of tumor tissue as if the primary were ovarian*
genes producing cancer	*oncogenes:* * derive from protooncogenes, * involved in the growth process

Table continued on following page

Table 4–1. OVERVIEW OF NEOPLASIA *Continued*

Most Common...	Answer and Explanation
function of suppressor genes	*prevent unregulated cell growth*
suppressor genes associated with human cancers	• **p53 suppressor gene**: * located on chromosome 17, * codes for proteins that control kinases involved in the movement of cells through the cell cycle, • *Rb-1 gene*: * chromosome 13, associated with * retinoblastoma, * osteogenic sarcoma, • *APC suppressor gene*: * chromosome 5, * associated with adenomatous polyposis coli, • *BRCA1*: * chromosome 17, associated with * breast, * ovarian, * colon, * prostate cancers, • *BRCA2*: * chromosome 13, * associated with breast cancers in males/females, • *WT1*: * chromosome 11, * Wilms' tumor
steps in oncogenesis	• *initiation*: irreversible mutation → • *promotion*: growth enhancement → • *tumor progression*: * subdivision of tumor cells into special functions, e.g., * resist drugs, * metastasis
oncogenes involved in human cancer	• **p53 suppressor gene**: * colorectal, * breast, * lung, * CNS cancers, • *ras oncogene*: * lung, * colon, * pancreas, * leukemia, * ovarian cancers [A point mutation inactivates the p53 suppressor gene and activates the ras oncogene.]
types of activation of protooncogenes	• **point mutation**: e.g., * ras oncogene, * p53 suppressor gene, • *translocation*: e.g., * t9;22 of the abl oncogene in CML, * t8;14 of the c-myc oncogene in Burkitt's lymphoma, * t14;18 of the bcl-2 oncogene leading to inactivation of an apoptosis gene on a B cell leading to a B cell follicular lymphoma, • *gene amplification*: e.g., erb-B2/neu oncogene in breast cancer
AD syndrome associated with inactivation of the p53 suppressor gene	*Li-Fraumeni multicancer syndrome*: increased incidence of * breast cancer, * sarcomas, * brain tumors, * leukemia
carcinogenic agent	*chemicals:* account for 80–90% of cancer, particularly those in cigarette smoke
chemicals linked to TCC of the bladder	• **polycyclic hydrocarbons in cigarette smoke**, • *aniline dyes*, • *cyclophosphamide*, • *benzidine*, • *phenacetin*

Table 4–1. **OVERVIEW OF NEOPLASIA** *Continued*

Most Common...	Answer and Explanation
chemicals linked to liver angiosarcoma	• **vinyl chloride**, • *arsenic*, • *Thorotrast*
chemicals linked to primary lung cancer	• **polycyclic hydrocarbons**, • *uranium: radon gas*, • *asbestos*: additive carcinogenic effect if combined with smoking, • *chromium*, • *arsenic*, • *nickel*, • *cadmium*
chemicals linked to HCC	• **aflatoxins**: especially in association with HBV, • *oral contraceptives*, • *Thorotrast*, • *alcohol*
chemicals linked to leukemia	• *benzene*, • *alkylating agents*: also predispose to malignant lymphoma
chemicals linked to esophageal cancer	• **polycyclic hydrocarbons**, • *nitrosamines*, • *alcohol*
chemicals linked to squamous cancer	• **polycyclic hydrocarbons**: * cervix, * larynx, * lung, * oral pharynx, • *arsenic*: skin, • *tar/soot/oils*: skin, • *immunosuppressive agents*: * skin, * squamous cancer of the skin is the most common cancer associated with immunosuppressive agents, • *chewing tobacco*: mouth
chemicals linked to pancreatic adenocarcinoma	• **polycyclic hydrocarbons**, • *alcohol*
chemical linked to clear cell adenocarcinoma of the vagina	*diethylstilbestrol* (DES)
oncogenic viruses linked to leukemia/lymphoma	• **EBV**: * primary CNS lymphoma, * polyclonal lymphoma, * Burkitt's lymphoma, • *HTLV-1*: adult T cell leukemia, • *HTLV-2*: ? hairy cell leukemia, • *HIV*: primary CNS lymphoma
oncogenic virus linked to nasopharyngeal carcinoma	*EBV*
oncogenic viruses linked to HCC	• **HBV**, • *HCV*
oncogenic virus linked to Kaposi's sarcoma	*herpesvirus 8*

Table continued on following page

Table 4–1. OVERVIEW OF NEOPLASIA *Continued*

Most Common...	Answer and Explanation
oncogenic virus linked to cervical and anal squamous cell carcinoma	**HPV type 16**, 18, 31
radiation-induced cancers	• **leukemia**, • *papillary carcinoma of the thyroid*, • *lung cancer*: radon gas from uranium, • breast cancer, • *liver angiosarcoma*: Thorotrast, • *UVB light-induced cancers*: * **BCC**, * SCC, * malignant melanoma, • *osteogenic sarcoma*
AR disease linked to cancer from UV radiation	*xeroderma pigmentosum*: deficiency of DNA repair enzymes
bacteria linked to cancer	*Helicobacter pylori*: * gastric adenocarcinoma, * low-grade mucosa-associated primary malignant lymphomas of the stomach
type of cancer linked with scars in the lungs	*adenocarcinoma*
type of cancer linked to chronic sinus tracts and third-degree burn sites	*squamous cell carcinoma*
cancer linked with immunosuppressive Rx	*squamous cell carcinoma of the skin*
terms applied to grading of cancer	• *low-grade*: well differentiated, • *intermediate-grade* moderately well differentiated, • *high-grade*: * poorly differentiated, * anaplastic [Grade refers to how closely the tumor resembles its parent tissue.]
elements involved in staging cancer	• *tumor size (T)*, • *lymph node status (N)*, • *presence or absence of other metastatic spread (M)* [Stage is more important than grade in prognosis.]
chemical factor associated with cachexia due to cancer	*tumor necrosis factor-α*. * secreted from host macrophages and cancer cells, * megestrol is an appetite stimulant commonly used in treating cachexia

Table 4–1. OVERVIEW OF NEOPLASIA *Continued*

Most Common...	Answer and Explanation
anemias associated with cancer	• **ACD**, • *iron deficiency*: e.g., colorectal cancer, • *macrocytic anemia*: secondary to folate deficiency from rapid tumor growth, • *autoimmune hemolytic anemia*: * CLL, * HTLV-1, • *microangiopathic hemolytic anemia*: * schistocytes, * RBCs damaged by tumor emboli in vessels, • *myelophthisic anemia*: metastasis to the marrow, • *marrow suppression*: * radiation, * chemotherapy
cause of a leukoerythroblastic peripheral smear	*metastasis to the BM:* metastasis to the bone marrow pushes hematopoietic elements into the peripheral blood (immature WBCs, nucleated RBCs)
coagulation abnormality in cancer	*hypercoagulability*
causes of hypercoagulability in cancer	• **increase in coagulation factors fibrinogen, V, VIII**, • *release of tissue thromboplastin*: activates the extrinsic coagulation system, • *thrombocytosis*: cancer accounts for 30% of all cases of thrombocytosis, • *decreased liver synthesis of antithrombin III and protein C*
overall COD in cancer patients	*infections:* most often secondary to gram-negative sepsis
malignancies associated with fever not related to infection	**HD**: Pel-Ebstein fever, • *renal adenocarcinoma*, • *osteogenic sarcoma*
term applied to remote effects of a tumor unrelated to metastasis	*paraneoplastic syndrome*: * occur in 10–15% of tumors, * may predate the onset of metastasis in the tumor
paraneoplastic syndrome	*hypercalcemia secondary to secretion of a PTH-like peptide*: * 40% of all cases of hypercalcemia, * cancer associations: ♦ primary squamous cancer of the lung, ♦ renal adenocarcinoma, ♦ breast cancer
mechanisms of hypercalcemia in cancer	• **metastasis to the marrow**: overall most common cause of malignancy-induced hypercalcemia, • *secretion of a PTH-like peptide*: increases calcium reabsorption from the kidneys, * see above discussion

Table continued on following page

Table 4–1. OVERVIEW OF NEOPLASIA *Continued*

Most Common...	Answer and Explanation
cause of the Eaton-Lambert syndrome	*small cell carcinoma of the lung*: see Table 12–5 and Table 15–4
cancer associated with Sweet syndrome	*acute leukemia*: fever, neutrophilic leukocytosis, red papular rash
phenotypic markers for gastric adenocarcinoma	• *Leser-Trélat sign*: multiple outcroppings of seborrheic keratoses, • *acanthosis nigricans*: black, verrucoid-appearing lesion usually located in the axilla
cancer associated with pulmonary osteoarthropathy	*primary lung cancer:* pulmonary osteoarthropathy refers to clubbing of the nails with an underlying periosteal reaction of bone
cancer associated with superficial migratory thrombophlebitis (Trousseau's sign)	*pancreatic adenocarcinoma*
collagen vascular disease associated with an underlying cancer	*dermatomyositis*: increased incidence of primary lung and breast cancer
renal disease associated with cancer	*nephrotic syndrome:* most commonly an immunocomplex-related diffuse membranous glomerulonephritis
cancers associated with granulocytosis (>8000 cells/μL)	• *primary lung cancer,* • *GI cancers*
cancer associated with subacute sensory peripheral neuropathy	*primary lung cancer:* may occur in 50% of lung cancers
adenocarcinomas associated with marantic vegetations	• *pancreas,* • *colon* [Marantic vegetations are sterile and are seen in mucus-secreting cancers.]
cancer associated with hyponatremia or ectopic Cushing's syndrome	*small cell carcinoma of the lung:* ectopic secretion of * ADH and * ACTH, respectively

Table 4–1. OVERVIEW OF NEOPLASIA *Continued*

Most Common...	Answer and Explanation
cancer associated with hypercalcemia or secondary polycythemia	*renal adenocarcinoma:* ectopic secretion of PTH-like peptide and erythropoietin, respectively
cancer associated with hypoglycemia or secondary polycythemia	*HCC:* ectopic secretion of an * insulin-like factor and * erythropoietin, respectively
cancer associated with hypocalcemia or hypercortisolism	*medullary carcinoma of the thyroid:* * production of calcitonin leads to hypocalcemia, * ectopic production of ACTH
cancers associated with gynecomastia	*gestationally or non-gestationally derived trophoblastic tumors that secrete β-hCG:* e.g., * hydatidiform moles (benign), * choriocarcinoma (malignant), * testicular cancers, * syncytiotrophoblast secretes β-hCG
cancers associated with secondary polycythemia	• **renal adenocarcinoma**: alone or in association with von Hippel-Lindau disease, • *Wilms' tumor,* • *HCC*
cancer and primary site associated with the carcinoid syndrome	*carcinoid tumor arising from the terminal ileum* [The majority of malignant carcinoid tumors that have the capacity to metastasize arise in the terminal ileum. When they metastasize to the liver, serotonin and other chemicals are directly released into the hepatic vein leading to signs and symptoms of the carcinoid syndrome. The appendix is the most common overall site for carcinoid tumors; however, they are too small to metastasize.]
cancers associated with secretion of AFP	• **HCC**, • *endodermal (yolk sac) sinus tumors:* most often located in the ovaries or testicles of young children [AAT is also increased in HCCs.]
tumor markers ordered in the evaluation of testicular tumors	• *AFP,* • *β-hCG*
tumor markers for multiple myeloma	• **Bence Jones protein**: light chains in the urine, • *β₂-microglobulin*
tumor marker for surface-derived ovarian cancers	*CA 125*

Table continued on following page

Table 4–1. OVERVIEW OF NEOPLASIA *Continued*

Most Common...	Answer and Explanation
tumor marker for small cell carcinoma of the lung	*CEA*
tumor marker for prostate cancer	*prostate-specific antigen* (PSA): * more sensitive than it is specific, since it is also elevated in prostate hyperplasia, * prostatic acid phosphatase is no longer used as a marker
tumor markers for breast cancer	• **CA 15-3**, • *CEA*
tumor marker for colorectal cancer	*CEA*: primarily used to detect recurrences rather than as a primary screen for colorectal cancer
tumor markers for pancreatic carcinoma	• **CA 19-9**, • *CEA*
enzyme elevated in malignant lymphomas	*LDH:* * particularly the LDH$_3$ isoenzyme fraction, * also increased in cystic teratomas
cancers in children	• **ALL**, • *CNS tumors*: * **cerebellar astrocytoma**, * medulloblastoma, • *malignant lymphoma*: Burkitt's lymphoma, • *neuroblastoma*, • *Wilms' tumor*, • *Ewing's sarcoma* [Cancer is second to accidents as the most common COD in children.]
cancers in decreasing order of incidence in men	• **prostate**, • *lung*, • *colorectal*
cancers in decreasing order of incidence in women	• **breast**, • *lung*, • *colorectal*
cancer mortalities in decreasing order in men	• **lung**, • *prostate*, • *colorectal*
cancer mortalities in decreasing order in women	• **lung**, • *breast*, • *colorectal*: colorectal cancer is the second most common cancer and cancer killer regardless of the sex of the individual
cancers that are decreasing in incidence in the United States	• **cervix**: due to Pap screens detecting cervical dysplasia and carcinoma in-situ, • *stomach:* * those involved with intestinal metaplasia and *Helicobacter pylori*, * does not include

Table 4–1. OVERVIEW OF NEOPLASIA *Continued*

Most Common...	Answer and Explanation
Continued	the signet ring type producing linitis plastica, • *endometrial:* Pap smears are not sensitive in detecting hyperplasia, the precursor of endometrial cancer
cancers that are increasing in incidence in the United States	• *breast*: due to early detection by mammography, • *prostate*: due to detection by PSA and DRE, • *lung*: particularly in women, incidence is decreasing in men, • *multiple myeloma*, • *malignant lymphoma*, • *pancreatic carcinoma*, • *malignant melanoma* [In general, cancer is more common in African Americans than whites, except for malignant melanoma and testicular cancer.]
cancer that is increasing at the fastest rate worldwide	*malignant melanoma*: Australia has the greatest increase in the incidence of malignant melanomas
cancer in Southeast China	*nasopharyngeal carcinoma secondary to EBV*
cancer in Northern China	*esophageal cancer*
cancers in Japan	**stomach adenocarcinoma**: due to smoked products, • *HTLV-1 adult T cell leukemia/ lymphoma*
cancer in Southeast Asia	*HCC secondary to HBV*: incidence is enhanced by aflatoxins
malignant lymphoma in Africa	*Burkitt's lymphoma:* due to EBV [In the United States, the relationship of EBV with Burkitt's lymphoma is less well defined. In Africa, Burkitt's is located in the jaw, while in the United States, it targets the terminal ileum, para-aortic lymph nodes, testicle, or ovary.]
cancer prevented by immunization	*HCC due to HBV*: HBV vaccination reduces not only liver cancer risk but also the risk for contracting HBV and HDV
cancer in Southeast Asia that is causally related to α-thalassemia	*choriocarcinoma:* Hb Bart's disease (deletion of all 4 α-globin genes) is associated with spontaneous abortions, which in turn predispose to choriocarcinoma

Table continued on following page

Table 4–1. OVERVIEW OF NEOPLASIA *Continued*

Most Common...	Answer and Explanation
cancers associated with parasitic diseases	• *cholangiocarcinoma:* due to *Clonorchis sinensis,* • *squamous cancer of the bladder:* due to *Schistosoma hematobium*
chromosome instability syndromes that predispose to cancer	• *ataxia telangiectasia:* * AR, * malignant lymphoma, • *Bloom's syndrome:* * AR, * acute leukemia, • *Fanconi's syndrome:* * AR, * acute leukemia
SXRs associated with cancer	• *Wiskott-Aldrich syndrome:* * triad of B and T cell immunodeficiency, eczema, thrombocytopenia, • increased risk for malignant lymphoma, • *sex-linked lymphoproliferative syndrome due to EBV:* increased risk for malignant lymphoma
trisomy associated with acute leukemia	*Down syndrome:* see Table 3–1
chromosome disorder associated with ovarian cancer	*Turner syndrome:* see Table 3–1
components of the MEN-I syndrome (AD inheritance)	*pituitary tumors,* • *parathyroid adenomas,* • *pancreatic tumors:* usually Zollinger-Ellison syndrome, followed by insulinoma
components of the MEN-IIa and IIb syndromes (AD inheritance)	• *MEN-IIa:* * medullary carcinoma of the thyroid, * parathyroid adenoma/hyperplasia, * pheochromocytoma, • *MEN-IIb:* * medullary carcinoma of the thyroid, * mucosal neuromas in the lips, pheochromocytoma
AD polyp syndrome associated with ovarian tumors	*Peutz-Jeghers syndrome:* increased incidence of sex cord tumors with annular tubules
AD syndrome associated with tumors and/or hamartomas in the CNS, heart, and kidneys	*tuberous sclerosis:* see Table 15–8
AD syndrome associated with acoustic neuromas and meningiomas	*neurofibromatosis*

Table 4–1. OVERVIEW OF NEOPLASIA *Continued*

Question: In which of the following organs is malignancy most often due to a primary cancer rather than metastasis? **SELECT 3**
- (A) CNS
- (B) Thyroid
- (C) Lymph node
- (D) Lung
- (E) Liver
- (F) Skin
- (G) Adrenal
- (H) Ovary
- (I) Bone

Answers: (B), (F), (H): Metastasis is more common than a primary cancer in the CNS **(choice A is incorrect,** most often a primary in the lung), lymph node **(choice C is incorrect,** lung), liver **(choice E is incorrect,** most often a primary in the breast), adrenal **(choice G is incorrect,** most often a primary in the lungs), and bone **(choice I is incorrect,** most often a primary in the breast). Primary cancers are more common than metastasis in the thyroid **(choice B,** papillary carcinoma), skin **(choice F,** BCC), and ovary **(choice H,** serous cystadenocarcinoma).

AAT = α¹-antitrypsin, ACD = anemia of chronic disease, ACTH = adrenocorticotropic hormone, AD = autosomal dominant, ADH = antidiuretic hormone, AFP = alpha-fetoprotein, ALL = acute lymphoblastic leukemia, APC = adenomatous polyposis coli, AR = autosomal recessive, BCC = basal cell carcinoma, BM = bone marrow, CEA = carcinoembryonic antigen, CLL = chronic lymphocytic leukemia, CML = chronic myelogenous leukemia, CNS = central nervous system, COD = cause of death, CT = computed tomography, DES = diethylstilbestrol, DRE = digital rectal examination, EBV = Epstein-Barr virus, ERA = estrogen receptor assay, GBM = glioblastoma multiforme, GI = gastrointestinal, Hb = hemoglobin, HBV = hepatitis B virus, HCC = hepatocellular carcinoma, hCG = human chorionic gonadotropin, HCV = hepatitis C virus, HD = Hodgkin's disease, HDV = hepatitis D virus, HIV = human immunodeficiency virus, HPV = human papillomavirus, HTLV = human T cell lymphotropic virus, Hx = history, IL-1 = interleukin-1, IVC = inferior vena cava, LDH = lactate dehydrogenase, MEN = multiple endocrine neoplasia, NHL = non-Hodgkin's lymphoma, Pap = Papanicolaou, PSA = prostate-specific antigen, PTH = parathormone, RBC = red blood cell, Rx = treatment, SCC = squamous cell carcinoma, SXRs = sex-linked recessive traits, TCC = transitional cell carcinoma, UV = ultraviolet, WBC = white blood cell.

Table 4–2. PRECURSOR LESIONS AND RISK FACTORS FOR CANCER

Most Common...	Answer and Explanation
precursor for squamous cancer of the skin	*actinic keratosis*: * UVB light induces the formation of thymidine dimers and cross-links, which distort the DNA molecule
precursor for squamous cancer of the lung	*squamous dysplasia secondary to smoking*
precursor for squamous cancer of the larynx	*squamous dysplasia secondary to smoking*
precursors for squamous cancer in the oral cavity	• **leukoplakia**: white patches, • *erythroplakia*: erythematous patches [Although leuko-, erythroplakia are descriptive terms for white or red patches that do not rub off, their presence is an indication for a biopsy to R/O dysplasia and/or cancer.]
precursor for distal adenocarcinoma of the esophagus	*Barrett's esophagus*: glandular metaplasia secondary to acid injury from GERD
precursor for gastric adenocarcinoma	*intestinal metaplasia*: secondary to *Helicobacter pylori*–induced chronic atrophic gastritis involving the antrum and pylorus
precursor lesion for colorectal cancer	*adenomatous polyps*: true neoplasms
factors suggesting malignant potential of adenomatous polyps	• **size**: >2 cm, • *percent villous component*: * surface mucosa looks like small intestine villi, * >50% is a high-risk polyp, • *presence of multiple polyps*
precursor for clear cell adenocarcinoma of the vagina	*vaginal adenosis in women whose mothers received DES during pregnancy:* DES inhibits müllerian differentiation, cancers may also occur in the cervix alone or cervix and vagina
precursor for cervical cancer	*cervical dysplasia*: most often associated with HPV types 16 (most common), 18, or 31
precursor for endometrial cancer	*endometrial hyperplasia*: * due to unopposed estrogen stimulation, * see Table 2–1
precursor for breast cancer	*atypical ductal hyperplasia*: * estrogen is responsible for division of the ductal epithelium, * see Table 2–1

Table 4–2. PRECURSOR LESIONS AND RISK FACTORS
FOR CANCER *Continued*

Most Common...	Answer and Explanation
precursor for vulvar cancer	*atypical squamous hyperplasia*: * squamous hyperplasia presents as a leukoplakia, * HPV 16, 18 relationship
IBD associated with colorectal cancer	*ulcerative colitis*: see Table 2–1
genetic precursor for colorectal cancer	*familial adenomatous polyposis:* * AD inheritance, * most common polyp syndrome in the GI tract, * see Table 2–1
precursor for medullary carcinoma of the thyroid	*C cell hyperplasia*: * C cells secrete calcitonin, * see Table 11–4
risk factor for breast cancer in women	*increasing age:* See Table 2–1 for more complete list
risk factor for prostate cancer	*increasing age:* See Table 2–1 for more complete list
risk factor for lung cancer	*cigarette smoking:* See Table 2–1 for more complete list
risk factor for colorectal cancer	*increasing age:* See Table 2–1 for more complete list
risk factor for endometrial cancer	*unopposed estrogen:* See Table 2–1 for more complete list
risk factor for ovarian cancer	*increasing age:* See Table 2–1 for more complete list
risk factor for cervical cancer	*early onset of sexual activity and/or multiple partners:* See Table 2–1 for more complete list
risk factor for BCC and SCC of the skin	*exposure to UVB light*
risk factors for SCC of the larynx	• **smoking**, • *alcohol*: * cocarcinogen with smoking or is a carcinogen by itself, * synergistic effect on producing laryngeal cancer if patient smokes, • *asbestos exposure*, • *squamous papillomas of the vocal cord*: HPV relationship
risk factors for malignant melanoma	*severe sunburn at an early age*: see Table 14–3 for a more complete list

Table continued on following page

Table 4–2. PRECURSOR LESIONS AND RISK FACTORS FOR CANCER *Continued*

Most Common...	Answer and Explanation
risk factor for mesothelioma	*exposure to asbestos*: asbestos exposure may be associated with * roofers (20 years plus), * pipe-fitters (Navy shipyards), * demolition of old buildings
risk factors for SCC of the nasal cavity and paranasal sinuses	• *nickel*, • *HPV*
risk factor for adenocarcinoma of the nasal cavity	*woodworking*
risk factors for SCC in the oral cavity	• **smoking**: see Table 2–3, • *alcohol:* see Table 2–4
risk factors for SCC of the esophagus	• **smoking**, • *alcohol:* synergistic with smoking, • *lye stricture*, • *achalasia*, • *Plummer-Vinson syndrome*, • *nitrosamines*
risk factors for adenocarcinoma of the stomach	• ***H. pylori* type B chronic atrophic gastritis involving the antrum and pylorus**, • *lack of fruits and vegetables*: deficiency of vitamin C, which normally prevents the formation of nitrosamines, • *smoking*, • *polycyclic hydrocarbons in smoked meats*, • *highly salted meats*, • *loss of gastric acidity*: achlorhydria, • *type A chronic atrophic gastritis*: secondary to PA, • *adenomatous polyps*, • *nitrosamines*, • *blood group A*
risk factors for malignant lymphoma of the stomach	• **immunosuppression**: high-grade immunoblastic lymphomas most common type, • *H. pylori*: low-grade mucosa-associated lymphomas
risk factors for small intestine malignant lymphoma	• **celiac disease**: usually a high-grade T cell lymphoma, • *IgA heavy chain disease*
risk factor for SCC of the anus	*unprotected anal intercourse among homosexual males*: * similar to cervical cancer, * there is a strong HPV relationship in anal carcinoma
risk factor for HCC	*HBV postnecrotic cirrhosis*: see Table 9–8

Table 4–2. PRECURSOR LESIONS AND RISK FACTORS
FOR CANCER *Continued*

Most Common...	Answer and Explanation
risk factor for angiosarcoma of the liver	• **vinyl chloride**, • *arsenic*, • *Thorotrast*
risk factors for gallbladder cancer	• **gallstones**: * presence of stone themselves may be carcinogenic, * bile salt degradation may result in the production of carcinogens, • *porcelain gallbladder*: dystrophic calcification of the wall of the gallbladder
risk factors for pancreatic adenocarcinoma	• **smoking**, • *chronic pancreatitis*: most commonly alcohol-related
risk factors for renal adenocarcinoma	• **smoking**, • *obesity*, • *APKD*, • *von Hippel-Lindau disease* (often bilateral)
risk factors for TCC of the bladder	• **smoking**, • *cyclophosphamide*, • *aniline dyes*, • *benzidine*, • *phenacetin*
risk factors for seminoma	• **cryptorchid testis**, • *testicular feminization*, • *maternal DES exposure during pregnancy*
risk factors for SCC of the penis	• **lack of circumcision**: * poor hygiene, * risk does not extend to cervical cancer, • *balanitis xerotica obliterans*, • *erythroplasia of Queyrat*, • *Bowen's disease*
risk factor for papillary carcinoma of the thyroid	*irradiation*
risk factor for primary malignant lymphoma of the thyroid	*Hashimoto's thyroiditis*
risk factor for osteogenic sarcoma	• **irradiation**, • *Paget's disease of bone*
risk factor for chondrosarcoma	*enchondromatosis:* Ollier's disease
risk factors for soft tissue sarcomas	• **previous history of radiation**: malignant fibrous histiocytoma, • *neurofibromatosis*: neurofibrosarcoma, • *trauma*: malignant fibrous histiocytoma, • *herpesvirus 8*: Kaposi's sarcoma, • *chronic lymphedema*: lymphangiosarcoma

Table continued on following page

Table 4–2. PRECURSOR LESIONS AND RISK FACTORS FOR CANCER *Continued*

Most Common...	Answer and Explanation
risk factors for astrocytoma	• *Turcot's syndrome*: AR polyposis syndrome, • *tuberous sclerosis*: AD disease
risk factors for primary CNS lymphoma	• **HIV**, • *EBV*
risk factors for acute leukemias	• **radiation exposure**, • *benzene*, • *Down syndrome*, • *chromosome instability syndromes*, • *alkylating agents*, • *CML*, • *MDS*, • *MPD*, • *smoking*
risk factor for CML	*radiation exposure*
risk factor for T cell leukemia/lymphoma	*HTLV-1*
risk factor for Burkitt's lymphoma	*EBV*

Question: Smoking and alcohol abuse are operative in which of the following types of cancer? **SELECT 4**
- (A) Lung cancer
- (B) Oral cavity cancer
- (C) Cervical cancer
- (D) Pancreatic cancer
- (E) Stomach cancer
- (F) Bladder cancer
- (G) Esophageal cancer
- (H) Laryngeal cancer
- (I) Acute leukemia

Answers: (B), (D), (G), (H): Smoking *alone* is a risk factor for lung (choice A is incorrect), cervical (choice C is incorrect), stomach (choice E is incorrect), bladder (choice F is incorrect), and acute leukemia (choice I is incorrect). Cancers of the oral cavity (choice B), pancreas (choice D), esophagus (choice G), and larynx (choice H) may be associated with smoking and/or alcohol abuse.

AD = autosomal dominant, APKD = adult polycystic kidney disease, AR = autosomal recessive, BCC = basal cell carcinoma, CML = chronic myelogenous leukemia, CNS = central nervous system, DES = diethylstilbestrol, EBV = Epstein-Barr virus, GERD = gastroesophageal reflux disease, GI = gastrointestinal, HBV = hepatitis B virus, HCC = hepatocellular carcinoma, HIV = human immunodeficiency virus, HPV = human papillomavirus, HTLV = human T cell lymphotropic virus, IBD = inflammatory bowel disease, MDS = myelodysplastic syndrome, MPD = myeloproliferative disorder, PA = pernicious anemia, R/O = rule out, SCC = squamous cell carcinoma, UVB = ultraviolet B.

Table 4–3. CONCEPTS OF CANCER THERAPY

Most Common...	Answer and Explanation
cancer Rx modalities	• **surgery**, • *radiation*, • *chemotherapy*
benefits of surgery	• **potential cure**, • *remove tumor burden*, • *staging*: e.g., ovarian cancer, • *Rx complications*: e.g., bowel adhesions secondary to previous surgery, radiation
benefits of radiation	• **potential cure**: may be the sole Rx in laryngeal cancer, oral cavity, certain CNS tumors, • *adjuvant to chemotherapy*, • *Rx of complications*: e.g., * SVC syndrome, * pain due to bone metastasis
tissue with the most tolerance to radiation	*brain*: necrosis is the most common complication
tissue with the least tolerance to radiation	*testes and ovaries*: sterilization is the most common complication
types of chemotherapy agents	• *cytotoxic drugs*: e.g., alkylating agents, • *hormones*: e.g., * DES in prostate cancer, * progesterone in endometrial cancer, • *cytokines:* e.g., recombinant α-interferon in CML, malignant melanoma, Kaposi's sarcoma, • *antihormones:* e.g., * tamoxifen is an antiestrogen used in the Rx of ERA-positive breast cancers, • *5-α reductase inhibitors:* block the effect of DHT in prostate cancer, • *biologic*: e.g., BCG in bladder cancer, • *plant products*: e.g., paclitaxel from the Pacific yew tree
benefits of chemotherapy	• **adjuvant Rx along with surgery/radiation**, • *potential cure*: e.g., * gestationally derived choriocarcinoma, * HD, • *palliation*, • *preoperative modality to shrink tumor*
terms applied to chemotherapy	• *induction*: try to induce complete remission, • *consolidation*: try to kill any remaining cancer cells in patients who enter remission, • *maintenance*: try to prolong remissions, • *adjuvant*: * similar in concept to consolidation therapy, * most important modality to destroy micrometastases
routes of administration of chemotherapeutic agents	• **oral**, • *intravenous*, • *intracavitary*: * bladder, * peritoneum, • *intrathecal*: * subarachnoid space, * methotrexate in Rx of ALL, • *intra-arterial*: * for administering high drug concentrations, e.g., * liver metastasis

Table continued on following page

Table 4–3. CONCEPTS OF CANCER THERAPY *Continued*

Most Common...	Answer and Explanation
cancers that are curable by chemotherapy	• **gestational choriocarcinoma,** • testicular cancer, • leukemias: e.g., * ALL, * AML, • lymphomas: e.g., * HD, * NHL
cancers that are usually resistant to chemotherapy	• *malignant melanoma,* • *astrocytomas,* • *prostate cancer,* • *Kaposi's sarcoma,* • *pancreatic cancer*
solid tumors sensitive to chemotherapy	• **gestationally derived choriocarcinoma,** • *germ cell tumors:* * ovary, * testis, • *breast cancer,* • *ovarian cancer,* • *small cell carcinoma of lung*
causes of failure of advanced cancers to respond to chemotherapy	• *tumor heterogeneity:* cell populations are resistant to chemotherapy, • *large numbers of neoplastic cells are not in the cell cycle:* malignant cells are in the resting phase
cell cycle–specific chemotherapy agents	• *antimetabolites,* • *bleomycin,* • *plant alkaloids:* e.g., * vinca alkaloids, * paclitaxel [The above drugs are only effective in cycling cells.]
cell cycle– nonspecific chemotherapy agents	• *alkylating agents,* • *antibiotics,* • *cisplatin,* • *nitrosourea,* • L-*asparaginase* [The above drugs kill cells either in the resting phase (G_0 phase, less toxic) or cycling cells (more toxic).]
antitumor mechanism of antimetabolites	• *compete with normal metabolites for the regulatory site of a key enzyme,* • *substitute for a metabolite normally incorporated into DNA or RNA* [Antimetabolites work best in the S phase (DNA replication) of the cell cycle, hence their usefulness in tumors with rapid cell proliferation.]
mechanism of action of methotrexate	*antimetabolite that inhibits dihydrofolate reductase in folic acid metabolism*
complications associated with methotrexate	• *megaloblastic anemia:* may be thwarted with leucovorin rescue, which bypasses the enzyme block, • *mucositis and GI ulceration,* • *liver toxicity:* fibrosis, • *interstitial pneumonitis:* potential for interstitial fibrosis, • *renal toxicity:* must keep urine alkaline to prevent crystal formation, • *marrow suppression:* * leukopenia, * thrombocytopenia

Table 4–3. CONCEPTS OF CANCER THERAPY *Continued*

Most Common...	Answer and Explanation
cancers treated with methotrexate	• *gestational choriocarcinoma*, • *ALL*, • *breast*, • *bladder*
mechanism of action of 6-mercaptopurine (6-MP)	*antimetabolite* (purine analog) *that blocks purine synthesis*
complications associated with 6-MP	• *6-MP toxicity associated with allopurinol*: * allopurinol is a xanthine oxidase inhibitor; therefore, lower doses of 6-MP must be administered, since it is metabolized as a purine, • *marrow suppression in high doses*
cancers treated with 6-MP	*maintenance phase of ALL*
mechanism of action of 5-fluorouracil (5-FU)	*antimetabolite* (pyrimidine analog) *that blocks the formation of thymidylic acid by inhibiting thymidylate synthetase*: effective throughout the cell cycle
complications associated with 5-FU	• *BM suppression*, • *mucositis*
cancers treated with 5-FU	• *colorectal*, • *breast*
mechanism of action of cytarabine (ara C)	*antimetabolite* (pyrimidine antagonist) *that blocks DNA and RNA*: effective in the S phase
complications associated with ara C	• **myelosuppression**, • *GI toxicity*, • *cerebellar ataxia*, • *hepatitis*, • *pancreatitis*
cancer treated with ara C	*AML*
mechanism of action of 2-chlorodeoxy-adenosine	*antimetabolite* (purine analog) *that resists degradation by adenosine deaminase*
complication associated with 2-chlorodeoxy-adenosine	*myelosuppression*
cancer treated with 2-chlorodeoxy-adenosine	*hairy cell leukemia*: replaced the previous therapy with splenectomy and α-interferon

Table continued on following page

Table 4–3. CONCEPTS OF CANCER THERAPY *Continued*

Most Common...	Answer and Explanation
mechanism of action of hydroxyurea	*antimetabolite that inhibits ribonucleotide reductase, which converts ribonucleotides to deoxyribonucleotides:* it crosses the blood-brain barrier
complications associated with hydroxyurea	• *GI toxicity*, • *leukopenia*, • *skin lesions*
cancers treated with hydroxyurea	• *chronic CML*, • *other MPDs:* e.g., PRV
mechanism of action of antitumor antibiotics	*interfere with DNA metabolism*: majority are derived from *Streptomyces* species
mechanism of action of bleomycin	• *antibiotic that breaks DNA by an oxidative process involving free radicals*, • *inhibits DNA ligase involved in DNA repair*: effective in the G2 phase—synthesis of the mitotic spindle
complications associated with bleomycin	• **pulmonary fibrosis**, • *stomatitis*, • *edema of the hands* [There is no BM suppression.]
cancers treated with bleomycin	• *testicular*, • *malignant lymphoma*, • *head and neck cancers*
mechanism of action of dactinomycin (actinomycin D)	*antibiotic that interferes with DNA synthesis*: * effective in the S phase, * inhibits topoisomerases, which are enzymes that repair single- or double-stranded DNA breaks
complications associated with dactinomycin	• **severe myelosuppression**, • *stomatitis*, • *alopecia*
cancers treated with dactinomycin	• *Wilms' tumor*, • *Ewing's sarcoma*, • *gestational choriocarcinoma*
mechanism of action of daunomycin	*antibiotic similar to dactinomycin*: see above
complications associated with daunomycin	• **dose-dependent cardiotoxicity**, • *marrow suppression*, • *alopecia*, • *red urine:* due to the drug
cancers treated with daunomycin	*acute leukemias*

Table 4–3. CONCEPTS OF CANCER THERAPY *Continued*

Most Common...	Answer and Explanation
mechanism of action of doxorubicin	*antibiotic similar to dactinomycin:* see above
complications associated with doxorubicin	*same as those listed for daunomycin:* see above
cancers treated with doxorubicin	• *breast cancer,* • *malignant lymphomas,* • *multiple myeloma,* • *Kaposi's sarcoma:* a liposomal doxorubicin is used
mechanism of action of mitomycin	*antibiotic similar to dactinomycin:* see above
complications associated with mitomycin	• *thrombocytopenia,* • *leukopenia,* • *hemolytic-uremic syndrome:* microangiopathic hemolytic anemia and renal failure, • *interstitial pneumonitis*
cancers treated with mitomycin	*GI malignancies*
mechanism of action of etoposide	*antibiotic* (plant alkaloid) *that inhibits topoisomerases*
complications associated with etoposide	• *BM depression,* • *alopecia*
cancers treated with etoposide	• *AML,* • *NHL,* • *ovarian,* • *lung,* • *testicular*
mechanism of action of paclitaxel	*antibiotic* (plant alkaloid) *that interferes with microtubules:* binds to microtubules and produces nonfunctional microtubules
complications associated with paclitaxel	• *neutropenia/thrombocytopenia,* • *fluid retention,* • *hypersensitivity reactions:* * flushing, * angioedema, * urticaria, • *peripheral neuropathy,* • *alopecia*
cancers treated with paclitaxel	• *ovarian,* • *breast,* • *lung,* • *malignant melanoma*
mechanism of action of vincristine/ vinblastine	*antibiotics* (plant alkaloids) *that disrupt the mitotic spindle:* * inhibit the M phase of the cycle, * they derive from the periwinkle plant
complications associated with vincristine/ vinblastine	• *neurotoxic:* * peripheral neuropathy, * muscle weakness, * areflexia, • *BM suppression,* • *alopecia,* • *SiADH,* • *Raynaud's phenomenon*

Table continued on following page

Table 4–3. **CONCEPTS OF CANCER THERAPY** *Continued*

Most Common...	Answer and Explanation
cancers treated with vincristine/vinblastine	• *vincristine:* * part of the MOPP regimen in treating HD and in treating ALL and NHL, * ALL, • *vinblastine:* used in treating * HD, * bladder, breast, and testicular cancers
mechanism of action of alkylating agents	*impair cell function by alkylating DNA, RNA, and other proteins*: alkylation primarily leads to breakage of DNA strands and cross-linking, which inhibits strand replication
complications associated with mechlorethamine (nitrogen mustard)	*alkylating agent that produces:* BM suppression
cancer treated with mechlorethamine	*part of the MOPP regimen in treating HD*
complications associated with cyclophosphamide	*alkylating agent that produces:* * hemorrhagic cystitis: blocked with mesna, * TCC of the bladder, * BM suppression, * SiADH [Cyclophosphamide is a nitrogen mustard that is changed by the cytochrome system into phosphamide, which interacts with DNA.]
cancers treated with cyclophosphamide	• *Burkitt's lymphoma,* • *breast cancer*
complications associated with the nitrosoureas (BCNU, CCNU)	*alkylating agents that produce*: * BM suppression with aplastic anemia, * pulmonary fibrosis: * inhibit both DNA and RNA replication, * effective in the S phase, * BCNU is administered with alcohol
cancers treated with nitrosoureas	• **brain tumors**: excellent concentration in the CNS due to their lipid solubility, • *HD,* • *NHL,* • *multiple myeloma*
complications associated with busulfan	*alkylating agent that produces*: * marrow suppression, * skin pigmentation similar to Addison's disease, * pulmonary fibrosis, * adrenal insufficiency, * gynecomastia, * sterility
cancer treated with busulfan	*myeloid leukemias:* particularly CML
complications associated with chlorambucil	*alkylating agent that produces:* * NHL, * myelosuppression

Table 4-3. CONCEPTS OF CANCER THERAPY *Continued*

Most Common...	Answer and Explanation
cancers treated with chlorambucil	• *CLL,* • *PRV,* • *Waldenstrom's macroglobulinemia*
complications associated with melphalan	*alkylating agent that produces:* * marrow suppression, * interstitial pneumonitis, * NHL
cancers treated with melphalan	• *multiple myeloma,* • *ovarian,* • *breast*
complications associated with streptozocin	*alkylating agent that produces:* * nephrotoxicity: proximal RTA, * hypoglycemia
cancers treated with streptozocin	• *islet cell cancers,* • *carcinoid syndrome*
complications associated with cisplatin	*alkylating agent that produces:* * nephrotoxicity, * magnesium wasting—hypomagnesemia, * acoustic nerve dysfunction, * peripheral neuropathy
cancers treated with cisplatin	• *TCC of the bladder,* • *cervical,* • *ovarian,* • *testicular,* • *osteogenic sarcoma*
complications associated with thiotepa	*alkylating agent that produces*: marrow suppression
cancers treated with thiotepa	• *breast,* • *ovarian*
mechanism of action of L-asparaginase	*hydrolyzes blood asparagine:* * tumor cells are deprived of the nutrient for protein synthesis, * only enzyme antitumor agent
complications associated with L-asparaginase	• *hypersensitivity reactions and anaphylaxis,* • *hepatitis,* • *encephalopathy,* • *prerenal azotemia,* • *hyperglycemia* [It is not associated with BM suppression.]
cancer treated with L-asparaginase	*ALL*
mechanism of action of procarbazine	*inhibits DNA and RNA*: monamine oxidase inhibitor that after oxidation by hepatic enzymes acts as an alkylating agent

Table continued on following page

Table 4–3. CONCEPTS OF CANCER THERAPY *Continued*

Most Common...	Answer and Explanation
complications associated with procarbazine	• *teratogenic*, • *neurotoxic*: peripheral neuropathy, • *may cause sterility* [It is contraindicated when taking foods with tyramine (cheese, wine), owing to its being an MAO inhibitor.]
cancers treated with procarbazine	• *HD*, • *astrocytomas*
mechanism of action of IL-2	• *increased T cell proliferation*, • *increases lymphokine-activated natural killer cells* [IL-2 is a cytokine derived from CD_4 T helper cells.]
complications associated with IL-2	• *vascular leak syndrome*, • *toxicities in all major organs*
cancers treated with IL-2	• *metastatic renal adenocarcinoma*, • *malignant melanoma*
mechanism of action of α-IF	• *inhibits cell proliferation*, • *increases the lytic potential of NK cells*, • *increases the expression of class I antigens:* this increases the cytotoxicity of CD_8 cytotoxic T cells [α-IF is produced by macrophages.]
complications associated with α-IF	• *fever*, • *headaches*, • *myalgia*, • *cardiovascular disturbances*
cancers treated with α-IF	• *CML*, • *HCL*, • *AIDS-related Kaposi's sarcoma*
mechanism of action of tamoxifen	*weak estrogen that acts as an estrogen antagonist that binds to estrogen receptors:* disrupts estrogen's effect on RNA synthesis
complication associated with tamoxifen	*endometrial hyperplasia/carcinoma*
cancer treated with tamoxifen	*adjuvant therapy in breast cancers that are ERA positive:* in addition, its weak estrogenic activity prevents osteoporosis and CAD
mechanism of action of DES	*estrogen compound that competes with androgens for intracellular receptor sites:* blocks the growth-promoting effect of estrogens
complications associated with DES	• *gynecomastia*, • *venous thrombosis*, • *clear cell adenocarcinoma of the vagina in female offspring*

Table 4–3. CONCEPTS OF CANCER THERAPY *Continued*

Most Common...	Answer and Explanation
cancer treated with DES	*prostate cancer*
mechanism of action of leuprolide	*analog of GnRH that when administered in a sustained fashion inhibits the release of LH and FSH*
complications associated with leuprolide	**hypogonadism**
cancer treated with leuprolide	*primarily used in the Rx of prostate cancer: reduces DHT levels*

Question: Which of the following chemotherapeutic drugs produce interstitial fibrosis? **SELECT 4**

- (A) 6-MP
- (B) Bleomycin
- (C) L-asparaginase
- (D) Methotrexate
- (E) 5-FU
- (F) Daunomycin
- (G) Cyclophosphamide
- (H) Melphalan

Answers: (B), (D), (G), (H) 6-MP is an antimetabolite that primarily produces hepatic cholestasis and marrow suppression **(choice A is incorrect).** L-asparaginase deprives neoplastic cells of asparagine and is primarily associated with hypersensitivity reactions and anaphylaxis **(choice C is incorrect).** 5-FU is an antimetabolite that produces marrow suppression **(choice E is incorrect).** Daunomycin is an antitumor antibiotic that primarily produces myelosuppression **(choice F is incorrect).** Bleomycin **(choice B)**, methotrexate **(choice D)**, cyclophosphamide **(choice G)**, and melphalan **(choice H)** are associated with pulmonary fibrosis.

AIDS = acquired immunodeficiency syndrome, ALL = acute lymphoblastic leukemia, AML = acute myelogenous leukemia, BCG = bacille Calmette-Guérin vaccine, BM = bone marrow, CAD = coronary artery disease, CLL = chronic lymphocytic leukemia, CML = chronic myelogenous leukemia, CNS = central nervous system, DES = diethylstilbestrol, DHT = dihdyrotestosterone, ERA = estrogen receptor assay, 5-FU = 5-fluorouracil, FSH = follicle stimulating hormone, GI = gastrointestinal, G_0 = resting phase of the cell cycle, GnRH = gonadotropin-releasing hormone, HD = Hodgkin's disease, α-IF = α-interferon, IL-2 = interleukin 2, LH = luteinizing hormone, MAO = monoamine oxidase inhibitor, 6-MP = 6-mercaptopurine, MPDs = myeloproliferative diseases, NHL = non-Hodgkin's lymphoma, PRV = polycythemia rubra vera, RTA = renal tubular acidosis, Rx = treatment, SiADH = syndrome of inappropriate antidiuretic hormone, SVC = superior vena cava, TCC = transitional cell carcinoma.

CHAPTER
5

CARDIOVASCULAR DISEASE

CONTENTS

Table 5–1. HISTORY, PHYSICAL EXAMINATION, AND DIAGNOSTIC PROCEDURES

Most Common...	Answer and Explanation
symptom of left-sided heart failure	*dyspnea:* sensation of difficulty with breathing. [Dyspnea is caused by stimulation of the J receptors (e.g., by fluid) innervated by the vagus nerve in the interstitium of the lung. *Orthopnea* is dyspnea in the recumbent position. *PND* is a choking sensation that awakens a patient at night and is relieved by sitting or standing.]
symptom of ischemic heart disease (IHD)	*chest pain* [Angina usually subsides in <15–30 minutes. An AMI is associated with more prolonged chest pain that is often described as pressure or tightness in the retrosternal area. It may radiate to the jaw, inner aspect of the arm, upper abdomen (simulating PUD or GERD), or shoulders. It is not relieved with nitroglycerin.]
cause of wheezing in left heart failure (LHF)	*peribronchiolar edema around the terminal bronchioles:* * produces small airway construction, * "cardiac asthma"

Table continued on following page

Table 5–1. HISTORY, PHYSICAL EXAMINATION, AND DIAGNOSTIC PROCEDURES *Continued*

Most Common...	Answer and Explanation
cause of calf claudication	*atherosclerotic PVD involving the femoral artery:* * claudication is crampy muscular pain occurring with exercise and relieved by resting, * similar pain in the buttocks is aortofemoral disease
cardiac cause of dependent pitting edema	*right heart failure* (RHF): blood builds up in the venous system behind the failed right heart with a subsequent increase in hydrostatic pressure leading to pitting edema
causes of an awareness of heart beat	• **anxiety**, • *increase in stroke volume:* e.g., * hyperthyroidism, * severe anemia, • *arrhythmia:* e.g., * sinus tachycardia, * ventricular premature beats ("skipped beat"), * atrial tachycardias
pathologic causes of cardiac-induced dizziness/syncope	• **postural hypotension**: e.g., drugs (beta-blockers) used in treating CVD or HTN, • *decrease in CO secondary to cardiac arrhythmias:* e.g., * sinus node arrest, * sinus bradycardia, * ventricular tachycardia, • atrioventricular conduction block, • *valvular disease:* e.g., * calcific AV stenosis (most common cause), * IHSS, *essential HTN:* headache or dizziness upon waking
pathophysiologic cause of cardiac-induced diaphoresis	• *hypotension*, • *baroreceptor stimulated release of catecholamines* [Diaphoresis refers to profuse perspiration.]
cardiac-induced cause of dysphagia for solids but not liquids	*LA enlargement secondary to MV stenosis* [LA is the most posteriorly located chamber in the heart and compresses the esophagus when enlarged. Transesophageal US is the best method of detecting LA enlargement. Both the LV and LA are enlarged in mitral regurgitation.]
factor responsible for systolic BP	*stroke volume* (SV): SV is the amount of blood ejected from the heart during systole
factors increasing SV	• **increase in cardiac contractility**: e.g., hyperthyroidism, • *increase in preload in the left ventricle*: e.g., aortic regurgitation. • *increase in venous return to the right heart*: e.g., arteriovenous fistula, • *left to right cardiac shunts*: e.g., VSD

Table 5–1. HISTORY, PHYSICAL EXAMINATION, AND DIAGNOSTIC PROCEDURES *Continued*

Most Common...	Answer and Explanation
factor responsible for the diastolic BP	*total peripheral resistance (TPR)*: * TPR is expressed in Poiseuille's equation—8 n $l/\pi r^4$, where n = viscosity of blood, l = length of the vessel, and r = radius of the arteriole, * peripheral arterioles are the resistance vessels, * the amount of blood remaining in the arterial vasculature during diastole represents the diastolic blood pressure
factors increasing TPR	• **arteriolar vasoconstriction**: e.g., * catecholamine effect—note that the r is to the 4th power, • *increase in blood viscosity (n)*: e.g., polycythemia
factors decreasing TPR	• **arteriolar vasodilatation**: e.g., * endotoxic shock—note that r is to the 4th power, • *decrease in viscosity (n)*: e.g., severe anemia
sites for auscultation of the MV, AV, TV, and PV	• *MV*: apex, • *AV*: 2nd right ICS, • *TV*: left parasternal, • *PV*: 2nd left ICS
heart sound corresponding with the carotid pulse	*SI heart sound*
cause of S1 heart sound	*closure of the MV and TV*: MV closes before the TV
causes of an accentuated S1	• **sinus tachycardia**: *short PR interval*, • *early MV stenosis*, • *increased cardiac output*: * *hyperthyroidism*, * *anemia*, * *exercise*
causes of a decreased S1	• *prolonged PR interval*: first-degree heart block, • *severe MV stenosis*, • *LHF*, • *IHD*
causes of a varying S1	• **atrial fibrillation**: • *complete heart block* [A variation in the closure of the MV is responsible for a varying S1 heart sound.]
cause of S2	*closure of the AV and PV during diastole*: AV normally closes before PV
S2 alterations with respiration	• *inspiration*: * split during inspiration, * more blood enters the right heart (negative intrathoracic pressure), * PV takes longer to close, • *expiration*: single sound
mechanism of a paradoxical S2	*P2 comes before A2*: * early closure of P2, * late closure of A2

Table continued on following page

Table 5–1. HISTORY, PHYSICAL EXAMINATION, AND DIAGNOSTIC PROCEDURES *Continued*

Most Common...	Answer and Explanation
causes of a paradoxical S2	• **LBBB**: * delayed activation of the left side of the heart, * AV closes later than the PV, • *AV stenosis:* late closure of AV, • *LHF:* late closure of AV, • *tricuspid regurgitation:* some blood enters the right atrium in systole, leading to early closure of P2
mechanism of fixed splitting of S2	*A2 closes earlier than normal or P2 closes later than normal:* S2 remains split in both inspiration and expiration
causes of fixed splitting of S2	• **left to right shunting of blood**: * constant volume overloading of the right heart, * late closure of PV, * e.g., **ASD**, VSD, • *right ventricular failure:* late closure of PV, • *RBBB:* late closure of PV, • *mitral regurgitation:* * some blood is redirected into the left atrium during systole, * A2 closes earlier
cause of an accentuated A2	*essential HTN*
cause of a decreased A2	*severe calcific AV stenosis*
cause of an accentuated P2	*pulmonary HTN*
cause of a decreased P2	*increased AP diameter of the chest:* most commonly due to COPD
mechanism of an S3	• *blood enters a volume overloaded ventricle in diastole,* • *vibration of the valves and ventricular wall produces the S3:* best heart with the bell of the stethoscope at the apex of the heart with the patient in the left lateral decubitus position
patient types in whom an S3 is normal	• *adults <40-y-old:* due to a hyperdynamic circulation, • *pregnant women in third trimester:* due to increased plasma volume
pathologic causes of an S3	• **LHF**: * LV is volume-overloaded, * left-sided S3 increases with expiration, • *RHF:* * RV is volume-overloaded, * right-sided S3 increases with inspiration, • *valvular regurgitation leading to volume overload:* e.g., * AV/PV regurgitation, * MV/TV regurgitation • *congestive cardiomyopathy*

Table 5–1. HISTORY, PHYSICAL EXAMINATION, AND DIAGNOSTIC PROCEDURES *Continued*

Most Common...	Answer and Explanation
heart sound initially heard in LHF	*S3*
mechanism of S4 heart sound	*atrium* (left or right) *contracting in late diastole against a noncompliant* (poorly filling) *ventricle* (left or right): * ventricles do not fill well in hypertrophy, when pericardial fluid restricts filling, or when volume overloaded * left-sided S4 increases with expiration, * right-sided S4 increases with inspiration
causes of a normal left-sided S4	*athlete with physiologic LVH*
causes of a pathologic left-sided S4	• **LVH secondary to essential HTN**, • *AV stenosis*: leads to LVH, • *restrictive cardiomyopathy*: e.g., amyloidosis, • *IHSS*, • *patients >60 years old,* • volume-overloaded LV
causes of a pathologic right-sided S4	• **RVH secondary to PH**, • *pulmonic stenosis*, • volume-overloaded RV
cause of an absent S4 heart sound	*atrial fibrillation*: AF interferes with late diastolic contraction of the atria
causes of a systolic ejection click	• **MVP**: click occurs as the MV balloons into the left atrium and is suddenly restrained by the chordae tendineae, • *congenital bicuspid aortic valve with AV stenosis*, • *aortic sclerosis*, • *TV prolapse*, • *pulmonic stenosis*
alterations of the click/murmur in MVP in relation to S1 and S2	• *click/murmur closer to S1*: * occurs when there is decreased venous return to the heart or less blood in the LV, * e.g., ♦ anxiety (increased heart rate decreases LV filling), ♦ standing up, ♦ Valsalva maneuver, • *click/murmur closer to S2*: * occurs when there is more blood in LV, * e.g., ♦ lying down (increased venous return to the heart), ♦ clenching the fists (increases LVEDV)
clinical findings in aortic sclerosis	• *normal in the elderly population,* • *AV is sclerotic but not hemodynamically abnormal,* • *murmur is shorter than in AV stenosis and does not radiate into the carotid artery*

Table continued on following page

Table 5–1. HISTORY, PHYSICAL EXAMINATION, AND DIAGNOSTIC PROCEDURES *Continued*

Most Common...	Answer and Explanation
mechanism of an OS	*atria* (left or right) *have difficulty in opening the MV or TV in diastole*: * valves thickened secondary to inflammation, * when the MV or TV finally open under increased pressure, the OS is produced, * high-pitched snap, * best heard with the diaphragm
causes of an OS	• **MV stenosis**, • TV stenosis
alterations of OS with severity of valvular stenosis	• *OS closer to S2*: sign of very severe valve stenosis, • *OS later in diastole*: sign of less severe valve stenosis
mechanism of a physiologic murmur	*temporary increase in blood flow through a valve*: it is not due to a structural abnormality in a valve
causes of a physiologic murmur	• **anemia**: decreased viscosity of blood increases the rapidity of blood flow through the PV, • *pregnancy*: due to increased plasma volume, • *fever*: due to increased heart rate and force of contraction, • *hyperthyroidism*: due to increased heart rate and force of contraction
causes of an innocent murmur	**aortic systolic ejection murmur**: * most often heard in children between 3 and 7 years old, * grade 1–2 murmur, * best heard in the 2nd left ICS with the patient supine, * disappears with sitting or standing up, • *turbulent blood flow through the PA*, • *venous hum:* turbulent blood flow throughout the jugular venous system
cause of a pathologic murmur	*structural disease*
causes of structural abnormalities leading to murmurs	• **partial obstruction of AV/PV**: e.g., AV stenosis is the most common pathologic murmur, • *blood flow across a valve irregularity*: e.g., congenital bicuspid AV, • *flow into an aneurysmally dilated vessel*: e.g., post-stenotic dilation of the aorta in a coarctation, • *regurgitant flow through an incompetent valve*: e.g., mitral regurgitation, • *shunting of blood from a high to low pressure chamber through an abnormal opening*: e.g., VSD

Table 5–1. HISTORY, PHYSICAL EXAMINATION, AND
DIAGNOSTIC PROCEDURES *Continued*

Most Common...	Answer and Explanation
method of grading heart murmurs	*grades 1 through 6:* * grades 1–2 are difficult to hear, * grade 3 murmurs are heard by most physicians, * grade 6 murmurs may be heard without a stethoscope
mechanism of stenosis murmurs	*murmur is due to problems in opening the valve:* * AV and PV open in systole, * MV and TV open in diastole
mechanism of regurgitation murmurs	*murmur is due to problems in closing the valve:* * MV and TV close in systole, * AV and PV close in diastole
types of stenosis murmurs	• **ejection type during systole**: * crescendo/decrescendo murmur due to flow under pressure through a narrow opening in the AV or PV, * ventricles hypertrophy due to increased afterload, * e.g., ♦ AV stenosis, ♦ PV stenosis, • *OS in diastole followed by a rumble:* * OS is due to sudden opening of a non-pliable MV or TV valve in diastole, * diastolic rumble is due to excess blood rushing into the ventricle from the volume-overloaded atrium, * e.g., ♦ **MV stenosis**, ♦ TV stenosis
types of regurgitation murmurs	• **pansystolic**: * even intensity murmur heard throughout systole, * murmur due to blood entering the atria during systole through an incompetent MV or TV, * S1 and S2 are often obliterated, * blood leaks back into the ventricles leading to volume overload and hypertrophy, * e.g., ♦ **MV regurgitation**, ♦ TV regurgitation, • *diastolic, high pitched blowing murmur after S2:* * murmur due to blood leaking back into the ventricles from an incompetent AV or PV, * ventricles become volume-overloaded and hypertrophied, * e.g., ♦ **AV regurgitation**, ♦ PV regurgitation
effect of squatting on heart murmurs	• **increases LV volume by increasing systemic vascular resistance**, • *increases venous return of blood to the right heart*
effect of inspiration/expiration on the intensity of heart murmurs/sounds	• *inspiration:* increases the intensity of right-sided murmurs/sounds due to the increased flow of blood into the right heart from the increase in negative intrathoracic pressure, • *expiration:* increases the intensity of left-sided murmurs/sounds as the positive intrathoracic pressure increases

Table continued on following page

**Table 5–1. HISTORY, PHYSICAL EXAMINATION, AND
DIAGNOSTIC PROCEDURES** *Continued*

Most Common...	Answer and Explanation
cause of a left parasternal heave	*RVH secondary to PH*: * the RV lies behind the sternum, * enlargement of the RV produces a palpable left parasternal heave
cause of a laterally displaced PMI	*LVH*: * LVH is most often associated with essential HTN, * there is a sustained PMI during systole
causes of LVH	• **essential HTN**: concentric hypertrophy due to increased afterload (TPR increased), • *AV stenosis*: concentric hypertrophy due to increased afterload (stenotic valve), • *AV regurgitation*: dilated and hypertrophied, • *MV regurgitation*: dilated and hypertrophied, • *left to right shunts:* * dilated and hypertrophied, as more blood returns to the left heart
causes of RVH	• **pulmonary HTN**: concentric hypertrophy due to increased afterload (hypertrophied pulmonary vessels), • *PV stenosis*: concentric hypertrophy due to increased afterload (stenotic valve), • *PV regurgitation*: dilated and hypertrophied, • *TV regurgitation*: dilated and hypertrophied, • *left to right shunts*: dilated and hypertrophied
cause of a pericardial knock	*constrictive pericarditis* [Owing to the small amount of room for expansion of the heart, when the cardiac chambers begin to fill up with blood during diastole, they prematurely impact on the thickened parietal pericardium before complete filling of the chambers. This produces a palpable knock. A knock does not occur if the pericardium is filled with fluid (e.g., a pericardial effusion).]
sound of a pericardial friction rub	• **scratchy sound heard best in the left parasternal area**, • *three components may be heard:* * one corresponding with ventricular systole (most common component), * the second occurs in early ventricular diastole, * the third occurs in atrial systole
causes of a pericardial friction rub	• **fibrinous pericarditis secondary to viral pericarditis**, • *AMI*: * first week, * autoimmune pericarditis in following weeks (Dressler syndrome), • *uremia*, • *rheumatic fever*, • *SLE*

Table 5–1. HISTORY, PHYSICAL EXAMINATION, AND DIAGNOSTIC PROCEDURES *Continued*

Most Common...	Answer and Explanation
method of calculating the pulse pressure	*difference between the systolic and diastolic pressure*: normally 30–40 mm Hg
valvular cause a narrow pulse pressure	*AV stenosis:* the SV is decreased in AV stenosis which decreases the systolic pressure and the pulse pressure
valvular cause of an increased pulse pressure	*aortic regurgitation:* * there is LV volume overload from an incompetent AV, * SV increases due to Frank-Starling forces, * diastolic pressure drops as well
cause of an increase in systolic BP in the elderly	*loss of compliance of the aorta:* * this is secondary to atherosclerosis, which decreases the elasticity of the vessel, * loss of compliance of the aorta produces systolic HTN in the elderly (same SV is compacted into a smaller diameter that does not expand)
effect of aging on heart rate	*decreased heart rate:* due to a diminished β-adrenergic response
effect of aging on cardiac output	*preserved both at rest and during exercise*
effect of aging on BP	*decreased blood pressure on standing:* due to an attenuated baroreceptor reflex
components of an arterial pulse wave	• *upstroke:* * due to systolic blood flow, * measure of vessel compliance (elasticity), * peak of the wave corresponds with the peak systolic pressure, • *downstroke*: * measure of vessel recoil (elasticity), • *dicrotic wave at the end of ventricular systole*: * due to blood refluxing back against the closed AV, * usually nonpalpable
cause of a bounding ("water hammer") pulse	• **increase in pulse pressure due to essential HTN:** there is a rapid upstroke and downstroke, • other causes: AV regurgitation
valvular cause of a weak pulse	*AV stenosis*
non-valvular causes of a weak pulse	• **hypovolemic/cardiogenic shock**, • *severe CHF*, • *congestive cardiomyopathy*

Table continued on following page

Table 5–1. HISTORY, PHYSICAL EXAMINATION, AND DIAGNOSTIC PROCEDURES *Continued*

Most Common...	Answer and Explanation
causes of a bisferiens (dicrotic) pulse	• **idiopathic hypertrophic subaortic stenosis**: * a bisferiens pulse has a double systolic peak, * a dicrotic wave is palpable, • *AV stenosis + regurgitation*
method of detecting pulsus paradoxus	*detecting a drop in blood pressure >10 mm Hg during inspiration* [Pulsus paradoxus is first suspected when the amplitude of the pulse is decreased during inspiration. Normally, there is a drop in systolic pressure of <10 mm Hg during inspiration. As the diaphragm contracts, the volume of the thorax increases, hence expanding the lungs and causing the intrapleural pressure to become even more negative than normal (normally −5 cm H_2O, usually −8 cm H_2O after inspiration). The drop in negative intrapleural pressure increases the inflow of venous blood into the right heart (decreases venous pressure, neck veins collapse), hence increasing RV volume and output into the pulmonary vasculature. Inspiratory expansion of the pulmonary vasculature easily accommodates the excess RV outflow leading to less blood delivered to the LV. In addition, the increase in RV volume pushes against the IVS, which diminishes the volume of the LV. The net effect is a slight drop in the systolic blood pressure on inspiration.]
mechanism of pulsus paradoxus	*restricted filling of the right heart with concomitant reduction in the stroke volume from the LV*: * restriction of blood flow into the right heart decreases the output of blood from the RV into the pulmonary vessels, * inspiratory expansion of the pulmonary vasculature containing less blood than usual leads to even less blood returned to the LV, * less volume of blood in the LV drops the systolic pressure >10 mm Hg

Table 5–1. HISTORY, PHYSICAL EXAMINATION, AND DIAGNOSTIC PROCEDURES *Continued*

Most Common...	Answer and Explanation
causes of pulsus paradoxus	• **pericardial effusion**: right heart cannot fill properly, • *decreased lung compliance in severe bronchial asthma:* * increased positive intrathoracic pressure drives water into the pulmonary interstitium, which reduces lung compliance, * increased positive pressure in the thorax compresses the thin-walled vena cava and right heart, hence further reducing blood entering the right heart
mechanism of Kussmaul's sign	*restricted filling of the right heart:* * blood that cannot enter the right heart regurgitates back into the neck veins on inspiration, * neck vein distention on inspiration is called Kussmaul's sign, * it is usually accompanied by pulsus paradoxus
causes of Kussmaul's sign	• **RHF**: blood builds up behind the failed heart, • *pericardial effusion*, • *TV stenosis*, • *PH*: blood from the right heart encounters increased afterload in the pulmonary vessels
method of detecting pulsus alternans	• *in the presence of a normal rhythm, there is an alteration in amplitude:* * high volume beat alternating with a low volume beat, * amplitude changes reflect SV changes in a heart with decreased contractility, * beat couplets are clearly separated from each other, * an S3 heart sound is usually present
cause of pulsus alternans	*severe LV failure*
pulse alteration confused with pulsus alternans	*bigeminal pulse:* * a bigeminal pulse has an *abnormal rhythm* with alternating high and low volume beats, * alternating low volume beats **occur earlier** than in pulsus alternans owing to incomplete emptying of the LV from recurrent premature ventricular contractions
JVP wave corresponding to RA contraction	*a wave:* * the *a wave* is a positive wave, * it represents the reflux of some blood back into the jugular vein when the RA contracts in late diastole

Table continued on following page

**Table 5–1. HISTORY, PHYSICAL EXAMINATION, AND
DIAGNOSTIC PROCEDURES** *Continued*

Most Common...	Answer and Explanation
JVP wave corresponding with S1	*c wave*: * the *c wave* is a positive wave that corresponds with RV contraction during systole, * RV contraction against the closed TV causes a positive deflection in the jugular vein
negative JVP wave following the *c wave*	*x wave*: * it is a negative wave following the *c wave*, * it corresponds to downward displacement of the TV as blood enters the PA
JVP wave corresponding with filling of the RA during systole	*v wave*: the *v wave* is a positive wave due to filling of the RA during systole while the TV is closed
negative JVP wave following the *v wave*	*y wave*: the *y wave* is a negative wave that occurs when the TV opens in diastole and empties blood into the RV
cause of a *giant a wave*	• **RVH**: atrial contraction in late diastole against increased resistance in the right ventricle leads to a *giant a wave*, • *TV and PV stenosis*, • *PH*
cause of a *giant c-v wave*	*RHF with TV regurgitation*: * in RHF, the volume-overloaded RV stretches the TV ring leading to TV regurgitation, * during systole, some blood is redirected into the RA owing to an incompetent valve, * this fuses the c and v wave together to form a *giant c-v wave*
uses of a chest x-ray in cardiology	• **LHF**: detect signs of pulmonary edema and cardiac enlargement, • *aortic abnormalities*: e.g., widening of the aortic shadow in a dissecting aortic aneurysm, • *PH*: e.g., pruning of the pulmonary vessels, • *calcifications*: e.g., * mitral annulus, * coronary atherosclerosis, * old healed infarct, • *heart and chamber size*: ECHO is a better test, • *pericardial effusion*: ECHO is a better test

Table 5–1. HISTORY, PHYSICAL EXAMINATION, AND DIAGNOSTIC PROCEDURES *Continued*

Most Common...	Answer and Explanation
diagnostic uses of an ECG	• **arrhythmias**, • *AMI*, • *LVH/RVH*, • *pericarditis*, • *atrial hypertrophy*, • *electrolyte abnormalities*: e.g., peaked T wave in hyperkalemia, • *effects of cardiac drugs*
use of a stress ECG	*evaluation of exercise-induced ischemia and hypotension*: it is not a good screen in an asymptomatic patient
use of a Holter monitor	• *detect arrhythmias in an ambulatory patient*, • *monitoring heart rate variations*
uses of an ECHO	• **assess heart and chamber size**, • *identify vegetations*: best performed via the esophagus, • *evaluate LV wall movement*: excellent method of evaluating IHD, • *measure the ejection fraction* (EF): * EF = SV ÷ LVEDV, * EF is a marker of prognosis after an AMI and distinguishes systolic from diastolic dysfunction, • *detection of mural thrombi*, • *detection of cardiac myxoma*, • *detection of pericardial effusion*, • *assess valve abnormalities*: e.g., MVP, • *Dx of IHSS*, • *detection of aortic dissection*: best performed via the esophagus, • *identification of intracardiac shunts*
test used to evaluate LA enlargement	*transesophageal US*: the LA is the most posteriorly located chamber
use of radioactive thallium scanning	*assess myocardial perfusion in exercise testing of ischemic heart disease*: diminished perfusion shows up as a "cold" spot
use of technetium pyrophosphate scintigraphy	*detect an acute AMI*: * radionuclide deposits in the area of infarction, * most useful 2–3 days post-AMI, * particularly valuable in detecting non-Q wave types, which are usually subendocardial
uses of cardiac catheterization	*evaluate both right and left heart disease*: e.g., * shunts, * valvular disease, * selective coronary arteriograms, * angioplasty

Table continued on following page

Table 5–1. HISTORY, PHYSICAL EXAMINATION, AND DIAGNOSTIC PROCEDURES *Continued*

Question: Which of the following would most likely be present in a patient with an acute anterior myocardial infarction who has inspiratory crackles in both lung fields and dependent pitting edema? **SELECT 5**

(A) Left-sided S4
(B) Accentuated P2
(C) Left parasternal heave
(D) Left-sided S3
(E) Systolic ejection murmur in 2nd right ICS
(F) Pansystolic murmur at the apex that increases with expiration
(G) Right-sided S3
(H) Orthopnea
(I) Normal central venous pressure

Answers: (A), (D), (F), (G), (H): In an AMI, there is a decrease in compliance of the infarcted muscle, hence the presence of a left-sided S4 (**choice A**). The increase in LVEDV stretches the MV annulus, resulting in mitral regurgitation (**choice F**, pansystolic murmur that increases on expiration) and a left-sided S3 heart sound (**choice D**). LHF is present in this patient, since inspiratory crackles are present. Orthopnea (**choice H**) commonly occurs in the setting of LHF. LHF is the most common cause of RHF. In RHF, the RVEDV is increased. This results in a right-sided S3 (**choice G**) and stretching of the TV ring, which could produce the murmur of TV regurgitation (pansystolic murmur heard best along the left parasternal border that increases with inspiration). The central venous pressure is increased (**choice I is incorrect**) owing to blood building up behind the failed right heart. An accentuated P2 indicates PH, which is not a complication of an AMI (**choice B is incorrect**). A left parasternal heave represents RVH, which is unlikely complication of an AMI (**choice C is incorrect**). A systolic ejection murmur indicates either AV or PV stenosis, which is not a feature of an AMI (**choice E is incorrect**).

AF = atrial fibrillation, AMI = acute myocardial infarction, ASD = atrial septal defect, AV = aortic valve, BP = blood pressure, CHF = congestive heart failure, COPD = chronic obstructive pulmonary disease, CVD = cardiovascular disease, Dx = diagnosis, ECG = electrocardiogram, ECHO = echocardiogram, EF = ejection fraction, GERD = gastroesophageal reflux disease, HTN = hypertension, ICS = intercostal space, IHD = ischemic heart disease, IHSS = idiopathic hypertrophic subaortic stenosis, IVS = interventricular septum, JVP = jugular venous pulse, LA = left atrium, LBBB = left bundle branch block, LHF = left heart failure, LV = left ventricle, LVEDV = left ventricular end-diastolic volume, LVH = left ventricular hypertrophy, MV = mitral valve, MVP = mitral valve prolapse, OS = opening snap, PA = pulmonary artery, PH = pulmonary hypertension, PMI = point of maximal impulse, PND = paroxysmal nocturnal dyspnea, PUD = peptic ulcer disease, PV = pulmonic valve, PVD = peripheral vascular disease, RA = right atrium, RBBB = right bundle branch block, RHF = right heart failure, RV = right ventricle,

RVEDV = right ventricular end-diastolic volume, RVH = right ventricular hypertrophy, SLE = systemic lupus erythematosus, SV = stroke volume, TPR = total peripheral resistance, TV = tricuspid valve, US = ultrasonography, VSD = ventricular septal defect.

Table 5–2. LIPID DISORDERS

Most Common...	Answer and Explanation
lipid fraction increased after eating a fatty meal	*chylomicrons*: see Table 1–3
lipid fraction containing endogenously synthesized TG	*VLDL*: * contains 55% TG and ~18% CH, * CHO in the diet increases VLDL, * inverse relationship with HDL, * LDL is derived from VLDL
functions of HDL	• *circulating reservoir for apo CII and E*: * apo CII activates capillary lipoprotein lipase, * apo E hooks into receptors on hepatocytes for uptake and removal of chylomicron remnants and IDL, • *reverse CH transport*: removes CH from fatty streaks
screen for CHD in people without CHD	*CH and HDL*: * see Table 2–1, * CH/HDL screens are not recommended for persons >75 years old
screen for CHD in people with CHD	*LDL*
formula used to calculate LDL	*LDL = CH − HDL − TG/5*: * TG/5 equals the VLDL fraction, * if TG is >400 mg/dL, a direct measurement of LDL is necessary
lipid ratio used as an indicator of CHD	*CH/HDL*: * an average risk for a M/F is a ratio of 5.0 and 4.4 or less, respectively, * 2× the average risk of CHD if M/F is 9.6 and 7.1, respectively, * 3× the average risk CHD if M/F is 23.4 and 11.0, respectively
lipid fraction known as the "good CH"	*HDL*: * an HDL <35 mg/dL is a major risk factor for CHD, * HDL >60 mg/dL is favorable (can subtract 1 major risk factor)
function of lipoprotein (a)	*enhances atherosclerosis*: * lipoprotein (a) combines LDL with an inhibitor of plasminogen, * plasmin levels are decreased, which impairs dissolution of fibrin clots, which contributes to plaque formation

Table continued on following page

Table 5–2. **LIPID DISORDERS** *Continued*

Most Common...	Answer and Explanation
"good" and "bad" apoliproproteins	• *apo A is good:* accompanies HDL, • *apo B is bad:* apo B100 accompanies LDL
risk factor for CHD in a woman during the childbearing age	*HDL:* * increased estrogen keeps the HDL levels higher in women than in men, * HDL is more important than LDL as a risk factor for CHD in this age bracket, * LDL is a risk factor for men at any age
recommendations for increasing HDL	• **estrogen**: for women only, • *exercise,* • *weight loss,* • *mild to moderate alcohol intake:* increases apo A synthesis, which increases HDL synthesis
medically significant CH level	*CH ≥240 mg/dL:* * if the CH is ≥200 mg/dL, it should be repeated two to three times after 1–8 weeks and the average taken to arrive at the true value, * CH <200 mg/dL is recommended, * CH 200–239 mg/dL is a moderate risk factor for CHD
medically significant LDL level	*LDL ≥160 mg/dL:* * an LDL value <130 mg/dL is desirable in a patient without a history of CHD, * LDL <100 mg/dL is desirable in a patient with a history of CHD/stroke, * LDL between 130 and 159 mg/dL is a moderate risk factor for CHD (dietary therapy and exercise are recommended)
clinical uses for LDL	• *screening test for patients with a previous history of CHD/stroke,* • *classification of hyperlipoproteinemias,* • *set points for dietary goals and whether drug Rx is indicated*
medically significant TG level	*TG >1000 mg/dL:* * a TG <250 mg/dL is desirable, * increased TG is an independent risk factor for CHD, * TG >1000 mg/dL is a risk factor for acute pancreatitis
components of a lipid profile	• *CH,* • *TG,* • *HDL,* • *calculated LDL*: measured LDL if TG is >400 mg/dL, • *standing chylomicron test*: * presence of a creamy supranate indicates an increase in chylomicrons, * presence of a turbid infranate indicates an increase in VLDL [Patients should be on their typical diets and fasting 9–12 hs prior to the test.]
effect of primary hypothyroidism on lipids	*increases CH*: hypothyroidism leads to a reduction in LDL receptor synthesis

Table 5–2. LIPID DISORDERS *Continued*

Most Common...	Answer and Explanation
effect of DM on lipids	• *high CH, TG, VLDL, LDL,* • *low HDL*
effect of the nephrotic syndrome on lipids	*high CH and LDL*
effect of intra- or extrahepatic cholestasis on lipids	*high CH:* bile is the primary mechanism of excreting CH
effect of CRF on lipids	• *high TG, CH* (LDL <160 mg/dL), *VLDL,* • *low HDL* [This profile is often associated with accelerated atherosclerosis and PVD.]
effect of excess alcohol intake on lipids	*high TG and VLDL:* * alcohol increases the liver synthesis of VLDL, * see Table 1–3
effect of an AMI on lipids	*CH decreases by ~40% after 48 hours and returns to normal after 2–3 months:* lipid profiles are not indicated in hospitalized patients
effect of obesity on lipids	• *high TG and CH,* • *low HDL*
effect of smoking on lipids	• *high LDL, CH, TG,* • *low HDL*
antihypertensive agents that adversely alter lipids	• *thiazide diuretics:* increase TG and CH, • *beta blockers:* increase CH and decrease HDL
effect of oral contraceptives on lipids	• *high CH, TG, LDL,* • *low HDL* [Progestins alter the lipids. Estrogen normally decreases TG and CH, and increases HDL.]
effect of corticosteroids on lipids	*high CH:* an increase in CH also occurs in Cushing's syndrome
major risk factor for CHD	*age > 45 in a man and > 55 in a woman:* see Table 2–1 for complete list
nomenclature used in hyperlipidemias	• *Fredrickson's original 5 phenotypes:* I through V, • *phenotypes correlate with seven distinct genotypes:* e.g., type II phenotype has three genotypes, familial, polygenic, and familial combined hypercholesterolemia

Table continued on following page

Table 5–2. **LIPID DISORDERS** *Continued*

Most Common...	Answer and Explanation
hyperlipidemias associated with eruptive xanthomas	• **familial hypertriglyceridemia**: types IV and V, • *familial lipoprotein lipase deficiency:* type I, • *familial apo CII deficiency:* types I and V [Eruptive xanthomas are painless yellow, papular deposits of chylomicrons at pressure points.]
hyperlipidemia associated with tendon xanthomas	*familial hypercholesterolemia* (FH): * tendon xanthomas (e.g., Achilles tendon) are painful deposits of CH, * they are pathognomonic of FH
hyperlipidemia associated with xanthelasmas	*all type II hyperlipidemias*: xanthelasmas are painless yellow deposits of CH in the eyelids that may occur in acquired or genetic hyperlipidemias associated with an increase in CH
hyperlipidemia associated with tuberous xanthomas	*type IIa and IIb hyperlipidemias*: tuberous xanthomas are nodular deposits of CH that develop in areas of trauma (e.g., elbows, knees.)
hyperlipidemia associated with plantar xanthomas	*familial dysbetalipoproteinemia:* plantar xanthomas are painless, yellow deposits of CH and TG in the flexor creases
hyperlipidemia associated with tuberoeruptive xanthomas	*familial dysbetalipoproteinemia:* tuberoeruptive xanthomas are painful deposits of CH and TG that are commonly located around the elbows
clinical/lab findings of polygenic hypercholesterolemia	• **most common type II hyperlipidemia**: 85%, • *multifactorial inheritance pattern*, • *lab*: * LDL >190 mg/dL and CH >260 mg/dL, • *clinical*: * no tendon xanthomas, * risk for premature CHD
clinical/lab findings of FH	• *AD disease*, • *deficiency of LDL receptors*, • *lab*: * CH and LDL elevated in cord blood, * homozygotes have LDL >220 mg/dL and CH >600 mg/dL, * heterozygotes have CH of 300–500 mg/dL, • *clinical*: AMIs occur at early age, * tendon xanthomas pathognomonic
clinical/lab findings in familial combined hyperlipidemia	• *AD inheritance*, • *premature CHD*, • *lab*: CH, LDL, and TG are not elevated at birth but increase around puberty

Table 5–2. LIPID DISORDERS *Continued*

Most Common...	Answer and Explanation
method of distinguishing type IIa phenotype from type IIb	• *IIa:* * LDL >190 mg/dL, * CH >260 mg/dL, * TG <300 mg/dL, * genotypes associated with IIa pattern include ♦ FH, ♦ polygenic, ♦ familial combined, • *IIb:* similar to IIa except TG >300 mg/dL, * genotypes with type IIb pattern are the same as for IIa, * IIb phenotypes are more likely to have obesity and glucose intolerance
clinical/lab findings of familial dysbetalipoproteinemia (type III, broad beta-disease, remnant disease)	• *AR disease or acquired,* • *deficiency of apo E or apo E3* (isoform), • *lab:* * chylomicron and IDL remnants increased in plasma (require apo E for hepatocyte uptake), * VLDL/TG ratio >0.3, * ultracentrifugation identifies remnants, * PCR identifies isoforms, • *clinical:* * plantar xanthomas, * DM, * obesity, * hypothyroidism, * hyperuricemia
clinical/lab findings in familial hypertriglyceridemia (type IV)	• *AD disease or acquired,* • *defect in either increased synthesis or decreased catabolism of VLDL,* • *lab:* * increased TG beginning at puberty, * TG >400 mg/dL, * LDL <190 mg/dL, * turbid infranate, • *clinical:* * eruptive xanthomas, * premature CHD and PVD, * obesity, * HTN, * glucose intolerance, * hyperuricemia
hyperlipidemia	*acquired type IV hyperlipoproteinemia:* causes include * DM, * alcohol excess, * CRF
clinical/lab findings in type V hyperlipidemia	• *most often acquired,* • *lab:* * normal or increased CH (>300 mg/dL), * TG >1000 mg/dL, * LDL <190 mg/dL, * supranate (chylomicrons) and infranate (VLDL) present, • *clinical:* * hyperchylomicronemia syndrome, * commonly seen in DKA and alcohol excess
S/S of the hyperchylomicronemia syndrome	• *may occur in both type IV and V hyperlipidemias,* • *abdominal pain,* • *acute pancreatitis,* • *lipemia retinalis:* * retinal vessels are milky, * produce blurry vision, • *dyspnea:* impaired oxygenation in the lungs, • *hepatomegaly:* fatty change, • *eruptive xanthomas,* • *hemolytic anemia:* called Zieve's syndrome and is more common in alcohol excess
cause of orange-colored tonsils	*Tangier's disease:* * absence of HDL, * accumulation of CH esters in the RES system (e.g., tonsils)

Table continued on following page

Table 5–2. LIPID DISORDERS *Continued*

Most Common...	Answer and Explanation
clinical/lab findings in abetalipoproteinemia	• *AD disease*, • *absence of apo B*: absence of B48 on chylomicrons and B100 on LDL, • *lab*: * chylomicrons trapped in intestinal cells, * VLDL trapped in hepatocytes, * low CH, LDL, and TG, • *clinical*: * malabsorption (macrophage filled with lipid interferes with absorption), * retinitis pigmentosum, * ataxia, * hemolytic anemia with thorny appearing RBCs (acanthocytes), • *Rx*: vitamin E
initial Rx of hyperlipidemia	*dietary therapy*: this also includes exercise and weight loss
features of step-1 and step-2 diets to lower CH	• *both diets recommend:* * total fat <30% of total calories, * CHO 50–60% of total calories, * protein 10–20% of total calories, * polyunsaturated fats (soybean, corn oil) <10% of total calories, * monounsaturated fats (canola, olive oils) 10–15% of the total calories, • *dietary differences:* * % saturated fat (step-1 <10%, step-2 <7%), * CH (step-1 <300 mg, step-2 <200 mg)
goals of dietary Rx	• **step-1 diet is started first**: * goal in patients without CHD and fewer than two major risk factors is LDL <160 mg/dL, * goal in patients without CHD and more than 2 major risk factors is LDL <130 mg/dL, * goal in patients with CHD is an LDL <100 mg/dL, • *step-2 diet*: begin diet if step-1 goals not attained by 3 months, • *drug Rx*: started after 6 months if the above goals are not obtained
role of dietary fiber in Rx of hyperlipidemia	• *soluble fiber:* greater effect in lowering LDL and CH than poly-, monounsaturated fats and insoluble fiber, • *dietary fiber should be at least 24 g/day*
role of margarine in dietary management of hyperlipidemia	*no role*: * margarine is hydrogenated vegetable oil containing trans fatty acids, * eliminate along with saturated fats
effects of Ω 3 polyunsaturated fats in fish oils	• *decrease LDL*, • *increase HDL*, • *decrease platelet aggregation*: important in preventing atherosclerosis

Table 5–2. LIPID DISORDERS *Continued*

Most Common...	Answer and Explanation
major first-line drugs used in Rx of hyperlipidemia	**HMG CoA reductase inhibitors:** statins, • *bile acid resins,* • *nicotinic acid*
second-line drugs used in Rx of hyperlipidemia	• *fibric acids,* • *probucol,* • *estrogen in post-menopausal women*
clinical use of statin drugs	*hypercholesterolemia:* drug of choice
MOA of statin drugs	*inhibit HMG CoA reductase:* * decrease synthesis of CH in the liver, * upregulate LDL receptors, * increase clearing of LDL from the blood
clinical/lab effects of statin drugs	• *lipid effects:* * decrease LDL ~15–40%, * decrease TG 10–20%, * increase HDL 5–10%, • *clinical:* * lower mortality due to CHD, * reduce the rate of revascularization in coronary artery bypass grafts used in CABG procedures
side-effects of statin drugs	• **liver toxicity:** increase serum transaminases, • *myopathy:* increase serum CK
clinical use of nicotinic acid (niacin)	*hypercholesterolemia with or without hypertriglyceridemia:* * least expensive of the lipid-lowering drugs, * Rx of choice for familial combined hypercholesterolemia
MOA of nicotinic acid	*inhibits lipolysis in adipose tissue:* this decreases the release of FAs and subsequent synthesis of LDL and VLDL
lipid effects of nicotinic acid	• *decreases LDL 10–20%,* • *decreases TG by ~40–50%,* • *increases HDL 15–20%*
side effects of nicotinic acid	• **flushing:** * prostaglandin-mediated vasodilatation, * reduced by pretreatment with aspirin, • *hepatitis:* * avoid sustained-release preparations, * use immediate-release preparations, • *hyperglycemia,* • *hyperuricemia*
clinical use of bile acid resins	*Rx of hypercholesterolemia:* particularly in pregnant women and those with liver disease

Table continued on following page

Table 5–2. LIPID DISORDERS *Continued*

Most Common...	Answer and Explanation
MOA of bile acid resins	*bind bile salts*: * bile is the primary excretory route of CH, * CH is the primary substrate for synthesizing bile acids/salts, * bile acid resins bind bile acids and reduce the total bile acid pool, * hepatocytes upregulate LDL receptor synthesis in response to the decrease in bile acids, * increased uptake of CH reduces the serum level of LDL
lipid effects of bile acid resins	• *decreases LDL 10–20%*, • *may increase TG*, • *increases HDL ~5%*
side-effects of bile acid resins	• **bloating and diarrhea**, • *heartburn*, • *malassimilation of drugs*: e.g., * digoxin, * warfarin, * L-levothyroxine
clinical use of fibric acid derivatives	*Rx of hypertriglyceridemia*
MOA of fibric acid derivatives	• **increase capillary lipoprotein lipase activity**: increase the breakdown of VLDL, • *decrease VLDL synthesis*
clinical/lipid effects of fibric acid derivatives	• *lipid effects*: * decreases LDL 0–15%, * decreases TG ~35%, * increases HDL 5–15%, • *clinical*: * reduces CHD incidence in men, * reduces mortality in men without a previous CHD Hx, * increases mortality in those with a previous CHD Hx
side-effects of fibric acid derivatives	• *GI cancer*: risk associated with both clofibrate (rarely used anymore) and gemfibrozil, • *potentiates warfarin activity*, • *myopathy*: increases serum CK, • *hepatitis*, • *gallstones*, • *SiADH*
clinical uses of probucol	• *Rx of hypercholesterolemia*, • *lipid effects*: * reduces the amount of oxidized LDL, * decreases LDL ~10–15%, * decreases HDL 15–30%
lipid effects of estrogen in postmenopausal women	• *decreases LDL ~15–20%*, • *increases HDL ~15%*
common drug combination used in Rx of hypercholesterolemia	*statin drug plus nicotinic acid*

Table 5–2. LIPID DISORDERS *Continued*

Question: In a 20-year-old man with a mass in the Achilles' tendon and a family history of premature CHD, you would expect which of the following laboratory abnormalities? **SELECT 1**
(A) HDL >35 mg/dL
(B) LDL >190 mg/dL
(C) Turbid supranate in a standing chylomicron test
(D) Turbid infranate in a standing chylomicron test
(E) VLDL:TG ratio >0.3

Answer: (B): The patient has a tendon xanthoma, which is pathognomonic of familial hypercholesterolemia. Expected lab findings would include an LDL >190 mg/dL **(choice B)**, HDL <35 mg/dL **(choice A is incorrect)**, CH <260 mg/dL, and no plasma turbidity, since only TG increases plasma turbidity **(choices C and D are incorrect)**. A VLDL:TG ratio >0.3 is suggestive of a familial dysbetalipoproteinemia **(choice E is incorrect)**.

AD = autosomal dominant, AMI = acute myocardial infarction, AR = autosomal recessive, CABG = coronary artery bypass graft, CH = cholesterol, CHD = coronary heart disease, CHO = carbohydrate, CK = creatine kinase, CoA = coenzyme A, CRF = chronic renal failure, DM = diabetes mellitus, DKA = diabetic ketoacidosis, F = female, FA = fatty acid, FH = familial hypercholesterolemia, GI = gastrointestinal, HDL = high density lipoprotein, HMG = 3-hydroxy-3 methylglutaryl, HTN = hypertension, Hx = history, IDL = intermediate density lipoprotein, LDL = low density lipoprotein, M = male, MOA = mechanism of action, PVD = peripheral vascular disease, RBC = red blood cell, RES = reticuloendothelial system, Rx = treatment, SiADH = syndrome of inappropriate antidiuretic hormone, S/S = signs and symptoms, TG = triglyceride, VLDL = very low density lipoprotein.

Table 5–3. SELECTED VASCULAR DISORDERS

Most Common...	Answer and Explanation
causes of endothelial damage leading to atherosclerosis	• **native and oxidized LDL**, • *products in cigarette smoke*: * CO, * ammonia, • *turbulence at vessel bifurcations*, • *immunologic injury*, * *viral/chlamydial injury*: e.g., Chlamydia pneumoniae, • *increased plasma homocysteine levels*: * most often due to folate deficiency (see Table 8–5), * less frequently due to B_{12} deficiency or heterozygote carriers for homocystinuria
antioxidants that neutralize oxidized LDL	• *vitamin E*, • *vitamin C*, • β-*carotenes*

Table continued on following page

Table 5-3. SELECTED VASCULAR DISORDERS *Continued*

Most Common...	Answer and Explanation
sites for atherosclerosis in descending order	• **abdominal aorta**, • *coronary artery*, • *popliteal artery*, • *descending thoracic aorta*, • *internal carotid*
complication of atherosclerosis in the abdominal aorta	• **aneurysm formation**, • *embolization*: * to SMA leading to small bowel infarction, * to vessels in the lower legs leading to digital infarction, • *small bowel infarction*: thrombosis over a plaque in the proximal SMA, • *renovascular HTN*
complications of atherosclerosis in the peripheral vascular system	• **gangrene**, • *claudication*: atherosclerosis of the superficial femoral artery in the adductor canal is the most common cause of leg claudication, • *aneurysm:* e.g., popliteal artery
complications of atherosclerosis in the coronary artery	• **angina**, • *AMI*, • *sudden cardiac death*, • *chronic ischemic heart disease*
complications of atherosclerosis in the internal carotid artery	• **TIA**, • *atherosclerotic stroke*, • *embolic stroke*, • *cerebral atrophy*
complication of atherosclerosis in the renal artery	*renovascular HTN*
aneurysm	*abdominal aortic aneurysm*: * aneurysms are caused by weakening of the vessel with subsequent outpouching of the vessel wall, * there is no vasa vasorum below the orifices of the renal arteries (most common location for abdominal aortic aneurysm)
complication of an abdominal aortic aneurysm	*rupture*: * size of the aneurysm is the most important factor that determines the risk of rupture, * aneurysms >5 cm have a 25–40% risk for rupture
test used to identify an abdominal aortic aneurysm	*ultrasonography*: gold standard test
S/S of a ruptured abdominal aortic aneurysm	• **sudden onset of left flank pain**: due to hemorrhage into the retroperitoneum, • *hypotension*: blood loss, • *pulsatile mass in the abdomen*

Table 5–3. SELECTED VASCULAR DISORDERS *Continued*

Most Common...	Answer and Explanation
aneurysm of the peripheral vascular system	*popliteal artery aneurysm*: * commonly associated with an abdominal aorta aneurysm (50% of cases), * commonly embolizes material to digital vessels leading to digital infarction, * commonly thrombose
cause of a berry aneurysm in the circle of Willis	*congenital absence of the internal elastic membrane and muscle wall at the bifurcation of the communicating arteries with their corresponding cerebral arteries*: potential for rupture leading to a subarachnoid hemorrhage
cause of an aortic arch aneurysm	*dissecting aortic aneurysm*
risk factors for a dissecting aortic aneurysm	• **HTN**: * the aortic arch is weakened by elastic tissue fragmentation and cystic medial necrosis in the middle and outer layers of the vessel, * HTN supplies the shearing force to produce an intimal tear, • *Marfan's syndrome*: most common COD, • *Ehlers-Danlos syndrome*: most common COD, • *pregnancy*: increased plasma volume
types of dissecting aortic aneurysm	• **type A**: * involves the ascending aorta, * greatest mortality, • *type B:* begins below the ligamentum arteriosum and extends distally
S/S of a dissecting aortic aneurysm	• **acute onset of severe chest pain in association with HTN**: often confused with an AMI, except HTN is uncommon in an AMI, • *radiation of pain down the back*, • *unequal pulses in the upper extremity*, • *aortic regurgitation*: due to widening of the aortic root
tests used to Dx a dissecting aortic aneurysm	• **chest radiograph**: widening of the superior mediastinum (dilated aortic knob) in ~80% of cases, • *transesophageal US:* greater sensitivity (~98%) than a chest radiograph, • *arteriography:* gold standard confirmatory test
initial step in management of a dissecting aortic aneurysm	• **lower the blood pressure with nitroprusside to prevent further dissection**: propranolol is also added to lower the pulse rate, • *type A dissections require surgical intervention*, • *type B dissections are usually managed medically*

Table continued on following page

Table 5–3. SELECTED VASCULAR DISORDERS *Continued*

Most Common...	Answer and Explanation
side-effect of nitroprusside	*increases thiocyanate levels:* * cyanide is a part of nitroprusside, * cyanide reacts with thiosulfate, * thiocyanate levels must be monitored to prevent toxicity
S/S of thiocyanate toxicity	• *weakness*, • *disorientation*, • *convulsions*
COD in a dissecting aortic aneurysm	• **hemopericardium due to rupture of the aneurysm into the pericardial sac**, • *other rupture sites*: * mediastinum, * peritoneum, * reentry into the aorta creating a double-barreled aorta (not a COD)
causes of Raynaud's phenomenon	• **PSS/CREST syndrome**: * vasospastic disorders of the digital vessels that produce color changes (white to blue to red), * it is the initial manifestation of both PSS and CREST syndrome, • *Takayasu's arteritis*, • *cold agglutinin disease*, • *cryoglobulinemia*, • *ergot poisoning*, • *Buerger's disease*
long-term effect of Raynaud's phenomena	*fibrosis of the digital vessels*
clinical findings of the CREST syndrome	• *calcinosis*, • *Raynaud's*, • *eosphageal motility dysfunction*, • *sclerodactyly*, • *telangiectasia*
AD hereditary vascular disease	*hereditary hemorrhagic telangiectasia, or Osler-Weber-Rendu disease*: * associated with small aneurysmal telangiectasias on the skin and mucous membranes, * produces nosebleeds and GI bleeds, the latter leading to iron deficiency
cause of spider angiomas on the skin	*hyperestrinism secondary to pregnancy or cirrhosis of the liver*: * spider angiomas are small AV fistulas, * may lead to increased intrapulmonary shunting of blood
mechanism of hyperestrinism in cirrhosis	• **decreased metabolism of estrogen**, • *decreased metabolism of DHEA and androstenedione*: * they are 17-ketosteroids (weak androgens), * they are aromatized in the adipose into estrogen
clinical findings in von Hippel-Lindau disease	• *AD inheritance*, • *cavernous hemangiomas in the cerebellum, skin, and eyes*, • *increased risk for bilateral renal adenocarcinomas*: an

Table 5–3. SELECTED VASCULAR DISORDERS *Continued*

Most Common...	Answer and Explanation
Continued	increase in EPO release causes secondary polycythemia, • *increased incidence of pheochromocytomas*
cause of calcification of the digital vessels	*DM*
cause of Kaposi's sarcoma in AIDS	*HSV-8*: * KS is the most common cancer in AIDS, * it is an AIDS-defining lesion
cause of lymphangiosarcoma in the United States	*chronic lymphedema secondary to radiation post-modified radical mastectomy*
cause of phlebothrombosis	*stasis of blood flow*: * phlebothrombosis is thrombosis of a vein without inflammation, * it commonly occurs in patients who are postpartum or postoperative (particularly after hip and pelvic surgery)
location for phlebothrombosis	*deep veins of the calf*: * most DVTs in this area resolve spontaneously, * ~20% propagate into the proximal vessels, * ~50% of DVTs that extend into the proximal vessels (femoral, popliteal, iliac veins) embolize to the lungs
primary site for embolization to the lungs	*iliofemoral venous system*: ~50% of DVTs in the iliofemoral system embolize to the lungs
tests used to Dx DVTs in the lower legs	• **duplex ultrasonography**: * it is a modification of Doppler ultrasonography, * detects femoral vein thrombi, • *impedance plethysmography*: detect DVTs in the femoral veins, • *invasive venography*: * gold standard test, * detects DVTs in the deep veins of the calf
nonpharmacologic technique used in preventing DVTs in the hospital	• **early ambulation**, • *graded stockings*: method of choice in low-risk elective surgery, • *intermittent pneumatic compression*: method of choice in GU surgery and neurosurgery
patient risk factors for DVTs	• **>40 years old**, • *previous DVTs*, • *malignancy*, • *CHF*, • *obesity*, • *DM*
surgery risk factors for DVTs	• **hip/knee replacement**, • *GU surgery*, • *neurosurgery*

Table continued on following page

Table 5–3. SELECTED VASCULAR DISORDERS *Continued*

Most Common...	Answer and Explanation
drug prevention for patients who are at risk for DVTs in the hospital	• **low dose heparin**: * *medical patients*—5000 units SC of low dose heparin q12-h, * *low to moderate risk* patients scheduled for major surgery—above dose is started 2-hs before surgery and continued q12-h postoperatively, * *high risk surgical patients* (not including hip/knee replacement)—as above for surgery but q8-h plus intermittent pneumatic compression, • *warfarin*: * patients undergoing *total hip/knee surgery* are started on warfarin from preoperative day one to the time of ambulation, * high risk of postoperative bleeding
initial anticoagulant used in Rx of proximal DVTs	• **intravenous heparin**: * initial dose is 5000–10,000 units, * aPTT kept between 50 and 80 seconds, • *warfarin*: * started along with heparin on day one, * continued for ~3 months, * heparin is D/C when INR used to follow warfarin is 2.0–3.0 for at least 48-hs, * requires ~3–4-d before a patient on warfarin is fully anticoagulated
cause of primary varicose veins in the legs	*congenital absence of the sentinel valve in the common femoral vein*: pregnancy is a common precipitating event
causes of secondary varicose veins	• **vessel obstruction**: e.g., DVT, • *vessel damage*: e.g., thrombophlebitis leading to dysfunctional penetrating branches between the superficial and deep system
cause of stasis dermatitis around the ankles	*DVT in the proximal venous system*: * venous blood around the ankles flows from the deep to the superficial saphenous vein system, * a proximal DVT increases the pressure in penetrating vessels in the ankles
clinical findings of stasis dermatitis	• **edema**: first sign, • *hemorrhage into subcutaneous tissue*: orange skin discoloration, • *ulceration*: due to ischemia, • *secondary varicose veins in the superficial saphenous veins*: deep vein pressure is transmitted into the superficial system
cause of the SVC syndrome	*obstruction of the SVC by a primary small cell carcinoma of the lung*
clinical findings of SVC syndrome	• **venous congestion in the face, neck, and shoulders**, • *distention of jugular veins*, • *headache*, • *conjunctival vessels engorged*, • *increased CSF pressure*

Table 5–3. SELECTED VASCULAR DISORDERS *Continued*

Most Common...	Answer and Explanation
Rx of SVC syndrome	*chemotherapy and radiation*
pathologic cause of a chylous effusion in the pleural cavity	• **malignant lymphoma**, • *surgical mishap*
lab findings in chylous effusions	• *mature lymphocytes*, • *increased TG*: * due to chylomicrons reabsorbed in the small bowel, * form supranate in a tube
cause of a pseudochylous effusion in the pleural cavity	*rheumatoid arthritis involving the lungs* [A pseudochylous effusion is milky but, unlike a true chylous effusion, it is not lymphatic fluid but an inflammatory exudate containing neutrophils and CH.]
lab findings of pseudochylous effusion	• *increased neutrophils*, • *increased CH*

Question: Atherosclerosis directly contributes to the pathophysiology of which of the following conditions? **SELECT 7**
- (A) Calf claudication
- (B) Dissecting aortic aneurysm
- (C) Aneurysm of the thoracic aorta
- (D) Raynaud's phenomenon
- (E) Cerebrovascular stroke
- (F) Abdominal aortic aneurysm
- (G) Berry aneurysm
- (H) Prinzmetal's angina
- (I) Renovascular hypertension
- (J) Leriche syndrome
- (K) Arteriovenous fistula
- (L) Small bowel infarction

Answers: (A), (C), (E), (F), (I), (J), (L): Calf claudication (**choice A**) is most often due to obstructive atherosclerosis involving the superficial femoral artery. Aortoiliac atherosclerotic disease is associated with claudication and impotence (Leriche syndrome, **choice J**). Occlusive atherosclerotic vascular disease is also operative in CVA (internal carotid disease, **choice E**), renovascular HTN (**choice I**), and small bowel infarction (thrombosis overlying an atherosclerotic plaque in the proximal SMA, **choice L**). Atherosclerosis is operative in both thoracic (**choice C**) and abdominal aortic aneurysms (**choice F**). Atherosclerosis is not operative in dissecting aortic aneurysms (elastic tissue fragmentation, **choice B is incorrect**), berry aneurysms (congenital, **choice G is incorrect**), Raynaud's phenomenon (digital vessel spasm, **choice D is incorrect**), Prinzmetal's angina (vasospasm of the coronary artery, **choice H is incorrect**), or an AV fistula (usually due to a knife injury, with communication of the arterial with the venous circulation, **choice K is incorrect**).

AD = autosomal dominant, AIDS = acquired immunodeficiency syndrome, AMI = acute myocardial infarction, aPTT = activated partial thromboplastin time, AV = arteriovenous, CH = cholesterol, CHF = congestive heart failure, COD = cause of death, CREST = calcinosis, Raynaud's phenomenon, esophageal motility dysfunction, sclerodactyly, telangiectasia, CSF = cerebrospinal fluid, CVA = cerebrovascular accident, D/C = discontinue, DHEA = dehydroepiandrosterone, DM = diabetes mellitus, DVT = deep venous thrombosis, Dx = diagnosis, EPO = erythropoietin, GU = genitourinary, HSV = herpes simplex virus, HTN = hypertension, INR = International Normalized Ratio, LDL = low density lipoprotein, PSS = progressive systemic sclerosis, Rx = treatment, SMA = superior mesenteric artery, S/S = signs and symptoms, SVC = superior vena cava, TG = triglyceride, TIA = transient ischemic attack, US = ultrasonography.

Table 5–4. HYPERTENSION (HTN)

Most Common...	Answer and Explanation
prescription disorder in the United States	*essential HTN*
cause of HTN	*essential HTN* (~90–95%): the average blood pressure of two or more separate readings per visit on at least three visits that are several weeks apart must be ≥140/90 mm Hg
classification used in defining blood pressure disorders	<table><tr><td></td><td>**Systolic**</td><td>**Diastolic**</td></tr><tr><td>Optimal</td><td><120</td><td><80</td></tr><tr><td>Normal</td><td><130</td><td><85</td></tr><tr><td>High normal</td><td>130–139</td><td>85–89</td></tr><tr><td>Hypertension</td><td></td><td></td></tr><tr><td>Stage 1 (mild)</td><td>140–159</td><td>90–99</td></tr><tr><td>Stage 2 (moderate)</td><td>160–179</td><td>100–109</td></tr><tr><td>Stage 3 (severe)</td><td>180–209</td><td>110–119</td></tr><tr><td>Stage 4 (very severe)</td><td>≥210</td><td>≥120</td></tr><tr><td>Systolic hypertension</td><td>≥160</td><td><90</td></tr></table> [A single measurement of ≥210/≥120 mm Hg or the presence of target organ disease (see below) is sufficient to diagnose HTN.]
target organs affected by HTN	• **heart**: * LVH, * CAD, * CHF, * dissecting aortic aneurysm, • *CNS:* * intracerebral bleed, * lacunar infarcts, • *kidneys:* * BNS, * malignant HTN, • *retina:* hypertensive retinopathy
cause of LVH	*essential HTN*: see Table 5–1
cause of RVH	*pulmonary HTN:* see Table 5–1
ethnic group with the highest prevalence of essential HTN	*African-Americans* (20–30%): * prevalence is 10–20% in white adults, * men affected more than women, * onset between 25–55 years, * uncommon in people <20 years old

Table 5–4. HYPERTENSION (HTN) *Continued*

Most Common...	Answer and Explanation
cause of a falsely elevated BP in elderly patients	*atherosclerotic involvement of the brachial artery*: hardened artery cannot be compressed by the cuff
BP effect of a cuff that is too small or too narrow for the circumference of the arm	*falsely high BP*: in obese individuals, a thigh cuff may be necessary to obtain an accurate BP in the arm
DOA producing HTN	*cocaine:* it stimulates the sympathetic nervous system
medications producing HTN	• **NSAIDs:** block the vasodilator effect of prostaglandins which leaves ATII unopposed, • *decongestants*, • *appetite suppressants*, • *excess thyroid hormone*
cause of HTN in young women	*birth control pills:* estrogen increases liver synthesis of angiotensinogen
effect of alcohol and cigarette smoking on BP	*elevate the BP:* due to stimulation of catecholamine release
factors predisposing to HTN	• **defects in natriuresis**: diminished ability to excrete a sodium load, • **genetic predisposition**, • *obesity:* increased intravascular volume, • *sedentary lifestyle*, • *race*: African-American > white, • *activation of the RAA system:* see below, • *congenital defects in the arterioles:* resistance arterioles controlling the diastolic BP have an increase in intracellular Na^+ concentration in the SMCs which opens up calcium channels, leading to an increase in vessel tone and resistance
effects of body position on the PRA	• *reclining:* decreases PRA by increasing volume return to the right heart → left heart → renal artery, • *upright:* increases PRA, which decreases venous return of blood to the right heart → left heart → renal artery
alteration in PRA in elderly and African-Americans hypertensives	*low plasma PRA*: a low plasma PRA indicates an increased intravascular volume with suppression of renin release

Table continued on following page

Table 5–4. HYPERTENSION (HTN) *Continued*

Most Common...	Answer and Explanation
alteration in PRA in young hypertensives	*high plasma PRA:* * an increase in plasma PRA is associated with sympathetic overactivity, * there is an increased incidence of CVAs in these patients
alteration in PRA in most hypertensives	*normal plasma PRA:* in general, * 50% of patients with HTN have a normal PRA, * 35% a low PRA, and * 15% a high PRA
symptoms of essential HTN	• *pulsating suboccipital headache occurring early in the morning and subsiding before noon,* • *dizziness,* • *blurry vision,* • *sweating,* • *chest pain,* • *dyspnea*
signs of essential HTN	• **increased amplitude and lateral displacement of the PMI:** due to LVH, • *accentuated A2,* • *early systolic ejection click,* • *retinopathy:* see below, • S4: due to LVH
findings in grade I hypertensive retinopathy	• *focal narrowing of the arterioles:* * 1:2 ratio, * normal ratio is of the arteriole to the venule is 3:4, • *mild AV nicking:* depression in the wall of the venule due to sclerosis of the overlying arteriole
findings in grade II hypertensive retinopathy	• *more diffuse narrowing of the arterioles:* 1:3 ratio, • *copper wiring of the arterioles:* sclerotic changes in the arteriole, but blood is still visible, • *more accentuation of AV nicking*
findings in grade III hypertensive retinopathy	• *more advanced arteriole narrowing:* 1:4, • *silver wiring of the arterioles:* no blood is visible in the lumen, • *flame hemorrhages:* due to ruptured microaneurysms, • *soft exudates:* * microinfarctions, * look like "cotton balls" with blurry borders, • *hard exudates:* * leakage of protein from the vessels, * sharp borders, • *advanced AV nicking:* vein under the arteriole disappears, • *normal disk*
findings in grade IV hypertensive retinopathy	*all of the above for grade III plus papilledema of the optic disk*

Table 5–4. HYPERTENSION (HTN) Continued

Most Common...	Answer and Explanation
initial tests in the work-up of HTN	• *CBC*: R/O polycythemia or anemia, • *serum electrolytes*: R/O primary aldosteronism (hypernatremia, hypokalemia, metabolic alkalosis), • *fasting blood glucose*: R/O * DM, * pheochromocytoma, • *urinalysis*: R/O primary renal disease (e.g., proteinuria), • *serum BUN and creatinine*: R/O renal disease, • *serum uric acid*: R/O urate nephropathy, • *serum CH and HDL*: secondary prevention screen for CHD, • *ECG*: R/O * LVH, * ischemia, • *chest radiography*: evaluate the heart and lungs
goal of Rx of HTN	*reduce the BP to <140/90 mm Hg*
goal of Rx in systolic HTN	*reduce the systolic BP to <160 mm Hg*
life-style change recommended to lower BP	*weight reduction*: see Table 2–1 for other modifications
nephron site targeted by loop diuretics	*blocks Na^+-K^+-2Cl^- cotransport pump in the TAL segment*: this pump is responsible for generation of free water (water not accompanied by solute)
nephron site targeted by carbonic anhydrase inhibitors	*block proximal reclamation of bicarbonate*: bicarbonate binds with Na^+ ions and is excreted in the urine (diuretic effect)
side-effects associated with CA inhibitors	*normal AG metabolic acidosis*: bicarbonate is lost in the urine and replaced by Cl^- anions
nephron site targeted by thiazides	*block Na^+ reabsorption at the Na^+/Cl^- pump in the proximal portion of the DCT*
MOA of thiazide/ loop diuretics in lowering BP	• **induce a natriuresis**, • *reduce plasma volume*, • *mild VD of arterioles*

Table continued on following page

Table 5–4. HYPERTENSION (HTN) *Continued*

Most Common...	Answer and Explanation
thiazide effect on calcium	*increases calcium reabsorption*: * Ca^{++} uses the same channel as Na^+ for reabsorption, * blocking Na^+ reabsorption opens the channel for increased PTH-enhanced Ca^{++} reabsorption, * this underscores the role thiazides have in the Rx of calcium stone formers
side-effects of thiazide diuretics	• **hypokalemia**: muscle weakness, • *hyponatremia*, • *metabolic alkalosis*, • *hypomagnesemia*: may produce hypocalcemia by interfering with PTH release, • *increase LDL and TG*, • *hyperglycemia*, • *hyperuricemia*, • *hypercalcemia*: * may indicate an underlying primary HPTH, * Na^+ channel is now open for PTH-enhanced Ca^{++} reabsorption, • *prerenal azotemia*, • *acute pancreatitis*
side-effects of loop diuretics that differ from thiazides	*absence of*: * hyperglycemia, * hyperuricemia, * hypercalcemia
loop diuretic effect on calcium	*block Ca^{++} reabsorption*: this underscores the use in the Rx of hypercalcemia
MOA of aldosterone blocker and Na^+/K^+ pump blockers	• *spironolactone:* * only true aldosterone blocker, * blocks the aldosterone-enhanced Na^+/K^+ pump in the late DT and collecting duct, • *triamterene/amiloride:* * they do not inhibit aldosterone, * they block Na^+ reabsorption and the secretion of K^+ in the aldosterone-enhanced Na^+/K^+ pump (K^+ sparing effect)
use of aldosterone blocker, Na^+/K^+ pump blockers	*adjuncts to thiazide/loop diuretics in patients who cannot take oral K^+ supplements*: K^+ sparers
side-effects of spironolactone	• **hyperkalemia**, • *normal AG metabolic acidosis*, • *gynecomastia:* block androgen receptors in breast tissue
MOA of β-blockers (e.g., propranolol) in lowering BP	• *decrease HR*, • *decrease CO*, • *stimulate prostaglandin release*: VD of arterioles

Table 5–4. **HYPERTENSION (HTN)** *Continued*

Most Common...	Answer and Explanation
side-effects of β-blockers	• *conduction disturbances*: e.g., AV block, • *block the adrenergic S/S of hypoglycemia in DM*: do not block sweating, • *induce bronchospasm*: particularly in those with asthma, • *depression*, • *lipid effects* (mainly in non-selective β-blockers): * increase TG, * decrease HDL, • *rebound angina*, • *HTN if abruptly withdrawn*: up-regulation of β-adrenergic receptors occurs when they are blocked
MOA of α-adrenergic blockers (e.g., prazosin) in lowering BP	*block post-synaptic α-adrenergic receptors:* * they VD arterioles/venules, * unlike β-adrenergic blockers, they lower TG and CH, and increase HDL
MOA of centrally acting adrenergic drugs (e.g., clonidine, methyldopa) in lowering BP	*stimulate α-adrenergic receptors in the CNS:* they reduce efferent peripheral sympathetic outflow
side-effects associated with methyldopa	• **positive direct Coombs in 20–25% of patients**: a hemolytic anemia occurs in ~1% of these patients, • *fulminant hepatitis*, • *positive serum ANA*
MOA of calcium channel blockers (e.g., verapamil, diltiazem) in lowering BP	• *VD of arterioles:* block L-type calcium channels, • *decrease cardiac contractility and heart rate:* negative inotropic and chronotropic effect, respectively
classes of calcium channel blockers	• *phenylalkylamines*: * e.g., verapamil, * produce a cardiac and peripheral vascular effect, • *benzothiazepines*: * e.g., diltiazem, * produce a cardiac and peripheral vascular effect, • *dihydropyridines*: * e.g., procardia, * primarily produces a peripheral vascular effect
side-effects of calcium channel blockers	• *increase mortality post-AMI:* primarily short-acting types like verapamil, diltiazem, • *flushing*, • *headache*, • *peripheral edema*, • *constipation*, • *postural hypotension*
MOA of hydralazine in lowering BP	*direct-acting arteriole VD*: it is mainly used in treating HTN in pregnancy and refractory HTN

Table continued on following page

Table 5–4. HYPERTENSION (HTN) *Continued*

Most Common...	Answer and Explanation
side-effect of hydralazine	*may produce drug-induced SLE with a positive ANA*
MOA of ACE inhibitors (e.g., captopril) in lowering BP	• *decrease ATII*: VD of arterioles/venules, • *decrease aldosterone*: natriuresis, • *increase bradykinins*: * VD of arterioles, * pathogenesis of cough with ACE inhibitors, • *stimulate renal synthesis of prostaglandins*: VD of afferent arterioles
clinical uses of ACE inhibitors in HTN	• **useful in hypertensives with CHF, LVH, hyperglycemia, hyperlipidemia, and hypokalemia**: best agent for reversing LVH, • *useful in high PRA HTN*
clinical usefulness of ATII receptor blockers (e.g., losartan)	*useful in patients who develop side-effects related to ACE inhibitors*
complications of ACE inhibitors	• **cough**: bradykinin effect, • *angioedema*: bradykinin effect, • *hyperkalemia*: due to hypoaldosteronism, • *skin rash*, • *dysgeusia*: taste abnormalities, • *ARF in patients with bilateral RAS*: * ATII controls renal blood flow in both kidneys when both the renal arteries are stenotic, * blocking ATII leaves the kidneys without any blood flow controlling factor
antihypertensive to avoid when eating tyramine-containing foods	*monoamine oxidase inhibitors:* tyramine-containing foods include wine and certain cheeses
MOA of parenteral nitroprusside in lowering BP	*direct acting VD of arterioles/venules:* nitroprusside contains * iron, * cyanide (combines with thiosulfate to produce thiocyanate), * nitro-moiety
clinical uses of nitroprusside in HTN	• **agent of choice in Rx of malignant HTN**, • **agent of choice in lowering BP in Rx of aortic dissection along with propranolol**
initial drugs used in Rx of HTN in African-Americans	• **diuretics**: most African-Americans have an increase in Na+ and plasma volume, • *calcium channel blockers:* added if the desired goal is not established, • *ACE inhibitors or ATII-receptor blockers*

Table 5–4. HYPERTENSION (HTN) *Continued*

Most Common...	Answer and Explanation
initial drug used in Rx of HTN in elderly patients	*diuretics*: reduce the incidence of strokes and fatal AMIs in this age group
initial drug used in Rx of systolic HTN	*diuretics*
Rx recommendation for HTN in obesity	*weight reduction*: diuretics may also be necessary owing to the increase in plasma volume in these patients
initial drug used in Rx of HTN in DM	*ACE inhibitors*: HTN control is the single most important factor in preventing a loss of renal function in DM
effect of drug Rx and weight loss on LVH	*reduction in LV mass*: * ACE inhibitors have the greatest overall effect on initiating regression of LVH, * direct-acting VD drugs do not reduce LV mass
initial drug used in Rx of HTN in CRF	*loop diuretics*: controlling HTN with loop diuretics also reduces the progression of chronic renal insufficiency
initial drug used in Rx of HTN in CHF	*ACE inhibitors*: * ACE inhibitors reduce afterload (decrease ATII) and preload (decrease aldosterone) in CHF, * decrease mortality in CHF
drugs used in Rx of HTN in (diastolic BP >100 mm Hg) in pregnancy	• **methyldopa**, • *hydralazine*: alternative drug choice
drug combinations used in treating HTN	• **diuretic + beta-blocker**, • *diuretic + ACE inhibitor*, • *diuretic + calcium channel blocker*, • *calcium channel blocker + ACE inhibitor*: useful if the patient has hyperlipidemia and is not a candidate for a diuretic + β-blocker
beneficial effects of controlling HTN	• **decrease mortality due to stroke**, • *decrease mortality due to CHD*
COD in HTN in decreasing frequency	• **AMI**, • *stroke*, • *renal failure*

Table continued on following page

Table 5–4. HYPERTENSION (HTN) *Continued*

Most Common...	Answer and Explanation
cause of secondary HTN	*unilateral renovascular HTN*
mechanisms of renovascular HTN	• **elderly men**: * atherosclerotic occlusion of the proximal renal artery, * activates RAA system, * high PRA, • *middle-aged women*: fibromuscular hyperplasia due to multifocal areas of SMC hyperplasia in the media of the renal artery
secondary causes of HTN in young people	• *renovascular HTN*, • *coarctation of the aorta*, • *birth control pills*: most common cause in women
renal disorders associated with secondary HTN	• **diabetic nephropathy**, • *chronic PN*, • *acute/chronic GN*, • *PSS*, • *Wilms' tumor*: secrete renin, • *renal adenocarcinoma*: secrete renin
adrenal disorders associated with secondary HTN	• **primary aldosteronism**, • *pheochromocytoma*: adult, • *neuroblastoma*: child, • *11-, 17-hydroxylase deficiency*: * AR diseases, * adrenogenital syndrome, * see Table 3–3, • *adrenal Cushing's syndrome*
neurogenic disorders associated with secondary HTN	• *increase in intracranial pressure*: e.g., * brain tumor, * encephalitis, • *bulbar poliomyelitis*
hematologic disorder associated with secondary HTN	*polycythemia*: an increase in blood viscosity decreases the TPR
obstetric disorder associated with secondary HTN	*pre-eclampsia/eclampsia*
parathyroid disorder associated with secondary HTN	*primary HPTH*
thyroid disorder associated with HTN	• *primary hypothyroidism*: diastolic HTN due to an increase in blood volume, • *Graves' disease*: systolic HTN due to an increase in SV

Table 5–4. HYPERTENSION (HTN) *Continued*

Most Common...	Answer and Explanation
clinical findings associated with renovascular HTN	• **abrupt onset of severe, uncontrolled HTN that is resistant to standard medical therapy**, • *HTN in a patient with severe atherosclerotic PVD*, • *presence of an abdominal bruit*
noninvasive screening test for renovascular HTN	*radionuclide scan of the kidneys followed by captopril* (ACE inhibitor): * the initial scan reveals a small kidney with decreased uptake and clearance of the radiotracer post-captopril, * captopril stimulation also leads to a marked increase in PRA activity over baseline values owing to the loss of the inhibitory effect of ATII on renin release
confirmatory test for renovascular HTN	• **renal arteriography**, • *evaluation of PRA in the renal veins draining the affected and unaffected side*
arteriogram findings in renovascular HTN	• *significant stenosis (>70%) within the proximal 2 cm of the artery secondary to atherosclerosis*, • *in FMH, there is a "string-of-beads" effect owing to multifocal vessel involvement*
renal vein PRA findings in renovascular HTN	• *increased renal vein PRA activity on the affected side*: due to decreased blood flow through the renal artery, • *suppressed renal vein PRA on contralateral side*: due to suppression of renin release by increased ATII from the affected kidney, * no suppression of PRA indicates that the contralateral kidney has suffered irreversible vascular damage from sustained HTN
Rx of unilateral RAS	• *aortorenal bypass in atherosclerotic occlusion*, • *angioplasty in FMH*, • *angioplasty is the Rx of choice in patients with significant bilateral RAS*
effect of bilateral RAS on PRA	*PRA is near normal owing to the inhibitory effects of ATII that are operative in both kidneys*
cause of primary aldosteronism (Conn's syndrome)	*unilateral adrenal adenoma involving the zona glomerulosa (~60–75% of cases):* primary adrenal hyperplasia occurs in ~25–35% of patients

Table continued on following page

Table 5–4. HYPERTENSION (HTN) *Continued*

Most Common...	Answer and Explanation
S/S suggesting primary aldosteronism	• **muscle weakness/paralysis**: * due to hypokalemia from augmented exchange of K^+ for Na^+ in the aldosterone-enhanced Na^+/K^+ pump, • *diastolic HTN*: combination of Na^+ retention and an increase in plasma volume, • *tetany*: alkalosis increases binding of ionized Ca^{++} to albumin, • *polyuria*: hypokalemic nephropathy renders the collecting ducts refractory to ADH (nephrogenic DI), • *absence of pitting edema*: * important negative finding, * increase in plasma volume inhibits proximal tubule reabsorption of Na^+ leading to natriuresis, * natriuresis is the "escape mechanism" that offsets Na^+ reabsorption by aldosterone, * total body Na^+ is not increased enough to produce pitting edema
screening tests for primary aldosteronism	• **plasma aldosterone/PRA ratio >20–25 after 4-h of standing upright**: * in normal people, standing upright is a stimulus for renin release, * patients with *primary hyperplasia* have an increase in both PRA and plasma aldosterone after standing upright for 4-hs, * patients with an *adenoma* have suppression of PRA and little change in plasma aldosterone, • *PRA <5 μg/dL*, • *urine aldosterone >20 μg in a 24h urine*, • *24h urine K^+ > 30 mEq/d*
confirmatory tests for primary aldosteronism	• **failure to suppress plasma aldosterone after an isotonic saline infusion**: in a normal person, infusion of isotonic saline should suppress PRA and aldosterone, • *failure to suppress plasma aldosterone after captopril administration or a synthetic mineralocorticoid* (fludrocortisone), • *CT scan*: identifies adenomas, • *elective venous sampling*: most sensitive test for localizing adenomas or defining primary hyperplasia, • *measuring precursor mineralocorticoids* (e.g., 18-hydroxycorticosterone): increased precursors are more likely present in an adenoma than in primary hyperplasia

Table 5–4. HYPERTENSION (HTN) *Continued*

Most Common...	Answer and Explanation
lab findings in primary aldosteronism	• **hypokalemia**, • *normal to slightly increased serum Na+*, • *marked kaluresis*: leads to hypokalemia, • *metabolic alkalosis*: * increased exchange of H+ ions with Na+ at the aldosterone-enhanced Na+/K+ pump occurs when K+ is depleted, * increased excretion of H+ leads to increased reclamation of HCO_3^-
Rx of primary aldosteronism	• *adenomas*: surgically removed, • *primary hyperplasia*: spironolactone
cause of mineralocorticoid excess without HTN	*Bartter's syndrome*
mechanism of mineralocorticoid excess in Bartter's syndrome	• **defect in Cl− reabsorption by the Na+-K+-2Cl− cotransport pump in the TAL segment of the nephron**: similar to a loop diuretic, • *excess Cl− anions in the urine increase K+ and H+ loss*: * kaluresis leads to hypokalemia, * H+ ions drawn out of the tubules by the negative charge increase reclamation of HCO_3^- (metabolic alkalosis), • *hypokalemia stimulates renal prostaglandin synthesis*, • *prostaglandins and volume depletion from loss of NaCl in the urine stimulate the JG apparatus and activate the RAA system*: * JG hyperplasia is noted on renal Bx specimens, * PRA is increased, * plasma aldosterone is increased, * volume depletion offsets the effect of aldosterone on increasing the BP
mineralocorticoid associated with HTN without an elevation in plasma aldosterone	*Liddle's syndrome*
mechanism of HTN in Liddle's syndrome	*increased sensitivity of the tubules to the normal action of aldosterone*: all the clinical/lab findings associated with primary aldosteronism occur except plasma aldosterone is normal
cause of HTN in a patient eating excessive amounts of licorice	*mineralocorticoid effect of glycyrrhizic acid in licorice*

Table continued on following page

Table 5–4. HYPERTENSION (HTN) *Continued*

Most Common...	Answer and Explanation
clinical findings in pheochromocytoma	• **classic triad of sustained HTN in a patient with excessive sweating, anxiety, and headaches**, • *palpitations*, • *orthostatic hypotension*: plasma volume is reduced owing to VC of arterioles/venules, *ileus:* catecholamines inhibit peristalsis, • *chest pain:* subendocardial ischemia, • *association with MEN IIa and IIb*, • *association with von Hippel-Lindau disease*, • *association with neurofibromatosis*, • *most tumors are benign, unilateral, and located in the adrenal medulla*
screening tests for a pheochromocytoma	*24-hour urine for metanephrine* (most sensitive test) *and vanillylmandelic acid* (VMA)
confirmatory tests for a pheochromocytoma	• *lack of suppression of catecholamines after administration of Clonidine*, • *CT scan*: most useful in localizing the tumor
effect of catecholamine excess on glucose and RBCs	• *hyperglycemia*: increased glycogenolysis in muscle and liver, • *secondary polycythemia*: contraction of the plasma volume
Rx for a pheochromocytoma	*surgical removal*: * preoperative preparation includes the use of an α-adrenergic blocker (phenoxybenzamine) to control HTN and restore plasma volume, * β-blockers are used to control tachycardias
Rx for hypertensive crisis during surgery for removal of a pheochromocytoma	• **nitroprusside**, • *phentolamine*
cause of a systolic pressure >240 mm Hg and diastolic pressure >130 mm Hg	*malignant HTN in a patient with pre-existing essential HTN*
S/S of malignant HTN	• **hypertensive encephalopathy**: * headache from intracranial HTN, * papilledema, * retinopathy (flame hemorrhages, soft/hard exudates), * potential for an intracerebral bleed, • *oliguric renal failure*, • *dyspnea secondary to pulmonary edema*, • *chest pain*: * angina, * subendocardial ischemia/infarction

Table 5–4. HYPERTENSION (HTN) Continued

Most Common...	Answer and Explanation
lab findings in malignant HTN	• *hematuria*, • *RBC casts*, • *proteinuria*, • *renal azotemia*: * increased serum BUN and creatinine, * BUN: creatinine ratio <15:1
Rx of malignant HTN	*intravenous sodium nitroprusside*: the goal of Rx is to reduce the diastolic pressure immediately to 100–110 mm Hg

Question: Which of the following are expected lab/clinical findings in essential HTN? **SELECT 4**
   (A) LVH
   (B) Elevated urine metanephrines
   (C) Hypokalemia
   (D) Retinal microaneurysms
   (E) Proteinuria
   (F) High PRA
   (G) S4 heart sound
   (H) Disparity in upper and lower extremity BP
   (I) Hyperglycemia
   (J) Epigastric bruit

Answers: (A), (D), (E), (G): Expected HTN findings in essential HTN target the heart [LVH, S4 heart sound, choices A and G], retina (retinal microaneurysms, choice D), and kidneys (proteinuria, choice E). Most cases of essential HTN have a normal PRA (elevated in ~15%, choice F is incorrect); normal electrolytes (hypokalemia may be seen in primary aldosteronism, Cushing's syndrome, renovascular HTN, choice F is incorrect); normal metanephrine levels (elevated in pheochromocytoma, choice B is incorrect), approximately equal BP readings between upper and lower extremities (upper > lower in coarctation of the aorta, choice H is incorrect); no epigastric bruits (feature of renovascular HTN, choice J is incorrect); and a normal serum glucose (elevated in pheochromocytoma and Cushing's syndrome, choice I is incorrect).

ACE = angiotensin converting enzyme, ADH = antidiuretic hormone, AG = anion gap, AMI = acute myocardial infarction, ANA = antinuclear antibody, AR = autosomal recessive, ARF = acute renal failure, ATII = angiotensin II, AV = arteriovenous, BNS = benign nephrosclerosis, BP = blood pressure, BUN = blood urea nitrogen, CAD = coronary artery disease, CBC = complete blood cell count, CH = cholesterol, CHD = coronary heart disease, CHF = congestive heart failure, CNS = central nervous system, CO = cardiac output, COD = cause of death, CRF = chronic renal failure, CT = computed tomography, CVA = cerebrovascular accident, DCT = distal collecting tubule, DI = diabetes insipidus, DM = diabetes mellitus, DOA = drug of abuse, DT = distal tubule, ECG = electrocardiogram, FMH = fibromuscular hyperplasia, GN = glomerulonephritis, HDL = high density lipoprotein, HTN = hypertension, HPTH = hyperparathyroidism, HR = heart rate, JG = juxtaglomerular apparatus, LDL = low density lipoprotein, LV = left ventricular, LVH

= left ventricular hypertrophy, MEN = multiple endocrine neoplasia, MOA = mechanism of action, NSAIDs = nonsteroidal anti-inflammatory drugs, PMI = point of maximal impulse, PN = pyelonephritis, PRA = plasma renin activity, PSS = progressive systemic sclerosis, PTH = parathormone, PVD = peripheral vascular disease, RAA = renin-angiotensin-aldosterone, RAS = renal artery stenosis, RBC = red blood cell, R/O = rule out, RVH = right ventricular hypertrophy, Rx = treatment, SLE = systemic lupus erythematosus, SMC = smooth muscle cell, S/S = signs and symptoms, TAL = thick ascending limb, TG = triglyceride, TPR = total peripheral resistance, VC = vasoconstriction, VD = vasodilatation, VMA = vanillylmandelic acid.

Table 5–5. HEART FAILURE

Most Common...	Answer and Explanation
causes of heart failure	• **reduced ventricular contractility**: e.g., * myocardial ischemia, * systolic dysfunction, • *restricted filling*: e.g., * LVH, * constrictive pericarditis, * diastolic dysfunction, • *increased workload*: * increase in afterload (increased TPR in essential HTN), * increase in preload (incompetent MV), * increased return of blood to the right heart (severe anemia)
pathophysiologic responses to heart failure	• *hypertrophy secondary to volume overload*, • *increased force of contraction*: Frank-Starling mechanism plus catecholamine stimulation of the β-receptors in the heart, • *increased TPR*: stimulation of the high pressure baroreceptors due to a low CO with increased sympathetic activity, • *activation of RAA system*: * catecholamine stimulation of the JG apparatus, * reduced renal artery blood flow, * increased production of ATII and aldosterone, • *increased HR*: sympathetic stimulation of the heart
causes of LHF	• **AMI**, • *essential HTN* • *IHD*, • *cardiomyopathies*, • *myocarditis*, • *valvular disease*
mechanism of systolic heart failure (systolic dysfunction)	*problem with LV contractility*: * ejection fraction is <0.40, * see Table 5–1
causes of systolic dysfunction	• **AMI**, • *congestive cardiomyopathy*, • *chronic IHD*

Table 5–5. HEART FAILURE *Continued*

Most Common...	Answer and Explanation
Rx of systolic dysfunction	• *reduce TPR*: * ACE inhibitors—see Table 5–4, • *increase contractility*: dobutamine (positive inotropic agent)
mechanism of diastolic failure (diastolic dysfunction)	*problem with LV filling*: * decreased LV compliance, * EF is >0.40 owing to an increase in left atrial pressure which is able to maintain the EF, albeit at the expense of pulmonary congestion
causes of diastolic dysfunction	• **severe LVH**: e.g., * essential HTN, * AV stenosis, • *IHSS*, • *restrictive cardiomyopathy*: e.g., amyloid heart, • *constrictive pericarditis*, • *high output failure*
Rx of diastolic dysfunction	*increase preload in the LV*: * decrease heart rate, * reduce the force of LV contraction, * e.g., negative inotropic agents, such as calcium channel blockers
causes of RHF	• **LHF**: blood accumulates behind the failed left heart, causing an increased afterload that the right heart must contract against, • *right-sided valvular disease*: e.g., tricuspid regurgitation, • *cor pulmonale*, • *cardiomyopathies*, • *myocarditis*, • *pulmonary embolus* (PE)
cause of acute RHF	*large PE*: a large PE (saddle embolus) produces right heart strain and failure
type of heart failure primarily manifested by symptoms	*LHF*
type of heart failure primarily manifested by signs	*RHF*
symptoms of LHF	**dyspnea**: see Table 5–1, • *pillow orthopnea*: see Table 5–1, • *PND*: see Table 5–1, • *exercise intolerance*, • *cough*, • *nocturia*: "normalization" of the GFR occurs when the patient lies down at night and venous return to the heart is increased, • *wheezing*: peribronchiolar edema
heart sounds associated with both LHF and RHF	• **S3**, • **S4** [see Table 5–1.]

Table continued on following page

Table 5–5. HEART FAILURE *Continued*

Most Common...	Answer and Explanation
murmur associated with LHF and RHF	*MV and TV regurgitation, respectively*: volume overload of the failed ventricles dilates the valve ring, producing pansystolic regurgitation murmurs and volume overload in the ventricular chambers
lab finding in LHF	*prerenal azotemia*: * increase in serum BUN and creatinine, * BUN:creatinine ratio >15:1, * see Table 10–1 for discussion
chest radiograph findings in LHF	• **prominent congestion of blood in the upper lobes**: pulmonary venous congestion in the lower lobes redirects extra-alveolar blood to the upper lobes, • *perihilar congestion*: "batwing" configuration, *Kerley lines*: * represent fluid in the interlobular septa, * *Kerley A* lines are diagonal lines in the upper lobes that radiate out from the hilum, *Kerley B* lines are linear lines that are perpendicular to the pleura in the lower lobes, * *Kerley C* lines are a mesh of linear markings in the middle portion of the lower lobes (most common type), • *patchy interstitial and alveolar infiltrates*: represent pulmonary edema, • *pleural effusion*: * increased hydrostatic pressure in the lungs decreases uptake of pleural fluid, * CHF is the most common cause of a pleural effusion
signs in RHF	• **jugular neck vein distention**: fluid builds up in the venous system behind the failed right heart, • *right-sided S3 heart sound*: see Table 5–1, • *giant c-v wave*: see Table 5–1, • *systolic pulsation of the liver*: TV regurgitation, • *HJ reflux*: hepatic congestion associated with hepatomegaly, • *dependent pitting edema*: increased venous hydrostatic pressure, • *ascites*: increased hydrostatic pressure, • *cyanosis*: low oxygen saturation due to increased amount of time for the tissue to extract oxygen
lab findings in RHF	*hyponatremia:* * hypotonic gain of more water than salt from the kidneys, * see Table 10–2, *prerenal azotemia*: see Table 10–1, • *elevated serum transaminases*: hepatic congestion with hepatic cell necrosis

Table 5–5. HEART FAILURE *Continued*

Most Common...	Answer and Explanation
nonpharmacologic treatments for LHF and RHF	• **restrict Na+ and water intake**: restricting Na+ (<2 g/day) and water (<1.5 liters/d) reduces preload, • *rotating tourniquets*: reduces preload, • *bedrest*, • *oxygen*
pharmacologic Rx of heart failure	• **ACE inhibitors**: * standard Rx in systolic dysfunction, * see Table 5–4 for mechanisms, * decrease both preload (decrease aldosterone) and afterload (decrease ATII), • *diuretics*: reduce preload by establishing a natriuresis, • β-*blockers*: used in chronic CHF due to diastolic dysfunction, • *calcium channel blockers*: * mainly used for diastolic dysfunction, * increases preload, • *nitroglycerin*: * used in the Rx of systolic dysfunction due to an AMI, * decreases afterload
MOA of digoxin	• **blocks the Na+/K+ ATPase pump**: entry of Na+ into cardiac muscle opens up Ca++ channels, leading to increased muscle contraction (inotropic effect), • *inhibits atrioventricular conduction*: increases the PR interval, which decreases the ventricular response to atrial arrhythmias, • *enhances vagal tone*: increases parasympathetic activity
ECG changes due to digoxin	• *P wave changes*, • *prolonged PR interval*, • *ST depression*, • *T wave inversion*
use of digoxin in Rx of CHF	*second-line drug that is used in treating systolic dysfunction associated with atrial fibrillation/flutter*
factors interfering with digoxin activity	• *electrolyte abnormalities*: e.g., * hyperkalemia, which reduces enzyme inhibition, • *drugs*: e.g., * cholestyramine (bile salt binder that also binds to digoxin), • *hormones*: hyperthyroidism increases the metabolism of digoxin
causes of digoxin toxicity	• *drugs*: e.g., * quinidine, * erythromycin, • *electrolyte abnormalities*: e.g., * hypokalemia, * hypomagnesemia, * hypercalcemia, • *renal insufficiency*: decreases excretion of digoxin, • *hypothyroidism*: decreases metabolism of digoxin, • *hypoxemia*, • *volume depletion*: concentrates digoxin

Table continued on following page

Table 5–5. HEART FAILURE *Continued*

Most Common...	Answer and Explanation
S/S of digoxin toxicity	• **AV conduction disturbances**: * first/second/third-degree blocks, * junctional tachycardia, • *sinus bradycardia*: <50 bpm, • *premature atrial beats*, • *atrial fibrillation* (AF), • *PAT*, • *ventricular premature depolarizations*, • *ventricular tachycardia*, • *GI disturbances*: * N/V, * diarrhea, • *blurring of vision with a yellowish overtone to colors*
Rx of digoxin toxicity	• **D/C drug**, • *correct electrolyte abnormalities*, • *administer oxygen*, • *Rx with digoxin-specific Fab antibody fragments:* * antibody fragments bind digoxin and are rapidly excreted in the urine, * digoxin levels are falsely increased while on this drug, • *atropine:* useful in patients with sinus bradycardia or heart block, • *lidocaine or phenytoin*: use in suppressing ventricular and atrial arrhythmias, • *cardioversion may precipitate lethal arrhythmias, hence it is contraindicated*
cause of high output failure due to increased contractility	*hyperthyroidism*: * high output cardiac failure is characterized by a normal to increased cardiac output, * hyperthyroidism leads to increased LV contractility
cause of high output failure due to decreased blood viscosity	*severe anemia*: * a decrease in blood viscosity decreases TPR (Poiseuille's law), * decreased TPR increases venous return to the right heart
causes of high output failure due to vasodilatation	• **endotoxic shock**: * increasing the radius of the peripheral resistance arterioles by vasodilatation decreases TPR (Poiseuille's law), * a decrease in TPR increases venous return to the right heart, * endotoxins stimulate the release of anaphylatoxins, nitric oxide, and PGI_2, all of which are potent vasodilators, • *thiamine deficiency*: vasodilatation of arterioles, • *arteriovenous fistula*: bypasses the microcirculation and increases return of blood to the heart

Table 5–5. HEART FAILURE *Continued*

Question: Which of the following characterize LHF rather than RHF?
SELECT 3
- (A) Dependent pitting edema
- (B) HJ reflux
- (C) Pulmonary venous hypertension
- (D) Decreased cardiac output
- (E) S3 heart sound
- (F) PND
- (G) Jugular neck vein distention
- (H) Pulmonary congestion in the upper lobes on chest radiograph

Answers: (C), (F), (H): In LHF, blood accumulates behind the failed left heart, causing pulmonary venous HTN (**choice C**) and congestion of pulmonary veins in the upper lobes (**choice H**). At night, increased venous return of blood to the left heart causes blood to reflux back into the lungs. This leads to a sudden awakening with the sensation of choking (PND), **choice F**). A decreased cardiac output and S3 heart sound are present in both LHF and RHF (**choices D and E are incorrect**). RHF is characterized by accumulation of blood behind the failed heart leading to jugular neck vein distention (**choice G is incorrect**), pitting edema (**choice A is incorrect**), and a congested liver, which is responsible for an HJ reflux (**choice B is incorrect**).

ACE = angiotension converting enzyme, AF = atrial fibrillation, AMI = acute myocardial infarction, ATII = angiotension II, AV = atrioventricular, BUN = blood urea nitrogen, CHF = congestive heart failure, CO = cardiac output, D/C = discontinue, ECG = electrocardiogram, EF = ejection fraction, GFR = glomerular filtration rate, GI = gastrointestinal, HJ = hepatojugular reflux, HTN = hypertension, HR = heart rate, IHD = ischemic heart disease, IHSS = idiopathic hypertrophic subaortic stenosis, JG = juxtaglomerular, LHF = left heart failure, LV = left ventricle, LVH = left ventricular hypertrophy, MOA = mechanism of action, MV = mitral valve, N/V = nausea and vomiting, PAT = paroxysmal atrial tachycardia, PE = pulmonary embolus, PGI_2 = prostaglandin I_2, PND = paroxysmal nocturnal dyspnea, RAA = renin-angiotensin-aldosterone, RHF = right heart failure, Rx = treatment, S/S = signs and symptoms, TPR = total peripheral resistance, TV = tricuspid valve.

Table 5–6. SELECTED ELECTROCARDIOGRAPHIC ABNORMALITIES

Most Common...	Answer and Explanation
electrophysiologic events causing the P wave	*atrial depolarization:* * the P wave initiates atrial contraction (atrial systole), * the PR interval is the time from initial atrial depolarization to initial depolarization of the ventricles (onset of QRS)

Table continued on following page

Table 5–6. SELECTED ELECTROCARDIOGRAPHIC ABNORMALITIES *Continued*

Most Common...	Answer and Explanation
P wave findings in atrial hypertrophy	• *LA hypertrophy:* ⋆ broad (≥0.12 sec), notched P wave, ⋆ best seen in leads I and II, • *RA hypertrophy:* ⋆ tall, peaked P waves, ⋆ best seen in leads II, III, aVF (≥2.5 mm in lead II), ⋆ peaked, diphasic P waves or inverted P waves in lead V1
electrophysiologic events producing the PR interval	• *atrial depolarization,* • *normal conduction delay through the AV node* (PR segment), • *passage of the conduction impulse through the bundle of His and bundle branches to the onset of ventricular depolarization* [The normal PR interval is 0.12–0.2 sec.]
drug causing a prolonged PR interval (first degree AV block)	*digoxin*
disorders that prolong the PR interval	• **bradycardia**, • *atrial enlargement:* e.g., MV stenosis
causes of a short PR interval	• **sinus tachycardia**, • *WPW syndrome*: pre-excitation syndrome associated with an accessory bypass tract (bundles of Kent) between the atria and ventricles, • *short PR interval syndromes other than WPW*
ECG findings in WPW syndrome	• *short PR interval with a normal P wave,* • *initial slurring of the upstroke of the R wave* (delta wave) *or of the downstroke of the Q wave,* • *ST depression and T wave inversion are also present*
mechanisms for a short PR interval syndrome other than WPW	• *intra-AV nodal bypass tract,* • *anatomically short AV node,* • *atrio-His connection, which bypasses the AV node*
electrophysiologic event causing the QRS complex	*ventricular depolarization*: upper limit of normal in the precordial leads is 0.11 sec
electrophysiologic event causing the T wave	*ventricular repolarization*

Table 5–6. SELECTED ELECTROCARDIOGRAPHIC ABNORMALITIES *Continued*

Most Common...	Answer and Explanation
abnormal T wave patterns	• *tall*: e.g., * hyperkalemia with tall, symmetrical T waves with a narrow base are the earliest ECG finding, * hyperacute tall T waves in an AMI, • *inverted*: occur after ST segment elevation in an AMI, • *prolonged*
electrophysiologic event producing a U wave	• *prolongation of ventricular polarization*: positive deflection following the T wave
causes of a U wave	• **hypokalemia**, • *quinidine*: giant U wave that is larger in amplitude than the T wave
method of determining the HR on an ECG	*HR = 1/cycle length in sec*: * the cycle length is represented by the R-R interval, or the time between two R intervals, * HR (beats/min) = 1/cycle length in sec, * e.g., R-R = 600 msec, HR = 1/0.6 sec = 1.66 beats/sec or 100 beats/min
cause of a new Q wave	*anterior AMI*: * a new Q wave represents the area of necrosis in an AMI, * it is pathologic if it is ≥0.04 sec in duration
causes of false positive Q waves	• **LVH**, • *IHSS*: simulates an AMI, • *COPD*, • *restrictive cardiomyopathy*: * amyloid, * iron overload, * myxedema heart, • *WPW syndrome*
AMI with an absent Q wave in a standard ECG	*posterior AMI*
Q wave locations in an anterior AMI	*leads V₂–V₆*
Q wave locations for an inferior AMI	*leads II and aVF*
Q wave locations for a lateral AMI	*leads I, aVL, and V₆*
Q wave location for a posterior AMI	*Q waves are only recorded from the posterior surface of the heart and are not present on the usual anterior leads*: there is a reciprocal ST depression in leads V₁–V₂

Table continued on following page

Table 5–6. SELECTED ELECTROCARDIOGRAPHIC
ABNORMALITIES *Continued*

Most Common...	Answer and Explanation
electrophysiologic events producing the QT interval	• *measured from the beginning of the Q wave to the end of the T wave,* • *represents electrical systole,* • *normally not >0.42 sec in men and >0.43 sec in women,* • *QT interval approximates the refractory period of ventricular tissue*
causes of a short QT interval	• **hypercalcemia**: ST wave is eliminated, • *digoxin*
causes of a prolonged QT interval	• **hypocalcemia**, • *quinidine,* • *tricyclic antidepressants,* • *procainamide,* • *amiodarone,* • *subarachnoid hemorrhage*
clinical findings in prolonged QT syndrome	• *family Hx of sudden death,* • *patient has a sudden loss of consciousness during exercise or stressful experiences,* • *onset is late in childhood or early adolescence,* • *prolonged QT interval is frequently evident in an ECG:* may have to be induced after carefully monitored exercise, • β-*blockers may be life saving*
method of measuring the ST segment	• *measured from the beginning of the ST segment* (J point) *to the onset of the T wave,* • *it is usually isoelectric but may vary from* − 0.5 *mm to* + 2 *mm in the precordial leads*
causes of ST depression	• **subendocardial ischemia in exertional angina**: * ST depression in subendocardial ischemia, * ST elevation in transmural ischemia, * typical ST wave depression in ischemia is accompanied by T wave inversion in LV epicardial leads, • *digitalis:* "scooped" ST configuration, • *hypokalemia,* • *hyperventilation in anxiety states*
causes of ST elevation	• **transmural AMI**: * convex upward elevation of the ST segment, * ST elevation represents the area of injury surrounding the infarcted tissue, * it is the most consistent ECG finding in an AMI, • *Prinzmetal's angina,* • *LBBB,* • *pericarditis*: concave upward, • *ventricular aneurysm*: elevated for months to years

Table 5–6. SELECTED ELECTROCARDIOGRAPHIC
ABNORMALITIES *Continued*

Most Common...	Answer and Explanation
criteria for Dx of LVH	• *R wave in lead 1 + S in lead III > 26 mm,* • *R wave in aVL >11 mm,* • *R wave in lead V_5 or V_6 >26 mm,* • *S wave in lead V_1 + R in V_5 or V_6 >35 mm*
criteria for Dx of RVH	• *right axis deviation is usually present:* greater than +90 degrees, • *R wave in lead V_1 >5 mm,* • *R/S ratio in lead V_1 >1,* • *additional findings:* ST depression and inverted T waves are noted in leads V_1–V_3
ECG findings associated with quinidine	• **prolongation of the QTU interval owing to the presence of a giant U wave**, • *ST depression,* • *flattening of the T waves*
side-effects of quinidine	• **cinchonism**: * tinnitus, * headache, • *autoimmune thrombocytopenia/hemolytic anemia*
MOA of amiodarone	*antiarrhythmic drug that blocks Na^+, Ca^{++}, K^+ channels* and β-adrenoreceptors: it is effective in most types of arrhythmias owing to its broad spectrum of activity
ECG findings associated with amiodarone	• *slowing of the sinus rate and AV conduction,* • *prolongation of the QT interval,* • *prolongation of the QRS interval,* • *increased atrial, AV, and ventricular refractory periods*
side-effects of amiodarone	• *interstitial fibrosis,* • *hyper- or hypothyroidism,* • *crystalline deposits in the cornea and skin*
criteria for Dx of sinus arrhythmia	*cyclic increase in normal HR with inspiration and decrease with expiration*
cause of a sinus arrhythmia	*reflex changes in the vagus nerve influence on the normal pacemaker:* * cyclic change decreases when holding the breath or in the presence of sinus tachycardia, * normal variation
criteria for Dx of sinus bradycardia	*HR <60 bpm*: * normal HR 60–100 bpm, * normal sinus bradycardia increases with exercise and slows with vagal stimulation, * may be a sign of excellent conditioning

Table continued on following page

Table 5–6. SELECTED ELECTROCARDIOGRAPHIC ABNORMALITIES *Continued*

Most Common...	Answer and Explanation
pathophysiologic causes of sinus bradycardia	• *increased vagal tone*: e.g., nausea, • *SA node disease*: e.g., * inferior AMI, * SA node firing rate is decreased in ♦ hypothermia, ♦ hyperkalemia, ♦ hypothyroidism, and with ♦ drugs (e.g., quinidine)
Rx of symptomatic sinus bradycardia	• **atropine**, • *cardiac pacing*: necessary in severe cases
criteria for Dx of sinus tachycardia	*HR >100 bpm*
mechanism of sinus tachycardia	*acceleration of the SA node*
pathophysiologic causes of sinus tachycardia	• **stress/fever**, • *hyperthyroidism*, • *hypovolemia*, • *pheochromocytoma*, • *decreased CO*: e.g., CHF, • *hypoxemia*, • *respiratory acidosis*, • *ischemia/necrosis*, • *hypokalemia*
chronic arrhythmia	*atrial fibrillation* (AF)
criteria for Dx of AF	*irregular pulse with an atrial rate of 400–600 bpm and a ventricular response usually between 80 and 100 bpm*: • rate may be regular in extreme bradycardic states (e.g., digoxin toxicity with an HR <60 bpm)
mechanism of AF	*multiple wandering wave fronts of depolarization impacting on the AV node*: * disorders increasing atrial size (e.g., MV stenosis), * disorders that interfere with atrial conduction
pre-existing conditions associated with AF	• **hypertensive heart disease**, • CHF, • RF, • *hyperthyroidism* [Patients with AF who lack an identifiable CVD are said to have "lone AF".]
valvular disease that causes AF	*MV stenosis secondary to RF*: due to dilatation of the LA
complication associated with chronic AF	*thrombosis with embolization into the systemic circulation*: * all patients with chronic AF should be anticoagulated, * embolic strokes and small bowel infarction commonly occur

Table 5–6. SELECTED ELECTROCARDIOGRAPHIC ABNORMALITIES *Continued*

Most Common...	Answer and Explanation
endocrine disorder associated with AF	*hyperthyroidism*: **always** order a TSH whenever an atrial tachyarrhythmia is present
Rx of acute AF	• **cardioconversion**, • *calcium channel blockers*: * diltiazem, * verapamil, • *IV beta-blockers*: * esmolol, * drug of choice in hyperthyroidism, • *digoxin*: slower action than those listed above, • *carotid sinus massage*: either has no effect or leads to an AV block, with a slowed ventricular rate
criteria for Dx of atrial flutter	• *regular atrial activity at a rate of 260–350 bpm*, • *ventricular rate of 125–175 bpm*: 2:1 to 4:1 AV conduction ratio, • *P waves with a "sawtooth" appearance*, • *above findings are best observed in leads II, III, aVF, and V1*, • *may convert into AF or normal sinus rhythm*
causes of atrial flutter	• **atrial enlargement**, • *COPD*, • *CHD*, • *RF*, • *ASD*
Rx of acute atrial flutter	• **cardioconversion**, • *similar drugs as those used in Rx of AF*, • *amiodarone is effective in chronic atrial flutter*, • *anticoagulation in chronic atrial flutter*: embolization less frequent than in AF, • *carotid sinus massage*: may produce an * AV nodal block, * have no effect, or * lead to AF
paroxysmal tachycardia	*paroxysmal supraventricular tachycardia* (PSVT)
criteria for Dx of PSVT	• *regular rhythm with a ventricular rate of 150–230 bpm*, • *QRS duration <100 msec*, • *abnormal P wave*: * may be superimposed on a T wave, * fixed relationship to each QRS
mechanism of PSVT	• *re-entry involving the SA node, AV node*, • *accessory pathway*: ~ one-third of cases
S/S of PSVT	*abrupt onset of palpitations with*: * dizziness, * syncope, * anginal pain
causes of PSVT	• **digoxin toxicity**, • *WPW syndrome*, • *hyperthyroidism*

Table continued on following page

Table 5–6. SELECTED ELECTROCARDIOGRAPHIC ABNORMALITIES *Continued*

Most Common...	Answer and Explanation
Rx of acute PSVT	• **vagal maneuvers**: e.g., * carotid sinus massage, * Valsalva maneuver is effective in ~90% of cases, • *drugs*: * adenosine, * calcium channel blockers (e.g., diltiazem, verapamil)
Rx of chronic PSVT	• **digoxin**: first line drug, • *calcium channel antagonists*, • *β-adrenergic antagonists*
Rx for re-entry tachycardias associated with accessory pathways	• **catheter ablation of accessory pathway**, • *amiodarone*: it delays conduction and prolongs the refractory period, hence abolishing transmission through the accessory pathway, • *WPW Rx*: should not treat with digoxin or verapamil, since they shorten the refractory period of the accessory pathway and increase the ventricular rate
cause of "skipped" beats	*ventricular premature beats* (VPB)
criteria for Dx of VPB	• *wide, notched, or slurred QRS complexes*, • *not preceded by a premature P wave*, • *fully compensatory pause is perceived by the patient as a "skipped" beat*, • *exercise abolishes these beats*, • *often confused with bigeminy*: when every other beat is a VPB, it is called bigeminy
causes of VPBs	• **common in young/old age, stress, excess caffeine**, • *drugs*: * digoxin, * quinidine, * tricyclic antidepressants, • *AMI*: strong association with the size of the infarct and precipitation of ventricular fibrillation, • *sudden death in those with pre-existing organic heart disease*
effect of the R-on-T VPB on ventricular tissue	*may precipitate an episode of ventricular tachycardia/fibrillation*: when a VPB occurs at the peak of the T wave or on its downstroke, it falls in the vulnerable period of ventricular tissue, which may initiate repetitive ventricular beating
Rx of symptomatic VPB	*β-adrenergic blockers*: IV lidocaine is used in the Rx VPBs after an AMI

Table 5–6. SELECTED ELECTROCARDIOGRAPHIC
ABNORMALITIES *Continued*

Most Common...	Answer and Explanation
effect of ventricular arrhythmias on S1 and the JVPs	• **variation in the intensity of S1**: * S1 varies owing to the asynchrony between atrial and ventricular contraction, * the MV/TV may be opened, partially closed, or fully closed with each ventricular contraction, • *giant a waves in the JVP*: when the RA contracts against a closed TV, a *giant a wave* occurs
life-threatening arrhythmia	*VT*
criteria for Dx of VT	• **three or more consecutive VPBs when the HR is ≥100–250 bpm**, • *QRS is usually >120 msec*
causes of VT	• **CHD**, • *cardiomyopathies*, • *infectious disease*: e.g., * Lyme's disease, * Chagas' disease, * viral myocarditis
Rx of acute VT	• **synchronized DC cardioversion** (100–360 J) **if sustained** (VT >30s), • *IV lidocaine if the patient is hemodynamically stable:* * other drugs that may be used include procainamide and bretylium, * Rx of chronic recurrent VT is controversial
drug toxicities/ metabolic disturbances	• **quinidine**, • *electrolyte abnormalities*: * hypokalemia, * hypomagnesemia, • *phenothiazines*, • *tricyclic antidepressants*, • *sotalol*: K^+ channel blocker, • *bepridil:* calcium channel blocker, • *terfenadine*: H_1 blocker
criteria for defining torsades de pointes	*type of polymorphic ventricular tachycardia*: * considerable variation in the QRS configuration that undulates around an isoelectric point, * usually self-terminates, * can progress into ventricular fibrillation, * prolonged QT interval is present
Rx of torsades of pointes	• **administer a β-adrenergic antagonist**, • *if present, correct the electrolyte abnormality*, • *remove the offending drug*
AV block	*first-degree AV block*: * PR interval is >0.21 sec, * patients are usually asymptomatic, * S1 heart sound is soft

Table continued on following page

**Table 5–6. SELECTED ELECTROCARDIOGRAPHIC
ABNORMALITIES** *Continued*

Most Common...	Answer and Explanation
mechanism of a first-degree AV block	*conduction delay in the AV node*
causes of first degree AV block	• **drugs**: e.g., * digoxin, * beta-blockers, • *IHD*
types of second-degree AV blocks	• **type I**: other names include * AV nodal block, * Wenckebach, * Mobitz type I, • *type II*: other names include * His-Purkinje bundle type, * Mobitz type II
criteria for Dx of type I block	*progressive lengthening of the PR interval until the P wave is not followed by a QRS complex:* usually narrow complexes that appear normal
criteria for Dx of type II block	• *block is in a regular sequence* (e.g., 2:1, 3:1) *or an irregular sequence* (e.g., 3:2, 4:3), • *PR interval is not followed by a QRS complex,* • *PR interval for conducted P waves is constant:* no conduction delay, • *may precede complete heart block,* • *often associated with ischemic disease in the LAD coronary artery and bundle branch disease*
mechanisms producing a third-degree block (complete heart block)	• *complete dissociation between the atrial and ventricular rhythms:* atrial rate exceeds the ventricular rate, • *site of block may be at the AV node* (usually congenital disease) *or within the His-Purkinje bundle system* (acquired disease)
criteria for third-degree block at AV node	• *HR of 50–60 bpm,* • *regular QRS rhythm and QRS appearance*
criteria for third-degree block involving His-Purkinje system	• *HR of 30–40 bpm,* • *broad, slurred, or notched QRS complexes*
causes of a third degree block	• **IHD**, • *AMI involving the LAD coronary artery*

Table 5–6. SELECTED ELECTROCARDIOGRAPHIC ABNORMALITIES *Continued*

Most Common...	Answer and Explanation
Rx for AV blocks	• *first-degree block:* no Rx, • *second-degree blocks:* * atropine (usually a poor response), * permanent pacemaker insertion is usually required, • *third-degree blocks:* permanent pacemaker

Question: Which of the following conditions produce ST depression? **SELECT 5**
- (A) Hypercalcemia
- (B) Hypokalemia
- (C) Hyperkalemia
- (D) Hypocalcemia
- (E) Pericarditis
- (F) Transmural AMI
- (G) Exertional angina
- (H) Ventricular aneurysms
- (I) Digoxin
- (J) Quinidine
- (K) WPW syndrome

Answers: (B), (G), (I), (J), (K): ST depression is present in hypokalemia (choice B), digoxin (choice I), quinidine (choice J), subendocardial ischemia (exertional angina, choice G), and WPW (choice K). Hypercalcemia is associated with a short QT interval and absence of the ST segment (choice A is incorrect). Hypocalcemia is not associated with any ST wave changes (choice D is incorrect). Hyperkalemia, pericarditis, ventricular aneurysms, and a transmural AMI are associated with ST elevation (choices C, E, F, and H are incorrect).

AF = atrial fibrillation, AMI = acute myocardial infarction, ASD = atrial septal defect, AV = atrioventricular, bpm = beats per minute, CHD = coronary heart disease, CHF = congestive heart failure, CO = cardiac output, COPD = chronic obstructive pulmonary disease, CVD = cardiovascular disease, DC = direct current, Dx = diagnosis, ECG = electrocardiogram, HR = heart rate, Hx = history, IHD = ischemic heart disease, IV = intravenous, JVP = jugular venous pulse, LA = left atrium, LAD = left anterior descending, LBBB = left bundle branch block, LVH = left ventricular hypertrophy, MOA = mechanism of action, MV = mitral valve, PSVT = paroxysmal supraventricular tachycardia, RA = right atrium, RF = rheumatic fever, RVH = right ventricular hypertrophy, Rx = treatment, SA = sinoatrial, S/S = signs and symptoms, TSH = thyroid stimulating hormone, TV = tricuspid valve, VPB = ventricular premature beat, VT = ventricular tachycardia, WPW = Wolff-Parkinson-White.

Table 5–7. ADULT CONGENITAL HEART DISEASE (CHD)

Most Common...	Answer and Explanation
differences between adult and childhood CHD	• *adults have less complex CHD*, • *adults have less cyanotic CHD* [~90% of children born with CHD survive until adulthood.]
adult CHDs	• **congenital bicuspid AV**, • *ostium secundum type of ASD*: * second most common type, * most commonly first noted in pregnant women (increased plasma volume), * more common in women than in men, • *pulmonic stenosis*, • *coarctation of the aorta*, • *PDA*
adult cyanotic CHD	*tetralogy of Fallot*: * infravalvular pulmonic stenosis (most important defect), * RVH, * VSD, * overriding aorta
clinical findings in tetralogy of Fallot	• **most patients have mild cyanosis and a systolic murmur**, • *those with a mild degree of infravalvular pulmonic stenosis are acyanotic*, • *echocardiography with color flow imaging and Doppler interrogation studies are diagnostic*
problems associated with a congenital bicuspid AV	**calcific AV stenosis and isolated AV regurgitation**, • *coarctation of the aorta*: 25% of patients, • *IE*
clinical findings in adult ASD	• **supraventricular atrial arrhythmias**: AF most common, • *PH secondary to left to right shunting of blood*, • *cyanosis with exercise*, • *hemoptysis*: pulmonary congestion from PH, • *RHF*, • *reversal of the shunt*: see below
cardiac findings in ASD	• **fixed splitting of S2**: see Table 5–1, • *midsystolic pulmonary flow murmur*: increased blood flow across the PV, • *left axis deviation*, • *accentuation of P2*: due to PH
late complication of left-to-right shunts	*Eisenmenger's complex*: refers to reversal of a left-to-right shunt to a right-to-left shunt owing to development of PH from volume overload of the right heart
cardiac findings in pulmonic stenosis	• *systolic ejection murmur in the second left ICS*, • *systolic ejection click*, • *fixed splitting of S2*, • *diminished P2 heart sound*, • *right-sided S4 heart sound*, • *parasternal heave*: due to RVH, • *giant a wave*, • *post-stenotic dilatation of the PA* [The majority of cases are mild to moderate. Many patients have a normal life expectancy.]

Table 5–7. ADULT CONGENITAL HEART DISEASE (CHD)
Continued

Most Common...	Answer and Explanation
mechanism of an adult coarctation	*defect in the media of the Ao*: * distal to the ligamentum arteriosum (postductal in adults), * preductal in children, * five times more common in men than in women, * develops after the third or fourth decade
S/S in a postductal coarctation	• **HTN in the upper extremities with diminished BP in the lower extremities**: surgical cause of diastolic HTN, • *greater upper body muscles than lower body,* • *systolic murmur heard best in the posterior left thorax*
complications associated with a coarctation	• *dissecting aortic aneurysm with rupture,* • *IE,* • *leg claudication with exercise*: due to ischemia, • *diastolic HTN*: due to reduced renal blood flow and activation of RAA, • *increased incidence of berry aneurysms*: increased pressure in the aortic arch vessels
chest radiograph findings in a postductal coarctation	• **rib notching due to erosion of bone by dilated collateral intercostal arteries,** • *figure of "3" sign*: due to pre- and post-stenotic dilation of the Ao
murmur associated with a PDA	*machinery murmur*: murmur occurs in systole and diastole
chest radiograph finding in a PDA	*calcification of the ductus in older adults*
late complication of a PDA	*Eisenmenger's complex with differential cyanosis*: with the reversal of the shunt, unoxygenated blood selectively reaches the feet as the blood enters the Ao below the subclavian artery
complications of cyanotic CHD	• **secondary polycythemia**: due to right to left shunting of blood and the stimulus for EPO release by hypoxemia, • *IE:* antibiotic prophylaxis is necessary, • *cerebral abscesses*: * vegetations cross directly into the systemic circulation, * usually multiple abscesses, • *platelet defect*: reduced large multimeric forms of VWF, • *clubbing*: increased collagen formation due to the release of PDGF from platelets shunted into the systemic circulation

Table continued on following page

Table 5–7. ADULT CONGENITAL HEART DISEASE (CHD)
Continued

Most Common...	Answer and Explanation
prophylaxis used to prevent IE in CHD	*amoxicillin:* not necessary for uncomplicated ASO
congenital malformation of the coronary artery	*coronary arteriovenous fistula*: most often recognized by the presence of an atypical continuous murmur

Question: A 38-year-old woman who experiences exertional dyspnea following exercise is noted to have an irregularly irregular pulse, fixed splitting of S2, an accentuated P2, a parasternal heave, and a soft systolic heart murmur in the second left ICS. She most likely has which of the following disorders? **SELECT 1**
- (A) Congenital bicuspid aortic valve
- (B) Patent ductus arteriosus
- (C) Pulmonary valve stenosis
- (D) Acyanotic tetralogy of Fallot
- (E) Atrial septal defect

Answer: (E): The patient has an ASD (**choice E**) with a significant left-to-right shunt leading to fixed splitting of S2. PH (accentuated P2), RVH (parasternal heave), a PV flow murmur, and AF (irregularly irregular pulse secondary to dilatation of the RA). None of the other CHDs listed have left-to-right shunts (**choices A, C, D are incorrect**) except a PDA. PDA has a machinery murmur (**choice B is incorrect**).

AF = atrial fibrillation, Ao = aorta, ASD = atrial septal defect, AV = aortic valve, BP = blood pressure, CHD = congenital heart disease, EPO = erythropoietin, HTN = hypertension, ICS = intercostal space, IE = infectious endocarditis, PA = pulmonary artery, PDA = patent ductus arteriosus, PDGF = platelet derived growth factor, PH = pulmonary hypertension, PV = pulmonic valve, RA = right atrium, RAA = renin-angiotensin-aldosterone, RHF = right heart failure, RVH = right ventricular hypertrophy, S/S = signs and symptoms, VSD = ventricular septal defect, VWF = von Willebrand's factor.

Table 5–8. ISCHEMIC HEART DISEASE (IHD)

Most Common...	Answer and Explanation
CHD in the United States	*CHD*: * accounts for ~25% of all deaths in the United States in spite of an overall decline in death rate of 40% since the 1990s, * four times more common in men than in women
distribution of the LAD coronary artery	• *anterior wall of the LV,* • *anterior two-thirds of the IVS* [It is the most common vessel thrombosed in an AMI.]

Table 5–8. ISCHEMIC HEART DISEASE (IHD) *Continued*

Most Common...	Answer and Explanation
clinical findings unique to LAD thrombosis	*most common cause of second- and third-degree AV nodal blocks requiring a permanent pacemaker*: due to the location of the bundles in the anterior one-third of the IVS
distribution of the RCA	• *posterior-inferior wall of the LV,* • *right ventricle (RV),* • *posterior one-third of the IVS,* • *supplies 90% of the blood to the AV node*
clinical findings unique to RCA thrombosis	• *sinus bradycardia*: supplies 90% of the blood to the AV node, • *papillary muscle dysfunction/rupture*: RCA supplies the posteromedial papillary muscle, • *right ventricular infarction*
distribution of the LCA coronary artery	*supplies the anteroposterolateral wall of the LV*
myocardial site susceptible to ischemia	*subendocardium*: * farthest away from the epicardial surface, * greatest amount of wall tension (limits coronary artery perfusion)
symptom of myocardial ischemia	*chest pain* (angina): angina occurs when the O_2 demand of the ventricles is greater than the O_2 supply
causes of angina	*coronary artery*: * **atherosclerosis**, * vasculitis, * embolization, * vasospasm
factors responsible for myocardial O_2 demand	• *HR:* * as HR increases, contractility increases (more action potential per unit time, more O_2 consumption, * reducing HR reduces O_2 consumption, * HR > 180 bpm decreases the length of diastole, which decreases filling of the coronary arteries, • *ventricular wall pressure:* * an increase in wall pressure increases O_2 consumption, * wall pressure increases when ventricles are hypertrophied (e.g., LVH, RVH) or when the radius of the ventricle is decreased owing to noncompliant muscle (most often the result of ischemia)
factor responsible for myocardial O_2 supply	*coronary artery blood flow*: flow is dependent on *coronary artery perfusion pressure* and *coronary artery resistance* to blood flow—resistance increases with fibrofatty plaques, thrombosis, vasospasm

Table continued on following page

Table 5–8. ISCHEMIC HEART DISEASE (IHD) *Continued*

Most Common...	Answer and Explanation
factors responsible for vasodilatation of the coronary artery	*regulated by the endothelium*: * endothelial cells contain NO, a potent vasodilator, * endothelial dysfunction decreases NO production (e.g., chemicals in cigarette smoke)
clinical manifestations of IHD	• **angina pectoris**, • AMI, • *sudden cardiac death (SCD)*: * death within 1 hour of chest pain, * accounts for ~50% of deaths due to CHD, • *chronic IHD*: severe fixed CAD with ischemic damage to the myocardium and replacement by fibrous tissue, • *cardiac arrhythmias*
causes of SCD	• **severe coronary artery atherosclerosis**: occlusive thrombi are not usually present at autopsy, • *MVP*, • *Marfan's syndrome*, • *IHSS*, • *AV stenosis*, • *prolonged QT interval syndrome*: see Table 5–6, • *conduction system defects*: * WPW, * see Table 5–6, • *cocaine abuse*
risk factors for SCD	• *cigarette smoking*, • *previous AMI*: particularly non-Q wave types, • *DM*, • *HTN*
COD in SCD	*VT/VF*
type of angina pectoris	*exertional angina*: associated with fixed atherosclerotic CAD
clinical findings in exertional angina	• *chest pain*: * precipitated by exercise, * relieved by rest and/or nitroglycerin, • *stress ECG*: ST segment depression
type of angina associated with vasospasm	*Prinzmetal's, or variant angina:* coronary artery vasospasm due to * platelet thrombi on top of the plaque's release of TXA_2 (vasoconstrictor) or * endothelial cell dysfunction
clinical findings in Prinzmetal's angina	• *primarily occurs in women <50 years old*, • *chest pain*: * occurs at rest, * usually occurs in the early morning, • *stress ECG*: ST segment elevation, • *coronary angiogram*: some atherosclerotic CAD, but not enough to cause the chest pain
type of angina associated with rest	*unstable angina*

Table 5-8. ISCHEMIC HEART DISEASE (IHD) *Continued*

Most Common...	Answer and Explanation
clinical findings of unstable angina	• *resting angina that usually arises out of pre-existing exertional angina or may be new onset*, • *chest pain*: occurs more frequently and may or not be relieved by rest, • *stress ECG*: * not usually recommended, * ST segment depression/elevation (less frequent), • *coronary angiogram*: * >50% have multivessel disease, * vessels have eccentric, irregular lumens, and rupture or fissuring of the plaques with the formation of nonocclusive thrombi, • *prognosis*: ~20% progress to an AMI in next 3 months
chest pain characteristics of angina pectoris	• *precipitating events*: * exertion (exertional type), * during meals, * stress/excitement, * may occur at rest (Prinzmetal's and unstable type), • *relieved by*: * rest (exertional type), • nitroglycerin, • *pain characteristics*: * tightness, * squeezing, * burning, * aching, • *pain location/radiation*: * retrosternal (90%), * radiation into the jaw, neck, left shoulder, or inner aspect of the arm, • *duration*: usually <3 minutes and rarely >20 minutes, • *time of day*: 6 AM–12 PM
signs of angina pectoris	• *increased HR and BP*, • *S4 heart sound*: decreased LV compliance due to ischemia, • *S3 heart sound*: if CHF is present, • *MV regurgitation murmur*: sign of CHF and/or papillary muscle dysfunction, • *inspiratory crackles*: sign of LHF
ECG findings in angina pectoris	• *downsloping depression of ST segment*: rarely ST segment elevation (Prinzmetal's type), • *T wave peaking or inversion*
screening test for angina pectoris	*stress ECG*
criteria for angina in a stress ECG	• *positive test*: 1–1.5 mm horizontal or downsloping ST segment depression at 0.08 sec after the J point of the ECG, • *radionuclide studies may be used in equivocal cases*: see Table 5–1, • *severe CHD*: * ST segment depression is an early event, * patient is unable to exercise, * hypotension, * ST segment depression >2 mm in multiple leads, • *severe CHD requiring coronary angiography*: stenosis ≥70% is clinically significant

Table continued on following page

Table 5–8. ISCHEMIC HEART DISEASE (IHD) *Continued*

Most Common...	Answer and Explanation
Rx of an acute attack of angina	*sublingual NG*
MOA of nitrates	• *decrease preload*: venodilators, • *decrease afterload*: vasodilate arterioles, • *vasodilate coronary arteries*: increase the blood flow and improve collateral blood flow, • *lower O_2 demand in the heart*
drug used in preventing angina	• **β-adrenergic blockers**: * initial drug of choice (see Table 5–4 for MOA), * decreases HR, BP, contractility, and myocardial O_2 demands, • *isosorbides*: * long-acting nitrates, * used in cases that are refractory to β-blockers, • *calcium channel blockers*: * direct coronary artery vasodilator, * decreases LV wall stress, * drugs of choice in Prinzmetal's angina or resistance to nitrates/β-blockers, • *aspirin*: * prevention of coronary artery thrombosis/strokes, * increases survival in unstable angina, • *Rx hyperlipidemias*: see Table 5–2, • *heparin*: * mainly used for unstable angina for ~2 days, * combined with aspirin, * angiography is recommended and patients are hospitalized with unstable angina
differences between PTCA and CABG for the Rx of occlusive CHD	• *PTCA advantages*: * less mortality than a CABG, * less post-AMI than a CABG, * procedure of choice for one- or two-vessel disease, * exception: left main coronary artery, • *PTCA disadvantages:* * higher rate of recurrence than CABG, * may require emergency CABG (4–5%), * risk of AMI 4–5% [Patients should be given aspirin before the procedure and heparin during and after the procedure.]
vessels used in the CABG procedure	• *internal mammary artery:* * graft patency is best with the internal mammary artery, * e.g., 90% patency rate after 10 years, • *saphenous veins*: * 40–50% patency rate after 10 years, * "arterialization" of the vessels, fibrosis, and occlusion
advantages of a CABG procedure over PTCA	• *greater rate of symptomatic relief from angina than PTCA*: however, longevity is not increased (exception: left main stem artery CABG), • *procedure of choice with two-vessel disease involving the proximal LAD and with three-vessel disease*, • *lower number of recur-*

Table 5–8. ISCHEMIC HEART DISEASE (IHD) *Continued*

Most Common...	Answer and Explanation
Continued	rences: * due to a longer graft patency, * PTCA has a 30–50% chance of restenosis after 3–6 months, • *diabetics have better outcomes with a CABG procedure than PTCA*
vessel thrombosed in an AMI in decreasing order	• *LAD,* • *RCA,* • *LCA*
clinical findings in a Q wave AMI	• *usually transmural*: ST segment elevation, • *occlusive thrombosis*: >90% of cases, • *large size,* • *increased early mortality*
clinical findings in a non-Q wave AMI	• *usually subendocardial*: * ST segment depression, * difficult to distinguish from unstable angina, • *occlusive thrombosis in 30% of cases,* • *small size,* • *increased risk of SCD within several months post-AMI*
cause of a silent AMI	*elderly patients and those with DM*: * due to autonomic neuropathy, * silent AMIs occur in ~25% of patients
cause of reperfusion injury of cardiac muscle in an AMI	*thrombolytic agents*: reperfusion injury refers to FR injury to injured cells by oxygen FRs and calcium
S/S with a high predictive value for an AMI	• *character of pain:* * crushing retrosternal chest pain lasting >30–45 min, * pain not relieved by nitroglycerin, • *radiation of pain*: down the ulnar aspect of the left arm, into the left shoulder, or jaw, • *pain associated with:* * diaphoresis, * dyspnea/tachypnea (signs of pulmonary congestion), * orthopnea (sign of LHF), • *negative predictors*: * pain produced with movement of the torso, * pain with tenderness over the chest wall
type of AMI associated with epigastric pain simulating GERD	*inferior wall AMI*: RCA thrombosis
factor influencing survival in an AMI	• **rapid transportation to a CCU**: * ~25% die before reaching the hospital, * most deaths occur in the first 2-hs after an AMI, • *ECG monitoring for arrhythmias in CCU,* • *thrombolytic therapy,* • *drug Rx for complications*

Table continued on following page

Table 5–8. ISCHEMIC HEART DISEASE (IHD) *Continued*

Most Common...	Answer and Explanation
criteria for thrombolytic Rx in an AMI	• *chest pain >30 minutes with new onset LBBB*, • *ST segment elevation >1 mm*, • *ST segment depression >2 mm in anterior leads* (posterior AMI) *within the last 12 hours*
clinical benefits of thrombolytic Rx in an AMI	• *initial choice for reperfusion after an AMI*: the earlier the initiation of Rx the greater the benefit, • *reduces mortality*, • *preserves LV function*, • *reduces the infarct size*
thrombolytic agents used for reperfusion	• *recombinant tPA*: * agents that are fibrin-specific are more expensive than SK, * greater incidence of intracranial hemorrhage than SK, * modest net clinical benefit in patient salvage (1%) over SK, * 60–90% patency rate, • *SK*: * less expensive, * 60% patency rate, • *use of heparin and aspirin*: * given concomitantly with the fibrin-specific thrombolytic agents (e.g., recombinant tPA), * controversial with SK, * recommended following Rx to prevent rethrombosis
signs of reperfusion	• *resolution of pain*, • *early peaking of CK-MB*: flushes the enzyme out of damaged tissue, • *precipitation of ventricular arrhythmias*, • *rapid evolution of Q waves*
complication of thrombolytic therapy	*bleeding*: intracranial hemorrhage is the most dangerous complication
lab parameters to follow thrombolytic Rx	• *aPTT*, • *Hb/Hct*, • *platelet count*
indications for PTCA in an AMI	• **contraindication for thrombolytic agent**, • *reperfusion failure with thrombolytic agents*, • *patients in cardiogenic shock*
initial management steps in Rx of an AMI	• *morphine sulphate for pain*: * vasodilates veins (decreases preload) and arterioles (decreases afterload), * decreases HR, • *oxygen*: treats the mild hypoxemia that may accompany an AMI, • *sublingual nitroglycerin*, • *aspirin*, • β-*blockers*: * limit infarct size, * reduces myocardial ischemia, • *ACE inhibitors*: particularly useful in * large infarcts, * LHF, * low EF (<0.40)
drugs used to limit infarct size	• **thrombolytic Rx**, • β-*blockers*, • *ACE inhibitors*

Table 5–8. ISCHEMIC HEART DISEASE (IHD) *Continued*

Most Common...	Answer and Explanation
complications in an AMI	• **arrhythmias**: VPD leading to VT and then to VF, • *LHF*, • *cardiogenic shock*, • *cardiac rupture*
time frame for cardiogenic shock and LHF in an AMI	*first 24-hs*: particularly if >40% of the LV is infarcted
Rx of shock and systolic dysfunction in an AMI	• *hypovolemic shock*: ∗ result of ♦ vomiting ♦ diaphoreses, ♦ previous diuretics, ∗ cautious infusion of isotonic saline until the PCWP (SGC measurement of LVEDP) reaches 15–18 mm Hg, • *pulmonary congestion* (edema): ∗ sign of noncompliant LV with back-up of blood into the lungs or volume overload, ∗ Rx with ♦ diuretics, ♦ IV nitroglycerin, • *systolic dysfunction*: ∗ recognized by a decrease in CO and an increase in PCWP (EF <0.40), ∗ may lead to hypoperfusion of the kidneys and ischemic ATN, ∗ Rx with ♦ IV nitroglycerin, ♦ ACE inhibitors, ♦ dobutamine
cause of cardiac tamponade in an AMI	*rupture of the anterior free wall of the LV*: ∗ 2nd–7th day post-AMI, ∗ ~10% deaths, ∗ frequents ♦ elderly women, ♦ patients with HTN, ♦ patients previously treated with NSAIDs or steroids (inhibit the repair process)
clinical findings in an IVS rupture	• *most common in LAD AMI*, • *pansystolic heart murmur*, • *hypotension/shock*, • *step-up of oxygen in the RV*
AMI associated with mural thrombosis	*anterior AMI*: ∗ usually LAD thrombosis, ∗ mixed venous and arterial clots, ∗ occur in ~2% of AMIs, ∗ danger of embolization
Rx to prevent mural thrombosis	• *heparin*, • *warfarin*, • *aspirin*
cerebral artery embolized to an AMI	*MCA:* results in an embolic stroke
causes of a mitral regurgitation murmur in an AMI	• **LHF**: dilatation of the MV ring due to volume overload in the LV, • *posteromedial papillary muscle dysfunction/rupture*: RCA thrombosis involving the inferoposterior part of the heart

Table continued on following page

Table 5–8. ISCHEMIC HEART DISEASE (IHD) *Continued*

Most Common...	Answer and Explanation
cause of reappearance of CK-MB after 3 days	*reinfarction*: * occurs in ~5–20% of patients, * frequently preceded by chest pain
cause of a friction rub during the first week of an AMI	*transmural infarction*: * increased vessel permeability leading to fibrinous pericarditis, * occurs in 15–25% of patients, * aspirin Rx of choice
late complication of an AMI	*ventricular aneurysm*: * occur in 10–20% of AMIs, * due to expansion in size of an infarct, * begin to develop after 1–2 weeks, * clinically recognized in 2–4 weeks
clinical/lab findings in ventricular aneurysms	• *precordial bulge noted during systole*, • *LHF*: correlates with size of the aneurysm, • *risk of thromboembolization*, • *rupture rarely occurs*, • *echocardiogram*: dyskinetic movement of the involved portion of LV, • *ECG*: persistence of ST segment elevation
mechanism of Dressler's syndrome	*autoimmune pericarditis:* • develops 2–10 weeks post-AMI, * thrombolytic Rx has reduced this compilation to <5%
clinical findings in Dressler's syndrome	• **fever**, • *pericarditis:* friction rub, • *pleuritis:* friction rub, • *effusions*: pericardial/pleural, • *arthralgias*, • *lab findings*: * neutrophilic leukocytosis, * elevated antimyocardial antibodies
Rx of Dressler's syndrome	*aspirin or indomethacin*
cause of an RV AMI	*RCA thrombosis*
S/S of an RV infarction	• *hypotension*, • *jugular venous distention*, • *right-sided S3 and S4*, • *positive Kussmaul sign*: see Table 5–1, • *preserved LV function*: PCWP measured by SGC shows normal to decreased pressure (PCWP increased in LV infarction)
sequential ECG findings in transmural AMI	• *peaked T waves*: area of ischemia, • *ST segment elevation*: * area of injury, * most consistent finding, * good indicator for thrombolytic Rx, • *symmetric T wave inversion*: area of ischemia, • *Q wave*: area of infarction [All of these changes occur in <70% of patients with an AMI. The lack of Q waves represents a non-Q wave infarction.]

Table 5–8. ISCHEMIC HEART DISEASE (IHD) *Continued*

Most Common...	Answer and Explanation
CK isoenzymes in cardiac tissue	• **CK-MM:** ~85%, • *CK-MB:* 10–15%
CK isoenzyme pattern in an AMI	• *initial increase in 4–6-hs,* • *peaks in 24-hs,* • *disappears in 1.5–3 days*
causes of FP CK-MB results	• **cross-reactivity with CK-BB**, • *delayed clearance of CK-MB from noncardiac sources*
LDH isoenzymes in cardiac tissue	$LDH_1 > LDH_2$: * normally, LDH_2 is > than LDH_1, * since heart muscle has a predominance of LDH_1, there is an LDH_1/LDH_2 flip
LDH_1/LDH_2 pattern in an AMI	• *peaks in 48–72 hs,* • *disappears in 7–14 d,* • *most useful for AMIs >24-h old,* • *troponin assays are replacing LDH isoenzymes:* see below
cause of an LDH_1/LDH_2 flip and increased LDH_5	• *AMI:* LDH_1/LDH_2 flip, • *RHF secondary to LHF leading to congestive hepatomegaly:* responsible for the increase in LDH_5, which is increased in liver tissue
time sequence of troponin-I in an AMI	• *initially increases in 2–12 hours after an AMI,* • *peaks in 24–48 hours,* • *returns to normal in 5–14 days* [Since it appears earlier and lasts longer than CK-MB, it is an excellent adjunct with CK-MB and replacement for LDH isoenzymes.]
COD in an AMI	*VT leading to VF and death*
factor determining the prognosis in an AMI	*degree of LV dysfunction:* LV dysfunction is evaluated with measurement of the EF by echocardiography or radionuclide techniques
discharge medications post-AMI	• *aspirin,* • *warfarin:* if the infarcts are large or AF is present, • β-*blockers:* * reduce mortality, * reduce rate of reinfarction, * reduce incidence of SCD, • *ACE inhibitors:* reduce mortality and incidence of CHF
non-drug–related recommendations post-AMI	• *submaximal stress ECG test before discharge,* • *cardiac rehabilitation program in 3–4 weeks,* • *resume sexual intercourse after 4 weeks,* • *return to work in 8 weeks*

Table continued on following page

Table 5–8. ISCHEMIC HEART DISEASE (IHD) *Continued*

Question: On day 4 of an AMI, a patient develops recurrent chest pain, hypotension, a pansystolic murmur heard best at the apex, left-sided S3/S4 heart sounds, and bibasilar rales. Both CK-MB and troponin-I are increased. Which of the following statements apply to this patient's complication? **SELECT 3**
  (A) Anterior AMI
  (B) Left heart failure
  (C) Papillary muscle dysfunction/rupture
  (D) Reinfarction
  (E) Ventricular aneurysm
  (F) Rupture of the anterior wall

Answers: (B), (C), (D): The patient has a reinfarction (reappearance of CK-MB after 3 days, **choice D**), papillary muscle dysfunction/rupture (pansystolic murmur at the apex, **choice C**) secondary to an inferior AMI (RCA supplies the posteromedial papillary muscle, **choice A is incorrect**), and LHF (bibasilar rales, S3/S4 heart sounds, **choice B**). The troponin-I levels are still elevated after 4 days. A ventricular aneurysm does not develop this early and is not associated with a heart murmur (**choice E is incorrect**). Rupture of the anterior wall implies an LAD thrombosis, which is not present in this patient (**choice F is incorrect**). Furthermore, in cardiac rupture, cardiac tamponade muffles the heart sounds and no murmur would be present.

ACE = angiotensin converting enzyme, AF = atrial fibrillation, AMI = acute myocardial infarction, aPTT = activated partial thromboplastin, ATN = acute tubular necrosis, AV = aortic valve, BP = blood pressure, CABG = coronary artery bypass graft, CAD = coronary artery disease, CCU = coronary care unit, CHD = coronary heart disease, CHF = congestive heart failure, CK = creatine kinase, CO = cardiac output, COD = cause of death, DM = diabetes mellitus, ECG = electrocardiogram, EF = ejection fraction, FP = false positive, FR = free radical, GERD = gastroesophageal reflux disease, Hb = hemoglobin, Hct = hematocrit, HTN = hypertension, HR = heart rate, IHD = ischemic heart disease, IHSS = idiopathic hypertrophic subaortic stenosis, IV = intravenous, IVS = interventricular septum, LAD = left anterior descending, LBBB = left bundle branch block, LCA = left circumflex artery, LDH = lactate dehydrogenase, LHF = left heart failure, LV = left ventricle, LVEDP = left ventricular end-diastolic pressure, LVH = left ventricular hypertrophy, MCA = middle cerebral artery, MOA = mechanism of action, MV = mitral valve, MVP = mitral valve prolapse, NG = nitroglycerin, NO = nitric oxide, NSAID = nonsteroidal anti-inflammatory drug, PCWP = pulmonary capillary wedge pressure, PTCA = percutaneous transluminal coronary angioplasty, RA = right atrium, RCA = right coronary artery, RHF = right heart failure, RV = right ventricle, RVH = right ventricular hypertrophy, Rx = treatment, SCD = sudden cardiac death, SGC = Swan-Gan catheter, SK = streptokinase, S/S = signs and symptoms, tPA = tissue plasminogen activator, TXA_2 = thromboxane A_2, VF = ventricular fibrillation, VPD = ventricular premature depolarizations, VT = ventricular tachycardia.

Table 5–9. VALVULAR HEART DISEASE

Most Common...	Answer and Explanation
immune-mediated valvular heart disease	*rheumatic heart disease* (RHD): peak age is 5–15 years of age
pathogenesis of RHD	• **immunologic damage due to cross-reactivity of antibodies directed against group A streptococci M protein with antigens also present in host tissue** [e.g., heart, synovial tissue], • *the initiating infection is usually a pharyngitis but may be a skin infection*
valves involved in RHD in descending order	• **MV:** 75–80%, • *AV:* 30%, • *TV,* • *PV* [Nonembolic vegetations develop along the line of closure of the MV • MV regurgitation initially occurs and progresses to MV stenosis if recurrent attacks occur.]
major criteria used for the Dx of ARF (Jones' criteria)	• **polyarthritis:** * 75%, * no joint deformity, • *carditis:* 35%, • *subcutaneous nodules:* * 10%, * similar to rheumatoid nodules, * located on extensor aspect of elbows, * more common in children, • *erythema marginatum:* 10%, • *chorea:* * 3%, * latest occurring manifestation
minor criteria used in Dx of acute ARF	• *arthralgia,* • *fever,* • *elevated ESR,* • *prolonged PR interval,* • *supporting evidence:* * positive throat culture for group A streptococcus, * elevated/rising ASO titers [Two major or one major and two minor are necessary to firm the diagnosis.]
COD in ARF	*myocarditis leading to heart failure*
chronic valvular diseases in RHD in descending order	• **MV stenosis:** most are discovered within 10 years of the initial attack, • *AV regurgitation,* • *MV regurgitation*
COD in chronic RHD	*heart failure secondary to MV stenosis*
Rx of ARF	• *IM benzathine penicillin G:* eradicate residual group A streptococci, • *salicylates:* reduce fever and joint pain, • *corticosteroids:* for patients with severe carditis and heart failure
recommendations for prophylaxis in RHD	*IM benzathine penicillin G:* q4 wks for at least 5 years from the most recent attack

Table continued on following page

Table 5–9. VALVULAR HEART DISEASE *Continued*

Most Common...	Answer and Explanation
valvular disease associated with hemoptysis	*MV stenosis:* * hemoptysis is secondary to pulmonary venous HTN, * anastomoses between the pulmonary and bronchial veins with subsequent development of submucosal varices in the bronchi
cause of MV stenosis	*chronic RHD*
cardiac signs in MV stenosis	• *accentuation of SI:* early in the disease when the valve is still pliable, • *OS:* see Table 5–1, • *mid-diastolic rumble:* heard best at the apex or along the left sternal border, • *increased P2:* if PH is present, • *parasternal heave:* RVH, if PH is present, • *hemoptysis:* see above, • *malar flush:* from chronic pulmonary congestion, • *Graham Steell murmur:* occurs in early diastole from PV regurgitation secondary to PH
clinical presentations of MV stenosis	• **dyspnea on exertion**, • *AF:* due to LA dilatation, • *dysphagia for solids:* due to LA enlargement pushing on esophagus, • *hoarseness:* due to LA enlargement and compression of left recurrent laryngeal nerve (Ortner's syndrome), • *evidence of systemic embolization:* 20% of cases, • *pulmonary edema,* • *RHF,* • *PH*
arrhythmia in MV stenosis	*AF:* * 50–80% of patients, * secondary to dilatation of the LA, * danger of clot formation and embolization, * requires long-term anticoagulation
cause of a left-to-right shunt in MV stenosis	*increased LA pressure in combination with an ASD:* called Lutembacher's syndrome
immune diseases associated with sterile valvular vegetations	• **RHD**, • *SLE:* * called Libman-Sacks endocarditis, * found in ~75% of autopsy cases, * usually no valve incompetence, * may be a site for IE
valvular disease associated with malignancy	*nonbacterial thrombotic endocarditis* (marantic vegetations): * MV most commonly involved, * associated with mucinous carcinomas of the colon, pancreas, or lungs, * paraneoplastic syndrome (see Table 4–1), * may embolize or become infected

Table 5–9. VALVULAR HEART DISEASE *Continued*

Most Common...	Answer and Explanation
valvular diseases associated with IE	• **MVP with regurgitation**: due to the high incidence of MVP in the United States, • *degenerative disease involving the AV and MV,* • *CHD:* * 10–20%, * PDA, * VSD, * coarctation, • *RHD*: 30%, • *prosthetic heart valves*
organisms producing infective endocarditis (IE)	• ***Streptococcus viridans***: 50–75%, • *Staphylococcus aureus*: 25%, • *Enterococci* [Blood cultures are positive in >85% of patients.]
organism involved with IE secondary to prosthetic heart valves	*Staphylococcus epidermidis* (coagulase negative): prosthetic heart valves are the most common predisposing cardiac lesion for nosocomial IE
source of bacteremia producing nosocomial IE	*intravenous catheters:* * *Staphylococcus aureus* is the most common organism associated with intravenous catheters, * indwelling urinary catheters are a common source of gram-negative IE
organism producing IE in a patient with colon cancer of IBD	*Streptococcus bovis*
procedures leading to bacteremia and IE	• *dental procedures inducing mucosal bleeding,* • *cystoscopy,* • *GB surgery,* • *vaginal hysterectomy,* • *urologic surgery*
organism producing IE after dental or upper respiratory procedures	*Streptococcus viridans*
prophylaxis recommended to prevent IE	*amoxicillin*: prescribed 1 hour before certain dental (e.g., dental extraction), esophageal (e.g., sclerotherapy of esophageal varices), respiratory tract procedures (e.g., bronchoscopy with a rigid scope)
organism producing IE after a GI or GU procedure	*Enterococcus:* amoxicillin is usually administered 1 hour before GI/GU procedures
cause of culture negative IE	*inadequate treatment of a prior IE*
investigative test used to diagnose and follow IE	*echocardiography:* including transthoracic and transesophageal echocardiography

Table continued on following page

Table 5–9. VALVULAR HEART DISEASE *Continued*

Most Common...	Answer and Explanation
valve involved in IE	*MV*: * vegetations are bulky and friable, * danger of septic embolization
organism producing IE in an IVDA	*Staphylococcus aureus*
valves involved in IVDA in descending order	• *TV*: * 44%, * usually an isolated lesion, * produces tricuspid regurgitation, • *MV*: 43%, • *AV*: 40%, • *two valves involved*: 16%
S/S of IE	• **fever**, • *arthralgias/myalgias*, • *heart murmurs*: changing murmurs are uncommon, • *CHF*, • *signs related to systemic embolization*: * hematuria, * embolic stroke, * friction rub over the spleen, • *metastatic abscesses*: CNS abscesses, • *splenomegaly*, • *IC-induced vasculitis findings*: * Roth's spot in the retina, * splinter hemorrhages of the nails, * Osler's nodes (painful nodules on the hands and feet), * Janeway's lesions (painless lesions on the hands and feet), * GN
complication of IE	*CHF*: most commonly occurs with left-sided valvular lesions
organisms producing IE that have the highest mortality	• **IE due to fungi and aerobic gram-negative enteric organisms**, • *Staphylococcus aureus*, • *Enterococcus*, • *Streptococcus viridans*
valves involved with the highest mortality in IE	• **AV**, • *early onset prosthetic valve IE has a greater mortality than native valve IE*
initial Rx for *Staphylococcus aureus* IE	*oxacillin + an aminoglycoside* (gentamicin or tobramycin)
initial Rx for *Streptococcus viridans* IE	*penicillin G*: vancomycin is used in penicillin-allergic patients
initial Rx for *Enterococcus* spp. IE	*ampicillin* (or penicillin) + *gentamicin*
initial Rx for *Staphylococcus epidermidis*	*vancomycin*

Table 5–9. **VALVULAR HEART DISEASE** *Continued*

Most Common...	Answer and Explanation
valvular lesion not requiring antibiotic prophylaxis	*MVP not complicated by MV regurgitation*
valvular heart disease	*mitral valve prolapse* (MVP): * occurs in ~5–10% of the population, * most occur in tall, thin women
cause of MVP	*myxomatous degeneration*: * leads to redundancy of the MV leaflets, * anterior and posterior (most common) valve leaflets involved, * AD inheritance pattern in some cases, * increased in ♦ Marfan's syndrome, ♦ Ehlers-Danlos syndrome, ♦ fragile X syndrome, ♦ APKD
cause of sudden death in Marfan's syndrome	*MVP*
S/S of MVP	• **most cases are asymptomatic**, • *chest pain:* **most common symptomatic presentation**, • *postural hypotension*, • *palpitations*, • *fatigue*
cardiac signs in MVP	*mid-systolic ejection click followed by a mid- to late systolic murmur of mitral regurgitation*: MV leaflets prolapse into the LA like a parachute during systole
maneuvers that move the click and murmur of MVP closer to S1	*see Table 5–1*
maneuvers that move the click and murmur of MVP closer to S2	*see Table 5–1*
complications associated with MVP	• **isolated MV regurgitation**: most common cause is MVP, • *rupture of the chordae*: acute MV regurgitation, • *SCD*: usually due to VT, • *autonomic dysfunction*: decreased parasympathetic and increased α-adrenergic tone lead to VT and the potential for sudden death, • *IE*

Table continued on following page

Table 5–9. VALVULAR HEART DISEASE *Continued*

Most Common...	Answer and Explanation
method of diagnosing MVP	*echocardiography*: * identifies the movement of the MV leaflets into the LA, * when the posterior leaflet prolapses into the LA in late systole it has an inverted ? mark appearance, * a hammock configuration occurs when the posterior leaflet prolapses into the LA throughout most of systole
Rx for symptomatic MVP	• **β-blockers**, • *calcium channel blockers* [These drugs have a negative inotropic effect, hence reducing the amount of stress on the chordae tendineae.]
causes of MV regurgitation	• **MVP**, • *RHD*, • *IE*, • *papillary muscle dysfunction/rupture*: AMI, • *CHF*
cardiac findings in MV regurgitation	• *apical pansystolic murmur radiating into the axilla and left parasternal border*, • *S1 and S2 often obscured by the murmur*, • *left-sided S3*, • *prominent PMI and displacement to the left mid-clavicular line*, • *AF*: commonly present (75%) due to LA dilatation
causes of AV stenosis	• **congenital bicuspid AV**: >50% of cases, • *degenerative disease of the AV*: most common cause in * patients >70 years old, * smokers, * hypertensives, • *RHD*
valvular lesion associated with syncope with exercise and angina	*AV stenosis*
mechanism for syncope/angina with exercise in AV stenosis	• *stenotic valve*: decreases cardiac output (less blood to the brain leads to syncope), • *concentric hypertrophy of LV*: hypertrophied muscle has a greater myocardial O_2 consumption (reason for angina)
valvular lesion associated with microangiopathic hemolytic anemia	*AV stenosis*: * RBCs hitting the calcified valve are damaged (produces schistocytes) leading to an intravascular hemolysis, * see Table 8–6

Table 5–9. VALVULAR HEART DISEASE *Continued*

Most Common...	Answer and Explanation
cardiac findings in AV stenosis	• *harsh systolic ejection type murmur heard best at the upper right or left sternal border*: sometimes heard best in the apex in elderly patients, • *radiation into the carotid arteries,* • *diminished S2,* • *prominent S4,* • *systolic ejection click,* • *prominent PMI,* • *delay in upstroke of the peripheral pulse,* • *narrow pulse pressure,* • *normal sized heart on chest x-ray:* * concentric hypertrophy does not enlarge the heart, * increased heart size and S3 indicate heart failure with volume overload, • *calcification of the AV on chest x-ray:* usually evident by 40–45 years of age
cardiac findings in aortic sclerosis	*see Table 5–1*
causes of AV regurgitation	• **long-standing HTN,** • *aortic root/annulus disease*: medial disease of the aorta (some authors state that this is the most common cause of AV regurgitation), • *bicuspid AV,* • *IE,* • *dissecting aortic aneurysm*: AV regurgitation is the most common valvular lesion, *coarctation of the aorta*: proximal dilatation of aortic valve ring, • *ankylosing spondylitis*: valve inflammation, • *tertiary syphilis*: AV ring dilatation
cause of acute AV regurgitation	*infective IE in IVDA*: in acute AV regurgitation, the LV is not as dilated as in chronic AV regurgitation, where it is dilated and has a laterally displaced PMI
cause of an Austin-Flint murmur	*AV regurgitation*: * the Austin-Flint murmur is a rumbling diastolic murmur secondary to blood dripping from the incompetent AV onto the anterior MV leaflet, * the murmur is preceded by an S3 heart sound, * it is heard best at the apex, * marker of severe regurgitant AV disease that requires valve replacement

Table continued on following page

Table 5–9. VALVULAR HEART DISEASE *Continued*

Most Common...	Answer and Explanation
heart murmur most often confused with the Austin-Flint murmur	*MV stenosis:* unlike MV stenosis, an Austin-Flint murmur does not have an OS and S1 is not accentuated
cardiac findings in AV regurgitation	• *high-pitched blowing murmur after S2,* • *soft S1 heart sound,* • *hyperdynamic PMI with lateral displacement beyond the mid-clavicular line,* • *wide pulse pressure:* see Table 5–1, • *bisferiens pulse:* see Table 5–1, • *Corrigan's water hammer pulse:* see Table 5–1 for other signs of a hyperdynamic circulation
cause of tricuspid stenosis	*chronic RHD:* tricuspid stenosis usually occurs in association with MV stenosis
cardiac findings in TV stenosis	• *heart murmur is similar to MV stenosis except that it increases in inspiration,* • *giant* a wave *in the JVP*
causes of TV regurgitation	• **RHF owing to stretching of the ring from RV dilatation,** • *carcinoid syndrome:* serotonin increases fibrosis of valve leaflets, • *IE in IVDA*
cardiac findings in TV regurgitation	• *pansystolic murmur that increases with inspiration:* heard best along the left parasternal border, • *giant* c-v *wave in the JVP,* • *hepatic pulsation during systole*
causes of PV stenosis	• *congenital:* infravalvular stenosis in tetralogy of Fallot, • *acquired:* carcinoid heart disease
cardiac findings in PV stenosis	• *systolic ejection murmur heard best in the left upper sternal border,* • *left parasternal heave:* RVH, • *right-sided S4,* • *giant* a wave *in the JVP*
causes of PV regurgitation	• **PH,** • *elevated PA pressure from MV stenosis*
cardiac findings in PV regurgitation	*early diastolic blowing murmur after P2:* when associated with PH, it is called the Graham Steell murmur

Table 5–9. VALVULAR HEART DISEASE *Continued*

Most Common...	Answer and Explanation
valve abnormalities in carcinoid heart disease	• *TV regurgitation*, • *PV stenosis*

Question: A 25-year-old man with a long history of IVDA presents with fever, neck vein distention, hepatomegaly, and a pansystolic murmur that increases with inspiration. Which of the following are additional findings you would expect in this patient? **SELECT 2**
- (A) Giant <u>a wave</u> in the JVP
- (B) Pulmonary edema
- (C) Right-sided S3 heart sound
- (D) Accentuated P2
- (E) *Staphylococcus epidermidis* septicemia
- (F) Pulsatile liver

Answers: (C), (F): The patient has TV regurgitation (pansystolic murmur that increases with inspiration) most likely secondary to acute IE due to *S. aureus* (not *S. epidermidis*; **choice E is incorrect**). Owing to RV volume overload, a right-sided S3 would be expected (**choice C**); a giant c-v wave (not a giant a wave, which is noted in TV stenosis; **choice A is incorrect**), and a pulsatile liver as increased venous pressure is transmitted back into the liver (**choice F**). Pulmonary edema would more likely occur in a left-sided valvular lesion (e.g., AV regurgitation, MV regurgitation; **choice B is incorrect**), and an accentuated P2 in PH secondary to MV stenosis rather than TV regurgitation (**choice D is incorrect**).

AD = autosomal dominant, AF = atrial fibrillation, AMI = acute myocardial infarction, APKD = adult polycystic kidney disease, ARF = acute rheumatic fever, ASD = atrial septal defect, ASO = anti-streptolysin O, AV = aortic valve, CHD = congenital heart disease, CHF = congestive heart failure, CNS = central nervous system, COD = cause of death, Dx = diagnosis, ESR = erythrocyte sedimentation rate, GB = gallbladder, GI = gastrointestinal, GN = glomerulonephritis, GU = genitourinary, HTN = hypertension, IBD = inflammatory bowel disease, IC = immuno-complex, IE = infective endocarditis, IM = intramuscular, IVDA = intravenous drug abuse, JVP = jugular venous pulse, LA = left atrium, LV = left ventricle, MV = mitral valve, MVP = mitral valve prolapse, OS = opening snap, PDA = patent ductus arteriosus, PH = pulmonary hypertension, PMI = point of maximal impulse, PV = pulmonic valve, RBC = red blood cell, RHD = rheumatic heart disease, RHF = right heart failure, RV = right ventricle, RVH = right ventricular hypertrophy, Rx = treatment, SCD = sudden cardiac death, SLE = systemic lupus erythematosus, S/S = signs and symptoms, TV = tricuspid valve, VSD = ventricular septal defect, VT = ventricular tachycardia.

Table 5–10. MYOCARDIAL AND PERICARDIAL DISORDERS

Most Common...	Answer and Explanation
cause of myocarditis	*viral infection:* coxsackievirus B
parasitic diseases causing myocarditis	• **Chagas' disease due to *Trypanosoma cruzi***: * common cause of myocarditis in Central and South America, * transmitted by the bite of a Reduviid bug, * leishmanial forms invade the cardiac muscle, • *trichinosis: Trichinosis spiralis:* may also invade cardiac tissue
toxin-induced myocarditis	*diphtheria exotoxin produced by Cornyebacterium diphtheriae*
collagen vascular diseases associated with myocarditis	• **progressive systemic sclerosis**, • *rheumatoid arthritis*, • *SLE*
causes of drug-induced myocarditis	• **doxorubicin**, • *tricyclic antidepressants*, • *α-interferon*, • *cocaine*, • *cyclophosphamide*
S/S of myocarditis	• **chest pain**, • *fatigue*, • *sinus tachycardia*, • *S3/S4 heart sounds*, • *pericardial friction rub*
confirmatory test for myocarditis	*endomyocardial biopsy:* * in viral myocarditis, there is a patchy lymphocyte infiltration with focal areas of necrosis, * echocardiography documents cardiomegaly
lab findings in myocarditis	• *ST/T wave changes*, • *CM-MB and troponin-I may be elevated*
type of cardiomyopathy	*congestive* (dilated) *cardiomyopathy*
causes of congestive cardiomyopathy	• **previous viral myocarditis**, • *idiopathic*, • *postpartum state*, • *alcohol*: * direct toxic effect, * thiamine deficiency, • *drugs*: doxorubicin, • *cocaine*, • *hypothyroidism*: myxedema heart
S/S of congestive cardiomyopathy	• **dyspnea secondary to CHF**, • *easy fatigability*, • *palpitations*, • *classic signs of both LHF/RHF*: see Table 5–5, • *pulsus alternans*: see Table 5–1, • *MV/TV regurgitation*
lab abnormalities in congestive cardiomyopathy	• *generalized cardiomegaly*, • *global myocardial dysfunction noted on echocardiography*: best means of diagnosis, • *EF <0.30*: normal ≥0.55, • *ECG*: low voltage QRS, • *endomyocardial biopsy*: generally not recommended

Table 5–10. MYOCARDIAL AND PERICARDIAL
DISORDERS *Continued*

Most Common...	Answer and Explanation
Rx of congestive cardiomyopathy	• **treat the underlying cause**, • *anticoagulation*: high incidence of LA mural thrombi, • *management of LHF/RHF*: see Table 5–5, • *partial left ventriculectomy*, • *cardiac transplantation in medically resistant cases*
cardiomyopathy associated with SCD, syncope, and angina with exercise	• *hypertrophic cardiomyopathy* (HCM): * SCD is secondary to abnormalities in the conduction system in the asymmetrically hypertrophied IVS (e.g., WPW, left anterior hemiblock), * syncope and angina with exercise is similar in pathogenesis to AV stenosis (see Table 5–9), • *~20–30% have an AD pattern of inheritance*: mutational defect of β-cardiac myosin heavy chains
cause of the obstruction in HCM	*sharp systolic anterior motion of the anterior MV leaflet against the asymmetrically hypertrophied IVS*: the rapid ejection of blood through the narrow outflow space sucks the anterior leaflet against the IVS wall
S/S of HCM	• **exertional dyspnea**, • *PND secondary to pulmonary congestion*, • *chest pain*, • *syncope*, • *dizziness with exercise*: see above, • *exercise-induced angina*: see above, • *palpitations*: atrial/ventricular arrhythmias
cardiac findings in HCM	• *systolic ejection murmur* • best heard along the left sternal border/apex, • *sharp upstroke of the carotid arterial pulse*, • *bisferiens peripheral pulse*: see Table 5–1, • *sustained PMI*: LVH, • *S4*: universally present, • *paradoxical split of S2*: * late closure of the AV, * see Table 5–1, • *MV regurgitation murmur*: anterior leaflet movement in systole interferes with proper closure of MV
drugs used in Rx HCM	• **β-blockers**, • *calcium channel blockers* [These drugs decrease myocardial contractility, which increases LVEDV and cardiac output and relieves the obstruction.]
maneuvers that decrease murmur intensity in HCM	*increase venous return to the heart*: * squatting, * lying down

Table continued on following page

Table 5–10. MYOCARDIAL AND PERICARDIAL DISORDERS *Continued*

Most Common...	Answer and Explanation
maneuvers/drugs that increase murmur intensity in HCM	• *positive inotropic agents*: * increased contraction increases the degree of obstruction, * e.g., digitalis, • *reduce venous return to the heart*: * venodilators (nitro drugs), • Valsalva maneuver
differences in the cardiac findings of AV stenosis and HCM	• *intensity of the murmur of HCM decreases with squatting*: * an increase in LVEDV decreases murmur intensity in HCM, * an increase in LVEDV increases the murmur of AV stenosis since more blood must be pushed through the stenotic valve, • *intensity of the murmur of HCM decreases with sustained hand grip exercises*: * hand grip exercises increase LVEDV, * the murmur of HCM decreases while the murmur of AV stenosis increases
method for diagnosing HCM	*echocardiography*: * demonstrates the asymmetric IVS and abnormal MV anterior leaflet motility, * there is a sharp upstroke of the carotid pulse
COD in HCM	*SCD*: usually secondary to VT
drug used to prevent SCD in HCM	*amiodarone*: * suppresses the majority of atrial and ventricular arrhythmias, * see Table 5–6
mechanisms of heart failure in restrictive cardiomyopathy	• *systolic dysfunction*: * due to reduced contractility, * decreased EF, • *diastolic dysfunction*: reduced compliance of the ventricles, • *ECG reveals a low voltage pattern and conduction disturbances*
causes of restrictive cardiomyopathy in adults	• *amyloidosis*: * low voltage ECG, * conduction disturbances, • *post-radiation therapy*, • *post-open heart surgery*, • *iron overload: e.g., hemochromatosis*
effect of digoxin in amyloid cardiomyopathy	*digoxin toxicity*: * amyloid in cardiac muscle absorbs digoxin, * sudden release of digoxin from muscle leads to toxicity
cardiac tumor in adults	*cardiac myxoma*: * most cardiac myxomas arise in the LA (80%), * ~15% arise from the RA

Table 5–10. MYOCARDIAL AND PERICARDIAL
DISORDERS *Continued*

Most Common...	Answer and Explanation
valvular lesion confused with a cardiac myxoma	*MV stenosis*: cardiac myxomas obstruct the MV orifice leading to a mid-diastolic rumble, syncope, sudden death, left-sided heart failure, chest pain, and dyspnea
S/S of cardiac myxomas	• *constitutional signs*: * fever, * fatigue, * weight loss, * elevated ESR, * arthralgia, * myalgias, * Raynaud's phenomenon, • *embolization*: * ~50% of patients, * embolize to ♦ CNS, ♦ coronary arteries, ♦ peripheral organs/viscera
method of diagnosing a cardiac myxoma	*transesophageal ultrasonography*
Rx of cardiac myxoma	*surgery*
cancers of the heart	• **metastatic disease from a primary in the lung or breast** • *metastatic malignant melanoma* • *metastatic malignant lymphomas*, • *metastatic Kaposi's sarcoma*
cause of pericarditis	*viral infection*: most commonly secondary to coxsackievirus B
causes of bacterial pericarditis	• *Streptococci spp*, • *Staphylococci spp*, • *gram-negative rods*
causes of metabolic pericarditis	• **uremia**: * pericarditis occurs in ~one-third of cases, * due to ♦ nondialyzable chemicals, ♦ autoimmune disease, ♦ infection, • *myxedema:* effusion sometimes contains CH, • *amyloidosis*
collagen vascular diseases associated with pericarditis	• **SLE**: * most common cardiac manifestation of SLE, * may also occur in drug-induced lupus erythematosus, • *rheumatoid arthritis*: one-third of cases
S/S of pericarditis	• *precordial chest pain*: * aggravated by lying down, * relieved by sitting up, • *friction rub*: see Table 5–1, • *effusion*
ECG findings in pericarditis	• **diffuse ST segment elevation with an upward concavity**, • *inversion of T waves*

Table continued on following page

Table 5–10. MYOCARDIAL AND PERICARDIAL DISORDERS *Continued*

Most Common...	Answer and Explanation
causes of constrictive pericarditis	• **tuberculosis**: * most common cause worldwide, * arises from hematogenous spread of primary TB, • **idiopathic**: most common cause in the United States, • *prior open heart surgery,* • *radiation of the mediastinum,* • *neoplastic disease,* • *previous pericarditis*
S/S of constrictive pericarditis	• **dyspnea**, • *JVP distention,* • *pericardial knock*: * there is some early diastolic filling of the chambers until the chambers encounter the thick pericardium (knock is produced), * in pericardial effusions, there is very little filling of the chamber in early or late diastole, • *ascites,* • *hepatosplenomegaly,* • *pitting edema,* • *Kussmaul's sign and pulsus paradoxus*: not usually evident (see Table 5–1), • *pericardial calcifications may be present on chest radiographs*
method of distinguishing constrictive pericarditis from restrictive cardiomyopathy	• *catheterization:* * equal elevation of all pressures in all four cardiac chambers in constrictive pericarditis, * differences in end-diastolic pressures are more variable with restrictive cardiomyopathy after volume loading and after exercise, * pericardial knock and an RVEDP that is more than one-third of the peak systolic pressure are more commonly seen in constrictive pericarditis than in restrictive cardiomyopathy, • *CT scan*: demonstration of pericardial thickening is a very useful test in distinguishing constrictive pericarditis from restrictive cardiomyopathy
S/S of a pericardial effusion	• **Beck's triad**: * hypotension, * elevated JVP, * muffled heart sounds, • *Kussmaul's sign and pulsus paradoxus*: see Table 5–1. • *all the chambers have restricted filling throughout diastole*: no pericardial knock
first step in the Dx and Rx of a pericardial effusion	*echocardiogram followed by a pericardial paracentesis*: a chest radiograph reveals a "water bottle" configuration
causes of cardiac tamponade	• *rupture of the heart in an AMI,* • *trauma,* • *neoplastic disease*

Table 5–10. MYOCARDIAL AND PERICARDIAL DISORDERS *Continued*

Most Common...	Answer and Explanation
pathogenesis of heart failure in tamponade	• *elevated intrapericardial pressure >15 mm Hg and equal elevation of atrial and pericardial pressures,* • *may be secondary to any of the causes of a pericardial effusion,* • *increase in intrapericardial pressure restricts venous return and filling of the ventricles, leading to a reduction in cardiac output and death*
Rx of cardiac tamponade	*pericardiocentesis*

Question: In a patient with HCM, which of the following reduce the intensity of the murmur and improve the cardiac output? **SELECT 3**
  (A) Squatting
  (B) β-blocker
  (C) Digoxin
  (D) Nitrates
  (E) Calcium channel blocker
  (F) Isoproterenol
  (G) Exercise

Answers: (A), (B), (E): any maneuver or drug that increases the LVEDV will diminish the intensity of the murmur and improve the cardiac output. Squatting **(choice A)**, β-blockers **(choice B)**, and calcium channel blockers **(choice E)** all increase LVEDV. Nitrates are venodilators that reduce venous return to the heart, hence decreasing the LVEDV **(choice D is incorrect)**. Isoproterenol and digoxin are inotropic agents that increase the force of contraction and reduce the LVEDV **(choices C and F are incorrect)**. Exercise increases the heart rate, hence reducing LVEDV **(choice G is incorrect)**.

AD = autosomal dominant, AMI = acute myocardial infarction, AV = aortic valve, CH = cholesterol, CHF = congestive heart failure, CK = creatine kinase, CNS = central nervous system, COD = cause of death, CT = computed tomography; ECG = electrocardiogram, EF = ejection fraction, ESR = erythrocyte sedimentation rate, HCM = hypertrophic cardiomyopathy, IVS = interventricular septum, JVP = jugular venous pulse, LA = left atrium, LHF = left heart failure, LVEDV = left ventricular end-diastolic volume, LVH = left ventricular hypertrophy, MV = mitral valve, PMI = point of maximal impulse, PND = paroxysmal nocturnal dyspnea, RA = right atrium, RHF = right heart failure, RVEDP = right ventricular end-diastolic pressure, Rx = treatment, SCD = sudden cardiac death, SLE = systemic lupus erythematosus, S/S = signs and symptoms, TB = tuberculosis, TV = tricuspid valve, VT = ventricular tachycardia, WPW = Wolff-Parkinson-White syndrome.

CHAPTER

6

PULMONARY DISEASE

CONTENTS

Table 6–1. SYMPTOMS AND SIGNS OF RESPIRATORY DISEASE

Most Common...	Answer and Explanation
symptom of respiratory disease	*dyspnea:* see Table 5–1
causes of dyspnea due to increased work of breathing	• *decreased compliance:* interstitial fibrosis, • *increased airway resistance:* e.g., bronchial asthma, • *chest bellows disease:* e.g., obesity
tests for evaluation of dyspnea	• **chest radiograph:** e.g., R/O COPD, • *bronchoscopy:* suspected airway obstruction
causes of cough with a normal chest radiograph	• **postnasal discharge,** • *acute inflammation*: viral URI, • *GERD*
cause of nocturnal cough	*GERD:* acid reflux into the tracheobronchial tree at night
causes of productive cough	• **cigarette smoking:** cough in CB is usually most prominent in the AM, • *bacterial pneumonia:* greenish-yellow sputum, • *bronchiectasis:* copious amounts of sputum

Table continued on following page

**Table 6–1. SYMPTOMS AND SIGNS OF
RESPIRATORY DISEASE** *Continued*

Most Common...	Answer and Explanation
infectious cause of nonproductive cough	*atypical pneumonia due to* Mycoplasma pneumoniae
drugs causing cough	• *ACE inhibitors:* bradykinin effect, • *aspirin*
cause of persistent cough	*bronchial asthma*: persistent cough often precedes wheezing
tests for chronic cough	• *sputum for cytology, culture, Gram stain, acid-fast stain:* R/O infection, cancer, • *chest radiograph:* R/O anatomic cause for cough, • *bronchoscopy:* suspected airway abnormality, • *sinus radiographs:* suspected sinusitis, • *esophageal pH monitoring:* suspected GERD
mechanism of hemoptysis	• **parenchymal necrosis,** • *vessel damage:* bronchial or pulmonary
causes of hemoptysis	• **CB,** • *pneumonia,* • *cancer* [Hemoptysis is coughing up blood-tinged sputum.]
upper respiratory cause of hemoptysis	*epistaxis* (nosebleed)
causes of massive hemoptysis	• *TB,* • bronchiectasis, • *cancer, aspergilloma* [Massive hemoptysis is coughing up of >600 mL/48-h.]
tests for evaluating hemoptysis	• *chest radiograph,* • *sputum cytology, Gram stain, acid-fast stain/culture,* • *ABGs,* • *UA:* R/O Goodpasture's, • *bronchoscopy:* first step in management to R/O cancer, if risk factors are present
causes of chest pain of respiratory origin	• **pleuritis secondary to pneumonia,** • *pleuritis due to a pulmonary infarction* [Pleuritis is a sharp inspiratory pain that increases in magnitude with breathing.]
causes of bradypnea	• **respiratory depressants:** e.g., DOA, • *uremia,* • intracranial HTN [Bradypnea is a slow, regular respiratory rate <14 cycles/minute (normal = 14–18 cycles/minute).]
causes of tachypnea	• **fever/anxiety,** • anemia, • *pulmonary infections,* • *pleuritic pain* [Tachypnea is rapid, shallow breathing (16–25 cycles/min).]
causes of Kussmaul breathing	• **DKA,** • *uremia* [Kussmaul's breathing is a regular, deep, sighing type of breathing.]

Table 6–1. SYMPTOMS AND SIGNS OF
RESPIRATORY DISEASE *Continued*

Most Common...	Answer and Explanation
causes of hyperpnea	• **emphysema,** • *hypoglycemia affecting the midbrain or pons,* • *tissue hypoxia* [Hyperpnea is rapid, deep breathing regardless of what the $PaCO_2$ is in the patient.]
type of periodic breathing	*Cheyne-Stokes breathing:* * periods of apnea (no breathing) followed regularly with periods of hyperpnea, * crescendo/decrescendo pattern
causes of Cheyne-Stokes breathing	• **normal during sleep in children and in the elderly,** • *LHF,* • *intracranial HTN*
causes of Biot's breathing	• **meningitis,** • *pontine disease* [Biot's breathing is a variant of Cheyne-Stokes breathing. Breathing is *irregular* and of *equal depth* and then ends abruptly *(lacks a crescendo/decrescendo pattern).* It is followed by a variable period of apnea.]
types of cyanosis	• **peripheral cyanosis:** * redistribution of oxygenated blood from the skin to internal organs, * dusky skin but normal mucous membranes, • *central cyanosis:* * decrease in SaO_2 (<85%), * dusky skin and mucous membranes
causes of peripheral cyanosis	• **cold temperature,** • *hypovolemic/cardiogenic shock*
causes of central cyanosis	• **lung disorders:** * V/Q defects in the lungs (COPD), * alveolar hypoventilation, * diffusion defects (interstitial fibrosis), • *cardiac disorders:* * right to left intracardiac shunts (tetralogy of Fallot), • *Hb disorders:* metHb ≥1.5 g/dL, • *hypoxemia ≤60 mm Hg*
causes of inspiratory stridor	*upper airway obstruction:* * food (cafe coronary), * epiglottitis [Stridor is a high-pitched inspiratory sound associated with upper airway obstruction.]
cause of inspiratory/ expiratory stridor	*fixed upper airway obstruction:* e.g., cancer
normal breath sound	*vesicular:* inspiration > expiration
abnormal breath sounds	• **wheezing:** * expiration longer than inspiration, * high-pitched sound, * occur in small

Table continued on following page

Table 6–1. SYMPTOMS AND SIGNS OF
RESPIRATORY DISEASE *Continued*

Most Common...	Answer and Explanation
Continued	airway disease, • *bronchial breath sounds:* * expiration longer than inspiration, * occur in pulmonary consolidations
causes of wheezing	• **bronchial asthma,** • *pulmonary edema:* peribronchiolar edema, • *bronchiolitis:* RSV, • **PE with infarction:** TXA$_2$ (bronchoconstrictor) released from platelets, • *carcinoid syndrome:* serotonin is a bronchoconstrictor
site for normal airway resistance	*segmental bronchi:* * airflow is turbulent in this location, * conducting airways proximal to the bronchioles exhibit turbulent breathing
site for laminar air flow	*terminal bronchioles:* * terminal and respiratory bronchioles are "small airways," * parallel branching increases the cross-sectional area of these airways and converts turbulent into laminar air flow, * inflammation of the terminal bronchiole causes air trapping, wheezing, and increased airway resistance
causes of crackles (rales)	• *reduced compliance in the small airways or alveoli due to fluid or fibrosis:* inspiratory crackles occur when there is a sudden opening of previously closed small airways (delayed elastic recoil) and alveoli, • *early inspiratory crackles:* * transmitted to the mouth and are not altered by coughing, * indicate severe obstruction (CB, emphysema, asthma), • *late inspiratory crackles:* * not transmitted to the mouth, * located at the lung bases, * indicate decreased compliance and increased elasticity (interstitial fibrosis)
cause of moist coarse rales (rhonchi)	*airflow through large bronchi encountering liquids of different viscosities:* * pulmonary edema, * bronchitis, * bacterial pneumonia
cause of moist fine rales	*alveolar fluid:* * pulmonary edema, * pneumonia
cause of dry rales	*movements of thick exudates:* bacterial pneumonia
signs of lung consolidation	• *decreased percussion,* • *increased tactile fremitus:* increased vibration of chest wall, • *egophony:* e sounds like a, • *whispered pectoriloquy:* whispered syllables become clear

Table 6–1. SYMPTOMS AND SIGNS OF
RESPIRATORY DISEASE *Continued*

Most Common...	Answer and Explanation
signs of a pleural effusion	• *decreased percussion*, • *absence of consolidation signs*, • *bronchial breath sounds heard above and through the fluid*
causes of hyper-resonance to percussion	• **increased AP diameter:** emphysema, • *pneumothorax:* collapse of the lungs
causes of clubbing	• **pulmonary disease:** * bronchiectasis, * CF, • *cyanotic CHD*, • *GI disease:* IBD [Clubbing refers to a bulbous enlargement of the ends of fingers and/or toes. There is loss of the normal angle ($\leq$160 degrees) between the skin and the nail ($\geq$180 degrees).]

Question: A 28-year-old man presents with an abrupt onset of spiking fever, cough productive of yellowish-green sputum, and pain on inspiration. A Gram stain of sputum reveals neutrophils with numerous gram-positive diplococci. Which of the following additional findings would you expect in the lungs? **SELECT 4**

    (A) Hyper-resonance to percussion
    (B) Uniform vesicular breathing
    (C) Fine rales/rhonchi
    (D) Egophony
    (E) Decreased tactile fremitus
    (F) Bronchial breath sounds
    (G) Inspiratory/expiratory wheezing
    (H) Whispered pectoriloquy

Answers: (C), (D), (F), (H): The patient has acute bronchopneumonia due to *Streptococcus pneumoniae* (gram-positive diplococci). Expected signs of consolidation include decreased percussion (**choice A is incorrect**), bronchial breath sounds (**choice F**), increased tactile fremitus (**choice E is incorrect**), whispered pectoriloquy (**choice H**), egophony (**choice D**), and fine rales/rhonchi (**choice C correct**; **choices B and G are incorrect**).

ACE = angiotensin converting enzyme, ABGs = arterial blood gases, AP = anteroposterior, CB = chronic bronchitis, CF = cystic fibrosis, CHD = congenital heart disease, CNS = central nervous system, COPD = chronic obstructive pulmonary disease, deoxyHb = deoxyhemoglobin, DKA = diabetic ketoacidosis, DOA = drugs of abuse, GERD = gastro-esophageal reflux disease, GI = gastrointestinal, Hb = hemoglobin, HTN = hypertension, IBD = inflammatory bowel disease, LHF = left heart failure, metHb = methemoglobin, PaO_2 = partial pressure of arterial oxygen, PE = pulmonary embolus, R/O = rule out, RSV = respiratory syncytial virus, SaO_2 = arterial oxygen saturation, TB = tuberculosis, TXA_2 = thromboxane A_2, UA = urinalysis, URI = upper respiratory infection.

Table 6–2. LABORATORY TESTING IN
RESPIRATORY DISEASE

Most Common...	Answer and Explanation
method of measuring lung volumes/ capacities	*spirometry*
volumes/capacities not directly measured by spirometry	• RV: volume of air left over after maximal expiration, • *TLC:* ∗ amount of air in a fully expanded lung, ∗ measured with a nitrogen or helium dilution method, • *FRC:* ∗ total amount of air in the lungs at the end of a normal expiration (end of the TV), ∗ obtained by a helium dilution technique or body plethysmography
outpatient method of evaluating FVC	*peak expiratory flow meter:* ∗ FVC is the total amount of air expelled after a maximal inspiration, ∗ RV is what is left over at the end of maximal expiration
method of measuring RV	*subtract the expiratory reserve volume (ERV) from the functional residual capacity (FRC):* ∗ ERV is the amount of air forcibly expelled at the end of a normal expiration (end of the TV), ∗ FRC encompasses the ERV + RV
method of measuring diffusion of air	DL_{CO}
dependent factors in DL_{CO}	• *CO reaching the alveoli:* impaired if airways blocked or collapsed, • *CO crossing alveolar/ capillary interface:* impaired if fibrosis/fluids are present, • *CO binding to Hb in RBCs:* ∗ depends on pulmonary capillary blood volume, ∗ impaired if ♦ perfusion is decreased (PE), ♦ capillaries destroyed (COPD), ♦ Hb is low or high (anemia, polycythemia)
causes of an increased DL_{CO}	• *pulmonary congestion:* increases the pulmonary capillary blood volume and uptake of CO, • *air trapping:* increases the overall cross-sectional area of lungs, • polycythemia
effect of restrictive disease on compliance/ elasticity	• *compliance decreased:* lungs cannot fully expand with air due to fibrosis, • *elasticity increased:* lung recoil increased on expiration [Restrictive disease is a problem with getting air into the lungs.]
effect of restrictive lung disease on PFTs	• *all lung volumes and capacities are equally reduced:* compliance problem, • FEV_{1sec}

Table 6–2. LABORATORY TESTING IN
RESPIRATORY DISEASE *Continued*

Most Common...	Answer and Explanation
Continued	(amount of air expelled in 1 sec after maximal inspiration) *and FVC are both decreased:* cannot lose more air than what is inspired, • *FEV$_{1sec}$/FVC ratio increased:* * increased elasticity results in similar values for FEV$_{1sec}$ and FVC, * most of the air is expressed in 1 sec (FEV$_{1sec}$ ≈ FVC)
effect of obstructive disease on compliance/ elasticity	• *compliance increased:* lungs easily expand since the elastic tissue support is destroyed, • *elasticity decreased:* elastic support is destroyed and airways collapse [Obstructive disease, unlike restrictive disease, is a problem with expelling air (air trapping).]
effect of obstructive disease on PFTs	• *RV increased:* air is trapped on expiration, • *TLC increased:* * due to increased RV, * lungs are like blown-up balloons, • *other volumes/capacities decreased:* compressed by the increase in RV, • *FEV$_{1sec}$, FVC, and FEV$_{1sec}$/FVC ratio are decreased:* * the reduction in these parameters is much greater than in restrictive disease, * e.g., FEV$_{1sec}$ in restrictive disease = 3 liters (normal 4 liters) compared to 1 liter in obstructive disease
mechanism of an A-a gradient	<u>A</u>lveolar P$_{O_2}$ never equals <u>a</u>rterial P$_{O_2}$: * V̇/Q̇ mismatches normally occur throughout the lungs, * some unoxygenated blood enters left atrium from coronary veins
formula used to calculate A-a gradient	P$_{AO_2}$ = % O$_2$ (713) − P$_{aCO_2}$/0.8 [Using normal values: P$_{AO_2}$ = 0.21 (713) − 40/0.8 = 100 mm Hg. If the patient is on a respirator, the % oxygen the patient is breathing is placed in the formula (e.g., 0.30 (713) − P$_{aCO_2}$/0.8). A medically significant value is an A-a gradient ≥30 mm Hg.]
causes of an increased A-a gradient	• **perfusion without ventilation:** * this causes intrapulmonary shunting, * e.g., ♦ atelectasis, ♦ ARDS, • *ventilation without perfusion:* * this increases dead space, * e.g., PE, • *diffusion abnormalities:* * problems with O$_2$ exchange at the alveolar/capillary interface, * e.g., interstitial fibrosis, pulmonary edema, • *right-to-left shunting in the heart:* unoxygenated blood enters systemic circulation

Table continued on following page

Table 6–2. LABORATORY TESTING IN
RESPIRATORY DISEASE *Continued*

Most Common...	Answer and Explanation
effect of 100% O_2 on PaO_2 in intrapulmonary shunts	*PaO_2 does not significantly increase when the patient is given 100% oxygen*
causes of hypoxemia with a normal A-a gradient	• **depression of the respiratory center in the medulla:** e.g., * barbiturates, * CNS injury, • *chest bellows dysfunction:* e.g., * paralyzed diaphragm, * neuromuscular disease, • *high altitude:* % O_2 is 21%, however atmospheric pressure is decreased, resulting in less O_2 in the alveoli for gas exchange*
uses of a chest radiograph	• *defines rib cage and diaphragmatic abnormalities:* e.g., * lytic rib lesions, * diaphragmatic hernia, • *detects parenchyma, vascular, and pleural space abnormalities:* e.g., * pneumonia, * PH, * pleural effusions, • *evaluates cardiac size and chamber contours*
uses of CT	• *detect pleural effusions/thickening,* • *fine definition of pulmonary lesions:* e.g., calcification in solitary nodules, • *staging primary lung cancer:* identification of hilar and mediastinal lymph nodes, • *sinus films in chronic sinusitis*
use of echocardiography	*detecting PH:* * estimates PA pressure, * right heart catheterization measures pressure and resistance
use of cytology	*gold standard in the Dx of primary lung cancer:* * cytology is most sensitive in centrally located cancers (sensitivity ~65%), * sensitivity ~60% in Dx of malignant pleural effusions
use of a Gram stain of sputum	• **work-up of pneumonia,** • *determine the adequacy of a sample for detecting bacterial pathogens*
criteria used to determine adequacy of a sputum sample	*satisfactory sputum:* * 25 or more PMNs and <10 epithelial cells per LPF, * 62% sensitivity/85% specificity in detecting/confirming *Streptococcus pneumoniae,* * sputum culture 50% sensitivity/100% specificity

Table 6–2. LABORATORY TESTING IN
RESPIRATORY DISEASE *Continued*

Most Common...	Answer and Explanation
use of bronchoscopy	• *evaluation of the airways,* • *Dx and staging of cancer,* • *work-up of hemoptysis,* • *obtain material for culture/cytology:* bronchoalveolar lavage, • *remove foreign bodies*
ABG components directly measured	• *pH,* • *PaCO_2,* • *PaO_2* [SaO_2, O_2 content, HCO_3^-, base excess/deficit are calculated.]
noninvasive method for measuring SaO_2	*pulse oximeter:* dependent on: * rate of blood flow (e.g., VC alters readings), * position of ODC, * type of Hb (e.g., cannot detect CO)
effect of air exposure on ABG	• *increased PaO_2:* O_2 higher in atmosphere than arterial blood, • *decreased PaCO_2:* CO_2 higher in arterial blood than atmosphere
acid base disorders	• **respiratory acidosis:** PaCO_2 >44 mm Hg, • *respiratory alkalosis:* PaCO_2 <33 mm Hg, • *metabolic acidosis:* HCO_3^- <22 mEq/L, • *metabolic alkalosis:* HCO_3^- >28 mEq/L
term applied when two or more ABG disorders occur simultaneously	*mixed ABG disorders*
clues suggesting a mixed ABG disorder	• **Hx and physical exam:** know what to expect, • *normal pH:* a normal pH implies full compensation (pH in normal range), which rarely occurs, • *markedly increased arterial pH:* * presence of two alkaloses, * e.g. respiratory/metabolic alkalosis, • *markedly decreased arterial pH:* * presence of two acidoses, * e.g., metabolic/respiratory acidosis, • *formulas:* see below, • *triple disorders:* * difficult to recognize, * Hx and exam most important
types of compensation	• *uncompensated:* * expected compensation is still in the normal range, * e.g., HCO_3^- = 24 mEq/L (22–28 mEq/L) in respiratory acidosis, • *partially compensated:* * expected compensation and pH are outside normal ranges, * e.g., in respiratory acidosis, pH = 7.33 (7.35–7.45) and HCO_3^- >28 mEq/L, • *fully compensated:* * when the pH is in the normal range, * rarely occurs

Table continued on following page

Table 6–2. LABORATORY TESTING IN
RESPIRATORY DISEASE *Continued*

Most Common...	Answer and Explanation
compensation for respiratory acidosis	*metabolic alkalosis*
compensation for respiratory alkalosis	*metabolic acidosis*
compensation for metabolic alkalosis	*respiratory acidosis:* dangerous, since an increase in $Paco_2$ decreases Pao_2
compensation for metabolic acidosis	*respiratory alkalosis*
causes of acute respiratory acidosis (pH <7.35, $Paco_2$ >44 mm Hg, HCO_3^- ≤30 mEq/L)	• **depression of the medullary respiratory center:** * drug overdose, * CNS trauma, * central sleep apnea, • *upper airway obstruction:* * cafe coronary, * laryngospasm, * obstructive sleep apnea, • *chest bellows disease:* * paralysis of diaphragms, * neuromuscular disease, • *primary lung disease:* * ARDS, * pneumothorax
causes of chronic respiratory acidosis (pH <7.35, $Paco_2$ >44 mm Hg, HCO_3^- >30 mEq/L)	• **primary lung disease:** e.g., COPD, • *chronic neuromuscular disease:* e.g., * ALS, * MD, * MG, • *kyphoscoliosis,* • *Pickwickian syndrome:* obesity prevents diaphragm movement on inspiration
S/S of respiratory acidosis	• **somnolence,** • *intracranial HTN:* high $Paco_2$ vasodilates and increases vessel permeability, • *pseudotumor cerebri:* * headache, * see Table 15–6, • *secondary polycythemia:* hypoxemic stimulus for EPO
electrolyte abnormalities in respiratory acidosis	• *hypochloremia:* * HCO_3^- moves out of cells as compensation and Cl^- ions move into the cells to maintain electroneutrality, * the exchange serum HCO_3^- increases ~3–4 mEq/L (≤30 mEq/L), • *hyperkalemia:* shift of H^+ into cells (buffer) in exchange for K^+ ions
renal response in respiratory acidosis	*reclaim/regenerate HCO_3^- as compensation:* requires 3–4 d
formula to calculate expected compensation in acute respiratory acidosis	• $\Delta HCO_3^- = 0.10 \times \Delta Pco_2$: * to calculate ΔPco_2, subtract normal Pco_2 (40 mm Hg) from measured Pco_2, * multiply ΔPco_2 by 0.10 to arrive at ΔHCO_3^-, * add ΔHCO_3^- to normal HCO_3^- (24 mEq/L), which equals expected

Table 6–2. LABORATORY TESTING IN
RESPIRATORY DISEASE *Continued*

Most Common...	Answer and Explanation
Continued	HCO_3^-, • *measured HCO_3^- approximates expected HCO_3^-*: acute, uncompensated respiratory acidosis
Dx if measured HCO_3^- > expected HCO_3^- in above ABG	*mixed disorder:* * there is an additional component of primary metabolic alkalosis, * retaining more HCO_3^- than required for compensation, * e.g., patient with COPD (respiratory acidosis) on a diuretic (metabolic alkalosis)
Dx if measured HCO_3^- >45 mEq/L in above ABG	*mixed disorder:* * additional primary metabolic alkalosis, * e.g., mixed respiratory acidosis and metabolic alkalosis
Dx if measured HCO_3^- < expected HCO_3^- in above ABG	*mixed disorder:* * there is an additional component of primary metabolic acidosis, * losing more HCO_3^- than required for normal compensation, * e.g., cardiopulmonary arrest (respiratory acidosis from not breathing + lactic acidosis from tissue hypoxia)
Dx if measured HCO_3^- <23 mEq/L in above ABG	*mixed disorder:* * primary metabolic acidosis present, * e.g., mixed respiratory acidosis and metabolic acidosis
formula to calculate expected compensation in chronic respiratory acidosis	• $\Delta HCO_3^- = 0.40 \times \Delta P_{CO_2}$: * to calculate ΔP_{CO_2}, subtract the normal P_{CO_2} (40 mm Hg) from measured P_{CO_2}, * multiply ΔP_{CO_2} by 0.40 to arrive at ΔHCO_3^-, * add ΔHCO_3^- to the normal HCO_3^- (24 mEq/L) to arrive at expected HCO_3^-, • *measured HCO_3^- approximates expected HCO_3^-*: chronic respiratory acidosis (or, partially compensated respiratory acidosis) is present, • *Dx of mixed disorders:* use the same criteria for acute respiratory acidosis
causes of acute respiratory alkalosis (pH >7.45, Pa_{CO_2} <33 mm Hg, HCO_3^- ≥18 mEq/L)	• **hyperventilation syndrome:** * **anxiety,** * tissue hypoxia (e.g., ♦ high altitude, ♦ severe anemia), • *stimulation of CNS respiratory medullary center:* * endotoxemia, * salicylates, * progesterone in pregnancy, * toxic

Table continued on following page

Table 6–2. LABORATORY TESTING IN
RESPIRATORY DISEASE *Continued*

Most Common...	Answer and Explanation
Continued	metabolites in liver failure, • *primary lung disease:* * initial phase of bronchial asthma (respiratory acidosis develops if patient tires), * PE, * ILD
causes of chronic respiratory alkalosis (pH >7.45, Paco$_2$ <33 mm Hg, HCO$_3^-$ <18 mEq/L but >12 mEq/L)	• **high altitude,** • *liver failure:* e.g., cirrhosis, • *chronic ILD:* e.g., sarcoidosis
S/S in respiratory alkalosis	• **lightheadedness,** • *tetany:* see Table 11–3
electrolyte abnormalities in respiratory alkalosis	• *hyperchloremia:* HCO$_3^-$ moves into cells as compensation and Cl$^-$ ions move out of cells to maintain electroneutrality, • *hypokalemia:* * K$^+$ moves into cells in exchange for H$^+$ ions, which enter the blood to lower the pH, * lowers HCO$_3^-$ 3–4 mEq/L
renal response in respiratory alkalosis	*loss of HCO$_3^-$ in urine as compensation*
formula to calculate expected compensation in acute respiratory alkalosis	*ΔHCO$_3^-$ = 0.20 × ΔP*co$_2$: * to calculate ΔPco$_2$, subtract measured Pco$_2$ from the normal Pco$_2$ (40 mm Hg), * multiply ΔPco$_2$ by 0.20 to arrive at ΔHCO$_3^-$, * subtract ΔHCO$_3^-$ from the normal HCO$_3^-$ (24 mEq/L) to arrive at expected HCO$_3^-$, • *measured HCO$_3^-$ approximates the expected HCO$_3^-$:* acute, uncompensated respiratory alkalosis
Dx if measured HCO$_3^-$ > expected HCO$_3^-$ in above ABG	*mixed disorder:* * there is an additional primary metabolic alkalosis, * retaining more HCO$_3^-$ than required for compensation, * e.g., pulmonary embolus + patient taking a diuretic
Dx if measured HCO$_3^-$ <12 mEq/L in above ABG	*mixed disorder:* * an additional primary metabolic acidosis is present, * HCO$_3^-$ is much lower than expected for compensation,

Table 6–2. LABORATORY TESTING IN RESPIRATORY DISEASE *Continued*

Most Common...	Answer and Explanation
Continued	* e.g., ♦ endotoxic shock (endotoxins overstimulate respiratory center → respiratory alkalosis + tissue hypoxia and lactic acidosis from shock → metabolic acidosis), ♦ salicylate intoxication (salicylates overstimulate respiratory center → respiratory alkalosis + increased salicylate anions → metabolic acidosis)
Dx if measured HCO_3^- < expected HCO_3^- in above ABG	*mixed disorder:* there is an additional primary metabolic acidosis present, * HCO_3^- is much lower than expected for compensation, * e.g., mixed respiratory alkalosis and metabolic acidosis
formula to calculate expected compensation in chronic respiratory alkalosis	• *$\Delta HCO_3^- = 0.50 \times \Delta PCO_2$:* * *to calculate* ΔPCO_2, subtract measured PCO_2 from the normal PCO_2 (40 mm Hg), * multiply ΔPCO_2 by 0.50 to arrive at ΔHCO_3^-, * subtract ΔHCO_3^- from the normal HCO_3^- (24 mEq/L) to arrive at expected HCO_3^-, • *measured HCO_3^- approximates expected HCO_3^-:* chronic respiratory alkalosis (partially compensated respiratory alkalosis), • *mixed disorder:* use the same criteria used above for acute respiratory alkalosis, • *measured HCO_3^- <12 mEq/L:* * mixed disorder with an additional primary metabolic acidosis
types of metabolic acidosis (pH <7.35, HCO_3^- <22 mEq/L)	• **increased anion gap,** • *normal anion gap metabolic acidosis*
formula used to distinguish increased from normal anion gap (AG) metabolic acidosis	*AG = serum Na^+ − (serum Cl^- + serum HCO_3^-):* using normal values: AG = 140 − (104 + 24) = 12 mEq/L ± 4, * the 12 mEq/L represents anions not represented in the formula (e.g., albumin, PO_4^{--}, SO_4^{--}), * an increase in AG is most often due to an excess of anions from acids (e.g., lactate, see below), * a normal AG indicates a loss of HCO_3^- ions (see below) and replacement by Cl^- ions in order to maintain electroneutrality

Table continued on following page

Table 6–2. LABORATORY TESTING IN
RESPIRATORY DISEASE *Continued*

Most Common...	Answer and Explanation
causes of increased AG metabolic acidosis	• **diabetic ketoacidosis:** increase in AcAc and β-OHB anions, • *alcoholic liver disease:* * increase in lactate and β-OHB anions, • see Table 1–3, • *starvation:* ketoacidosis with an increase in AcAc and β-OHB anions, • *tissue hypoxia:* increase in lactate anions, • *salicylate intoxication:* increase in salicylate and lactate ions (uncouples phosphorylation in the mitochondria), • *methyl alcohol poisoning:* increase in formate ions from the metabolism of methyl alcohol (windowshield wiper fluid), • *ethylene glycol poisoning:* increase in oxalate ions from the metabolism of ethylene glycol (antifreeze), • *chronic renal failure:* increase in phosphate and sulfate anions
causes of a normal AG metabolic acidosis	• **loss of HCO_3^- in the GI tract:** * diarrhea, * loss of pancreatic fluid, • *loss of HCO_3^- in the GU tract:* * proximal/distal RTA, * carbonic anhydrase inhibitor (blocks the reclamation of bicarbonate)
S/S of metabolic acidosis	• **hyperventilation:** * respiratory alkalosis is compensation, * called Kussmaul breathing, • *negative inotropic effect on the heart:* decreased response of cardiac muscle to catecholamines, • *osteoporosis:* bone buffers excess H^+ ions, • *warm shock:* acidosis vasodilates peripheral arterioles
electrolyte findings in metabolic acidosis	• **low HCO_3^-:** primary abnormality in metabolic acidosis, • *hyperkalemia:* * shift of K^+ out of cells, * mainly inorganic types of increased AG metabolic acidosis (phosphate, sulfate), • *hypokalemia:* diarrhea and type I/II RTA have a greater loss of K^+ than gain by transcellular shifting, • *hyperglycemia:* acidosis inhibits glycolysis, • *hyperuricemia:* above acids compete with uric acid for excretion in the kidneys
pulmonary response for metabolic acidosis	*blow off CO_2* (hyperventilation): it requires 12–24 hours for the lungs to reach a steady state of compensation in primary metabolic disorders

Table 6–2. LABORATORY TESTING IN
RESPIRATORY DISEASE *Continued*

Most Common...	Answer and Explanation
formula used to calculate expected compensation in metabolic acidosis	• $\Delta PCO_2 = 1.2 \times \Delta HCO_3^- \pm 2$: * to calculate ΔHCO_3^-, subtract measured HCO_3^- from the normal HCO_3^- (24 mEq/L), * multiply ΔHCO_3^- by 1.2 to arrive at ΔPCO_2, * subtract ΔPCO_2 from the normal PCO_2 (40 mm Hg), * express the range of expected PCO_2 as $\pm$ 2 mm Hg, • *measured PCO_2 is within the range of the expected PCO_2:* simple metabolic acidosis is present
Dx if measured PCO_2 > expected PCO_2 in above ABG	*mixed disorder:* * there is an additional primary respiratory acidosis, * retaining more CO_2 than required for compensation, * e.g., DKA (metabolic acidosis) + COPD (respiratory acidosis), * e.g., cardiopulmonary arrest
Dx if measured PCO_2 < expected PCO_2 in above ABG	*mixed disorder:* * there is an additional primary respiratory alkalosis, * blowing off more CO_2 than required for normal compensation, * e.g., ♦ endotoxic shock, ♦ salicylate intoxication
Dx is measured PCO_2 <10 mm Hg in above ABG	*mixed disorder:* there is an additional component of primary respiratory alkalosis, * e.g., mixed disorder with metabolic acidosis and respiratory alkalosis
causes of metabolic alkalosis (pH >7.45, HCO_3^- >28 mEq/L)	• **diuretics:** see Table 5–4 discussion, • *vomiting:* loss of acid in the gastric juice with retention of HCO_3^-, • *loss of anions in the urine:* * e.g., HCO_3^-, * anions of drugs like penicillin, ticarcillin, * strong negative charge in urine draws H^+ ions out of the tubules, • *mineralocorticoid excess:* e.g., * primary aldosteronism (see Table 5–4), * Cushing's syndrome (see Table 11–4)
S/S of metabolic alkalosis	• **arrhythmias:** particularly ventricular arrhythmias due to tissue hypoxia, • *tetany:* not as common as in respiratory alkalosis (see above)

Table continued on following page

**Table 6–2. LABORATORY TESTING IN
RESPIRATORY DISEASE** *Continued*

Most Common...	Answer and Explanation
electrolyte abnormalities in metabolic alkalosis	• **increased HCO_3^-:** primary alteration in metabolic alkalosis, • *hypokalemia:* shift of K^+ into cells in exchange for H^+ ions, which enter the blood to lower pH
pulmonary response for metabolic alkalosis	*retain CO_2* (hypoventilation) *as compensation:* an increase in alveolar P_{CO_2} is always accompanied by a corresponding decrease in alveolar P_{O_2} and Pa_{O_2}
formula to calculate expected compensation in metabolic alkalosis	• $\Delta P_{CO_2} = 0.7 \times \Delta HCO_3^- \pm 2:$ * to calculate ΔHCO_3^-, subtract the normal HCO_3^- (24 mEq/L) from measured HCO_3^-, * multiply ΔHCO_3^- by 0.7 to arrive at ΔP_{CO_2}, * add the ΔP_{CO_2} to the normal P_{CO_2} (40 mm Hg), * express the range of expected P_{CO_2} as $\pm$ 2 mm Hg, • *measured P_{CO_2} is within the range of the expected P_{CO_2}:* metabolic alkalosis is present
Dx if measured P_{CO_2} > expected P_{CO_2} in above ABG	*mixed disorder:* * there is an additional primary respiratory acidosis, * retaining more CO_2 than required for compensation, * e.g., patient with COPD (respiratory acidosis) who is vomiting (metabolic alkalosis), * e.g., patient with COPD who is on a diuretic (metabolic alkalosis)
Dx is measured P_{CO_2} < expected P_{CO_2} in above ABG	*mixed disorder:* * there is an additional component of primary respiratory alkalosis, * blowing off more CO_2 than required for normal compensation, * e.g., patient on a diuretic (metabolic alkalosis) who has an anxiety attack (respiratory alkalosis)
Dx if measured P_{CO_2} >55 mm Hg in above ABG	*mixed disorder:* * there is an additional primary respiratory acidosis, * see above

Table 6–2. LABORATORY TESTING IN RESPIRATORY DISEASE *Continued*

Question: You would expect a patient with long-standing chronic bronchitis who is on a loop diuretic for congestive heart failure to have which of the following abnormalities? **SELECT 5**

(A) Normal arterial pH
(B) Normal $PaCO_2$
(C) Increased HCO_3^-
(D) Decreased FEV_{1sec}/FVC ratio
(E) Normal DL_{CO}
(F) Low PaO_2
(G) Normal SaO_2
(H) Increased TLC

Answers: (A), (C), (D), (F), (H): A patient with chronic bronchitis on a loop diuretic will very likely have a mixed disorder consisting of chronic respiratory acidosis and metabolic alkalosis, respectively. Since this is a mixed ABG disorder, the pH is normal **(choice A)**. The $PaCO_2$ is markedly elevated **(choice B is incorrect)**, due to a combined effect of the increase in $PaCO_2$ from respiratory acidosis and compensation for metabolic alkalosis. The serum HCO_3^- is elevated **(choice C)** owing to the combined effect of metabolic alkalosis plus compensation from respiratory acidosis (both have an increase in bicarbonate). Hypoxemia **(choice F)** should be present in chronic bronchitis and retention of CO_2. A low SaO_2 **(choice G is incorrect)** is expected, since the PaO_2 is decreased. Normally, O_2 moves from the lungs, through the alveolar-capillary interface, into the plasma. Some dissolves in plasma to increase PO_2, diffuses through the RBC membrane, and attaches to Hb, which has four heme groups to bind O_2 (increases SaO_2). Hence, hypoxemia (low PaO_2) automatically lowers the SaO_2. The DL_{CO} should be decreased, since there is obstruction to airflow in the lungs **(choice E is incorrect)**. The PFTs in chronic bronchitis reveal obstructive findings including an increase in TLC **(choice H)** secondary to an increase in RV. There is a decrease in the FEV_{1sec}/FVC ratio **(choice D)**.

A-a = alveolar-arterial, ABG = arterial blood gas, AcAc = acetoacetic acid, AG = anion gap, ALS = amyotrophic lateral sclerosis, ARDS = adult respiratory distress syndrome, β-OHB = β-hydroxybutyric acid, CHF = congestive heart failure, Cl^- = chloride ions, CNS = central nervous system, CO = carbon monoxide, COPD = chronic obstructive lung disease, CT = computed tomography, DKA = diabetic ketoacidosis, DL_{CO} = diffusion capacity using carbon monoxide, Dx = diagnosis, EPO = erythropoietin, ERV = expiratory reserve volume, FRC = functional residual capacity, FEV_{1sec} = forced expiratory volume in 1 second, FVC = forced vital capacity, GI = gastrointestinal, GU = genitourinary, H^+ = hydrogen ions, Hb = hemoglobin, HCO_3^- = bicarbonate, HTN = hypertension, Hx = history, ILD = interstitial lung disease, LPF = low-power field, MD = muscular dystrophy, MG = myasthenia gravis, ODC = oxygen dissociation curve, $PaCO_2$ = partial pressure of arterial carbon dioxide, PaO_2 = partial pressure of arterial oxygen, PA = pulmonary artery, PaO_2 = partial pressure of alveolar oxygen, PE = pulmonary embolus, PFT = pulmonary function test, PH = pulmonary hypertension, PMNs = polymorphonuclear cells (neutrophils), P_{O_2} = partial pressure of oxygen, RBC = red blood cell, RTA = renal tubular acidosis, RV = residual volume, Sa_{O_2} = arterial oxygen saturation, S/S = signs and symptoms, TLC = total lung capacity, TV = tidal volume, VC = vasoconstriction, $\dot{V}/\dot{Q}$ = ventilation/perfusion.

Table 6–3. UPPER RESPIRATORY TRACT DISORDERS

Most Common...	Answer and Explanation
causes of rhinitis	• **rhinovirus infection,** • *allergies*
cause of chronic rhinitis	*allergies*
S/S of allergic rhinitis	• **seasonal nasal stuffiness/sneezing,** • *boggy, bluish-white nasal mucosa,* • *positive nasal smear for eosinophils*
Rx of allergic rhinitis	• **antihistamines/decongestants,** • *inhaled nasal steroids*
causes of nasal polyps	• **allergic rhinitis,** • *traid asthma:* aspirin/NSAID sensitivity leading to asthma, • *cystic fibrosis:* polyps noted in children
causes of epistaxis	• **bleeding from Kiesselbach's plexus on the anterior nasal septum secondary to trauma:** * nose picking, * impact sports, • *allergic rhinitis/polyps,* • *thrombocytopenia:* epistaxis most common symptom, • *hemorrhagic telangiectasia*
causes of olfactory dysfunction	see Table 15–3
causes of acute sinusitis	• **blockage of the sinus ostia due to inflammation:** e.g., * viral URI, * deviated nasal septum, • *barotrauma,* • *smoking,* • *immotile cilia syndrome*
site for acute sinusitis in adults	*maxillary sinus:* complain of pain over the cheeks
pathogens causing sinusitis	• ***Streptococcus pneumoniae,*** • *Haemophilus influenzae,* • *rhinoviruses,* • *anaerobes:* chronic sinusitis
method of Dx of acute sinusitis	• *CT scan:* most sensitive test, • *transillumination:* helpful in differentiating sinusitis from other causes of facial pain

Table 6–3. UPPER RESPIRATORY TRACT DISORDERS
Continued

Most Common...	Answer and Explanation
Rx of acute sinusitis	• **amoxicillin:** * TMP/SMX, * cefuroxime, * newer macrolides, • *decongestants:* topical and systemic
causes of fungal sinus infections	• *Aspergillus fumigatus,* • *Candida,* • *Mucor:* * especially in DM, * invades frontal lobes
sinus infection responsible for orbital cellulitis in children	*ethmoid sinusitis: Haemophilus influenzae* is the most common cause
clinical findings in orbital cellulitis	• **fever,** • *proptosis,* • *periorbital swelling,* • *ophthalmoplegia,* • *normal retinal exam:* papilledema is present if cavernous sinus thrombosis is the cause
Rx of orbital cellulitis	*IV cefuroxime*
causes of saddle nose deformity	• **Wegener's granulomatosis,** • *congenital syphilis*
malignancy of the nasal cavity and paranasal sinuses	*squamous cell carcinoma*
malignancy associated with woodworking	*adenocarcinoma of the nasal cavity*
malignant tumor of the nasopharynx	*nasopharyngeal carcinoma:* * causal relationship with EBV, * metastasizes to the cervical lymph nodes
types of sleep apnea	• **obstructive sleep apnea,** • *central sleep apnea:* * total absence of ventilatory effort during apnea, * Cheyne-Stokes breathing [Apnea refers to breath cessation for at least 10 seconds.]
causes of obstructive sleep apnea (OSA)	• **upper airway obstruction:** loss of normal pharyngeal muscle tone causes pharyngeal collapse on inspiration, • *tonsillar hypertrophy,* • *obesity,* • *hypothyroidism*

Table continued on following page

Table 6–3. UPPER RESPIRATORY TRACT DISORDERS
Continued

Most Common...	Answer and Explanation
S/S of OSA	• **snoring at night and inordinate daytime somnolence,** • *headaches,* • *personality* changes: irritability, • loud *snoring followed by periods of apnea with increasing strong ventilatory efforts failing to produce adequate airflow,* * *loud snort is coincident with the first breath after a period of apnea*
lab abnormalities in OSA	• **low SaO_2/PaO_2 during apneic episode:** drop of ~4% in SaO_2, • *respiratory acidosis,* • *polycythemia:* hypoxemic stimulus for EPO
complications in OSA	• **PH:** secondary to vasoconstrictive effects of chronic hypoxemia/respiratory acidosis, • *cor pulmonale:* PH + RVH, • *secondary polycythemia,* • *cardiac arrhythmias*
confirmatory test for OSA	*polysomnography:* also helps in determining what level of continuous positive airway pressure (CPAP) is necessary to keep the airways open
Rx for OSA	• **nasal CPAP:** O_2 may sometimes prolong periods of apnea (loss of hypoxemic drive to breathe), • *weight loss,* • *surgery:* * correction of nasal septum deviation, * uvulopalatopharyngoplasty, * tracheostomy (last resort)
cause of acute epiglottitis in adults	• ***Haemophilus influenzae,*** • *group A streptococcus*
S/S of epiglottitis	*inspiratory stridor*
radiographic finding in acute epiglottitis	*lateral radiograph of the neck reveals swelling of the epiglottis:* resembles a "thumbprint"
antibiotic used in Rx of acute epiglottitis	*IV cefuroxime or ceftriaxone*
causes of hoarseness	• **viral infection,** • *smoking,* • *allergies,* • *vocal cord nodule,* • *GERD*
causes of recurrent hoarseness	*smoking/allergies*
causes of vocal cord paralysis	• **injury to the recurrent laryngeal nerve during thyroidectomy,** • *Pancoast tumor:* see Table 6–7, • *tumors involving the vagus nerve in the jugular foramen:* e.g., schwannoma

Table 6-3. UPPER RESPIRATORY TRACT DISORDERS
Continued

Most Common...	Answer and Explanation
sign of unilateral vocal cord paralysis	*hoarseness*
sign of bilateral vocal cord paralysis	*stridor*
benign tumor of vocal cords	*squamous papillomas:* * due to HPV types 6/11, * due to passage through infected birth canal
Rx of squamous papillomas of the vocal cord	*laser therapy:* * recurrence is common, * risk for squamous carcinoma of the larynx
cause of true vocal cord polyps	*voice abuse:* vocal cord polyps are treated with laser or resection by direct laryngoscopy
causes of laryngeal cancer	• **cigarette smoking,** • *alcohol*
symptom of laryngeal cancer	*hoarseness*
site for squamous carcinoma of the larynx	*supraglottic area above the false vocal cords:* most proximal location directly impacted upon by the carcinogens in cigarette smoke
Rx for carcinoma of the larynx	• *lesions <2 mm:* radiation, • *lesions >2 mm:* radiation and surgery
indications for tracheostomy	• **respiratory failure requiring prolonged mechanical ventilation,** • *airway obstruction at or above the level of the larynx*

Question: A 56-year-old man has a history of loud snoring at night and daytime somnolence. Physical exam reveals an accentuated P2 and left parasternal heave. Which of the following would most likely be present? **SELECT 4**
- (A) Respiratory alkalosis
- (B) Chronic hypoxemia
- (C) PH
- (D) ECG evidence of LVH
- (E) Polycythemia
- (F) Abnormal polysomnogram

Answers: (B), (C), (E), (F): The patient has obstructive sleep apnea complicated by cor pulmonale (accentuated P2 is PH + RVH, which causes left parasternal heave, **choice D is incorrect**). PH (**choice C**) is secondary to hypoxemia (**choice B**) and respiratory acidosis (**choice A is incorrect**). Polycythemia (**choice E**) is secondary to hypoxemia (low PaO_2). Polysomnography (**choice F**) is the gold standard for confirming the diagnosis.

CPAP = continuous positive airway pressure, CT = computed tomography, DM = diabetes mellitus, Dx = diagnosis, ECG = electrocardiographic, EPO = erythropoietin, EBV = Epstein-Barr virus, GERD = gastroesophageal reflux disease, HPV = human papillomavirus, IV = intravenous, LVH = left ventricular hypertrophy, NSAID = nonsteroidal anti-inflammatory drug, OSA = obstructive sleep apnea, P2 = pulmonic component of the second heart sound, PaO_2 = partial pressure of arterial oxygen, PH = pulmonary hypertension, RVH = right ventricular hypertrophy, Rx = treatment, SaO_2 = oxygen saturation of hemoglobin, S/S = signs and symptoms, TMP/SMX = trimethoprim sulfamethoxazole, URI = upper respiratory infection.

Table 6–4. ATELECTASIS, ASPIRATION, PNEUMOTHORAX, VASCULAR DISORDERS

Most Common...	Answer and Explanation
causes of atelectasis	• **small airway obstruction by mucus plugs with resorption of alveolar air:** atelectasis is collapse of lung tissue, • *lung compression:* e.g., pleural effusion, • *lack of surfactant:* ARDS, • *luminal obstruction:* cancer
S/S of atelectasis	• **fever:** not related to infection, • *cyanosis:* if widespread, • *dyspnea,* • *ipsilateral elevation of diaphragm:* loss of lung mass, • *inspiratory lag on the affected side*
cause of fever in the first 24 h post-surgery	*atelectasis:* RUQ surgery is notorious for this complication
causes of postoperative atelectasis	• **anesthesia,** • *systemic analgesic effects,* • *painful upper abdominal incisions*
complications of postoperative atelectasis	• **pneumonia,** • *intrapulmonary shunting with hypoxemia*
method of preventing postoperative atelectasis	• **cough/deep breaths,** • *humidification,* • incentive spirometry
cause of the right middle lobe syndrome	*atelectasis:* * syndrome is due to recurrent or persistent atelectasis of the right middle lobe, cancer is often responsible
causes of persistent atelectasis	*bronchial obstruction:* * enlarged hilar lymph nodes, * foreign body, * cancer

Table 6–4. ATELECTASIS, ASPIRATION, PNEUMOTHORAX, VASCULAR DISORDERS *Continued*

Most Common...	Answer and Explanation
causes of ARDS	• **gram-negative sepsis,** • *aspiration of gastric contents,* • *trauma/shock,* • *acute pancreatitis,* • *near-drowning,* • *multiple blood transfusions,* • *drug overdose*
pathophysiologic abnormality in ARDS	*massive intrapulmonary shunting from widespread atelectasis:* atelectasis is due to neutrophil-related injury of type II pneumocytes (contain surfactant)
S/S of ARDS	• **rapid onset of dyspnea/tachypnea within 24–48 hours of the initiating event,** • *inspiratory crackles*
chest radiograph findings in ARDS	• **bilateral pulmonary infiltrates with an initial interstitial pattern followed by an alveolar pattern,** • *air bronchograms* (80%), • *absence of vessel redistribution:* no upper lung venous engorgement as in CHF, • *normal heart size,* • *absence of pleural effusions*
lab abnormalities in ARDS	• **severe hypoxemia,** • *increased A-a gradient:* * intrapulmonary shunting, * diffusion abnormalities, • *PCWP ≤18 mm Hg:* >18 mm Hg is noted in cardiogenic pulmonary edema, • *respiratory acidosis*
Rx of ARDS	• **PEEP + oxygen:** * improves oxygenation, * no improvement in survival, • *placement of an SG catheter:* * measure MVOC (detects tissue hypoxia), * find the lowest PCWP that maintains an adequate CO, • *drugs:* * ? inhalation of NO (potent vasodilator), * ? ketoconazole inhibiting lipoxygenase/TXA$_2$
COD in ARDS	*nonpulmonary multiple organ failure:* * mortality rate >50, * >90% if sepsis is the cause of ARDS
causes of spontaneous pneumothorax	• **rupture of a subpleural bulla at the apex of the lung:** * most patients are tall, slender smoking men between the ages of 30 and 40, * recurrent disease is the rule, • *COPD:* most common secondary cause, • *penetrating chest injuries,* • *Marfan's syndrome,* • *mechanical ventilation,* • *CF,* • *insertion of a subclavian catheter,* • *menstruation:* catamenial pneumothorax, • *ruptured esophagus*

Table continued on following page

Table 6–4. ATELECTASIS, ASPIRATION,
PNEUMOTHORAX, VASCULAR DISORDERS *Continued*

Most Common...	Answer and Explanation
S/S of a spontaneous pneumothorax	• **sudden onset of severe pleuritic chest pain with dyspnea,** • *hyper-resonance,* • *absent tactile fremitus,* • *ipsilateral tracheal deviation,* • *elevation of hemidiaphragm* [Pleural cavity pressure is similar to atmospheric pressure causing lung collapse.]
mechanism of a tension pneumothorax	• **air enters the pleural cavity through a tear on the pleura (e.g., knife wound) that has a check valve mechanism,** • *air moves into the cavity on inspiration and flap closes on expiration,* • *pleural cavity pressure higher than atmospheric pressure,* • *compression atelectasis as lung is pushed to contralateral side*
S/S of a tension pneumothorax	**more severe respiratory embarrassment than spontaneous pneumothorax,** • *hypotension due to decreased venous return,* • *bulging intercostal muscles,* • *depression of hemidiaphragm,* • *tracheal deviation to contralateral side*
radiographic appearance of a pneumothorax	*pleural shadow separates from the chest wall in a spontaneous pneumothorax* [The diagnosis of a tension pneumothorax is clinically made (see above S/S)].
Rx of a spontaneous pneumothorax	• *lung collapse <15%:* * hospitalized if in respiratory distress, * sent home if mildly symptomatic, • *symptomatic pneumothorax >15%:* chest tube inserted through 2nd ICS in mid-clavicular line under water seal drainage with suction to re-expand the lung, • *recurrent pneumothoraces:* * pleural sclerosis by ♦ surgery, ♦ thoracoscopy, ♦ chemical pleurodesis
Rx of a tension pneumothorax	• **large-bore needle with fluid in a syringe is inserted into the 2nd ICS in the mid-clavicular line to relieve the pressure,** • *followed by chest tube insertion*
body position for aspiration into the posterobasal segment of RLL	*sitting or standing*

Table 6–4. ATELECTASIS, ASPIRATION,
PNEUMOTHORAX, VASCULAR DISORDERS *Continued*

Most Common...	Answer and Explanation
body position for aspiration into superior segment of RLL	*lying down on the back*
body position for aspiration into right middle lobe and/or posterior segment of RUL	*lying down on the right side*
body position for aspiration into the lingula	*lying down on the left side*
causes of aspiration of gastric contents	• **trauma patients who are unconscious post-anesthesia,** • *strokes*
cause of endogenous lipoid pneumonia	*obstruction of an airway by tumor*
site of origin of a PE	*proximal deep veins of the thigh* (femoral, iliac, popliteal): see Table 5–3
lung site of a PE	*right lower lobe:* perfusion is greater than ventilation in this area
risk factors for a PE	see Table 5–3
cause of acute cor pulmonale	*large PE blocking the majority of PA orifices:* called a saddle embolus
pathophysiologic effects of a PE	• *initial perfusion defect:* leads to increased dead space, • *hypoxemia:* * causes generalized vasoconstriction of pulmonary vessels, * decreased surfactant synthesis, • *after 24–48 hours:* segmental atelectasis leading to intrapulmonary shunting
initial S/S of a PE	• **tachypnea and dyspnea,** • *pleuritic chest pain,* • *fever,* • *cough,* • *leg pain* (DVT), • *hemoptysis,* • *wheezing,* • *syncope/acute cor pulmonale/cardiorespiratory arrest:* if massive PE
complications of a PE	• *hemorrhagic infarction:* * 10–15%, * more likely in presence of pre-existing lung disease, • *secondary PH:* loss of the capillary bed over time with recurrent PE

Table continued on following page

**Table 6–4. ATELECTASIS, ASPIRATION,
PNEUMOTHORAX, VASCULAR DISORDERS** *Continued*

Most Common...	Answer and Explanation
chest radiograph findings in a PE	• **parenchymal infiltrate with or without a pleural effusion:** * ~45%, * 10% have a normal chest radiograph, • *area of hypovascularity:* * Westermark's sign, * area of hyperlucent lung, • *pleural-based wedge-shaped density:* Hampton's hump
initial step in the Dx of a PE	*ventilation/perfusion scan:* * normal scan R/O PE, * high-probability scan has high predictive value for PE, * low-probability scan does not exclude PE, * pulmonary angiography in equivocal cases (gold standard test)
lab and ECG abnormalities in a PE	• *respiratory alkalosis,* • *PaO$_2$ <80 mm Hg:* * 85%, * perfusion defect, • *increased A-a gradient,* • *D-dimers:* cross-linked fibrin monomers indicate plasmin breakdown of fibrin, • ECG: * RV strain pattern (S$_1$Q$_3$T$_3$), * sinus tachycardia (~80%)
Rx of a PE	• **anticoagulation:** * heparin (aPTT 1.5–2.5 control value), * warfarin (INR 2.0–3.0), • *supplemental oxygen,* • *thrombolytic Rx:* patients with massive emboli and hypotension
clinical findings in primary PH	• *uncommon cause of PH,* • *young/middle-aged women with primary pulmonary vascular disease*
causes of secondary PH	• **reduction in cross-sectional area of the PA bed:** e.g., * recurrent PE, * emphysema, • *persistent PA vasoconstriction due to hypoxemia/respiratory acidosis:* e.g., * high altitude, * COPD, * OSA, * amphetamine/cocaine abuse, • *increased left-to-right shunting of blood:* e.g., * VSD, * ASD, • *increased pulmonary venous pressure:* e.g., mitral stenosis, • *increased blood viscosity:* e.g., polycythemia
S/S of PH	• **progressive dyspnea/fatigue,** • *chest pain,* • *syncopal episodes,* • *accentuation of P2,* • *left parasternal heave:* RVH, • *paradoxical split of S2:* PV closes early due to PH

Table 6–4. ATELECTASIS, ASPIRATION, PNEUMOTHORAX, VASCULAR DISORDERS *Continued*

Most Common...	Answer and Explanation
lab/radiographic abnormalities in PH	• *chest radiograph:* * enlarged right/left main/lobar pulmonary arteries, * tapering of vessels as they reach the periphery (called pruning), * RVH, * right atrial enlargement, • *Doppler ultrasonography:* increased PA systolic pressure, • *PFTs:* decreased DL$_{CO}$, • *PA catheterization:* increased PA pressure, • *ABGs:* hypoxemia
Rx of PH	• **vasodilator therapy:** * IV epoprostenol (PGI$_2$), * inhaled NO, * calcium channel blockers, • *anticoagulation:* warfarin, • *supplemental O$_2$,* • *surgery:* * single/double lung transplant, * heart-lung transplant
complication of lung transplantation	*bronchiolitis obliterans*
causes of cor pulmonale	• **COPD:** * cor pulmonale specifically refers to PH + RVH, * PH either primary PA or secondary to non-cardiac disease, • *CF,* • *ILD*

Question: Approximately 24 hours after a total hip replacement, a 62-year-old woman develops a sudden onset of dyspnea and pleuritic chest pain in the lower right lung. A chest radiograph reveals an area of lucency in the RLL and a small pleural effusion. Which of the following would you expect in this patient? **SELECT 2**

(A) Hypocapnia
(B) Normal A-a gradient
(C) Abnormal ventilation scan/normal perfusion scan
(D) Mild hypoxemia
(E) Normal ECG

Answers: (A), (D): The patient has an acute PE involving the RLL, most likely secondary to a clot originating in the iliofemoral venous system. Expected findings in a PE include respiratory alkalosis (choice A, hypocapnia), mild hypoxemia (choice D), normal ventilation scan but abnormal perfusion scan (choice C is incorrect), an increased A-a gradient (perfusion defect, choice B is incorrect), and an abnormal ECG (choice E is incorrect).

A-a = alveolar-arterial, ABGs = arterial blood gases, aPTT = activated partial thromboplastin time, ARDS = adult respiratory distress syndrome, ASD = atrial septal defect, CF = cystic fibrosis, CHF = congestive heart failure, CO = cardiac output, COD = cause of death, COPD = chronic obstructive pulmonary disease, DL$_{CO}$ = diffusion capacity with carbon monoxide, DVT = deep venous thrombosis, Dx = diagnosis, ECG = electrocardiogram, ICS = intercostal space, ILD = interstitial lung disease, INR = International Normalized Ratio, IV = intravenous, MVOC

= mixed venous oxygen content, NO = nitric oxide, OSA = obstructive sleep apnea, P2 = pulmonic component of the second heart sound, PA = pulmonary artery, PCWP = pulmonary capillary wedge pressure, PE = pulmonary embolus, PEEP = positive end-expiratory pressure, PFTs = pulmonary function tests, PGI_2 = prostaglandin I_2, PH = pulmonary hypertension, PV = pulmonary valve, RDS = respiratory distress syndrome, RLL = right lower lobe, R/O = rule out, RUL = right upper lobe, RUQ = right upper quadrant, RVH = right ventricular hypertrophy, Rx = treatment, S/S = signs and symptoms, S2 = second heart sound, TXA_2 = thromboxane A_2, VSD = ventricular septal defect.

Table 6–5. RESPIRATORY TRACT INFECTIONS

Most Common...	Answer and Explanation
cause of a cold in fall and winter	*rhinovirus:* person-to-person by droplet infection and hand contamination
cause of a cold in the spring/summer	*adenovirus:* infects * pharynx, * conjunctiva (viral "pink-eye")
viral cause of increased morbidity/ mortality in people >55 years of age	*influenzavirus:* • only influenza A (most common) and B cause human disease, • more common during the winter months
cause of pandemics in influenza	*antigenic shift usually by reassortment of genome segments of hemagglutinin or neuraminidase*
S/S of influenza	• **fever**, • *retro-orbital headache*, • *myalgias*, • *productive cough*, • *upper respiratory signs*
prevention/Rx of influenza A	*see Tables 2–1 and 2–2*
COD in influenza	*influenzae pneumonia:* superinfection with *Staphylococcus aureus* or *S. pneumoniae*
serious childhood complication of influenza	*Reye's syndrome*
causes of acute bronchitis	• **rhinovirus**, • *influenza*, • *parainfluenza viruses*
causes of exacerbations in CB	• ***Streptococcus pneumoniae***: ABGs reveal a further increase in the $PaCO_2$ over the usual baseline value, • *Haemophilus influenzae*, • *Moraxella catarrhalis*, • *Mycoplasma pneumoniae*

Table 6–5. RESPIRATORY TRACT INFECTIONS *Continued*

Most Common...	Answer and Explanation
Rx for exacerbations of CB	• **antibiotics:** TMP/SMX, • *bronchodilators:* inhaled β_2-adrenergic agonists or ipratropium bromide, • O_2: keep SaO_2 between 88–90%
S/S of a typical community-acquired pneumonia	• **sudden onset of high fever/productive cough,** • *signs of consolidation in the lungs:* see Table 6–1
S/S of an atypical community-acquired pneumonia	• *insidious onset,* • *low-grade fever,* • *nonproductive cough,* • *interstitial pattern in the lungs*
types of typical pneumonia	• **bronchopneumonia:** bronchitis leading to patchy areas of pneumonia, • *lobar*
tests to diagnose typical pneumonia	• **chest radiograph,** • *Gram stain of sputum,* • *sputum culture,* • *CBC*
complications associated with a typical pneumonia	• **septicemia,** • *lung abscesses,* • *metastatic abscesses,* • *empyema:* pus in pleural cavity
causes of nosocomial pneumonia (hospital-acquired)	• ***Escherichia coli,*** • *Pseudomonas aeruginosa:* * respirator patients, * greenish sputum, • *Staphylococcus aureus:* yellow sputum [The above organisms colonize the airways and then spread into the lungs.]
cause of ICU pneumonia	*Pseudomonas aeruginosa*
Rx of *P. aeruginosa* pneumonia	*piperacillin or mezlocillin + gentamicin or tobramycin*
cause of community-acquired atypical pneumonia	*Mycoplasma pneumoniae:* common in crowded conditions
complications of *Mycoplasma pneumoniae* infections	• **bullous myringitis,** • *sinusitis,* • *otitis media*
Rx of *M. pneumoniae* pneumonia	• **erythromycin,** • *tetracycline*
Chlamydia causing atypical pneumonia	*Chlamydia pneumoniae:* * accounts for 5–10% of atypical pneumonias, * possible causal role in CAD

Table continued on following page

Table 6–5. RESPIRATORY TRACT INFECTIONS *Continued*

Most Common...	Answer and Explanation
Rx of *Chlamydia pneumoniae*	*erythromycin*
cause of pneumonia in handlers of psittacine birds or those in poultry industry	*Chlamydia psittaci:* * cause of ornithosis (or psittacosis), * psittacine birds include parrots and parakeets
cause of pneumonia in a people exposed to sheep manure	*Coxiella burnetii:* * cause of Q fever, * primarily transmitted by inhalation, * occurs in dairy farmers, veterinarians, those who clean up sheep, goat, cattle manure
Rx of Q fever	*doxycycline*
cause of community-acquired typical pneumonia	*Streptococcus pneumoniae*
risk factors for *Streptococcus pneumoniae* pneumonia	• **old age,** • *splenectomy,* • *smoking,* • *alcoholism,* • *HIV infection,* • *HbSS disease*
empiric Rx of community-acquired pneumonia	• **penicillin V potassium: 500 mg orally, qid for 7–10 d, azithromycin if allergic to penicillin,** • *tetracycline*
Rx of *S. pneumoniae* pneumonia	• **penicillin G,** • *macrolide* [Rx penicillin-resistant strains with IV vancomycin.]
infectious cause of tension pneumothorax	*Staphylococcus aureus:* * produces tension pneumatocysts in the pleura, * commonly occur in CF
cause of pneumonia in nursing homes	*Klebsiella pneumoniae:* * fat, gram-negative rod with a thick capsule, * commonly occurs in alcoholics and diabetics, * tends to involve the upper lobes and cavitate
Rx of *K. pneumoniae*	*cefazolin + gentamicin or tobramycin*
cause of pneumonia due to water coolers	*Legionella pneumophila:* * water-loving gram-negative rod, * commonly occurs in smoking men >40 years of age
lung findings in Legionellosis	• **striking fever,** • *rapidly progressive pneumonia with a dry cough,* • *flu-like S/S,* • *bloody sputum,* • *calcifications in infiltrates*

Table 6–5. RESPIRATORY TRACT INFECTIONS *Continued*

Most Common...	Answer and Explanation
extrapulmonary manifestations of Legionellosis	• *CNS:* * ataxia, * confusion, • *kidneys:* * interstitial nephritis, * type IV RTA (♦ hyponatremia, ♦ hyperkalemia, ♦ metabolic acidosis), • *heart:* * pericarditis, * endocarditis
methods to Dx *Legionellosis*	• *stains:* * Dieterle silver stain (best stain), * Gram stains often negative, • *culture:* media supplemented with iron and cysteine
Rx of *Legionellosis*	*erythromycin with rifampin*
partially acid-fast organism producing pneumonia	*Nocardia asteroides:* partially acid-fast gram-positive filamentous bacteria
clinical findings in nocardiosis	• *primarily infects immunocompromised hosts:* common in heart transplants, • *associated with pulmonary alveolar proteinosis,* • *produces granulomatous microabscesses:* cavitary lesions, • *simulates TB:* * fever, * night sweats, * hemoptysis
Rx of nocardiosis	*sulfisoxazole*
organism producing draining sinuses in the jaw, thorax, and abdominal cavity	*Actinomyces israelii:* * gram-positive filamentous bacteria (best seen in sulfur granules), • *produces sinus tracts extending to skin surface:* * jaw (♦ most common site, ♦ post dental abscess), * thorax, * abdomen
Rx of actinomycosis	*penicillin G*
screening test for TB	*see Table 2–1*
location for primary TB	*subpleural location:* * upper part of the lower lobes or lower part of the upper lobes, * most commonly seen in children
COD due to an infectious disease in the world	*TB:* * rapid increase in TB parallels HIV, * resistant strains are beginning to surface
cause of secondary (reactivation) TB	*reactivation of a previous primary TB site*
risk factors for reactivation TB	*see Table 2–1*
site of reactivation TB	*apex of the lungs:* * O_2 concentration is highest in the apex, * cavitation occurs

Table continued on following page

Table 6–5. RESPIRATORY TRACT INFECTIONS *Continued*

Most Common...	Answer and Explanation
S/S of TB	• **fever**, • *drenching night sweats*, • *weight loss*, • *hemoptsis:* <25%
extrapulmonary sites for TB	• **kidneys:** * sterile pyuria, * hematuria, • *CNS:* * meningitis, * tuberculoma, • *epididymis,* • *pericardium:* constrictive pericarditis, • *adrenals:* Addison's disease • *vertebral column:* Pott's disease
complications of TB in the lungs	• *miliary spread in lungs*: invasion into the bronchus or PA, • *systemic miliary spread:* invasion of pulmonary vein, • *scar carcinoma:* usually an adenocarcinoma, • *massive hemoptysis,* • *bronchiectasis:* most common cause world-wide, • *secondary amyloidosis,* • *cavity often the site for fungus ball*
methods to diagnose TB	• *fluorochrome and acid-fast stains*: only presumptive evidence of TB, • *use gastric aspirate if patients cannot cough,* • *culture:* * definitive Dx, * radiometric color systems reduce the time for obtaining positive cultures, • *DNA probes*
first-line antituberculous agents	• **INH**, • *rifampin,* • *ethambutol,* • *pyrazinamide,* • *streptomycin* [Initial Rx: INH, RIF, PZA, EMB or streptomycin. Adults (not children/pregnant patients) should receive pyridoxine (deficiency common in INH Rx). Screen with serum transaminases for INH Rx (hepatotoxic drug). Screen visual acuity/red-green color perception for EMB Rx. Screen hearing for streptomycin Rx.]
criteria indicating nontransmissability of TB	*three consecutive sputum smears negative for acid-fast bacilli on separate days*
criteria for INH prophylaxis	*see Table 2–1*
type of TB in AIDS	*Mycobacterium avium-intracellulare* (MAI)
clinical findings of MAI in AIDS	• *infection occurs when CD_4 T helper count <50 cells/μL,* • *persistent fever, night sweats, weight loss,* • *blood culture best for confirming the Dx,* • *clarithromycin for prophylaxis*

Table 6–5. RESPIRATORY TRACT INFECTIONS *Continued*

Most Common...	Answer and Explanation
atypical mycobacteria producing lung disease	• **MAI,** • *M. kansasii:* * *M. kansasii* resembles TB, * sensitive to the same drugs as TB, • TST is frequently ≥5 mm in atypical mycobacterial infections
atypical mycobacteria producing cervical adenitis in children	*M. scrofulaceum:* * fever is frequently absent, * surgery is Rx of choice, * adults with cervical adenitis usually have *M. tuberculosis*
systemic fungal infection involving the lungs	*Histoplasma capsulatum:* * most commonly contracted in the Ohio/Mississippi valley states, * transmission: ♦ starlings, ♦ chickens, ♦ bats (hazardous to cave explorers [spelunkers]), ♦ inhalation of the spores
clinical findings of histoplasmosis	• *similar to TB:* * consolidations, * coin lesions, * miliary spread, • *striking dystrophic calcification in lungs and extrapulmonary sites,* • *erythema nodosum* (painful nodules) *commonly occurs on the lower extremities*
methods to diagnose histoplasmosis	• **culture,** • direct visualization: yeast forms in macrophages, • *skin tests,* • *serologic tests*
Rx of histoplasmosis	• *itraconazole:* moderate disease, • *amphotericin B:* severe disease
systemic fungal infection in the Southwest	*Coccidioides immitis:* * transmitted by inhalation of arthrospores in dust (increased with earthquakes, 4–5 d after a rain), * called "valley fever"
clinical findings in coccidioidomycosis	• **flu-like syndrome with a dry, nonproductive cough,** • *erythema nodosum:* common, • *lung:* * localized "egg-shell" cavity in the lower lobes, * miliary spread (lung, systemic), * solitary coin lesion
methods to diagnose coccidioidomycosis	• **culture,** • *direct visualization of spherules with endospores,* • *skin tests,* • *serologic tests*
Rx of coccidioidomycosis	*fluconazole*
fungal pneumonia related to exposure to pigeon excreta	*Cryptococcus neoformans*

Table continued on following page

Table 6–5. RESPIRATORY TRACT INFECTIONS *Continued*

Most Common...	Answer and Explanation
clinical findings in cryptococcosis	*lungs:* * granulomatous reaction if cellular immunity is intact, * no inflammatory response if patient is immunocompromised
methods to diagnose cryptococcosis	• **culture,** • *direct visualization:* yeast has a narrow-based bud, • *serologic tests*
Rx of cryptococcosis	*amphotericin B*
fungus associated with hemoptysis, pneumonia, and asthma	*Aspergillus fumigatus:* * colonizes abandoned TB cavities (♦ fungus ball, ♦ cause of massive hemoptysis), * hemorrhagic pneumonia with infarctions (invades blood vessels), * asthma (see below).
clinical findings in acute bronchopulmonary aspergillosis	• occurs in patients with pre-existing asthma, • *sudden worsening of wheezing is characteristic,* • *symptoms wax and wane*
lab findings in acute pulmonary aspergillosis	• *fleeting pulmonary infiltrates on chest radiographs,* • *eosinophilia,* • *high IgE levels,* * *increased precipitins in blood*
Rx of acute pulmonary aspergillosis	*Rx:* * avoid *Aspergillus* mold, * intermittent steroids
methods to diagnose aspergillosis	• **culture,** • *direct visualization:* fruiting bodies
Rx of aspergillosis	• *aspergillomas:* surgery, • *amphotericin B:* invasive disease
fungus primarily associated with lung, skin, and bone lesions in men	*Blastomyces dermatitidis:* * endemic infection in the Ohio/Mississippi valley/southeastern states, * predilection for inland waterways and beaver dams, * granulomatous reaction, * skin lesions resemble squamous cancer
methods to diagnose blastomycosis	• **culture,** • *direct visualization:* yeast has a broad-based bud
Rx of blastomycosis	*itraconazole*
fungus that targets the lungs, nasal sinuses, and CNS	*Mucor:* * associated with fungi in the genera *Mucor, Rhizopoda, Absidia,* * vessel invader causing hemorrhagic infarctions, * in DKA, it extends from the sinuses into the frontal lobes (frontal lobe abscesses)

Table 6–5. **RESPIRATORY TRACT INFECTIONS** *Continued*

Most Common...	Answer and Explanation
methods to diagnose *Mucor*	• **culture,** • *direct visualization:* wide-angled, non-septate hyphae
Rx of *Mucor*	*amphotericin B*
fungus associated with sepsis secondary to intravascular catheters	*Candida albicans:* * present in the mouth and feces of most normal people, * invasive disease develops secondary to intravascular catheters, * risk factors: ♦ HIV, ♦ neutropenia, ♦ broad-spectrum antibiotic therapy, * pulmonary involvement secondary to fungemia
methods to diagnose candidiasis	• **culture blood and catheter tip,** • *direct visualization,* • *serologic tests*
Rx of candidiasis	• *remove the catheter,* • *Rx: amphotericin B*
AIDS-defining pneumonia	*Pneumocystis carinii:* see Table 13–2
S/S of PCP	• **severe dyspnea/tachypnea,** • *fever,* • *dry cough*
methods to diagnose PCP	• **induced sputum:** * best initial test, * Giemsa/silver stains identify cysts, • *bronchoalveolar lavage:* if induced sputum is unsuccessful, • *lung biopsy:* if lavage is unsuccessful
radiographic findings in PCP	• *chest radiograph:* diffuse interstitial infiltration, • *gallium scan:* lungs light up
lab findings in PCP	• *respiratory alkalosis,* • *increased A-a gradient,* • *severe hypoxemia,* • *single breath DL_{CO}:* markedly impaired diffusion, • *elevated serum LDH:* very characteristic
Rx of PCP	• **TMP/SMX,** • *prophylaxis to prevent PCP:* TMP/SMX when CD4 T helper count ≤200 cells/μL
parasitic diseases involving the lungs	• *larval phases of helminths:* * ascaris, * hookworms, * strongyloides when they migrate through the lungs, * *lung tapeworm: Paragonimus westermani,* • *Dirofilaria immitis:* pulmonary infarction, • *Entamoeba histolytica:* pleurocavitary disease

Table continued on following page

Table 6–5. RESPIRATORY TRACT INFECTIONS *Continued*

Most Common...	Answer and Explanation
causes of a pulmonary abscess	• **aspiration of infected oropharyngeal material/infected teeth,** • *lobar pneumonia:* * Staphylococcus aureus, * Klebsiella pneumoniae, • hematogenous spread: * sepsis, * infected thromboembolic material
clinical findings of lung abscess from aspirated oropharyngeal material	• *most aspirations occur at night while sleeping,* • *oropharyngeal material contains a mixed population of anaerobes:* e.g., * Prevotella melanogenicus, * Fusobacterium nucleatum, * anaerobic streptococci, • sputum foul smelling, • Dx: * Gram stain reveals a mixture of rods and cocci, * sputum cultures are useless, * specimens for culture obtained by protected bronchoscopy*
Rx of anaerobic lung abscesses	*IV aqueous penicillin G*

Question: A 53-year-old smoker and alcoholic presents with a sudden onset of spiking fever, cough productive of blood-streaked, mucoid-appearing sputum, decreased percussion in the left upper lobe of lung, and increased tactile fremitus. He has a history of a positive TST measuring 12 mm for which he refused follow-up. A Gram stain of sputum reveals encapsulated, fat gram-negative rods, abundant neutrophils, and RBCs. A chest radiograph exhibits a lobar consolidation in the left upper lobe with early cavitation. Which of the following is the most likely diagnosis at this stage in his investigation?
SELECT 1
- (A) Reactivation TB
- (B) *Escherichia coli* pneumonia
- (C) *Pseudomonas aeruginosa* pneumonia
- (D) *Klebsiella pneumoniae* pneumonia
- (E) Cavitary bronchogenic carcinoma

Answer: (D): The patient has *Klebsiella pneumoniae* (choice D) with early abscess formation. Alcoholics commonly develop this type of pneumonia. The abrupt history essentially rules out reactivation TB (choice A is incorrect). However, the lobar consolidation in the LUL may be concealing an additional component of TB that must await acid-fast stains and culture, especially with the history of a 12 mm TST. The Gram stain characteristics are not typical of *Escherichia coli* (choice B is incorrect) or *P. aeruginosa* (choice C is incorrect), both of which are gram-negative rods without capsules. Furthermore, both of the latter organisms are more often associated with nosocomial rather than community-acquired pneumonia. Cavitary bronchogenic carcinoma (choice E is incorrect) would not explain the abrupt onset and the Gram stain findings.

A-a = Alveolar-arterial, ABG = arterial blood gas, AIDS = acquired immunodeficiency syndrome, CAD = coronary artery disease, CB = chronic bronchitis, CBC = complete blood cell count, CF = cystic fibrosis, CNS = central nervous system, COD = cause of death, DKA = diabetic ketoacidosis, DL_{CO} = diffusion capacity with carbon monoxide, Dx = diagnosis, EMB = ethambutol, HIV = human immunodeficiency virus, ICU = intensive care unit, IgE = immunoglobulin E, INH = isoniazid, IV = intravenous, LDH = lactate dehydrogenase, LUL = left upper lobe, MAI = *Mycobacterium avium-intracellulare*, PA = pulmonary artery, $PaCO_2$ = partial pressure of arterial carbon dioxide, PCP = *Pneumocystis carinii* pneumonia, PZA = pyrazinamide, RBC = red blood cell, RIF = rifampin, RTA = renal tubular acidosis, Rx = treatment, SaO_2 = arterial oxygen saturation, S/S = signs and symptoms, TB = tuberculosis, TMP/SMX = trimethoprim/sulfamethoxazole, TST = tuberculosis skin test.

Table 6–6. INTERSTITIAL LUNG DISEASE, PULMONARY VASCULITIS, AND OBSTRUCTIVE LUNG DISEASE

Most Common...	Answer and Explanation
causes of ILD	• **pneumoconioses:** dust diseases, • *sarcoidosis,* • *drugs,* • *radiation,* • *infections,* • *lymphangitic spread of tumor,* • *hypersensitivity reactions,* • *pneumonitis,* • *collagen-vascular disease,* • *Goodpasture's syndrome*
pathophysiologic abnormalities in ILD	• *functional loss of alveolar/capillary units,* • *increase in interstitial fibrosis as a reaction to injury*
symptoms of ILD	• **dry cough,** • *exertional dyspnea*
signs of ILD	• **late inspiratory crackles in lower lungs,** • *digital clubbing,* • *accentuated P2:* sign of PH • *left parasternal heave:* RVH due to PH
lab findings of ILD	• *PFT findings:* see Table 6–2, • *ABG findings:* * hypoxemia, * chronic respiratory alkalosis, * increased A-a gradient
chest radiograph findings in ILD	• **diffuse bilateral reticular infiltrates:** described as "ground glass" in appearance, • *nodular infiltrates:* particularly in silicosis, • *reticulonodular infiltrates,* • *"honeycomb" lung:* Hamman-Rich lung
diagnostic tests used to evaluate ILD	• *fiberoptic bronchoscopy with biopsies,* • *bronchoalveolar lavage:* useful in excluding PCP, • *PFTs,* • *ABGs*

Table continued on following page

Table 6–6. INTERSTITIAL LUNG DISEASE, PULMONARY VASCULITIS, AND OBSTRUCTIVE LUNG DISEASE
Continued

Most Common...	Answer and Explanation
types of inhaled pollutants	*soluble pollutants:* e.g., * Farmer's lung, * exudative response with a large number of T lymphocytes in lavage specimens, • *insoluble pollutants:* * e.g., silica, * fibrogenic reaction
pollutants that are very fibrogenic	• *asbestos:* * roofers, * shipyard pipefitters, * insulation installation, • *talc:* mining, • *silicon dioxide:* * foundry workers (casting metal), * quarry workers, * sandblasters, • *beryllium:* aerospace industry
pollutants that are not very fibrogenic	• *coal:* mining, • *fiberglass:* insulation, • *iron:* mining
cause of "black lung disease"	*inhalation of anthracotic pigment:* * coal worker's pneumoconiosis (CWP), * involves the upper lobes
subtypes of CWP	• *simple CWP:* * fibrotic opacities <1 cm, * mild ventilatory dysfunction, * alveolar macrophages contain anthracotic pigment (called "dust cells"), • *progressive massive fibrosis* (PMF): * opacities ≥1 cm, * crippling ILD, * produces centrilobular emphysema
complications in CWP	• **increased risk for typical/atypical TB:** no risk of primary lung cancer, • *cor pulmonale:* PH + RVH, • *Caplan syndrome:* CWP + large cavitating rheumatoid nodules
cause of "egg shell" calcifications in centrally located hilar lymph nodes	*silicosis:* * silica, unlike other fibrogenic substances, is cytotoxic to macrophages, * inhalation produces nodulation in all lung fields after ~20 years of exposure, * simple and PMF types, * "egg shell" calcifications may also occur in sarcoidosis
complications of silicosis	• **increased risk for typical and atypical TB:** * macrophages lysed by silica (cannot kill TB), * no risk of primary lung cancer, • *cor pulmonale,* • *Caplan syndrome*
cause of ferruginous bodies in sputum	*inhalation of asbestos minerals, which become coated by iron:* * asbestos is a crystalline silicate, * two subfamilies— ♦ serpentines (e.g., chrysotile, most common type) and ♦ amphiboles (crocidolite)

Table 6–6. INTERSTITIAL LUNG DISEASE, PULMONARY VASCULITIS, AND OBSTRUCTIVE LUNG DISEASE
Continued

Most Common...	Answer and Explanation
lung lesions associated with asbestos	• **benign pleural plaque,** • *primary lung cancer:* all types, • *mesothelioma,* • *benign effusions,* • *laryngeal cancer*
complication of asbestos exposure plus smoking	*primary lung cancer:* * smoking + asbestos is synergistic, * 60- to 90-fold increase in primary lung cancer, * fivefold increase in nonsmokers, * most common cancer in asbestosis in smokers/nonsmokers
malignant pleural lesion associated with asbestos exposure	*mesothelioma:* * no smoking relationship, * crocidolite fibers implicated in pathogenesis, * require 20–40 years to develop, * must find asbestos fibers in lung parenchyma (none present in pleura) to confirm its causal relationship to asbestos exposure, * malignant effusions are common, * very poor prognosis
clinical findings in chronic berylliosis	• **exertional dyspnea,** • *predisposes to lung cancer but not TB*
cause of Farmer's lung	*inhalation of thermophilic actinomycetes:* * present in moldy hay, * hypersensitivity pneumonitis (extrinsic allergic alveolitis)
clinical findings in Farmer's lung	• *first exposure:* precipitating IgG antibodies develop (present in serum), • *second exposure:* antibodies combine with inhaled allergens to form localized ICs (type III Arthus reaction) in lung tissue, • *chronic exposure:* granulomatous inflammation (type IV hypersensitivity)
cause of silo filler's disease	*inhalation of nitrous oxide fumes:* hypersensitivity pneumonitis
cause of bagassosis	*exposure to moldy sugar cane:* hypersensitivity pneumonitis
cause of "Monday morning blues"	*byssinosis:* * hypersensitivity pneumonitis due to exposure to cotton/hemp/linen, * respiratory illness occurs when patients return to work on Monday

Table continued on following page

Table 6–6. INTERSTITIAL LUNG DISEASE, PULMONARY VASCULITIS, AND OBSTRUCTIVE LUNG DISEASE
Continued

Most Common...	Answer and Explanation
types of noninfectious interstitial pneumonias	• **UIP:** * associated with collagen-vascular diseases, * e.g., RA, PSS, SLE, • *DIP:* desquamated type II pneumocytes, • *LIP:* * lymphoid infiltrate commonly progresses into a malignant lymphoma, * common in children with AIDS, * may be EBV/HIV-related
long-term complication of noninfectious interstitial pneumonias	*Hamman-Rich lung:* alveolar fibrosis leads to proximal dilatation of the small airways, providing a honeycomb appearance of the lung
noninfectious granulomatous lung disease	*sarcoidosis:* * 10 times more common in blacks than whites, * women > men, * activated T cells target the lungs and produce an alveolitis
S/S in sarcoidosis	• **dyspnea,** • *fever,* • *uveitis:* * blurry vision, * uveitis + parotid enlargement is Hereford's syndrome, • CN *palsies:* Bell's palsy, • *polyuria:* central DI, • *hepatomegaly:* granulomatous hepatitis, • *myocarditis:* * conduction disturbances, * arrhythmias, • *erythema nodosum:* * indicator of acute sarcoidosis in combination with hilar adenopathy, * good prognostic sign, • *arthritis:* punched out lytic lesions in phalangeal/metacarpal bones are characteristic, • *renal stones*
chest radiograph findings in sarcoidosis	• **bilateral hilar node lymphadenopathy:** * called "potato nodes", * nodes contain granulomas, • *reticulonodular densities*
lab findings in sarcoidosis	• **increased ACE:** ~90%, • *hypercalcemia:* 20%: lymphocytes in granulomas synthesize 1-α-hydroxylase: increased vitamin D synthesis, • *hypercalciuria:* renal stones, • *polyclonal gammopathy,* • *cutaneous anergy:* * decreased CD_4 helper cells in PB, * cells are used up in granulomas, • *positive Kveim test:* intradermal injection of sarcoid antigens
diagnostic tests used to confirm sarcoidosis	*fiberoptic bronchoscopy with transtracheal biopsy:* * mainly used to R/O other diseases, * document noncaseating granulomas

Table 6–6. INTERSTITIAL LUNG DISEASE, PULMONARY VASCULITIS, AND OBSTRUCTIVE LUNG DISEASE
Continued

Most Common...	Answer and Explanation
Rx for sarcoidosis	*corticosteroids for extrapulmonary disease:* * does not improve outcome in lung disease, * improves outcome in extrapulmonary disease (e.g., heart, CNS), * drop in ACE levels correlates with improvement, * ketoconazole blocks synthesis of vitamin D
COD in sarcoidosis	*heart disease*
drugs causing ILD	• **amiodarone,** • *methotrexate,* • *bleomycin/busulfan,* • *cyclophosphamide,* • *methysergide,* • *nitrosourea/nitrofurantoin*
collagen vascular causes of ILD	• **PSS:** ILD most common COD, • *SLE:* 50%, • *RA:* 20%
types of lung disease in RA	• **chronic pleuritis,** • *exudative pulmonary effusions:* characteristic pseudochylous effusions with a low glucose, • *rheumatoid nodules + CWP/silicosis:* Caplan's syndrome, • *diffuse interstitial fibrosis,* • *nodules,* • *vasculitis,* • *PH*
ILD causing hemoptysis and renal failure	*Goodpasture's syndrome:* * begins in the lungs, * usually progresses into renal failure, * anti-basement membrane antibodies directed against pulmonary/glomerular capillary basement membranes
clinical findings in idiopathic hemosiderosis	*unlike GS, idiopathic hemosiderosis—* * primarily affects young women, * has no renal involvement
ILD associated with *Nocardia*	*pulmonary alveolar proteinosis:* * protein-rich fluid derived from type II pneumocytes/macrophages, * usually resolves, * patients are prone to *Nocardia* infections
ILD associated with a previous flu-like illness	*BOOP*
clinical findings in BOOP	• *patients 40–60 years old,* • *presentation:* previous Hx of flu-like syndrome leading to progressive dyspnea

Table continued on following page

Table 6–6. INTERSTITIAL LUNG DISEASE, PULMONARY VASCULITIS, AND OBSTRUCTIVE LUNG DISEASE
Continued

Most Common...	Answer and Explanation
histologic findings in BOOP	• *specific histologic Dx:* polypoid protrusions in RB, AD, alveoli, • *associations:* * adenovirus pneumonia, * toxic inhalants, • *Rx:* corticosteroids halt its progression into ILD
causes of pulmonary infiltrates with eosinophilia (PIE)	• *Loeffler's syndrome:* benign disorder with fleeting pulmonary infiltrates and eosinophilia • *acute eosinophilic pneumonia:* lung infiltrates + pleural effusion, • *chronic eosinophilic pneumonia:* infiltrates occur at the lung periphery, • *ABPA in patients with bronchial asthma,* • *parasitic infestations*
angiocentric vasculitides involving lung	• **Wegener's granulomatosis,** • *Churg-Strauss vasculitis* [see Table 12–3.]
angiocentric T cell lymphoma involving lung	*lymphomatoid granulomatosis*
cause of COPD	*smoking:* * ~10–15% of smokers develop COPD, * fourth most common COD
types of COPD	• **CB,** • *emphysema,* • *bronchial asthma,* • *bronchiectasis,* • *CF*
clinical features of CB	• **productive cough for ~3 months for 2 consecutive years,** • *airway obstruction due to inflammation/bronchoconstriction in terminal bronchioles,* • *segmental bronchi have increased mucus production*
pathophysiologic abnormality in CB	*V/Q mismatch:* * site of obstruction is more proximally located than emphysema, * affects large area of gas exchange
site of damage in emphysema	*functional respiratory unit:* unit consists of the RB, AD, alveoli
effects of smoking in respiratory unit	• *smoke attracts neutrophils into the lungs,* • *neutrophils release elastases that destroy tissue support in respiratory unit,* • *smoke inactivates AAT:* elastases left unneutralized
types of emphysema	• **centrilobular emphysema:** * involves upper lobes, * associated with **smoking**/CWP, * RB targeted for destruction, • *panacinar:* entire

Table 6–6. INTERSTITIAL LUNG DISEASE, PULMONARY VASCULITIS, AND OBSTRUCTIVE LUNG DISEASE
Continued

Most Common...	Answer and Explanation
Continued	respiratory unit destroyed, • *paraseptal:* targets AD and alveoli for destruction
type of emphysema due to AAT deficiency	*panacinar emphysema:* predilection for the lower lobes
clinical findings in AAT deficiency	• *AR disease,* • *deficiency of liver synthesis of AAT,* • *PiZZ phenotype most prone to lung disease,* • *smoking further enhances disease*
changes in the lungs in old age	*see Table 3–3*
S/S of COPD	• **persistent chronic productive cough with slowly progressive exertional dyspnea:** * EMP, * CB, • *hyperaerated lungs:* EMP, • *increased AP diameter:* EMP, • *flattened diaphragms:* EMP, • *diminished breath sounds:* EMP, • *normal/pink skin:* * EMP, * "pink puffer",* • *weight loss/cachectic:* EMP, • *sibilant rhonchi/expiratory wheezing:* CB, • *cyanosis:* * CB, * "blue bloater",* • *obese/stocky:* CB
chest radiograph findings in COPD	• *hyperlucent lung fields:* EMP, • *increased AP diameter:* EMP, • *vertical heart:* EMP, • *bullae/blebs:* EMP, • *low diaphragms:* EMP, • *large, horizontally oriented heart:* CB, • *increased bronchial markings:* CB
lab findings in COPD	• *increased TLC:* EMP, • *increased lung compliance:* EMP, • *decreased DL_{CO}:* EMP, • *respiratory alkalosis/normal ABG:* EMP, • *polycythemia:* CB, • *hypoxemia:* CB > EMP, • *respiratory acidosis:* CB, • *right axis deviation/RVH/cor pulmonale:* CB
Rx of acute exacerbations of COPD	• **metered-dose inhalation of selective β_2-adrenergic receptor agonists:** e.g., albuterol, • **O_2 therapy:** maintain SaO_2 ~90% (~PaO_2 60 mm Hg), • *inhaled anticholinergics:* * ipratropium bromide, * first-line drug that blocks vagally mediated bronchospasm, • *methylxanthines:* * controversial in acute Rx, * useful for long-term management, • *IV glucocorticoids:* benefit in some patients, • *antibiotics:* e.g., TMP/SMX (least expensive)

Table continued on following page

Table 6–6. INTERSTITIAL LUNG DISEASE, PULMONARY VASCULITIS, AND OBSTRUCTIVE LUNG DISEASE
Continued

Most Common...	Answer and Explanation
long-term Rx of COPD	• **stop smoking,** • *inhaled ipratropium bromide:* longer duration of action than β_2-agonists, • *oral theophylline,* • O_2 *Rx:* keep SaO_2 ~90%, • *glucocorticoids:* effective in 10–25%, • *yearly influenza vaccine,* • *pneumococcal vaccine:* every 6 years
chronic respiratory disease in children	*bronchial asthma:* * episodic, hyper-reactive, reversible, small airway disease that primarily targets the terminal bronchioles, * incidence increases with age, * multifactorial inheritance pattern noted in IgE-mediated asthma
cause of bronchial asthma	*exposure to allergens:* IgE-mediated type I hypersensitivity
mechanisms of IgE-mediated asthma	• *inhaled allergens activate previously sensitized mast cells covered by allergen-specific IgE antibodies:* * causes early mast cell release reaction, * mediators: ♦ histamine, ♦ eosinophil chemotactic factor, ♦ major basic protein, • *late phase reaction in mast cells:* synthesis/release of bronchoconstricting agents (♦ PGD_2, ♦ leukotrienes C_4, D_4, E_4)
nonimmunologic causes of asthma	• *aspirin/NSAID sensitivity:* drug-induced asthma + nasal polyps, • *cold temperature,* • *exercise,* • *environmental pollutants,* • *smoke*
S/S in asthma	• **episodic wheezing,** • *cough:* night and early AM, • *increased AP diameter:* air trapping, *pulsus paradoxus:* * see Table 5–1, * occurs in severe asthma, * decreased lung compliance due to excess water in interstitial tissue
lab findings in bronchial asthma	• **respiratory alkalosis:** * may progress into respiratory acidosis if bronchospasm is not relieved, * respiratory acidosis is an indication for ♦ hospitalization, ♦ intubation, ♦ mechanical ventilation, • *hypoxemia,* • *decreased FEV_{1sec}:* values <30% indicate need for hospitalization, • *eosinophilia,* • *positive skin tests for allergens,* • *precipitin antibodies if ABPA is present*
Rx for an acute bronchial asthmatic attack	• **metered-dose inhaler with a β_2-agonist:** e.g., albuterol, • O_2 *to keep SaO_2 >90%* • *IV corticosteroids:* severe cases

Table 6–6. INTERSTITIAL LUNG DISEASE, PULMONARY VASCULITIS, AND OBSTRUCTIVE LUNG DISEASE
Continued

Most Common...	Answer and Explanation
Rx for daily management of asthma	• *avoid known allergens,* • *inhaled β₂-agonist:* mild episodic asthma, • *inhaled corticosteroids:* mild/moderate persistent asthma, • *inhaled cromolyn sodium:* mild asthma/exercise-induced asthma, • *oral sustained-release β₂-agonist:* if nocturnal asthma is present
Rx for severe asthma	• *use of more potent inhaled corticosteroids:* e.g., fluticasone, • *systemic corticosteroids:* if not responding to inhaled preparation
causes of bronchiectasis in the United States	• **CF:** *Pseudomonas aeruginosa* most responsible for damage to bronchi/bronchioles leading to dilatation, • *infections:* * TB, * most common cause worldwide, * adenovirus, * *Staphylococcus aureus,* * histoplasmosis, • *bronchial obstruction:* e.g., tumor, • *B cell ID,* • *immotile cilia syndrome:* * Kartagener's syndrome, * absent dynein arm, * situs inversus
mechanisms causing bronchiectasis	*obstruction/infection:* * obstruction/infection lead to weakening of the bronchial wall and dilatation, * bronchi/bronchioles fill with pus and extend to the lung periphery, * most commonly occurs in the left lower lobe
S/S in bronchiectasis	• **cough productive of copious sputum:** sputum settles out in three layers, • *hemoptysis:* sometimes massive, • *fever,* • *cerebral abscess,* • *digital clubbing,* • *accentuated P2:* PH with or without cor pulmonale
chest radiograph findings in bronchiectasis	• *crowded bronchial markings extending to the lung periphery,* • *high resolution CT:* excellent in defining bronchiectasis
defect in cystic fibrosis	*defective gene on chromosome 7 that codes for CF transmembrane regulator* (CFTR): * CF is the most lethal genetic (AR inheritance) disease in the United States, * CFTR normally controls transport of Cl^- ions through certain epithelial cells
DNA defect in CF	*deletion of three nucleotide bases on chromosome 7:* * normally codes for phenylalanine, * leads to synthesis of a defective CFTR

Table continued on following page

Table 6–6. INTERSTITIAL LUNG DISEASE, PULMONARY VASCULITIS, AND OBSTRUCTIVE LUNG DISEASE
Continued

Most Common...	Answer and Explanation
abnormality in sweat glands/respiratory epithelium in CF	• *sweat glands:* * neither Cl^- or Na^+ ions are reabsorbed out of the lumen, * basis of the sweat test, • *respiratory epithelium:* * Cl^- ions are not secreted into the lumen, * Na^+ ions and water are reabsorbed out of the lumen leading to thick secretions
respiratory findings in CF	• *bronchiolitis:* initial infection in the terminal bronchioles, • *pneumonia:* * *Staphylococcus aureus* is most common pathogen in children, * *Hemophilus influenzae* and *Pseudomonas aeruginosa* (particularly the mucoid strain) are more common pathogens in later years, * *Burkholderia cepacia* infections produce rapidly progressive disease, • *cor pulmonale,* • *bronchiectasis*
S/S of CF	• **recurrent pulmonary infections,** • *malabsorption:* duct obstruction with subsequent exocrine gland atrophy, • *DM:* late manifestation, • *meconium ileus in newborns:* impacted meconium, • *secondary biliary cirrhosis:* thick bile secretions, • *productive cough:* * bronchiectasis, * pneumonia, • *bleeding diathesis:* vitamin K deficiency from malabsorption, • *ataxia/hemolytic anemia:* vitamin E deficiency from malabsorption, • *nasal polyps,* • *atresia of vas deferens:* males sterile, • *women may bear children but have fertility problems:* due to thick cervical mucus
lab test findings in CF	• **abnormal sweat chloride test:** * >60 mEq/L in children, * >80 mEq/L in adults, * pilocarpine iontophoresis is gold standard, • *increased serum immunoreactive trypsin in newborns:* due to obstructed pancreatic ducts, • *chronic respiratory acidosis,* • *hypoxemia,* • *obstructive type of PFTs,* • *hyperglycemia:* DM, • *prolonged PT/PTT:* vitamin K deficiency, • *hypocalcemia:* vitamin D deficiency from malabsorption, • *folate/iron deficiency:* * malabsorption, * mixed anemia
Rx of CF	• *IV antibiotics directed against Pseudomonas aeruginosa in acute exacerbations:* ceftazidime + tobramycin, • *aerosolized tobramycin:* reduces *Pseudomonas aeruginosa*

Table 6–6. INTERSTITIAL LUNG DISEASE, PULMONARY VASCULITIS, AND OBSTRUCTIVE LUNG DISEASE
Continued

Most Common...	Answer and Explanation
Continued	population, • *postural drainage,* • *anti-inflammatory agents:* intermittent use of * corticosteroids, * ibuprofen, • *recombinant DNAase:* decreases sputum viscosity, • *pancreatic enzyme replacement,* • *fat soluble vitamins,* • *medium chain triglycerides:* do not require enzyme degradation for absorption, • *double lung transplants:* patients with FEV_{1sec} of <1 liter
COD in CF	*progressive respiratory failure:* median survival for CF is ~30 years old

Question: Which of the following would more likely occur in emphysema than in sarcoidosis? **SELECT 4**
- (A) Increased TLC
- (B) Decreased RV
- (C) Hypoxemia
- (D) Hilar adenopathy
- (E) FEV_{1sec}/FVC ratio >80%
- (F) Prolonged expiratory phase
- (G) Low diaphragm on chest radiograph
- (H) Hypercalcemia
- (I) Hyperlucency of the lungs
- (J) Decreased DL_{CO}

Answers: (A), (F), (G), (I): Emphysema is an example of an obstructive lung disease and sarcoidosis a restrictive lung disease. Emphysema is associated with an increase in TLC **(choice A)**, increase in RV **(choice B is incorrect)**, and a prolonged expiratory phase **(choice F)**. Emphysema is more likely to have a low diaphragm on a chest radiograph **(choice G)** and hyperlucency of the lungs **(choice I)**. Sarcoidosis is more likely to have an increased FEV_{1sec}/FVC ratio **(choice E is incorrect)**, hilar adenopathy **(choice D is incorrect)**, and hypercalcemia **(choice H is incorrect)**. Both conditions have hypoxemia **(choice C is incorrect)**, and a decreased DL_{CO} **(choice J is incorrect)**. Sarcoidosis is associated with a decreased TLC and RV, hilar adenopathy, FEV_{1sec}/FVC ratio > 80% (increased elasticity), normal to decreased expiratory phase, reticulonodular densities in the lung, hypercalcemia, and a decreased DL_{CO}.

AAT = α_1-antitrypsin, ABG = arterial blood gas, ABPA = acute bronchopulmonary aspergillosis, ACE = angiotensin converting enzyme, AD = alveolar duct, AIDS = acquired immunodeficiency syndrome, AP = anteroposterior, AR = autosomal recessive, BOOP = bronchiolitis obliterans organizing pneumonia, CB = chronic bronchitis, CF = cystic fibrosis, CFTR = cystic fibrosis transmembrane regulator, CN = cranial nerve, CNS = central nervous system, COD = cause of death, COPD =

chronic obstructive pulmonary disease, CT = computed tomography, CWP = coal worker's pneumoconiosis, DI = diabetes insipidus, DIP = desquamative interstitial pneumonitis, DL_{CO} = diffusion capacity using carbon monoxide, DM = diabetes mellitus, Dx = diagnosis, EBV = Epstein-Barr virus, EMP = emphysema, FEV_{1sec} = forced expiratory volume in 1 second, FVC = forced vital capacity, GS = Goodpasture's syndrome, HIV = human immunodeficiency virus, Hx = history, IC = immunocomplex, ID = immunodeficiency, Ig = immunoglobulin, ILD = interstitial lung disease, IV = intravenous, LIP = lymphoid interstitial pneumonitis, NSAID = nonsteroidal anti-inflammatory drug, PaO_2 = partial pressure of arterial oxygen, PB = peripheral blood, PCP = *Pneumocystis carinii* pneumonia, PFT = pulmonary function test, PH = pulmonary hypertension, PIE = pulmonary infiltrates with eosinophilia, PMF = progressive massive fibrosis, PSS = progressive systemic sclerosis, PT = prothrombin time, PTT = partial thromboplastin time, RA = rheumatoid arthritis, RB = respiratory bronchiole, R/O = rule out, RV = residual volume, RVH = right ventricular hypertrophy, Rx = treatment, SaO_2 = oxygen saturation, SLE = systemic lupus erythematosus, S/S = signs and symptoms, TB = tuberculosis, TLC = total lung capacity, TMP/SMX = trimethoprim/sulfamethoxazole, UIP = usual interstitial pneumonitis, V/Q = ventilation/perfusion.

Table 6–7. LUNG TUMORS, MEDIASTINAL DISORDERS, AND DISEASES OF THE PLEURA

Most Common...	Answer and Explanation
COD due to cancer in men and women	*primary lung cancer:* * incidence decreasing in men and increasing in women, * adenocarcinoma is the most common type
lung cancer	• **metastasis from breast cancer,** • *other common metastases:* * renal adenocarcioma, * choriocarcinoma: both gestationally derived and testicular, * GI cancers: ♦ esophagus, ♦ stomach, ♦ pancreas, ♦ colorectal, * sarcomas in general, * malignant melanoma
sites of metastasis in the lung	• **parenchyma,** • *pleura/pleural space,* • *endobronchial mucosa,* • *lymphatics,* • *chest wall,* • *mediastinum*
primary lung cancers	• **adenocarcinoma:** * ~35%, * most are peripherally located, • *squamous cell carcinoma:* * ~30%, * centrally located, • *small cell carcinoma:* * ~20%, * centrally located, • *large cell undifferentiated:* ~10% [Most lung cancers are simply divided into small cell and non-small cell cancer.]
causes of primary lung cancer	*cigarette smoking:* * ~90%, * see Table 2–1 for a more extensive list

Table 6–7. LUNG TUMORS, MEDIASTINAL DISORDERS, AND DISEASES OF THE PLEURA *Continued*

Most Common...	Answer and Explanation
primary lung cancer with no relationship to smoking	*bronchioloalveolar carcinoma:* peripherally located cancer derived from Clara cells (non-ciliated epithelium)
oncogenes involved in small cell cancer	*point mutations leading to inactivation of the p53 suppressor gene and ras oncogene*
centrally located primary lung cancers	• **squamous carcinoma,** • *small cell carcinoma* [These cancers also have the greatest relationship with cigarette smoking.]
peripherally located primary lung cancers	*adenocarcinoma*
primary lung cancer in nonsmokers	*adenocarcinoma*
primary lung cancer confused with a lobar pneumonia	*bronchioloalveolar carcinoma*
primary lung cancer to cavitate	• **squamous carcinoma,** • *large cell undifferentiated cancers*
primary lung cancer detected by cytologic examination of sputum	*squamous cell carcinoma:* * Pap stains reveal deeply eosinophilic staining of squamous cell cancers, * small cell cancer is least likely detected by cytologic exam of sputum (often confused with lymphocytes)
S/S of primary lung cancer	• **cough that has changed in character:** 75%, • *dyspnea:* 60%, • *hemoptysis:* 50%, • *weight loss:* 40%, • *chest pain:* 40%, • *hypertrophic osteoarthropathy/Eaton-Lambert syndrome:* see Table 4–1
symptom of lung metastasis	*dyspnea:* hemoptysis is uncommon
ectopic hormone secreting primary lung cancers	• **small cell carcinoma:** * secretes ACTH (ectopic Cushing's syndrome), * *ADH* (~50%) resulting in SIADH, • *squamous carcinoma:* PTH-like peptide (hypercalcemia)
sites of metastasis of primary lung cancer outside the lungs	• **adrenal glands:** 50%, • *liver:* 30%, • *brain:* * 20%, * small cell most commonly, • *bone:* predominantly lytic metastases

Table continued on following page

Table 6–7. LUNG TUMORS, MEDIASTINAL DISORDERS, AND DISEASES OF THE PLEURA *Continued*

Most Common...	Answer and Explanation
cause of the superior vena caval syndrome	*primary small cell carcinoma with invasion and compression of the superior vena cava* [see Table 5–3]
cause of the Pancoast syndrome	*primary squamous cell carcinoma:* * invasion of the brachial plexus (T1/T2) and cervical sympathetic ganglion, * the latter associated with Horner's syndrome (ipsilateral lid lag, miosis, absence of sweating).
diagnostic tests used in working up lung cancer	• **cytologic evaluation of sputum:** * sensitivity 30% in asymptomatic patients, * 50% if cough is present, * 70% if hemoptysis is present, • *fiberoptic bronchoscopy:* sensitivity 85–95% when brushings, lavage, and biopsies are collected, • *FNA:* sensitivity 90–95% with CT guidance, • *examination of PF, if an effusion is present:* sensitivity 60–80%, • *chest radiograph:* * 95% of peripheral tumors and 70% of central tumors are visible, * CT further evaluates size, extent, and presence of additional lesions
staging guidelines used to determine Rx options in primary lung cancer	*cell type determines the approach to staging:* * TNM system is used for non-SCLC, * stages I and II are operable, * stage III is usually inoperable, * anatomic extent, nodal involvement, and extrathoracic spread dramatically reduce the prognosis
Rx options of non-SCLC and SCLC	• *non-SCLC:* surgery Rx of choice, • *SCLC:* * TNM system is not beneficial (85% stage III), * chemotherapy/prophylactic cranial irradiation to prevent CNS metastasis are the mainstays of Rx
factors indicating inoperability of a primary lung cancer	• *predicted postoperative FEV_{1sec} <0.8 liters,* • *previous history of IHD,* • *evidence of intrathoracic spread:* * CT scans of hilum/mediastinum lymph nodes evaluate intrathoracic spread, * contralateral lymph node disease/mediastinal disease are contraindications for surgery, • *distance of tumor from carina $\leq$2 cm,* • *presence of extrathoracic spread:* * CT of adrenal gland, * blood chemistry evaluation used to R/O bone/liver metastasis

Table 6–7. LUNG TUMORS, MEDIASTINAL DISORDERS, AND DISEASES OF THE PLEURA *Continued*

Most Common...	Answer and Explanation
primary neuroendocrine tumor of lung with a low grade malignant potential	*bronchial carcinoid:* * like SCLCs, they are neurosecretory tumors, * unlike SCLCs, there is no smoking relationship, * clinical: ♦ cough, ♦ hemoptysis, ♦ postobstructive lipoid pneumonias, ♦ ~40% locally metastasize, ♦ rarely produce carcinoid syndrome
risk factors for a solitary nodule to be malignant	• **age of the patient:** * patients <35 years old have 1% risk (most are granulomas, usually histoplasmosis), * patients ≥50 years old have 50–60% risk (most are primary lung cancer, not metastasis), • *smoking,* • *patterns of calcification:* think benign if: * diffuse speckled calcification, * "popcorn" calcification (hamartoma), * concentric calcifications (granulomas), • *size of nodule:* * doubling time of lung cancer 15–450 days, * doubling of nodule size in this time frame suspicious for malignancy, * lack of size change over 2 years is benign
tests used in evaluating solitary nodules	• **comparing previous chest radiographs,** • *skin testing for TB/systemic fungi,* • *FNA,* • *high resolution CT scans,* • *bronchoscopy*
clinical findings in bronchial hamartomas	• *peripherally located solitary nodule,* • *"popcorn" calcifications*
presentations for mediastinal disease	• **asymptomatic,** • *compression of vessels:* SVC syndrome, • *destruction of nerves:* hoarseness with recurrent laryngeal nerve involvement, • *Horner's syndrome:* see above, • *cough,* • *paraneoplastic syndrome:* ectopic hormones
mediastinal site for disease	*anterior mediastinum:* * thymoma (most common), * malignant lymphoma (nodular sclerosing Hodgkin's disease)
cause of a "mediastinal crunch" (Hamman's sign)	• **ruptured esophagus from endoscopy/retching,** • *pneumothorax* [The crunch occurs with each systole. It is due to subcutaneous emphysema.]
cause of sclerosing mediastinitis	*Histoplasma capsulatum*

Table continued on following page

Table 6–7. LUNG TUMORS, MEDIASTINAL DISORDERS, AND DISEASES OF THE PLEURA *Continued*

Most Common...	Answer and Explanation
tumor in the mediastinum	*neurogenic tumors:* * include ♦ neuroblastoma in children and ♦ ganglioneuroma in adults, * most commonly occur in posterior mediastinum
mediastinal tumor associated with MG and pure RBC aplasia	*thymoma:* * thymic hyperplasia (germinal follicles synthesize antibodies against acetylcholine receptors) is more common than thymomas in MG, * pure RBC aplasia is due to destruction of the RBC stem cell
mediastinal site for nodular sclerosing HD	*anterior mediastinum:* see Table 8–9
mediastinal site for germ cell tumors	*anterior mediastinum:* most germ cell tumors localize to the midline
disorders in the middle mediastinum	• **pericardial cyst,** • *bronchogenic cyst,* • *lymphadenopathy:* due to * sarcoidosis, * malignancy, * granulomatous disease, • *aortic arch aneurysms*
factors determining fluid movement in the pleural cavity	*hydrostatic pressure difference between the parietal and visceral pleura* [The net pressure in the parietal pleura is +9 cm H_2O (high hydrostatic pressure from the intercostal arteries). Net pressure in the visceral pleura is −11 cm H_2O (low hydrostatic pressure from the pulmonary circulation). Fluid moves from the parietal pleura into the pleural space and is taken up by the visceral pleura. The colloid osmotic pressure (oncotic pressure) is roughly equal between the parietal and visceral pleura and is not normally responsible for the fluid movements.]
mechanisms for fluid accumulation in the pleural cavity	• *alterations in the hydrostatic pressure:* in CHF, the high pulmonary vessel hydrostatic pressure reduces the uptake of fluid from the visceral pleura, • *alterations in oncotic pressure:* hypoalbuminemia causes a greater movement of fluid into the pleural space and less uptake by the visceral pleura due to a low oncotic pressure, • *increased vessel permeability:* e.g., * pneumonia, * pulmonary infarction, • *lymphatic blockage:* * blocks uptake of fluid from the pleural space, * e.g., lymphangitic spread of tumor in the lungs, •

Table 6–7. LUNG TUMORS, MEDIASTINAL DISORDERS, AND DISEASES OF THE PLEURA *Continued*

Most Common...	Answer and Explanation
Continued	*leakage of ascitic fluid through openings in the diaphragm:* ascites in cirrhosis
tests used to separate transudates from exudates in PF	• **ratios favoring an exudate:** * PF protein/serum protein ratio >0.5, * PF LDH/serum LDH >0.6, * PF LDH >0.45 × the upper limit of normal of serum LDH, * values less than the above indicate a transudate, • *PF protein:* * >3 g/dL = exudate, * <3 g/dL = transudate, • *cells:* * exudates have a cellular infiltrate, * transudates do not
cause of a pleural effusion	*CHF:* transudate
causes of a PF exudate	• **pneumonia,** • *pulmonary infarction:* hemorrhagic exudate, • *cancer:* hemorrhagic exudate, • *pancreatitis:* contains amylase
causes of a PF pH <7.3	• **malignancy:** primary or secondary, • *empyema:* e.g., *Staphylococcus aureus* pneumonia, • *TB,* • *collagen-vascular disease:* e.g., * RA, * PSS, * SLE
collagen vascular disease with a PF glucose <20 mg/dL	*RA:* selective block of glucose reabsorption
role of cytology of PF	*detection of primary/metastatic disease:* cytology has a greater sensitivity (60–80%) than a pleural Bx in detecting malignancy
PF findings in TB	*exudate with a lymphocyte dominant cell count:* culture of a pleural biopsy has a higher yield than culture of PF in detecting TB
causes of increased amylase in the PF	• **acute pancreatitis:** left-sided PF effusion, • *Boerhaave's syndrome:* rupture of the esophagus
primary pleural malignancy	*mesothelioma:* see Table 6–6
PF pH cutoff requiring tube drainage of a parapneumonic effusion	*pH <7.0*

Table continued on following page

Table 6–7. LUNG TUMORS, MEDIASTINAL DISORDERS, AND DISEASES OF THE PLEURA *Continued*

Most Common...	Answer and Explanation
physical findings in a pleural effusion	*see Table 6–1*
Rx for recurrent malignant effusions	*pleurodesis with injection of an irritant into the pleural cavity*
chest radiograph findings in a pleural effusion	• **blunting of the costophrenic angle with a concave meniscus,** • *loss of definition of the hemidiaphragm,* • *increased density in the hemithorax* [A minimum of 150–300 mL of fluid must be present to detect it on a routine chest radiograph.]
radiographic position used to detect effusions	*lateral decubitus views:* * suspected side in the dependent position, * detects smaller amounts of fluid, * generally more accurate in detecting effusions than upright films

Question: A 62-year-old woman with a history of a modified left radical mastectomy 10 years ago presents with dyspnea, persistent cough and a sharp, stabbing pain in the left posterior chest particularly aggravated by coughing. Physical examination reveals tachypnea, dullness to percussion at the base of the posterior left lung, and decreased breath sounds. An upright chest radiograph exhibits loss of definition of the hemidiaphragm on the left and a patchy interstitial infiltrate throughout both lung fields. Which of the following laboratory abnormalities would you expect in this patient? **SELECT 4**
- (A) Arterial pH <7.35
- (B) PaO₂ <80 mm Hg
- (C) PF protein <3 g/dL
- (D) PF glucose <40 mg/dL
- (E) PaCO₂ <33 mm Hg
- (F) PF cytology positive for malignant cells

Answers: (B), (D), (E), (F): The patient has recurrence of breast cancer with metastasis to the pleural cavity (malignant effusion) and pleura (pleuritic chest pain) along with lymphangitic spread throughout her lungs (interstitial infiltrate) producing cough and dyspnea. Owing to the presence of tachypnea, respiratory alkalosis is likely with a pH >7.45 **(choice A is incorrect)** and a PaCO₂ <33 mm Hg **(choice E).** Hypoxemia **(choice B)** is likely owing to a diffusion defect **(choice E).** PF analysis is likely to reveal an exudate with a PF protein >3 g/dL **(choice C is incorrect),** and a PF glucose <40 mg/dL **(choice D).** Malignant cells are likely to be identified in a cytologic specimen **(choice F).**

ACTH = adrenocorticotropic hormone, ADH = antidiuretic hormone, Bx = biopsy, CHF = congestive heart failure, CNS = central nervous system, COD = cause of death, CT = computed tomography, FEV_{1sec} = forced expiratory volume in 1 second, FNA = fine needle aspiration, GI = gastrointestinal, HD = Hodgkin's disease, IHD = ischemic heart disease, LDH = lactate dehydrogenase, MG = myasthenia gravis, $PaCO_2$ = partial pressure of arterial carbon monoxide, PaO_2 = partial pressure of arterial oxygen, PF = pleural fluid, PSS = progressive systemic sclerosis, PTH = parathormone, RA = rheumatoid arthritis, RBC = red blood cell, R/O = rule out, Rx = treatment, SCLC = small cell lung cancer, SIADH = syndrome of inappropriate antidiuretic hormone, SLE = systemic lupus erythematosus, S/S = signs and symptoms, SVC = superior vena cava, TB = tuberculosis, TNM = tumor/nodes/metastasis.

7

CRITICAL CARE MEDICINE

CONTENTS

Table 7–1. ACUTE RESPIRATORY FAILURE (ARF)

Most Common...	Answer and Explanation
types of ARF	• **hypercapnic-hypoxic ARF (HHARF):** defined as a * PaO_2 <60 mm Hg, * $PaCO_2$ >44 mm Hg, * pH <7.35 (respiratory acidosis), • *hypoxic ARF (HARF):* * defined as a PaO_2 <60 mm Hg (hypoxemia) not corrected after breathing 50% O_2, * $PaCO_2$ normal/decreased
causes of HARF	• **cardiogenic pulmonary edema,** • *cardiopulmonary arrest,* • *pneumonia,* • *ARDS,* • *sepsis*
pathophysiologic mechanisms of HARF	• **intrapulmonary shunting:** e.g., ARDS, • *diffusion abnormality:* e.g., ILD, • *V/Q mismatch:* e.g., * pneumonia, * PE
pathophysiologic mechanisms of HHARF	• **respiratory center depression:** e.g., * barbiturates, * primary intracranial disease, • *upper airway obstruction:* e.g., * foreign body, * angioedema, • *chest bellows disease:* e.g., * obesity–hypoventilation syndrome, * neuromuscular disease, • *increased dead space:* e.g., * asthma, • *metabolic derangements:* e.g., * sepsis, * hypokalemia,* hypophosphatemia
S/S of HARF	• **dyspnea,** • *cyanosis,* • *tachypnea:* >35 breaths/minute, • *tachycardia,* • *hypotension/HTN,* • *confusion,* • *lactic acidosis*
S/S of HHARF	• **dyspnea,** • **headache:** cerebral edema produced by vasodilatation from respiratory acidosis, • *conjunctival hyperemia,* • *papilledema,* • *lethargy,* • *coma,* • *asterixis:* flapping tremor

Table continued on following page

Table 7–1. ACUTE RESPIRATORY FAILURE (ARF)
Continued

Most Common...	Answer and Explanation
S/S of partial versus complete upper airway obstruction	• *partial:* * patient can cough, talk, and breathe, * let patient dislodge foreign body with forceful coughing, • *complete:* * cannot cough, talk, or breathe, * perform a Heimlich maneuver, * results in cardiac arrest in 4 min and irreversible brain injury in 3–5 min
causes of upper airway obstruction without ventilation	• **food:** cafe coronary, • *angioedema*
lab findings in ARF	• **low Pao_2:** * HARF, * HHARF, • *low $PaCO_2$:* * respiratory alkalosis, * *HARF,* • *high $PaCO_2$:* * respiratory acidosis, * HHARF, • *lactic acidosis:* HARF, • *increased A–a gradient:* primary lung disease in HARF/HHARF
factors to consider in Rx of ARF	• *ventilation:* O_2 inhaled and CO_2 expired, • *arterial oxygenation:* e.g., how well Pao_2 is transferred into mixed venous blood in the pulmonary capillaries in exchange for CO_2, • *O_2 transport:* e.g., * cardiac output, * Hb concentration, * Sao_2, * Pao_2, • *O_2 extraction/ utilization at tissue level:* e.g., * ODC, * mitochondrial function (e.g., oxidative/phosphorylation)
method of assessing ventilation	*measure $Paco_2$*
method of assessing arterial oxygenation	*measure Pao_2:* * calculation of A–a gradient (see Table 6–2) determines whether hypoxemia is due to lung disease (increased A-a) or CNS, upper airway, chest bellows disease (normal A-a)
methods of assessing O_2 transport/ extraction	• *measure/calculate the Sao_2:* measure directly with a pulse oximeter or calculate from the Pao_2, * pulse oximeter is a noninvasive method of assessing the Sao_2 (see Table 6–2) • *measure MVo_2 with an SGC:* * best index of tissue hypoxia, * blood sample taken from PA, * assesses adequacy of O_2 delivery to tissue O_2 extraction by tissue, and adequacy of cardiac index and systemic arterial O_2 content

Table 7–1. ACUTE RESPIRATORY FAILURE (ARF)
Continued

Most Common...	Answer and Explanation
general management principles in Rx of ARF	• *improve ventilation:* * mechanical ventilation (see below), * endotracheal intubation (e.g., provides a closed system for mechanical ventilation and delivery of high fractions of inspired O_2), * reduce dead space (e.g., remove secretions), * naloxone (reverses effects of respiratory depression from narcotic overdose), • *improve arterial oxygenation:* * encourage deep breathing (prevent atelectasis), * antibiotics (pneumonia, sepsis), * upright position (prevent atelectasis), * administer O_2—e.g., ♦ nasal prongs, ♦ Venturi mask, ♦ CPAP, ♦ PEEP, ♦ transfuse packed RBCs (anemia)
general types of mechanical ventilation	• *volume ventilators:* set for * tidal volume, * ventilation rate, * inspired O_2 concentration (FIO_2), * level of end-expiratory pressure (PEEP), • *pressure ventilators:* deliver a preset pressure to determine: * flow,* tidal volume, * inspiratory time, * frequency
indications for mechanical ventilation	• **acute hypoxemia or acute hypercapnia** (increased $PaCO_2$) **not responding to appropriate Rx,** • *clinical instability,* • *apnea*
goals for mechanical ventilation	• $FIO_2 \leq 0.50$, • $SaO_2 > 90\%$: equivalent to $PaO_2 \geq 60$ mm Hg, • *airway pressure ≤ 40 cm H_2O,* • *mean airway pressures ≤ 30 cm H_2O,* • *pH between 7.35 and 7.50*
use of continuous positive airway pressure (CPAP)	*decrease work of breathing:* positive pressure is maintained throughout the breathing cycle
use of PEEP therapy	*improves oxygenation*
mechanism of PEEP therapy	• **keeps terminal bronchioles open during the expiration cycle:** decreases intrapulmonary shunting, • *maintains or increases FRC:* * FRC is volume of air remaining in the lung after resting expiration, * FRC consists of ERV (part of FRC that is expelled with forceful deflation of the lung) + residual volume (part not expelled with forceful deflation)

Table continued on following page

Table 7-1. ACUTE RESPIRATORY FAILURE (ARF)
Continued

Most Common...	Answer and Explanation
complications of PEEP therapy	• **decreases CO:** * positive intrathoracic pressures compress thin-walled RV/RA and SVC entering right heart (reduces venous return), * expands lungs (increases lung compliance) leading to compression of interalveolar blood vessels (decreases emptying of LV); • *barotrauma,* • *hypotension,* • *pneumothorax*
cause of barotrauma with mechanical ventilation	*increasing TV:* if more ventilation is required, it is safer to increase rate of breathing than TV
effects of increasing or decreasing the minute volume (ventilatory rate per minute × TV)	• *increasing minute volume:* * produces respiratory alkalosis, * vasoconstricts cerebral vessels (useful in Rx of cerebral edema), • *decreasing minute volume:* * produces respiratory acidosis, * vasodilates cerebral vessels, * vasoconstricts pulmonary arterioles
complications associated with barotrauma	• **subcutaneous emphysema:** Hamman's crunch heard with a stethoscope, • *pneumomediastinum,* • *pneumothorax,* • *systemic gas embolization*
danger of an FiO_2 ≥0.50	*oxygen free radical damage of lung tissue*
cause of chronic respiratory failure	*COPD with end-stage fibrosis:* honeycomb lung

Question: Which of the following are common to both HARF and HHARF? **SELECT 2**
- (A) Hypoxemia
- (B) Increased $PaCO_2$
- (C) Intracranial hypertension
- (D) Respiratory alkalosis
- (E) Dyspnea

Answers: (A), (E): An increase in $PaCO_2$ and intracranial pressure is primarily seen in HHARF (**choices B and C are incorrect**). Respiratory alkalosis is commonly present in HARF (**choice D is incorrect**). Both HARF and HHARF are associated with hypoxemia (**choice A**) and dyspnea (**choice E**).

A–a = alveolar-arterial gradient, ARDS = adult respiratory distress syndrome, ARF = acute respiratory failure, COPD = chronic obstructive pulmonary disease, CPAP = continuous positive airway pressure, ERV = expiratory reserve volume, FiO_2 = inspired oxygen concentration, FRC

= functional residual capacity, HARF = hypoxic acute respiratory failure, Hb = hemoglobin, HHARF = hypercapnic-hypoxic acute respiratory failure, HTN = hypertension, ILD = interstitial lung disease, LV = left ventricle, MVO_2 = mixed venous oxygen content, ODC = oxygen dissociation curve, $PaCO_2$ = partial pressure of arterial carbon dioxide, PaO_2 = partial pressure of arterial oxygen, PA = pulmonary artery, PAO_2 = partial pressure of alveolar oxygen, PE = pulmonary embolus, PEEP = positive end-expiratory pressure, RA = right atrium, RBC = red blood cells, RV = right ventricle, Rx = treatment, SaO_2 = oxygen saturation in arterial blood, SGC = Swan-Ganz catheter, S/S = signs and symptoms, SVC = superior vena cava, TV = tidal volume, V/Q = ventilation/perfusion ratio.

Table 7–2. SHOCK

Most Common...	Answer and Explanation
types of shock	• **hypovolemic:** e.g., * **hemorrhage,** * fluids and electrolyte loss (e.g., diarrhea/vomiting, pancreatitis, hyperosmolar states, sweating) • *cardiogenic:* e.g., * **AMI,** * dysrhythmia, * valve dysfunction, • *distributive:* e.g., * **sepsis,** • neurogenic, • anaphylactic, • *obstructive:* e.g., * **acute cardiac tamponade,** * saddle embolus, * tension pneumothorax
pathophysiologic effect of shock	*tissue hypoxia secondary to microcirculatory insufficiency*
findings in stage I shock (compensated shock)	• *arterial pressure:* * normal to −1, * catecholamine release causes peripheral vasoconstriction, which may "normalize" BP, • *heart rate:* +1, • *narrow pulse pressure:* −1, • *respiratory rate:* normal, • *cardiac output:* * −1, * may be +1 in septic shock, • *mental status:* restlessness (inadequate perfusion of the brain), • *urine output:* normal to −1, • *skin:* cool, • *Rx:* vigorous Rx often reverses this stage
findings in stage II shock (decompensated shock)	• *arterial pressure:* −2, • *heart rate:* +2, • *pulse pressure:* −2, • *respiratory rate:* +2, • *cardiac output:* −2, • *mental status:* obtunded, • *urine output:* −2, • *skin:* mottled, • *pathophysiology:* * compensatory mechanisms (peripheral vasoconstriction, RAA activation, increased renal reabsorption of salt/water) are insufficient to maintain perfusion of vital organs, * myocardial depressant factor is released from underperfused pancreatic tissue

Table continued on following page

Table 7–2. SHOCK *Continued*

Most Common...	Answer and Explanation
findings in stage III shock (irreversible shock)	• *arterial pressure:* −3, • *heart rate:* +3 to −3, • *pulse pressure:* −3, • *respiratory rate:* +3 to − 3, • *cardiac output:* −3 • *mental status:* comatose, • *urine output:* anuric, • *skin:* cold/cyanotic, • *pathophysiology:* irreversible organ injury due to * mitochondrial dysfunction (decreased), * intracellular release of lysosomal enzymes, * complement system activation, * release of TNF from macrophages, * generation of FRs, * endothelial cell damage, * cellular swelling (impaired Na^+/K^+ ATPase pump)
cause of septic shock	*gram-negative sepsis:* e.g., * *Escherichia coli,* * *Klebsiella pneumoniae,* * *Pseudomonas aeruginosa*
causes of gram-negative sepsis	• **GU tract:** indwelling urinary catheters, • *GI tract,* • *wounds,* • *indwelling vascular catheters*
causes of gram-positive septic shock	• ***Staphylococcus aureus,*** • *Streptococcus species*
S/S of endotoxic shock	• *fever,* • *tachycardia,* • *variable blood pressure,* • *warm, dry skin,* • *shaking chills,* • *mental confusion*
mechanisms of endotoxic shock	• *endotoxins activate alternative complement pathway:* release of anaphylatoxins (C3a and C5a) leading to arteriolar vasodilatation (warm skin), • *endotoxins damage endothelial cells:* release * nitrous oxide (vasodilator), * PGI_2 (vasodilator), • *arteriolar vasodilatation increases venous return to heart:* * increases cardiac output (high output failure), * increases MVO_2
stages of septic shock	• **warm shock** → • *cold shock* → • *MOSF:* see below
clinical complications of shock	• **ischemic ATN:** decreased renal perfusion (renal medulla has the least blood supply), • *DIC:* * most commonly occurs in gram-negative sepsis, * leads to generalized ischemic damage of organs, bleeding, renal cortical necrosis, consumption of coagulation factors, • *ARDS:* most commonly occurs in gram-negative sepsis (see Table 6–4), • *stress bleeding from GI tract,* • *gut-mucosal function abnor-*

Table 7–2. SHOCK *Continued*

Most Common...	Answer and Explanation
Continued	malities: bacteria from GI tract enter blood stream, leading to sepsis, • *hepatic dysfunction*
COD in shock	*MOSF:* * post-shock syndrome, * multiple organ dysfunctions: ♦ ARDS, ♦ GI bleeding, ♦ sepsis, ♦ hepatic dysfunction, * 75% mortality rate
SGC measurements used in monitoring shock	• *central venous pressure:* CVP = 0–4 mm Hg, • *PA systolic pressure:* 15–30 mm Hg, • *PA diastolic* pressure: 3–12 mm Hg, • *mean arterial pressure:* MAP = 85–95 mm Hg, • MVO_2: * see Table 7–1, * 15 mL/dL, • *CO:* 4–8 L/min, • *cardiac index:* * CI = CO ÷ body surface area, * 2.5–4 L/min/m², • *PCWP:* * assesses preload in LV, * 12–15 mm Hg, • *SVR:* * calculated value, * indicates afterload LV must contract against, * SVR = [MAP − CVP ÷ CO] × 80 = 900 − 1400 dynes/sec/cm²
hemodynamic pattern in hypovolemic shock	• *CVP:* decreased, • *CI:* decreased, • *SVR:* increased, • *PCWP:* decreased, • MVO_2: decreased
hemodynamic pattern in cardiogenic shock	• *CVP:* increased, • *CI:* decreased, • *SVR:* increased, • *PCWP:* increased, • MVO_2: decreased
hemodynamic pattern in early septic shock	• *CVP:* increased, • *CI:* increased, • *SVR:* decreased, • *PCWP:* decreased, • MVO_2: increased
hemodynamic pattern in late septic shock	• *CVP:* decreased, • *CI:* decreased, • *SVR:* increased, • *PCWP:* decreased, • MVO_2: increased or decreased
lab findings in shock	• *increased anion gap metabolic acidosis:* lactic acidosis (anaerobic glycolysis), • *hyperglycemia:* release of * cortisol, * glucagon, * catecholamines increase glycogenolysis, • *elevated/decreased WBC count:* * in hypovolemic/cardiogenic shock, cortisol/catecholamines decrease adhesion molecule synthesis (leukocytosis), * endotoxins increase adhesion molecule synthesis leading to neutropenia

Table continued on following page

Table 7–2. SHOCK *Continued*

Most Common...	Answer and Explanation
initial effect of acute blood loss on Hb/Hct	*no effect:* * equal loss of plasma/RBCs does not alter Hb/Hct concentration, * RBC deficit is uncovered first as fluid enters the vascular compartment
effect of acute blood loss when crystalloids are infused	*drop in Hb/Hct concentration:* crystalloid solutions (isotonic saline, Ringer's lactate), remain in the ECF compartment and uncover the RBC deficit
factors to monitor in all types of shock	• *cerebral status:* sensitive indicator of cerebral perfusion, • *urine output:* * **most important parameter of adequate tissue perfusion,** * should be at least 0.5 mL/kg body weight each hour, • *arterial pH/serum lactate:* * lactic acidosis indicates tissue hypoxia, * lactate in Ringer's lactate is metabolically converted into HCO_3^-, * lactate in tissue hypoxia produces metabolic acidosis, • *Sao_2:* * evaluates oxygenation, * O_2 goal is to maintain $Sao_2 \geq 90\%/Pao_2 \geq 60$ mm Hg, • *Hb concentration:* ≥ 10 g/dL, • *volume status:* * Ringer's lactate is mainstay in treating hypovolemic shock, * packed RBCs are used if Hb falls <10 g/dL or Hct <30%, • *heart rate:* ECG monitoring, • *cardiac output:* use cardiotonic agents (see below)
problem associated with infusing isotonic (normal) saline in shock	*hyperchloremic normal anion gap metabolic acidosis:* * normal saline contains 154 mEq/L of NaCl, * infusion of large quantities dilutes HCO_3^-
cardiotonic agents used in treating shock	• **dopamine:** * doses 2–3 μg/kg/min increase renal/splanchnic blood flow, * doses of 4–5 μg/kg/min increase cardiac contractility, • *dobutamine:* inotropic vasodilator, • *amrinone:* * noncatecholamine that inhibits phosphodiesterase III, * inotropic vasodilator, • *nitroprusside:* vasodilator (decreases SVR)

Table 7–2. SHOCK *Continued*

Question: Which of the following distinguish early septic shock from cardiogenic and hypovolemic shock? **SELECT 3**
- (A) CI
- (B) SVR
- (C) Cold, clammy skin
- (D) MVO_2
- (E) PCWP
- (F) CVP

Answers: (A), (B), (D): In early septic shock, the CI (**choice A**) is increased (low in other types of shock), SVR (**choice B**) decreased (increased in other types of shock), and MVO_2 (**choice D**) increased (decreased in other types of shock). The skin is cold and clammy in hypovolemic and cardiogenic shock (**choice C is incorrect**). The PCWP is decreased in early septic and hypovolemic shock and increased in cardiogenic shock (**choice E is incorrect**). The CVP is increased in early septic and cardiogenic shock and decreased in hypovolemic shock (**choice F is incorrect**).

AMI = acute myocardial infarction, ARDS = adult respiratory distress syndrome, ATN = acute tubular necrosis, BP = blood pressure, CI = cardiac index, CO = cardiac output, COD = cause of death, CVP = central venous pressure, DIC = disseminated intravascular coagulation, ECF = extracellular fluid, ECG = electrocardiogram, FR = free radical, GI = gastrointestinal, GU = genitourinary, Hb = hemoglobin, Hct = hematocrit, LV = left ventricle, MAP = mean arterial pressure, MOSF = multiple organ system failure, MVO_2 = mixed venous oxygen content, PA = pulmonary artery, PCWP = pulmonary capillary wedge pressure, PGI_2 = prostaglandin I_2, RAA = renin-angiotensin-aldosterone system, RBC = red blood cell, Rx = treatment, SaO_2 = oxygen saturation of arterial blood, SGC = Swan-Ganz catheter, S/S = signs and symptoms, SVR = systemic vascular resistance, TNF = tumor necrosis factor, WBC = white blood cell.

Table 7–3. MISCELLANEOUS MECHANICAL AND PHYSICAL INJURIES

Most Common...	Answer and Explanation
steps in initial management of trauma	• **A = airway maintenance with cervical spine control,** • *B = breathing/ventilation,* • *C = circulation with hemorrhage control* [A brief neurologic exam should also be performed.]
maneuver to open the airway in the absence of head/neck trauma	*head tilt–chin lift*

Table continued on following page

Table 7–3. MISCELLANEOUS MECHANICAL AND PHYSICAL INJURIES *Continued*

Most Common...	Answer and Explanation
danger of a head tilt–chin lift in a patient with RA	*atlanto-axial instability:* * subluxation may occur, leading to decreased vertebral artery blood flow and stroke, * cervical hyperextension may injure the spinal cord
airway maneuver in a patient who is a suspect for a head/neck injury	*modified jaw thrust*: leaves out the head tilt component of the above procedure
cause of immediate death from trauma	• **head trauma**, • *massive hemorrhage*
cause of upper airway obstruction	*posterior displacement of the tongue:* jaw thrust maneuver moves tongue anteriorly
indications for tracheostomy	• *airway obstruction at/above level of the pharynx*, • *ARF requiring prolonged mechanical ventilation*
cause of accidental death from 1–24 years of age	*MVAs:* * most often associated with drunk driving, most common COD in white males between 25 and 44 yrs of age, * AIDS is the most common COD in black males and women between 25 and 44 years
fracture associated with the greatest blood loss	*complex pelvic fracture:* * ≥2 liters may be lost, * femoral fracture ranks second (up to 1 liter)
types of drowning	• **wet drowning** (90%): initial laryngospasm on contact with water followed by relaxation/aspiration of water into lungs, • *dry drowning:* intense laryngospasm prevents aspiration of water into lungs [Drowning is the fifth leading cause of accidental death in United States. *Near-drowning* is survival for at least 24 hrs after water submersion.]
pathophysiologic effects of drowning	• *hypoxemia from intrapulmonary shunting:* perfusion of poorly ventilated alveoli, • *respiratory/metabolic acidosis*, • *cerebral hypoperfusion*, • *death from cerebral edema* [Either fresh or salt water in the lungs destroys surfactant, leading to massive atelectasis, and intrapulmonary shunting of blood.]

Table 7–3. MISCELLANEOUS MECHANICAL AND PHYSICAL INJURIES *Continued*

Most Common...	Answer and Explanation
effect of salt water on plasma volume and sodium concentration	*volume depletion and hypernatremia:* * salt water draws fluid into the lungs from the pulmonary capillaries, * theoretically, death should be faster in salt water than in fresh water drowning
effect of fresh water on plasma volume and serum sodium	*volume overload and hyponatremia:* * hypotonic water moves into pulmonary capillaries by osmosis, * RBC hemolysis
COD in a fire	*smoke inhalation*
types of poisonings in a house fire	• **carbon monoxide,** • *cyanide poisoning:* cyanide gas arises from polyurethane in upholstery
S/S of heat cramps	• **leg cramps:** * salt loss from excessive sweating in hot environment, * replacement of sweat losses (hypotonic salt solution) with water alone may precipitate muscle cramps, • *absence of fever/volume depletion*
Rx of heat cramps	*oral, balanced salt solution*
S/S of heat exhaustion	• **fever:** rectal temperature 37.8°C, • *signs of volume depletion:* salt loss, • *N/V,* • *headache,* • *muscle cramps,* • *moist skin*
Rx of heat exhaustion	*IV normal saline administered in cool environment*
patient types at risk for classic heat stroke	• *>50 years old,* • *chronically ill patients who are obese and taking drugs that prevent sweating* (e.g., anticholinergics), • *cocaine abuse*
S/S of classic heat stroke	• **fever ≥40.5°C:** * ≥105°F, * usually occurs after several days of high ambient temperatures with high humidity, • *absence of sweating,* • *severe volume depletion,* • *comatose*
Rx of classic heat stroke	• **immediate cooling:** * tepid water, * ice packs, • *chlorpromazine if shivering,* • *crystalloid replacement of volume deficits*
patients at risk for exertional heat stroke	*unacclimatized people* (* **athletes,** * laborers, * soldiers) *working in a high ambient temperature/high humidity environment:* impaired thermoregulatory system

Table continued on following page

Table 7-3. MISCELLANEOUS MECHANICAL AND PHYSICAL INJURIES *Continued*

Most Common...	Answer and Explanation
S/S of exertional heat stroke	• **fever <40°C:** <104°F, • *sweating,* • *conscious,* • *muscle pain from rhabdomyolysis:* * myoglobinuria may occur, * danger for developing ♦ ATN, ♦ DIC, ♦ hyperkalemia, ♦ lactic acidosis
Rx of exertional heat stroke	*similar to classic heat stroke:* use mannitol if rhabdomyolysis is present
mechanism of malignant hyperthermia	• *AD disorder,* • *precipitated in surgery when patients receive halothane or muscle relaxants,* • *defect in calcium release channels in the muscle sarcoplasmic reticulum*
Rx of malignant hyperthermia	*dantrolene*
causes of hypothermia	• **intoxicated alcoholic exposed to cold temperatures,** • *cold water immersion* [Hypothermia is a core temperature <35°C (95°F).]
mechanism of injury in hypothermia	*uncoupling of oxidative phosphorylation (↓ ATP):* progression into circulatory failure
cardiovascular effects associated with hypothermia	• *decreased CO,* • *prolonged QT interval,* • *sinus bradycardia,* • *classic Osborne waves on ECG:* J-point elevation
Rx of hypothermia	• **rewarming patient:** * heated O_2, * warm blankets, • *IV thiamine* (alcoholic)
type of compensation for high altitudes	*respiratory alkalosis:* * FIO_2 is 21%, * barometric pressure decreased, * PAO_2 decreased, * hyperventilation lowers $PACO_2$, which raises PAO_2 and PaO_2
S/S of acute mountain sickness (AMS)	• **headache,** • *fatigue,* • *sleep disturbances,* • *N/V,* • *inability to concentrate* [AMS may occur in nonacclimatized hikers who ascend more than 2000 meters (6560 feet) in 1–2 days. *High-altitude pulmonary edema* and *cerebral edema* are more serious conditions and require immediate descent.]
Rx of AMS	• **immediate descent,** • *fluids,* • O_2, • *acetazolamide:* excellent preventive measure as well, • *dexamethasone if symptoms persist*

Table 7–3. MISCELLANEOUS MECHANICAL AND
PHYSICAL INJURIES *Continued*

Most Common...	Answer and Explanation
cause of decompression sickness (Caisson's disease)	*rapid ascent from water depths >9 meters* (~30 feet): * atmospheric pressure increases by 1 for every 33 feet of descent, * nitrogen gas dissolves in blood/tissue, * rapid ascent, depth/duration of submersion, and fitness determine presence/absence of S/S
S/S of decompression sickness	• **joint pains:** nitrogen gas released into joints, • *confusion,* • *dyspnea,* • *aphasia,* • *coma,* • *sequelae:* * hemiparesis, * neurologic dysfunction, * aseptic necrosis of bone
Rx of decompression sickness	• **recompression,** • *hyperbaric O$_2$,* • *volume replacement*

Question: A 45-year-old man at a restaurant is clutching at his throat and is unable to cough or speak. What is your first step in the management of this patient? **SELECT 1**
- (A) Encourage the patient to cough
- (B) Call an ambulance
- (C) Perform a head tilt and chin lift
- (D) Perform a jaw thrust
- (E) Perform a Heimlich maneuver

Answers: (E): The patient has complete obstruction of his upper airway (cannot cough or talk), most likely due to food. A Heimlich maneuver is the most appropriate therapy (**choice E**). Patients with partial airway obstruction (can cough and talk) should be encouraged to forcefully cough (**choice A is incorrect**). Head tilt–chin lift and a jaw thrust will not remove a foreign body from the upper airway (**choices C and D are incorrect**). Waiting for an ambulance is ill advised, since cardiac arrest and permanent brain damage may occur in only a few minutes (**choice B is incorrect**).

AD = autosomal dominant, AIDS = acquired immunodeficiency syndrome, AMS = acute mountain sickness, ARDS = adult respiratory distress syndrome, ARF = acute respiratory failure, ATN = acute tubular necrosis, ATP = adenosine triphosphate, CO = cardiac output, COD = cause of death, DIC = disseminated intravascular coagulation, ECG = electrocardiogram, F$_{IO_2}$ = fraction of inspired oxygen, IV = intravenous, MVAs = motor vehicle accidents, N/V = nausea/vomiting, P$_{ACO_2}$ = partial pressure of alveolar carbon monoxide, P$_{AO_2}$ = partial pressure of alveolar oxygen, P$_{aO_2}$ = partial pressure of arterial oxygen, RA = rheumatoid arthritis, RBC = red blood cell, Rx = treatment, S/S = signs and symptoms.

Table 7–4. MISCELLANEOUS ACUTE POISONINGS
(SEE Tables 2–4 and 2–5 FOR ALCOHOL AND
DRUGS OF ABUSE, RESPECTIVELY)

Most Common...	Answer and Explanation
age bracket associated with poisonings	*<5 years old*
causes of poisoning death in the United States	• **CO,** • *cocaine:* most common COD from an illicit drug, • *tricyclic antidepressants:* most common COD from a prescription drug
cause of cardiovascular drug death in the United States	*calcium channel blocker overdose:* recently surpassed digitalis as the most common cardiovascular drug COD
initial steps in the management of acute poisonings	• *100% O_2:* for inhalation of CO, hydrogen sulfide, smoke, chlorine gas, • *syrup of ipecac:* contraindications— * ingestion of caustic or petroleum distillate, * coma, * seizures, • *copious amounts of saline:* eye contamination, *lukewarm water or saline:* skin contamination, • *gastric lavage:* * effective in first hour of ingestion of most poisons, * contraindicated in caustic ingestion, • *activated charcoal:* * useful for most drug ingestions, * exceptions— ♦ lithium, ♦ cyanide, ♦ ferrous sulfate, ♦ alkalis, ♦ carbamate, ♦ mineral acids, ♦ alcohols, ♦ organophosphates, ♦ heavy metals, • *alkaline diuresis:* enhance renal excretion of drug— * salicylates, * barbiturates, * lithium, INH (use $NaHCO_3$), • *hemodialysis:* * methyl alcohol/ethylene glycol, * lithium, * salicylate, * theophylline, * valproic acid, • *specific antidotes:* see below, • *immunotherapy:* digoxin-specific antibody fragments for digitalis toxicity
tests used in the work-up of poisonings	• *toxicologic assays:* e.g., acetaminophen, • *general studies:* * CBC, * UA, * glucose/electrolytes, * ECG, * chest radiograph, * BUN/creatinine, • *specific studies:* * abdominal radiograph (iron tablets, Pb, Hg), * liver function tests (acetaminophen), * ABGs, • *osmotic gap:* * difference between calculated POsm $(2Na^+ + glucose/18 + BUN/2.8)$ and measured POsm, * if >10 mOsm/kg, suggests ♦ alcohol, ♦ methanol, ♦ ethylene glycol, * isopropyl alcohol, • *AG calculation:* increased AG— * iron, * salicylates, * methanol, * ethylene glycol, * CN, * CO, * phenformin

Table 7–4. MISCELLANEOUS ACUTE POISONINGS
(SEE Tables 2–4 and 2–5 FOR ALCOHOL AND DRUGS OF ABUSE, RESPECTIVELY) *Continued*

Most Common...	Answer and Explanation
body fluids used in toxicologic assays	• **urine,** • *serum,* • *gastric contents*
initial management steps in Rx of coma	• **A = airway control,** • *B = breathing,* • *C = circulation control,* • *D = drugs:* • naloxone for opioid overdose, * thiamine for alcohol intoxication, * dextrose for hypoglycemic coma
COD in coma	*ARF*
mechanism of injury of acetaminophen poisoning	*formation of acetaminophen FRs in liver cytochrome system:* GSH is used up in neutralizing the FRs
S/S of acetaminophen poisoning	• **N/V in first 24 hrs after ingestion,** • *jaundice,* • *hepatic encephalopathy,* • *lab:* serum levels >200 μg after 4 hrs indicate significant hepatotoxicity
target site for acetaminophen poisoning	• **liver:** * massive hepatocellular necrosis, * transaminase elevation begins in 1–2 days and peaks in 3–4 days, • *kidneys:* renal failure
Rx of acetaminophen poisoning	*N-acetylcysteine:* * substrate to replenish GSH, * best results occur if given in first 8 hrs
esophageal effect after ingestion of strong alkalis/acids	• *strong alkalis:* * 85%, * lye/ammonia, * liquefactive necrosis, * danger of perforation/stricture formation, • *strong acids:* * 15%, * toilet bowl cleaner, * coagulation necrosis, * less penetration and stricture formation
Rx of corrosive ingestion	*immediate esophagoscopy to assess damage*
S/S of *Amanita* mushroom poisoning	• *GI tract:* * abdominal pain, * bloody diarrhea, • *liver:* * hepatic necrosis, * fatty change, * hepatic encephalopathy, • *kidneys:* oliguric renal failure, • *CNS:* * seizures, * coma, • *toxin:* blocks RNA polymerase, • *Rx:* supportive
S/S of atropine/anticholinergic poisoning	• *mydriasis,* • *flushing of skin,* • *fever,* • *tachycardia,* • *dry mouth,* • *blurry vision*
Rx of anticholinergic poisoning	*physostigmine*

Table continued on following page

Table 7–4. MISCELLANEOUS ACUTE POISONINGS
(SEE Tables 2–4 and 2–5 FOR ALCOHOL AND
DRUGS OF ABUSE, RESPECTIVELY) *Continued*

Most Common...	Answer and Explanation
S/S of arsenic poisoning	• *poisoning:* * pet dips, * pesticides, * Fowler's solution, • *garlic odor to breath,* • *N/V,* • *abdominal pain,* • *gray skin,* • *watery diarrhea,* • *coma:* most common COD, • *cancer:* * squamous cancer of skin, * lung, * liver angiosarcoma
Rx of arsenic poisoning	*dimercaprol followed by penicillamine*
Rx of β-adrenergic antagonist poisoning	*glucagon:* stimulates cAMP synthesis in the heart, leading to increased cardiac contractility
Rx of calcium channel blocker poisoning	*calcium chloride*
causes of CO poisoning	• **automobile exhaust:** contains 5% CO, • *gas space heaters,* • *smoke in fires,* • *cigarette smoking,* • *wood stoves,* • *methylene chloride exposure:* common in painters, • *CO characteristics:* * colorless, * odorless, * incomplete combustion of carbon material
target organs susceptible to CO poisoning	*heart/brain:* * hypoxic injury, * blocks cytochrome oxidase, * left-shifts ODC, * decreases SaO_2 (number of heme groups occupied by O_2)
S/S of CO poisoning	• **headache:** 10–20% concentration, • *dizziness:* 20–40%, • *syncope, dyspnea, coma:* 40–60%, • *chest pain,* • *arrhythmias,* • *AMI,* • *cherry red discoloration,* • *death:* * >60% concentration, * respiratory/cardiac arrest
lab findings in CO poisoning	• **low SaO_2:** * if directly measured, * normal when calculated from PaO_2 (PaO_2 is normal in CO poisoning), * normal with pulse oximeter, • *increased AG metabolic acidosis:* lactic acidosis, • *increased carboxyHb:* direct measurement
chronic effect of CO poisoning	*Parkinson's disease:* necrosis of globus pallidus, • *accelerates atherosclerosis*
Rx of CO poisoning	*100% O_2*

Table 7–4. MISCELLANEOUS ACUTE POISONINGS
(SEE Tables 2–4 and 2–5 FOR ALCOHOL AND
DRUGS OF ABUSE, RESPECTIVELY) *Continued*

Most Common...	Answer and Explanation
causes of CN poisoning	• **smoke inhalation in house fire,** • *acrylic nail remover,* • *fumigant rodenticide,* • *apricot pits,* • *nitroprusside*
S/S cyanide poisoning	• *mechanism:* reversibly inhibits cytochrome oxidase, • *almond smell to breath,* • *headache,* • *dizziness followed by seizures → coma → death*
lab findings in cyanide poisoning	*increased AG metabolic acidosis:* lactate from tissue hypoxia, *increased MVo₂:* cytochrome oxidase block also blocks tissue uptake of oxygen
Rx for CN poisoning	*nitrites:* * crushed amyl nitrite pearls followed by IV sodium nitrite, * first step in Rx, * produces metHb, which competes with cytochrome oxidase for CN to form cyanmetHb, • *thiosulfate:* combines with CN in cyanmetHb to form harmless thiocyanate
antidote for digitalis toxicity	*digoxin specific Fab fragment antibodies:* falsely increases digoxin levels
mechanism of ethylene/diethylene glycol poisoning	• *present in antifreeze,* • *converted into oxalic acid:* oxalic acid combines with calcium to form calcium oxalate/hippurate crystals in kidneys (ATN), heart, lungs (CHF)
S/S of ethylene/ diethylene glycol poisoning	• **altered mental status,** • *seizures,* • *tetany → • CHF → renal failure*
lab findings in ethylene/diethylene glycol	• **increased AG metabolic acidosis:** * oxalate, * hippurate, • *increased osmolal gap (Δosm):* see above, • *hypocalcemia:* oxalates bind calcium, • *fluorescein added to antifreeze detected in urine with UVA light,* • *estimated serum concentration = Δosm × 6.2*
Rx for ethylene/ diethylene glycol poisoning	• **IV infusion of ethyl alcohol:** ethyl alcohol competes with ethylene glycol for ALDH, • *pyridoxine/thiamine:* pyridoxine + thiamine convert glyoxylate into glycine, • *hemodialysis:* for severe poisonings

Table continued on following page

Table 7–4. MISCELLANEOUS ACUTE POISONINGS
(SEE Tables 2–4 and 2–5 FOR ALCOHOL AND
DRUGS OF ABUSE, RESPECTIVELY) *Continued*

Most Common...	Answer and Explanation
clinical findings of iron poisoning	• **gastritis:** corrosive effect → • *shock, coma, metabolic acidosis, liver cell necrosis* → • *fulminant liver failure* → • *death,* • *important cause of mortality in children:* ingest mother's ferrous sulfate, • *mechanism:* ✶ depresses myocardial tissue, ✶ disrupts TCA cycle enzymes, • *radiograph:* undigested pills visible
lab findings of iron poisoning	• **high serum iron:** levels >300–500 μg/dL are toxic, • *metabolic acidosis*
Rx of iron poisoning	• *gastric lavage with sodium bicarbonate,* • *deferoxamine:* chelates free iron in blood to form ferroxamine (eliminated in urine)
S/S of isopropyl (rubbing) alcohol poisoning	• *N/V,* • *fruity odor to breath:* 15% converted to acetone, • *abdominal pain,* • *hypotension,* • *hyporeflexia, coma,* • no increased AG metabolic acidosis
lab findings in isopropyl alcohol poisoning	• *hypoglycemia,* • *increased osmolal gap* (Δosm), • *estimated serum concentration = Δosm × 5.9*
Rx of isopropyl alcohol poisoning	*hemodialysis if hypotension present*
clinical findings of lithium poisoning	• *stupor,* • *excessive thirst,* • *polyuria,* • *seizures,* • *respiratory depression,* • *mechanism:* ✶ competes with Na$^+$, K$^+$, Mg^{++}, and Ca^{++} (tetany, seizures) at cellular sites, ✶ inhibits adenyl cyclase (nephrogenic DI), ✶ inhibits release and augments reuptake of NOR at nerve endings
Rx of lithium poisoning	• **hemodialysis,** • *alkaline diuresis:* controversial
clinical findings of Hg poisoning	• *poisoning:* ✶ eating contaminated fish, ✶ ? dental amalgams, ✶ interior latex paints, ✶ industrial exposure, • *clinical:* ✶ metallic taste/burning in mouth, ✶ abdominal pain, ✶ bloody diarrhea, ✶ CNS findings— ♦ ataxia, ♦ intention tremors, ♦ constricted visual fields, ✶ oliguric renal failure (nephrotoxic ATN), • *radiograph:* densities in GI tract, lungs

Table 7–4. MISCELLANEOUS ACUTE POISONINGS
(SEE Tables 2–4 and 2–5 FOR ALCOHOL AND
DRUGS OF ABUSE, RESPECTIVELY) *Continued*

Most Common...	Answer and Explanation
Rx of Hg poisoning	*dimercaprol*
causes of metHb poisoning	*nitrates/nitrites:* * present in well water, industry, agriculture, drugs, * +2 iron (ferrous) oxidized to +3 iron (ferric), which cannot bind O_2 (decreases SaO₂ leading to cyanosis)
S/S of metHb poisoning	• **cyanosis:** no response to 100% O_2 (iron still +3), • *headaches,* • *dizziness,* • *tachypnea,* • *seizures,* • *coma*
lab findings in metHb poisoning	• **low SaO₂:** chocolate-colored blood from increase in deoxyhemoglobin, • *increased metHb levels:* 10% KCN to a tube of blood causes metHb to turn red
Rx of metHb poisoning	• **IV methylene blue:** activates an NADPH-dependent reductase in HMP that is normally nonfunctional, • *ascorbic acid:* reducing agent
hemolytic anemia that will not respond to methylene Rx of metHb poisoning	*G6PD deficiency:* NADPH-dependent reductase system is blocked by enzyme deficiency
clinical findings of methyl alcohol (wood alcohol) poisoning	• *poisoning:* * paint solvent, * windshield wiper fluid, * Sterno, • *mechanism:* methyl alcohol converted by ALDH into formic acid (irritates optic nerve), • *clinical:* * **"drunk" appearance,** * *tachypnea,* * *blurry vision*— ♦ "like being in a snowstorm," ♦ optic neuritis, * *coma*
lab findings in methyl alcohol poisoning	• **increased AG metabolic acidosis,** • *increases osmolal gap (Δosm), • estimated serum concentration = Δosm × 2.6*
Rx of methyl alcohol poisoning	**IV infusion of ethanol** + *folinic acid followed by folic acid:* * ethanol competes with methyl alcohol for ALDH, * unmetabolized methyl alcohol removed by hemodialysis, * folinic and folic acid increase metabolism of formate anions
causes of insecticide poisoning	• **organophosphates,** • *carbamates:* reversible ACh esterase inhibitors

Table continued on following page

Table 7–4. MISCELLANEOUS ACUTE POISONINGS
(SEE Tables 2–4 and 2–5 FOR ALCOHOL AND
DRUGS OF ABUSE, RESPECTIVELY) *Continued*

Most Common...	Answer and Explanation
mechanism of injury of organophosphates	• **irreversibly block ACh esterase,** • *ACh levels increase at synapses and myoneural junctions,* • *initially excite and then paralyze cholinergic receptor sites,* • *receptor sites in central/parasympathetic nervous systems* (both muscarinic) *and striated muscle/sympathetic ganglia* (both nicotinic)
S/S of organophosphate poisoning	• *initial signs* (primarily muscarinic): * salvitation, * lacrimation, * urination, * diarrhea, * bradycardia, * miotic pupils, * sweating, * blurry vision, • *later signs* (primarily nicotinic); * muscle fasiculations, * paralysis, * HTN, * weakness, * tachycardia, * mydriasis
lab findings in organophosphate poisoning	• **decreased RBC cholinesterase:** 25% reduction is confirmatory, • *decreased serum cholinesterase levels*
Rx of organophosphate poisoning	• **atropine:** reverses the muscarinic parasympathetic effects and many of the central effects, • *pralixdoxime* (2-PAM): * cleaves organophosphate from cholinesterase enzyme and allows it to hydrolyze excess ACh, * must be given before irreversible acetylation occurs
causes of Pb poisoning	• *children:* eating Pb-based paint, • *adults:* * incineration of batteries, * moonshine whiskey (Pb-based radiators), * welding, * painting pottery
mechanism of injury of Pb	• **denature enzymes:** * ferrochelatase (decreases production of heme causing sideroblastic anemia), * ALA dehydrase (increases Δ-aminolevulinic acid), * ribonuclease (produces coarse basophilic stippling of RBCs), • *increases uric acid reabsorption in the kidneys:* * gout, * HTN, • produces *coagulation necrosis of proximal tubules:* * proximal RTA, * nephrotoxic ATN, • *increases vessel permeability in brain:* cerebral edema
clinical findings of Pb poisoning	• **colicky abdominal pain,** • *constipation,* • *headache,* • *Pb line along gum margin,* • *peripheral neuropathy:* e.g., wrist drop, • *gout,* • *HTN,* • *convulsions,* • *radiograph:* * only heavy metal that deposits in the epiphyses, * visible in abdominal radiographs

Table 7–4. MISCELLANEOUS ACUTE POISONINGS
(SEE Tables 2–4 and 2–5 FOR ALCOHOL AND
DRUGS OF ABUSE, RESPECTIVELY) *Continued*

Most Common...	Answer and Explanation
lab findings in Pb poisoning	• **increased blood Pb levels:** best screen/confirmatory test, • *microcytic anemia,* • *increased FEP:* block in ferrochelatase increases FEP behind the block, • *iron overload:* * increased serum iron, percent saturation, ferritin, * decreased TIBC, • *increased Δ-aminolevulinic acid*
Rx of Pb poisoning	*EDTA:* dimercaprol and penicillamine are also used by some clinicians
S/S of salicylate poisoning	• *poisoning:* * excess salicylates, * oil of wintergreen, • *mechanism of injury:* * uncoupling agent in mitochondria, * irreversibly blocks cyclooxygenase, * produces increased AG metabolic acidosis, * *clinical:* * tinnitus, * hearing loss, * diaphoresis, * flushing, * hyperpyrexia (more common in children), * hyperventilation (primary respiratory alkalosis), * abdominal pain (gastritis), fulminant hepatitis
lab findings of salicylate intoxication	**increased AG metabolic acidosis:** * salicylic acid, * lactic acid (tissue hypoxia from mitochondrial damage), • *ABG abnormalities:* * adults have mixed primary metabolic acidosis and primary respiratory alkalosis, * children usually have metabolic acidosis
Rx of salicylate poisoning	• **forced alkaline diuresis:** promotes ionization of weak acids (prevents renal reabsorption), • *hemodialysis in severe cases*
clinical findings of strychnine poisoning	• *mechanism of injury:* * CNS stimulant, * interferes with neurotransmission at spinal synapses of inhibitory neurons (resembles tetanus), * lactic acidosis, • *clinical:* * tetanic muscle contractions, * opisthotonus, * hyperactive reflexes, * ARF
poisonings with a garlic breath	• *arsenic,* • *yellow phosphorus*
clinical findings of a black widow spider bite *(Latrodectus mactans)*	*sharp prick followed by muscle spasms in the thighs and abdomen:* * neurotoxin, * occur when picking up wood from a wood pile, moving boxes in a cellar, sitting in an outdoor outhouse*

Table continued on following page

Table 7–4. MISCELLANEOUS ACUTE POISONINGS
(SEE Tables 2–4 and 2–5 FOR ALCOHOL AND
DRUGS OF ABUSE, RESPECTIVELY) *Continued*

Most Common...	Answer and Explanation
Rx of black widow envenomation	• **antivenin,** • *calcium gluconate:* reduce the muscle spasms, • *tetanus prophylaxis*
clinical findings of a brown recluse spider bite *(Loxosceles reclusa)*	• *painless bite followed by intense local pain in 2–6 hrs:* necrotoxin, • *followed by a bulla or pustule surrounded by erythema:* "bull's eye" lesion, • *followed by a necrotic ulcer that expands,* • *complications:* * ATN, * hemolytic anemia
Rx of brown recluse spider envenomation	• *débride/excise ulcer,* • *colchicine and dapsone may have a beneficial effect,* • *tetanus prophylaxis is recommended*
S/S associated with poisonous scorpion bites	• *paresthesias at envenomation site,* • HTN, • respiratory paralysis: (most common COD) • *only one species is poisonous in United States: Centruroides species seen in Arizona*
COD due to a venomous bite	*anaphylaxis secondary to a bee sting*
poisonous snake envenomation in the United States	• *rattlesnake envenomation:* rattlesnakes, copperheads, water moccasins are pit vipers (heat-sensing organ), • *coral snake:* * red and yellow colors abut each other, * cobra family, * potent neurotoxin
S/S or rattlesnake envenomations	• *localized pain, swelling, redness:* due to cytolytic nature of venom, • *hypotension,* • *DIC*
"do nots" in rattlesnake envenomations	• *tight tourniquets,* • *running or excessive movement,* • *ice application,* • *cutting into the wound to remove venom:* often does more damage than good
Rx of rattlesnake envenomations	• **get patient to the hospital ASAP,** • *polyvalent crotalin antivenin:* * administer if systemic signs appear, * type I hypersensitivity reaction may initially occur with horse serum antivenin (should skin test prior to administering the antivenin), * serum sickness (type III IC disease) is a late complication, • *ceftriaxone,* • *tetanus prophylaxis*
poisonous lizard in the United States	*Gila monster in Southwestern United States*

Table 7–4. MISCELLANEOUS ACUTE POISONINGS
(SEE Tables 2–4 and 2–5 FOR ALCOHOL AND
DRUGS OF ABUSE, RESPECTIVELY) *Continued*

Question: A 43-year-old man presents in a stuporous state. His calculated POsm is 290 mOsm/kg (275–295 mOsm/kg) and measured POsm is 350 mOsm/kg. Serum electrolytes are as follows: serum Na^+ = 132 mEq/L (136–145 mEq/L), serum K^+ = 5.8 mEq/L (3.5–5.0 mEq/L), serum Cl^- = 94 mEq/L (95–105 mEq/L), serum HCO_3^- = 15 mEq/L (22–28 mEq/L). The urinalysis is normal. What should your differential include? **SELECT 2**

  (A) Isopropyl alcohol poisoning
  (B) Ethyl alcohol poisoning
  (C) Methyl alcohol poisoning
  (D) Salicylate poisoning
  (E) Ethylene glycol poisoning

Answers: (B), (C): The patient has a Δosm of 60 mOsm/kg (350 − 290 mOsm/kg = 60 mOsm/kg, normal Δosm <10 mOsm/kg], an increased AG metabolic acidosis (AG = Na^+ − [Cl^- + HCO_3^-] = 132 − [94 + 15] = 23 mEq/L (12 ± 4 mEq/L), indicating the presence of an alcohol in the patient's serum. Since the UA is normal, ethylene glycol is excluded (should be oxalate and hippurate crystals present, **choice E is incorrect**). This leaves ethyl alcohol (**choice B,** increase in lactate + β-OHB anions) and methyl alcohol (**choice C,** increase in formate anions), as the most likely suspects. Isopropyl alcohol increases Δosm, but does not produce metabolic acidosis (**choice A is incorrect**). Salicylates lead to an increased AG metabolic acidosis (increased lactate + salicylate anions); however, the Δosm is not increased (**choice D is incorrect**).

ABG = arterial blood gas, ACh = acetylcholine, AG = anion gap, ALA = aminolevulinic acid, ALDH = alcohol dehydrogenase, AMI = acute myocardial infarction, ARF = acute renal failure, ASAP = as soon as possible, ATN = acute tubular necrosis, β-OHB = β-hydroxybutyric acid, BUN = blood urea nitrogen, cAMP = cyclic adenosine monophosphate, CBC = complete blood count, CHF = congestive heart failure, CN = cyanide, CNS = central nervous system, CO = carbon monoxide, COD = cause of death, cyanmetHb = cyanmethemoglobin, DI = diabetes insipidus, DIC = disseminated intravascular coagulation, ECG = electrocardiogram, EDTA = ethylenediaminetetraacetic acid, FEP = free erythrocyte protoporphyrin, FR = free radical, GI = gastrointestinal, G6PD = glucose 6-phosphate dehydrogenase, GSH = glutathione, Hb = hemoglobin, Hg = mercury, HMP = hexose monophosphate shunt, HTN = hypertension, IC = immunocomplex, INH = isoniazid, IV = intravenous, KCN = potassium cyanide, metHb = methemoglobin, MVo_2 = mixed venous oxygen content, NADPH = nicotinamide adenine dinucleotide phosphate (reduced form), NOR = norepinephrine, N/V = nausea/vomiting, ODC = oxygen dissociation curve, Δosm = Δosmolality, 2-PAM = pralidoxime, Pao_2 = partial pressure of oxygen in arterial blood, Pb = lead, POsm = plasma osmolality, RBC = red blood cell, RTA = renal tubular acidosis, Rx = treatment, Sao_2 = oxygen saturation of arterial blood, S/S = signs and symptoms, TCA = tricarboxylic acid, TIBC = total iron binding capacity, UA = urinalysis, UVA = ultraviolet A.

CHAPTER

8

HEMATOLOGY

CONTENTS

Table 8–1. HISTORY AND PHYSICAL FINDINGS IN ANEMIA

Most Common...	Answer and Explanation
anemia	*iron deficiency*
anemia in alcoholics	*folate deficiency*
anemia in vegans	*B_{12} deficiency*
anemia in women <35 y old	*iron deficiency:* menorrhagia
anemia in men <50 y old	*iron deficiency:* duodenal ulcer
anemia in men/ women >50 y of age	*iron deficiency:* colon cancer
anemias associated with pregnancy	• **iron,** • *folate deficiency*

Table continued on following page

Table 8–1. HISTORY AND PHYSICAL FINDINGS IN ANEMIA *Continued*

Most Common...	Answer and Explanation
anemia in non-beer-drinking alcoholics	*folate deficiency:* beer is high in folate
anemia in African-Americans	*iron deficiency*
genetic anemias in African-Americans	• **sickle cell disease,** • α-/β-*thal,* • *G6PD deficiency,* • *hereditary persistence of HbF*
genetic anemias in Asians	• **HbE disease,** • α-*thal*
genetic anemias in Greek/Italians	• **β-thalassemia,** • *G6PD deficiency*
anemia with pica for clay, ice, starch	*iron deficiency:* pica is a craving for something unusual
anemia with pica for plaster/paint	*Pb poisoning*
anemia in malignancy	*ACD*
anemia in SLE	AIHA
anemia in CRF	*normocytic anemia:* deficiency of EPO
drugs precipitating AIHA	• **penicillin,** • *methyldopa,* • *quinidine*
drugs precipitating hemolysis in G6PD deficiency	• **primaquine,** • *dapsone*
anemia associated with INH therapy	*sideroblastic anemia:* pyridoxine deficiency
drugs associated with folate deficiency	• **methotrexate,** • *BCP,* • *phenytoin,* • *TMP/SMX* [methotrexate and TMP/SMX block dehydrofolate reductase.]
drugs associated with aplastic anemia	• *chloramphenicol,* • *phenylbutazone,* • *gold*
hepatitis associated with aplastic anemia	*NANB hepatitis*
anemias with calcium bilirubinate stones	*extravascular hemolytic anemias;* e.g., * sickle cell disease, * congenital spherocytosis

Table 8–1. HISTORY AND PHYSICAL FINDINGS
IN ANEMIA *Continued*

Most Common...	Answer and Explanation
anemias associated with malabsorption	• **iron deficiency,** • *folate deficiency,* • *B_{12} deficiency*
anemias associated with jaundice	*extravascular hemolytic anemias:* e.g., * sickle cell, * congenital spherocytosis, * AIHA
anemias associated with hemoglobinuria	*intravascular hemolytic anemias:* e.g., * PNH, * microangiopathic, * G6PD deficiency
anemia with family Hx of splenectomy	*congenital spherocytosis*
anemias beginning in childhood	• **sickle cell disease,** • *severe β-thalassemia,* • *congenital spherocytosis,* • *G6PD deficiency*
anemias associated with a Billroth II	• **iron deficiency,** • *B_{12} deficiency* [Billroth II is subtotal gastrectomy with anastomosis of stomach to jejunum. Duodenum (where iron is absorbed) left as blind loop. Decreased acid interferes with B_{12} release from meat.]
anemia with terminal ileal disease	*B_{12} deficiency:* site of B_{12} absorption
symptom of anemia	• **exertional dyspnea,** • *dizziness,* • *palpitations,* • *insomnia,* • *angina:* uncovers CAD, • *headache* [Hb <7 g/dL is symptomatic.]
skull abnormalities in severe hemolytic anemias	• *"chipmunk face":* zygomatic arch, • *frontal bossing* [Skull abnormalities are due to expansion of marrow cavity from RBC hyperplasia. Skull radiograph with "hair on end."]
anemia with spoon nails (koilonychia)	*iron deficiency*
cardiovascular signs of anemia	• *pulmonic flow murmur,* • *wide pulse pressure:* reduced viscosity produces high output failure, • *hypotension,* • *tachycardia*
skin signs of anemia	• *pallor palmar creases,* • *jaundice:* extravascular hemolytic anemia, • *telangiectasia:* Osler-Weber-Rendu disease, • *petechia/ecchymoses:* thrombocytopenia with GI blood loss, • *spider angiomas:* cirrhosis

Table continued on following page

Table 8–1. HISTORY AND PHYSICAL FINDINGS
IN ANEMIA *Continued*

Most Common...	Answer and Explanation
anemia with gray gum discoloration	*Pb poisoning*
anemias with glossitis	• **iron deficiency,** • *B_{12}/folate deficiency*
anemias with peripheral neuropathy	• *Pb poisoning,* • *B_{12}*
anemia with decreased vibratory sensation	*B_{12} deficiency*

Question: Drugs assume an important role in the pathogenesis of which of the following types of anemia? **SELECT 5**
- (A) Macrocytic anemia due to pernicious anemia
- (B) Macrocytic anemia due to folate deficiency
- (C) Aplastic anemia
- (D) Hemolytic anemia due to G6PD deficiency
- (E) AIHA
- (F) Sideroblastic anemia
- (G) Microcytic anemia due to α- or β-thalassemia

Answers: (B), (C), (D), (E), (F): Pernicious anemia is an anemia associated with autoimmune destruction of parietal cells in the stomach, leading to a deficiency of intrinsic factor and inability to reabsorb B_{12} **(choice A is incorrect).** The thalassemias are AR diseases with no direct drug relationship **(choice G is incorrect).** Folate deficiency **(choice B)** may be due to phenytoin, BCPs, and methotrexate. Aplastic anemias **(choice C)** are commonly due to drugs suppressing hematopoiesis in the bone marrow (e.g., chloramphenicol). Primaquine and dapsone are drugs that commonly precipitate hemolysis in G6PD deficiency **(choice D).** Penicillin and methyldopa are associated with AIHA **(choice E).** Pyridoxine deficiency secondary to INH therapy is a common cause of sideroblastic anemia **(choice F).**

ACD = anemia of chronic disease, AIHA = autoimmune hemolytic anemia, AR = autosomal recessive, BCP = birth control pill, CAD = coronary artery disease, CRF = chronic renal failure, EPO = erythropoietin, GI = gastrointestinal, G6PD = glucose 6-phosphate dehydrogenase, HbE = hemoglobin E, HbF = hemoglobin F, Hx = history, INH = isoniazid, NANB = non-A, non-B hepatitis, Pb = lead, PNH = paroxysmal nocturnal hemoglobinuria, RBC = red blood cell, SLE = systemic lupus erythematosus, thal = thalassemia, TMP/SMX = trimethoprim/sulfamethoxazole.

Table 8–2. DIAGNOSTIC TESTS IN HEMATOLOGY

Most Common...	Answer and Explanation
test to evaluate erythropoiesis	*PB blood reticulocyte count:* * retics are young RBCs requiring 24 h to become mature RBCs, * supravital stains identify RNA filaments, * retic count is best test to evaluate BM response to anemia
formula to correct PB retic count for anemia	*(patient Hct ÷ 45) × % reticulocyte count:* e.g., * Hct 30%, reticulocyte count 15%: (30 ÷ 45) × 15 = 10%, * good BM response to anemia (effective erythropoiesis) >3%, * poor response (ineffective erythropoiesis) <2%, * normal retic count 0.5–1.5%
formula to correct PB retic count for presence of polychromasia	*same formula as above, except final answer is divided by 2:* * polychromatic cells are marrow retics (bluish discoloration), * indicate accelerated erythropoiesis from EPO stimulated BM, * require 2–3 d to mature, * similar supravital stain findings as 24-h-old PB retic, * falsely increase retic response to anemia, * additional correction called *retic index*
method of calculating absolute reticulocyte count	*absolute reticulocyte count = (% retics ÷ 100) × RBC count:* * e.g., normal adult with 5 million/mm³, retic count 1.5%: absolute retic count = 0.015 × 5 = 75,000 cells/mm³, * anemia correction already included, * absolute retic count >100,000 cells/mm³ good response
parameters reported in CBC (complete blood cell count)	• *cell counts:* RBC, WBC, platelets, • *Hb/Hct:* Hb × 3 = Hct, • *RBC indices:* * MCV (Hct ÷RBC × 10 = 80–100 μm³), * MCH (not useful), * MCHC (Hb ÷ Hct × 100 = 31–36% Hb/cell), • *RDW:* estimate of RBC size variation, e.g., small/large cells versus uniform cells, • *RBC shape abnormalities:* poikilocytosis, • *RBC size abnormalities:* anisocytosis, • *platelet morphology,* • *WBC morphology,* • *100 WBC differential count:* % neutrophils, eosinophils, basophils, monocytes, lymphocytes
use of MCV	*classify anemia:* * normocytic, microcytic, macrocytic, * microcytic + macrocytic RBCs produces normal MCV (RDW high: > 16%)

Table continued on following page

Table 8–2. DIAGNOSTIC TESTS IN HEMATOLOGY
Continued

Most Common...	Answer and Explanation
use of MCHC	*HB concentration in RBCs:* * decreased in microcytic anemias (decreased Hb synthesis), * increased in spherocytosis (loss of cell membrane increases Hb concentration)
anemia with normal/ high RBC count and decreased Hb/Hct	α-/β-*thalassemia*
microcytic anemia with high RDW	*iron deficiency:* * normocytic before becoming microcytic, * normal/microcytic cells increase RDW >16%
parameters reported BM aspirate/core Bx	• *cellularity:* normally 30% fat, 70% cells, • *myeloid/erythroid* (M/E), *ratio:* normally 3/1, • *cell morphology,* • *megakaryocytes,* • estimate iron stores:* use Prussian blue stain, • *detect metastasis,* • *culture for FUO,* • *stage lymphomas*
anemias requiring iron studies	• *iron deficiency,* • *ACD,* • *sideroblastic anemias*
iron studies	• *serum iron:* 50–170 μg/dL, • *TIBC:* * transferrin, * normal 250–425 μg/dL, * high/low iron stores, increases/decreases liver transferrin synthesis→increases/decreases TIBC, • *% saturation:* * (serum Fe ÷ TIBC) × 100, * normal 20–50%, • *serum ferritin:* * 20–250 ng/mL, * storage form of iron, * normally stored in BM macrophages, * small circulating fraction correlates with BM stores, * best iron screening test
anemias requiring a Hb electrophoresis for confirmation	*hemoglobinopathies:* * e.g., ♦ thal, ♦ sickle cell trait/disease, * reports percentage of normal Hbs: ♦ HbA >97%, ♦ HbA$_2$ <2.5%, HbF <1%), * identifies abnormal HbS: e.g., ♦ HbH, ♦ HbE
anemias with an increase in FEP	• **iron deficiency,** • *ACD,* • *Pb poisoning* [Heme composed of iron + protoporphyrin. In iron deficiency/ACD, iron lack increases mitochondrial protoporphyrin. Ferrochelatase binds iron to protoporphyrin. Enzyme denatured in Pb poisoning causing protoporphyrin increase behind enzyme block. Serum Pb levels replaced FEP as screen.]

Table 8–2. DIAGNOSTIC TESTS IN HEMATOLOGY
Continued

Most Common...	Answer and Explanation
anemias requiring an enzyme assay for confirmation	• **G6PD deficiency,** • *PK deficiency*
causes of high EPO	• **decreased Hb:** e.g., * iron deficiency, * *tissue hypoxia:* e.g., high altitude, • *ectopic production:* e.g., HCC
causes of low EPO	• **CRF,** • *PRV,* • *RA,* • *HIV infection*
confirmatory test when B_{12} levels are nondiagnostic	*urine for methylmalonic acid:* * in propionate metabolism, B_{12} catalyzes reaction between methylmalonyl CoA → succinyl CoA, * deficiency causes an increase in methylmalonyl CoA, which is converted into methylmalonic acid
test to localize cause of B_{12} deficiency	*Schilling's test*
Schilling's test results in PA	*absorption of orally administered radioactive B_{12} corrected by addition of IF*
Schilling's test results in bacterial overgrowth	*absorption of orally administered radioactive B_{12} corrected after a course of antibiotics*
Schilling's test results in pancreatic dysfunction	*absorption of orally administered radioactive B_{12} after addition of pancreatic enzymes*
Schilling's test results in small bowel disease	*no absorption of orally administered radioactive B_{12} after IF, antibiotics, pancreatic enzymes*
anemias with an increase in plasma homocysteine levels	**folate**/B_{12} *deficiency:* * normally, methyl-THF donates methyl group to B_{12}, * methyl-B_{12} donates methyl group to homocysteine, which becomes methionine, * deficiency of B_{12}/folate increases homocysteine
confirmatory test when serum/RBC folate levels are nondiagnostic	*urine FIGLu:* * normally, FIGLu (histidine derivative) supplies one-carbon derivatives to replenish THF, * folate deficiency causes FIGLu accumulation
hemolytic anemias with an increase in UCB	*extravascular hemolytic anemias:* * see above, * severe intravascular hemolysis also raises UCB (haptoglobin-Hb complex phagocytosed by macrophages)*

Table continued on following page

Table 8–2. DIAGNOSTIC TESTS IN HEMATOLOGY
Continued

Most Common...	Answer and Explanation
hemolytic anemias with low serum haptoglobin	*intravascular hemolytic anemias:* * see above, * haptoglobin synthesized by liver, * binds free Hb to form haptoglobin-Hb complex (phagocytosed by macrophages), * low hapto-globin indicates ♦ intravascular hemolysis, ♦ liver disease, ♦ severe extravascular hemoly-sis (macrophages leak out Hb)
hemolytic anemia with an increase in urine hemosiderin	*intravascular hemolytic anemias:* * see above, * haptoglobin consumed → hemoglobinuria → hemosiderinuria (chronic intravascular he-molysis)
sickle cell screening tests.	**sodium metabisulfite test:** Na^+ metabisulfite reduces O_2 tension → induces visible sickling on slide, * high sensitivity/specificity, • *solu-bility test:* * deoxygenated HbS insoluble, * good specificity/poor sensitivity
confirmatory test for hemoglobinopathy	*Hb electrophoresis*
test to confirm congenital spherocytosis	*RBC osmotic fragility of RBCs:* * RBCs incu-bated in tubes with decreasing salt concentra-tion, * spherocytes hemolyze at 0.65% con-centration (normal RBCs hemolyze at 0.50%)
test to confirm PCH	*Donath-Landsteiner test:* * detects bithermal antibody of PCH, * IgG antibody has anti-P specificity → attaches to RBCs at 15°C/fixes C → upon warming, C causes RBC hemolysis
screening test for PNH	*sugar water test:* * sugar water enhances C attachment to RBCs susceptible to C destruc-tion (owing to absence of DAF, the defect in PNH), * DAF normally enhances C degrada-tion on RBCs
confirmatory test for PNH	*Ham's acidified serum test:* * duplicates PNH mechanism of RBC hemolysis, * RBCs lacking DAF incubated in acidified serum → C at-taches to RBCs → hemolyze
screening test for warm/cold AIHA	*direct Coombs' test:* * Coombs' reagent is rab-bit anti-human-IgG or anti-C3b, * RBCs coated by IgG/C3b visibly clump when re-agent containing specific rabbit anti-human antibodies are added (antibody forms bridge between IgG/C3b on subjacent cells)

Table 8–2. DIAGNOSTIC TESTS IN HEMATOLOGY
Continued

Most Common...	Answer and Explanation
serum test to identify antibodies	*indirect Coombs' test:* commonly used in working up AIHA and in the blood bank to identify antibodies in patient serum
screening test to identify G6PD deficiency during acute hemolytic episode	*Heinz body preparation:* * absence/defective G6PD lowers RBC GSH levels, * GSH neutralizes peroxide in RBCs during infections or when exposed to oxidizing drugs, * peroxide denatures Hb → clump up into Heinz bodies (visible with supravital stains), * positive Heinz body prep is confirmed with enzyme assay after hemolysis has subsided
WBC test to distinguish neutrophilic leukemoid reaction (>30,000 cells/μL) from CML	*leukocyte alkaline phosphatase* (LAP) *score:* * mature neutrophils contain LAP (neoplastic neutrophils in CML do not), * high LAP score (sum total of graded stain intensity from 0–4$^+$ in 100 cell count) R/O CML, which has a very low score
disorders with low LAP score	• **CML,** • *PNH,* • *IM,* • *aplastic anemia,* • *hypophosphatasia:* hereditary deficiency of alkaline phosphatase
test to evaluate respiratory burst of neutrophils/ monocytes	*NBT dye test* [O_2-dependent MPO system of killing bacteria by neutrophils/monocytes requires NADPH oxidase + NADPH to convert molecular O_2 into superoxide. Energy released by this reaction is called respiratory burst. Superoxide converted by SOD into peroxide. MPO combines peroxide with Cl^- to form bleach. To test system, a yellow-colored NBT dye is phagocytosed by patient leukocytes. Neutrophils/monocytes producing superoxide convert NBT into a blue color (intact respiratory burst). Abnormal NBT test in CGD of childhood (deficient NADPH oxidase).]
test for Dx of infectious mononucleosis	*heterophile antibody test:* patients with IM have IgM heterophile antibodies that react against beef/horse RBCs (basis of Monospot agglutination test)
EBV serologic test to document IM	*anti-viral capsid antigen IgM:* diagnostic of acute IM

Table continued on following page

Table 8–2. DIAGNOSTIC TESTS IN HEMATOLOGY
Continued

Most Common...	Answer and Explanation
test to identify lymphocyte subtypes	*immunophenotyping:* membrane receptors (e.g., CD_{21} receptor for EBV on B cells) or antigens (e.g., CD_4 antigen marking helper T cells) are located on lymphocytes by monoclonal antibodies when cells are run through a flow cytometer
MPD requiring an ABG	*PRV:* * ABG classifies type of polycythemia-appropriate/inappropriate, * SaO_2 ≤88% is appropriate (EPO mediated, e.g., COPD), * SaO_2 ≥92% inappropriate (e.g., PRV, ectopic production of EPO)
MPD requiring RBC mass studies	*PRV:* * RBC mass is actual number of RBCs reported in mL/kg (e.g., men = 26–34 mL/kg, women = 21–29 mL/kg), * RBC count is number of RBCs/µL, * increased RBC mass indicates absolute polycythemia, * RBC mass normal if plasma volume is low (relative polycythemia) but RBC count is high
use of cytogenetic studies	*Dx leukemia/malignant lymphomas:* e.g., * t(9;22) in CML, * t(8;14) Burkitt's lymphoma, * t(15;17) acute promyelocytic leukemia
stain to identify neoplastic B cells in HCL	*tartrate-resistant acid phosphatase* (TRAP) *stain*
stains to identify neoplastic cells of neutrophil origin	• *specific esterase,* • *peroxidase,* • *Sudan black stains*
stains to identify neoplastic cells of monocyte origin	• *nonspecific esterase,* • *muramidase*
stain to identify neoplastic cells of lymphocyte origin	*periodic acid–Schiff* (PAS): lymphoblasts contain PAS-positive chunks of material in cytosol
screening test for multiple myeloma	*SPE:* * detects monoclonal spike (M spike in 85%) in γ-globulin region, * spike from single clone neoplastic plasma cells producing one Ig/light chain (κ or λ), * excess light chains excreted in urine as Bence-Jones protein
confirmatory test for multiple myeloma	• **serum/urine IEP,** • *immunofixation* [Specifically identify Ig/light chain involved.]

Table 8–2. DIAGNOSTIC TESTS IN HEMATOLOGY
Continued

Most Common...	Answer and Explanation
test to evaluate platelets	*platelet count:* * 150,000–400,000 cells/μL, * 10–15 platelets/OIF in peripheral smear ~normal platelet count
platelet function test	*bleeding time (BT):* * normally 2–7 min, * evaluates vessel/platelet function up to primary hemostatic plug–platelet clump held together by fibrinogen (see Table 8–11), * does not evaluate coagulation factors
factors tested in BT	• *vessel integrity,* • *number/function of platelets,* • *VWF,* • *VWF receptors on platelets,* • *platelet release of ADP,* • *platelet synthesis of TXA₂,* • *platelet receptors for fibrinogen*
cause of prolonged BT	*NSAIDs:* inhibit platelet production of TxA₂ by inhibiting cyclooxygenase
tests measuring VWF (von Willebrand's factor)	• **ristocetin cofactor assay:** * ristocetin aggregates platelets containing GPIb platelet receptor for VWF or VWF itself, * in presence of ristocetin, absence of either component interferes with platelet aggregation, * best test for Dx classical VWD, • *agar gel electrophoresis:* identifies circulating VWF multimers (polymers of increasing molecular weight/size), which are important in diagnosing less common variants of VWD
tests of coagulation system	• **prothrombin time (PT),** • *partial thromboplastin time* (PTT)
test of extrinsic coagulation system	*PT:* * measures extrinsic system down to fibrin clot: VII → X → V → II → I → clot (normally 11–15 sec), * does not evaluate platelets, * prolonged if any one or more of above factors <40% of normal, * not sensitive for factor XIII deficiency, protein C or S
use of PT	• **follow patients on warfarin,** • *severity of liver disease,* • *detecting factor VII, X, V, II deficiencies*
use of International Normalized Ratio (INR) for reporting the PT	*follow warfarin anticoagulation:* * INR standardizes PT regardless of protein-lipid tissue reagents used in test kits, * INR = (patient PT ÷ control PT) × International Sensitivity Index (value assigned to protein-lipid tissue factor used in test kit), * INR should be between 2 and 3 for adequate anticoagulation

Table continued on following page

Table 8–2. DIAGNOSTIC TESTS IN HEMATOLOGY
Continued

Most Common...	Answer and Explanation
test of intrinsic coagulation system	*PTT:* * evaluates intrinsic system to fibrin clot: XII → XI → IX → VIII → X → V → II → I → clot (normal 25–35 sec), * does not evaluate platelets, * not sensitive to factor XIII deficiency, * prolonged if one or more of above factors, HMWK, or prekallikrein are <30–40% of normal
use of PTT	• **follow patients on heparin anticoagulation,** • *PTT >150 sec:* highly predictive of contact factor deficiency (XII, XI, HMWK, prekallikrein), • *less prolonged PTT:* factor IX, VIII, X, V, II, I deficiencies
test to evaluate final stage of clotting	*thrombin time* (TT): detects abnormalities in conversion of fibrinogen into fibrin clot by adding thrombin to test system
use of TT	• *fibrinogen deficiency,* • *dysfibrinogenemia:* structurally abnormal fibrinogen in liver disease, • *heparin therapy:* heparin via AT III inhibits thrombin added to test system
test for detecting circulating anticoagulants	*mixing studies:* * distinguishes coagulation factor deficiencies from decreased production/consumption of factors versus antibody destruction of factors (called inhibitors/circulating anticoagulants), * mix 0.5 mL of patient plasma together with 0.5 mL normal plasma: ♦ correction of previously prolonged PT and/or PTT → true factor deficiency (normal plasma added missing factor), ♦ no correction → antibody destroying factor in both patient and normal plasma
screening test to detect factor XIII deficiency	*clot solubility in 5 molar urea:* * factor XIII (fibrin stabilizing factor) produces covalent cross-links between urea-soluble fibrin strands to produce urea-insoluble fibrin strands of stable clot, * clot solubility → factor XIII deficiency, * factor XIII assay confirms Dx
use of Reptilase test	*fibrinogen abnormalities:* * prolonged test in patients with ♦ hypofibrinogenemia, ♦ dysfibrinogenemia, or ♦ FDPs associated with DIC, * serum protease from venom of *Bothrops atrox* cleaves fibrinopeptide A from fibrinogen (thrombin cleaves both fibrinopeptide A

Table 8–2. DIAGNOSTIC TESTS IN HEMATOLOGY
Continued

Most Common...	Answer and Explanation
Continued	and B from fibrinogen), * RT normal in patients on heparin, which neutralizes thrombin via AT III (TT is prolonged in patients on heparin)
use of Stypven time (Russell viper venom)	*screening test that distinguishes factor VII deficiency* (normal) *from factor X deficiency* (prolonged): * uses Russell's viper venom, which has factor VII activity, * normal time with factor VII deficiency, * prolonged time with factor X deficiency
tests of fibrinolytic system	• *fibrin(ogen) degradation (split) products (FDPs):* * FDPs are X, Y, D, E fragments of plasmin degradation of ♦ fibrinogen alone, ♦ clot-associated fibrinogen, or ♦ clot-associated fibrin, * fragments D/E detected with LA test, • *D-dimer assay:* * D-dimers are cross-linked FDPs (cross-links indicate factor XIII activity) associated with a fibrin clot, * not present when plasmin acts on fibrinogen alone or clot-associated fibrinogen, * positive FDP with negative D-dimer assay → primary fibrinolysis (see below), * positive results in both assays → intravascular clotting (e.g. DIC)
test to identify ABO blood groups	• *forward type:* * *forward type* identifies blood group antigen (e.g., A, B, AB) on RBC surface by reacting patient cells with anti-A/anti-B test sera, * O RBCs have no reaction (lack A/B antigens), * RBCs with A antigen react with anti-A test sera, * RBCs with B antigen react with anti-B sera, RBCs with AB antigens react with anti-A/anti-B test sera, • *back type:* * identifies isohemagglutinins corresponding with each blood group, * patient plasma mixed with A and B test RBCs, * O patients have ♦ anti-A-IgM, ♦ anti-B-IgM, ♦ anti-A,B-IgG isohemagglutinins, * A patients have anti-B-IgM, * B patients have anti-A-IgM, * AB patients lack isohemagglutinins
test to identify Rh antigens	*agglutination reactions using test antiserum that reacts against patient RBCs to detect D, C, c, E, or e Rh antigens on their surface:* * there is no d antigen, * Du is a weak variant of D (requires further testing), * D or Du+ patients are considered Rh positive

Table continued on following page

Table 8–2. DIAGNOSTIC TESTS IN HEMATOLOGY
Continued

Most Common...	Answer and Explanation
tests to detect antibodies in patient serum that may react against antigens in donor RBCs	• *indirect Coombs' test:* antibody screen of patient serum, • *major cross-match:* * patient serum mixed with RBCs from each donor unit in separate tubes, * lack of agglutination/hemolysis indicates compatibility
test to identify antibody specificity if the antibody screen is positive	*antibody panel:* * panels of 10 or more O test RBCs that contain different antigen profiles are individually mixed with patient serum to identify patient antibodies, * patient must receive donor RBCs that are negative for antigens corresponding with patient antibodies
tests used in a transfusion reaction	• *check for clerical error,* • *visual inspection of patient serum in pre- and post-transfusion specimen:* check for free Hb in plasma to R/O intravascular hemolysis of donor RBCs, • *direct Coombs' test:* R/O antibody destruction of donor RBCs, • *urine check for Hb:* check for hemoglobinuria

Question: Which of the following test result/interpretation associations is correctly matched? **SELECT 4**
(A) Prolonged BT:platelet defect
(B) Prolonged PT:hemophilia A
(C) Increased corrected reticulocyte count:iron deficiency
(D) Positive indirect Coombs' test:positive antibody screen
(E) Low plasma haptoglobin level:anemia of chronic disease
(F) Increased serum UCB:extravascular hemolytic anemia
(G) Increased TIBC:increased iron stores
(H) Abnormal ristocetin cofactor assay:VWD

Answers: (A), (D), (F), (H): A prolonged BT **(choice A)** indicates vessel and/or platelet abnormalities. A prolonged PT indicates a coagulation deficiency in the extrinsic system down to a clot, hence hemophilia A (factor VIII deficiency) would not have a prolonged PT but a prolonged PTT **(choice B is incorrect)**. An increased reticulocyte count indicates effective erythropoiesis, hence iron deficiency is incorrect, since iron is necessary for Hb synthesis **(choice C is incorrect)**. A positive indirect Coombs' test **(choice D)** indicates the presence of antibodies against RBC antigens. A low plasma haptoglobin is a marker of intravascular hemolysis, hence ACD, which is not a hemolytic anemia, is not associated with reduced levels of haptoglobin **(choice E is incorrect)**. Increased UCB is a marker for extravascular hemolysis by macrophages **(choice F)**. An increased TIBC indicates an increase in transferrin synthesis owing to low bone marrow iron stores **(choice G is incorrect)**. An abnormal ristocetin cofactor deficiency represents either a deficiency of VWF (VWD) or the receptor for VWF **(choice H)**.

ABG = arterial blood gas, ACD = anemia of chronic disease, ADP = adenosine diphosphate, AIHA = autoimmune hemolytic anemia, AT III = antithrombin III, BM = bone marrow, BT = bleeding time, Bx = biopsy, C = complement, C3 = complement component 3, CBC = complete blood count, CRF = chronic renal failure, CGD = chronic granulomatous disease, CML = chronic myelogenous leukemia, CoA = coenzyme A, COPD = chronic obstructive pulmonary disease, DAF = decay accelerating factor, DIC = disseminated intravascular coagulation, Dx = diagnosis, EBV = Epstein-Barr virus, EPO = erythropoietin, FDP = fibrin(ogen) degradation products, FEP = free erythrocyte protoporphyrin, FIGLu = formiminoglutamic acid, FUO = fever of unknown origin, G6PD = glucose 6-phosphate dehydrogenase, GSH = glutathione, Hb = hemoglobin, HbA = adult hemoglobin A, HbF = fetal hemoglobin, HbS = sickle hemoglobin, HCC = hepatocellular carcinoma, HCL = hairy cell leukemia, HcT = hematocrit, HIV = human immunodeficiency virus, HMWK = high molecular weight kininogen, IEP = immunoelectrophoresis, IF = intrinsic factor, Ig = immunoglobulin, IgG = immunoglobulin G, IgM = immunoglobulin M, IM = infectious mononucleosis, INR = International Normalized Ratio, LA = latex agglutination, LAP = leukocyte alkaline phosphatase, MCH = mean corpuscular hemoglobin, M/E = myeloid/erythroid ratio, MCHC = mean corpuscular hemoglobin concentration, MCV = mean corpuscular volume, MPD = myeloproliferative disease, MPO = myeloperoxidase, NBT = nitroblue tetrazolium, NSAIDs = nonsteroidal anti-inflammatory drugs, OIF = oil immersion field, PA = pernicious anemia, PAS = periodic acid–Schiff, Pb = lead, PB = peripheral blood, PCH = paroxysmal cold hemoglobinuria, PK = pyruvate kinase, PNH = paroxysmal nocturnal hemoglobinuria, PRV = polycythemia rubra vera, PT = prothrombin time, PTT = partial thromboplastin time, RA = rheumatoid arthritis, RBC = red blood cell, RDW = RBC distribution width, R/O = rule out, RT = reptilase time, SPE = serum protein electrophoresis, t = translocation, THF = tetrahydrofolate, TIBC = total iron binding capacity, TRAP = tartrate-resistant acid phosphatase, TT = thrombin time, TXA_2 = thromboxane A_2, UCB = unconjugated bilirubin, VWD = von Willebrand's disease, VWF = von Willebrand's factor, WBC = white blood cell.

Table 8–3. GENERAL CONCEPTS IN HEMATOPOIESIS AND ANEMIA

Most Common...	Answer and Explanation
sequence of development of marrow stem cells beginning with the pluripotential stem cell	• *pluripotential stem cell* (PPSC) → lymphoid stem cell (CFU-L) → B lymphocyte (bone marrow), • *pluripotential stem cell* (PPSC) → lymphoid stem cell (CFU-L) → T lymphocyte (thymus), • *pluripotential stem cell* (PPSC) → multipotential stem cell (CFU-GEMM) → committed stem cells (CFU-E, CFU-Meg, CFU-M, CFU-G) → mature/nonproliferating cells (RBC, platelets, macrophage/monocyte, neutrophil, eosinophil, basophil)

Table continued on following page

Table 8–3. GENERAL CONCEPTS IN HEMATOPOIESIS AND ANEMIA *Continued*

Most Common...	Answer and Explanation
stem cell involved in the pathogenesis of aplastic anemia and PRV	*myeloid stem cell* (CFU-GEMM): * derived from the PPSC, this stem cell divides into committed stem cells that produce granulocytes, RBCs, macrophages, and megakaryocytes, * suppression leads to aplastic anemia and overactivity to PRV
sites for extramedullary (outside the marrow) hematopoiesis	• **spleen,** • *liver* [this alteration is due to marrow replacement by fibrosis (myelofibrosis) or hematopoiesis beyond the marrow's capacity to produce cells (e.g., severe hemolytic anemia like sickle cell disease)]
site for EPO synthesis	*kidneys:* EPO stimulates burst forming unit–erythroid stem cell to produce RBCs
stimuli for accelerated erythropoiesis	• *tissue hypoxia:* secondary to * **hypoxemia** (PaO_2), * severe anemia, * left shifted ODC
causes of ineffective erythropoiesis	• **B$_{12}$/folate deficiency,** • severe thal, • *MDS* [Increase in serum LDH and UCB commonly occur due to macrophage destruction of RBCs in marrow = ineffective erythropoiesis.]
mechanism for removal of senescent, abnormally shaped, or IgG/C3 coated RBCs	*extravascular hemolysis by macrophages in the* **spleen,** *liver* (C3 coated), *bone marrow:* end-product of macrophage destruction is UCB → jaundice
enzyme marker of intra- or extravascular hemolysis	*LDH:* * present in RBCs, * released when RBCs destroyed
cells in mitotic, postmitotic, PB granulocyte pools	• *mitotic pool:* * myeloblasts, * progranulocytes, * myelocytes, • *postmitotic pool:* * metamyelocytes, * band/segmented neutrophils, • *PB pool:* * segmented/band neutrophils, * 50% circulating, * 50% adhere to endothelium (marginating pool)

Table 8–3. GENERAL CONCEPTS IN HEMATOPOIESIS AND ANEMIA *Continued*

Most Common...	Answer and Explanation
cause of left-shifted neutrophil count	*release of postmitotic pool into PB by interleukin-1:* * left shift is a shift to immature neutrophils (>10% bands/stabs or younger cells), * feature of ♦ acute bacterial infections, ♦ sterile inflammation (e.g., blood in peritoneal cavity)
cause of neutropenia in blacks	*normal increase in PB marginating pool:* no susceptibility to infection
cause of neutrophilic leukocytosis in patients on corticosteroids	*decrease in adhesion molecule synthesis:* * peripheralization of marginating neutrophil pool (doubling of neutrophil count), * other causes ♦ catecholamines, ♦ lithium, ♦ alcohol
lymphocyte in PB	*see Table 13–1*
control mechanism of iron uptake by BM RBC precursors	*intracellular levels of heme:* * heme = iron + protoporphyrin, * low heme increases iron uptake into RBC (unless iron stores decreased), * increased heme decreases iron uptake, * intracellular heme has negative feedback on δ-ALA synthase (rate-limiting enzyme of heme synthesis)
storage form of iron in macrophages	*ferritin:* * ~iron stores in BM, * also stored in hepatocytes (heme for cytochrome system)
effect of inflammation on ferritin	*increases serum ferritin:* * released by hepatocytes, * inflammation limits accuracy of ferritin levels representing BM iron stores
adult Hbs in decreasing concentration	**HbA** $(2\alpha2\beta)$, *HbA$_2$* $(2\alpha2\delta)$, *HbF* $(2\alpha2\gamma)$
Hb levels used to define anemia in adult men/women	• *adult man: Hb <13 g/dL,* • *adult women: Hb <12 g/dL* [Anemia is a sign of an underlying disease rather than a specific diagnosis.]
effect of anemia on PaO$_2$ and SaO$_2$	*no effect:* * PaO$_2$ and SaO$_2$ are normal, since gas exchange is normal, * O$_2$ content decreased: O$_2$ content = (1.34 × **Hb** g/dL) × SaO$_2$ + (0.003 × PaO$_2$), * Hb has greatest effect on amount of O$_2$ available for delivery to tissue

Table continued on following page

Table 8–3. GENERAL CONCEPTS IN HEMATOPOIESIS AND ANEMIA *Continued*

Question: A 63-year-old woman presents with weakness, scleral icterus, sore tongue, and decreased vibratory sensation in her lower extremities. A CBC reveals a severe macrocytic anemia, pancytopenia, corrected reticulocyte count <2%, decreased plasma haptoglobin, and an increased serum LDH. The bone marrow is hypercellular and megaloblastic. Iron stores are increased. Which of the following apply to this case? **SELECT 2**
- (A) Effective erythropoiesis
- (B) Macrophage destruction of RBCs
- (C) Folate deficiency
- (D) Destruction of the myeloid stem cell
- (E) B$_{12}$ deficiency
- (F) Intravascular hemolysis
- (G) Conjugated hyperbilirubinemia

Answers: (B), (E): The patient has B$_{12}$ deficiency. This is based on the macrocytic anemia, pancytopenia, megaloblastic bone marrow, ineffective erythropoiesis (low corrected reticulocyte count, hypercellular marrow, pancytopenia [macrophage destruction of RBCs, WBCs, and platelets in the marrow]; **choice A is incorrect**), increased LDH from macrophage destruction of RBCs **(choice B)**, and neurologic abnormalities consistent with dorsal column disease (rules out folate deficiency; **choice C is incorrect**). B$_{12}$ deficiency is not a stem cell disorder **(choice D is incorrect)**. An extravascular (within the bone marrow) rather than intravascular hemolysis **(choice F is incorrect)** is present. The jaundice is an unconjugated rather than a conjugated hyperbilirubinemia **(choice G is incorrect)** due to macrophage destruction of RBCs. Leakage of Hb out of the macrophages into the blood is responsible for the low plasma haptoglobin levels.

BM = bone marrow, CBC = complete blood cell count, CFU-E = colony-forming unit–erythroid, CFU-G = colony-forming unit–granulocyte, CFU-GEMM = colony-forming unit–granulocyte, erythroid, macrophage, megakaryocyte, CFU-L = colony-forming unit–lymphoid, CFU-M = colony-forming unit–macrophage, CFU-Meg = colony-forming unit–megakaryocyte, EPO = erythropoietin, Hb = hemoglobin, Ig = immunoglobulin, LDH = lactate dehydrogenase, MCC = most common cause, MDS = myelodysplastic syndrome, ODC = oxygen dissociation curve, PaO$_2$ = partial pressure of oxygen in arterial blood, PB = peripheral blood, PPSC = pluripotential stem cell, PRV = polycythemia rubra vera, RBC = red blood cell, SaO$_2$ = oxygen saturation in arterial blood, UCB = unconjugated bilirubin, WBC = white blood cell.

Table 8–4. MICROCYTIC ANEMIAS

Most Common...	Answer and Explanation
mechanism causing microcytic anemias	*reduced Hb synthesis:* * low Hb concentration in RBC precursors is stimulus for cells to undergo extra divisions, leading to microcytosis, * Hb is combination of heme (iron + protoporphyrin) + globin chains
microcytic anemias due to a reduction in heme synthesis	• **iron deficiency,** • *ACD,* • *sideroblastic anemias* [Both *iron deficiency* and *ACD* have low serum iron levels → decreased heme synthesis. *Sideroblastic anemias* have problems in combining iron with protoporphyrin (e.g., ferrochelatase enzyme is denatured in Pb poisoning) or in synthesis of protoporphyrin (e.g., pyridoxine deficiency, mitochondrial damage due to alcohol).]
microcytic anemia due to reduction in globin chain synthesis	*thalassemia:* α/β-thalassemia are AR diseases
cause of iron deficiency in women <35 y old	*menorrhagia:* * average menstrual loss per mth is 40–50 mL, * blood loss >80 mL/per mth called menorrhagia
cause of iron deficiency in men <50 y old	• **PUD:** duodenal ulcers > gastric ulcers, • *GERD,* • *Meckel's diverticulum:* MC cause in children, • *malabsorption:* e.g., celiac disease, • *chronic NSAID use,* • *diverticulosis,* • *hookworm infestation,* • *angiodysplasia*
cause of iron deficiency men/women >50 y old	*GI cancer:* left-sided colon cancers obstruct, right-sided cancers bleed
cause of iron loss in urine as Hb	• **calcific aortic stenosis:** * RBCs destroyed intravascularly after hitting calcified valves, * hemoglobinuria leads to iron losses, • *PNH:* chronic hemoglobinuria
cause of iron loss from increased utilization	• **pregnancy/lactation:** * net iron loss in pregnancy without supplements ~500 mg, * lactation adds 2.5–3 mg iron loss/d, • *Rx B$_{12}$ folate deficiency:* increased erythropoiesis
lab stages of iron deficiency	• **loss of BM iron** → • *low serum ferritin:* best test → • *low serum iron, increased TIBC, low % saturation* → • *normocytic anemia* → • *microcytic anemia* [Reverse sequence occurs when patient is treated with iron.]

Table continued on following page

Table 8–4. MICROCYTIC ANEMIAS *Continued*

Most Common...	Answer and Explanation
effect of acute hemorrhage on lab stages of iron deficiency	*Hb concentration decreased <u>before</u> loss of iron stores in BM*
Rx of iron deficiency	*oral ferrous sulfate* (325 mg, tid): * Rx should not be started until cause of iron deficiency identified, * expect an ~0.5–1 Hct point/d after lag period of ~1 wk, * black stools, * ~3 wks, Hct ~50% of normal, * Rx ~6 mths after Hct has normalized
cause of no reticulocyte response or increase in Hct after iron Rx	• **noncompliance,** • *poor GI absorption,* • persistent GI bleed, • *wrong Dx*
mechanisms of anemia in ACD	• **decreased EPO synthesis:** * macrophage release of IL-1/TNF block EPO synthesis, * also block iron release by macrophages (decreased iron to BM RBC precursors), • *reduced transferrin synthesis in liver:* see above, • *decreased RBC survival*
causes of ACD	• **chronic inflammation:** e.g., * RA, * liver disease, • *malignancy:* ACD MC anemia, • *hospitalization:* MC anemia in hospitalized patients
lab findings in ACD	• *low serum iron,* • *low TIBC:* high in iron deficiency, • *low % saturation,* • *high ferritin:* low in iron deficiency, • *normal RDW:* high in iron deficiency, • *MCV:* usually normal or slightly decreased in ACD
Rx of ACD	• **Rx underlying disease,** • *EPO*
mechanism of reduced globin chain synthesis in α-thal	*gene deletions on chromosome 16:* * four genes control α-globin chain synthesis, * one gene deletion: normal MCV, * two gene deletions: mild microcytic anemia, * three gene deletions: HbH disease (HbH = four β-chains, hemolytic anemia), * four gene deletions: Hb Bart's disease (incompatible with life, Hb Bart = four γ-chains), • *prenatal studies available*
mechanism of reduced globin chain synthesis in β-thal	• **splicing defect of β-globin chains on chromosome 11,** • *point mutations leading to defects in transcription or translation* [Absence of β-chain synthesis is designated β°, reduc-

Table 8–4. MICROCYTIC ANEMIAS *Continued*

Most Common...	Answer and Explanation
Continued	tion in β-chain synthesis is β$^+$, and normal β-chain synthesis is β. Clinical severity ranges from minor (β$^+$/β), to intermediate (β°/β), to major (β$^+$/β$^+$ or β°/β°).]
clinical findings in severe β-thal	• *facial enlargement:* * frontal bossing, * chipmunk appearance, • *growth retardation,* • *hepatosplenomegaly:* extramedullary hematopoiesis, • *heart failure:* restrictive cardiomyopathy from iron overload, • *miscellaneous:* * massive ineffective erythropoiesis, * extravascular hemolysis in spleen/liver (hemolytic component unlike thal minor), * excess α-chains in RBC precursors are toxic (contribute to intra-marrow RBC destruction of RBCs), * prenatal studies available
Hb electrophoresis findings in mild α-thal	*no abnormalities are noted in one and two gene deletion types of α-thalassemia:* HbA, A$_2$, and F all need α-chains (all equally decreased), * Hb H/Hb Barts are identified, * mild disease: ♦ normal iron studies, ♦ normal RDW, ♦ RBC count >5.0 cells/μL
Hb electrophoresis/ iron studies in β-thal	• *thal minor Hb studies:* * β-chains decreased, * α, δ, γ-chains normally produced, * α-chains + δ-chains → Hb A$_2$, * α-chains + γ-chains → Hb F, decreased HbA, • *thal major (Cooley's anemia) Hb studies:* * Hb F predominates, * small amounts of HbA$_2$, * trace HbA, • *thal minor iron studies:* normal iron studies, • *thal major iron studies:* * iron overload from transfusions, * high serum iron, * low TIBC, * high % saturation, * high serum ferritin
Rx of mild α- and β-thalassemia	*no Rx*
Rx of severe α- and β-thal	• **blood transfusion,** • *splenectomy:* severe β-thalassemia, • *bone marrow transplantation in severe β-thalassemia patients without iron overload,* • *iron chelation*
effect of iron deficiency on Dx of mild β-thal	*HbA$_2$ and HbF levels are normal, owing to decreased production of Hb related to iron deficiency:* * in mild β-thal, correction of iron deficiency causes increase in HbA$_2$/HbF, * lack of full response to iron Rx in iron deficiency usually indicates mild β-thal

Table continued on following page

Table 8–4. MICROCYTIC ANEMIAS *Continued*

Most Common...	Answer and Explanation
cause of a hemoglobinopathy with 100% HbF	*hereditary persistence of HbF:* * benign variant of β-thal, * occurs in 0.1% of African Americans, * either a deletion or inactivity of β and δ structural gene complex → excess production of HgF throughout life
lab findings in HPFH	• **100% HbF with no HbA or HbA₂,** • *no anemia,* • *slightly reduced MCV,* • *erythrocytosis:* HgF left shifts ODC
cause of sideroblastic anemia	• **alcohol abuse,** • *pyridoxine* (B₆) *deficiency:* INH Rx, • *Pb poisoning,* • *drugs:* * cycloserine, • *multiple myeloma,* • *MDS,* • *hereditary types* [Sideroblasts are nucleated RBC precursors with excess iron trapped in mitochondria. PB RBCs with iron are called siderocytes (iron inclusions called Pappenheimer bodies).]
BM findings in sideroblastic anemias	*increased iron stores/ringed sideroblasts*
lab findings in sideroblastic anemias	• *high serum iron,* • *low TIBC:* increased iron stores, decreased transferrin synthesis, • *high % saturation,* • *high serum ferritin*
Rx of sideroblastic anemias	• *pyridoxine:* * hereditary types, * INH-related, • *transfusion:* often in combination with chelation Rx to prevent iron overload
cause of Pb poisoning in children and adults	• *children:* eating Pb-based paint/plaster, • *adults:* * incineration of car batteries, * working with pottery, drinking moonshine whiskey (old radiators are Pb-based)
defects associated with Pb-poisoning	• *denatured enzymes:* ferrochelatase: iron + protoporphyrin → heme, * ALA dehydrase: δ-ALA → porphobilinogen, * ribosomes not degraded → coarse basophilic stippling, • *nephrotoxic to proximal tubule epithelial cells:* proximal RTA, • *increases renal reabsorption of uric acid:* association with gout/HTN, • *deposits in epiphysis:* * densities visible on radiograph, * growth retardation, • *CNS/peripheral nerve abnormalities:* demyelination in CNS/PNS
S/S of Pb poisoning in children and adults	• *children:* targets * brain (edema, learning defects), * bone (epiphyseal densities), * GI tract (colic, radiographs identify Pb), • *adults:*

Table 8–4. MICROCYTIC ANEMIAS *Continued*

Most Common...	Answer and Explanation
Continued	targets * peripheral nerves (claw hand, wrist drop), * gums (Pb line), * kidneys (proximal RTA, urate nephropathy)
lab findings in Pb poisoning	• **high blood lead level:** best screening/confirmatory test, • *iron overload,* • *coarse basophilic stippling,* • *high FEP,* • *increased urine δ-ALA,* • *normal AG metabolic acidosis:* proximal RTA, • *hyperuricemia*
Rx of Pb poisoning	• **EDTA,** • BAL • penicillamine in some cases
lab findings in sideroblastic anemias other than Pb poisoning	• *ringed sideroblasts:* necessary for Dx, • *iron overload*

Question: In iron deficiency, ACD, and Pb poisoning, which of the following test results are present in only one of the three anemias? **SELECT 4**
- (A) Low MCV
- (B) High serum iron
- (C) Low TIBC
- (D) Ringed sideroblasts in the BM
- (E) High serum FEP
- (F) Low % saturation of iron
- (G) High RDW
- (H) High TIBC

Answers: (B), (D), (G), (H): A low MCV is present in all the anemias (choice A is incorrect). A high serum iron is present only in Pb poisoning (low in iron deficiency and ACD, choice B). A low TIBC is present in both ACD and Pb poisoning (choice C is incorrect). Ringed sideroblasts (choice D) are present only in Pb poisoning. A high serum FEP is present in all three anemias (choice E is incorrect). A low % saturation of iron is present in iron deficiency and ACD (choice F is incorrect). A high RDW (choice G) and high TIBC (choice H) are present only in iron deficiency.

ACD = anemia of chronic disease, AG = anion gap, δ-ALA = aminolevulinic acid, AR = autosomal recessive, BAL = British-anti-Lewisite (dimercaprol), BM = bone marrow, CNS = central nervous system, Dx = diagnosis, EDTA = ethylenediamine tetraacetic acid, EPO = erythropoietin, FEP = free erythrocyte protoporphyrin, GERD = gastroesophageal reflux disease, GI = gastrointestinal, Hb = hemoglobin, Hct = hematocrit, HTN = hypertension, IL = interleukin, INH = isoniazid, MC =

most common, MCV = mean corpuscular volume, MDS = myelodysplastic syndrome, NSAID = nonsteroidal anti-inflammatory drug, ODC = oxygen dissociation curve, Pb = lead, PB = peripheral blood, PNH = paroxysmal nocturnal hemoglobinuria, PNS = peripheral nervous system, PUD = peptic ulcer disease, RA = rheumatoid arthritis, RBC = red blood cell, RDW = RBC distribution width, RTA = renal tubular acidosis, Rx = treatment, S/S = signs and symptoms, TIBC = total iron binding capacity, TNF = tumor necrosis factor.

Table 8–5. MACROCYTIC ANEMIAS

Most Common...	Answer and Explanation
cause of macrocytic anemia	**folate deficiency in alcoholic,** • B_{12} *deficiency:* PA MCC, • *reticulocytosis:* large RBCs, • *hypothyroidism,* • *toxic effect of alcohol:* * increased RBC membrane, * round target cell, • *zidovudine:* * unrelated to B_{12}/folate deficiency, * toxic effect on BM, * EPO effective Rx
sources of folate B_{12}	• *folate in plant/animal products,* • B_{12} *only animal products* [Both are required for DNA synthesis. Deficiency results in large, immature nucleus and *megaloblastic anemia.*]
drugs interfering with absorption of folate in the jejunum	*phenytoin/birth control pills:* * phenytoin inhibits intestinal conjugase (converts polyglutamate to monoglutamate form for absorption), * BCPs/alcohol block uptake monoglutamates
factor required for absorption of B_{12}	*intrinsic factor* (IF): * synthesized in parietal cells of body/fundus, * R factor in saliva combines with B_{12} to prevent acid destruction, * R factor cleaved off B_{12} in duodenum by pancreatic enzymes, * IF binds B_{12} and complex is reabsorbed in terminal ileum
function of B_{12} in relation to folate metabolism	*see Table 8–2*
drugs that block dihydrofolate reductase	*see Table 8–1*
method to circumvent drugs blocking dihydrofolate reductase	*leucovorin rescue* (citrovorum factor, folinic acid): leucovorin replaces $N^{5,10}$ methylene FH_4 (substrate required for deoxythymidine monophosphate synthesis)

Table 8–5. MACROCYTIC ANEMIAS *Continued*

Most Common...	Answer and Explanation
function of B$_{12}$ in propionate metabolism	*see Table 8–2*
causes of folate deficiency	• **nutritional deficiency:** e.g., **alcohol abuse** (excluding beer), • *goat's milk,* • *small bowel disease:* e.g., celiac disease, • *drugs:* see above, • *overutilization:* e.g., * pregnancy, * cancer, * hemolytic anemia
causes of B$_{12}$ deficiency	• **pernicious anemia** (PA), • *pure vegan diet,* • *achlorhydria:* acid required to free B$_{12}$ from food, • *fish tapeworm,* • *bacterial overgrowth,* • *gastrectomy,* • *chronic pancreatitis,* • *terminal ileal disease:* e.g., * surgical resection, * Crohn's disease
S/S folate/B$_{12}$ deficiency	• *glossitis:* smooth, sore tongue, • *malabsorption:* small bowel epithelial cells cannot reabsorb nutrients
S/S of B$_{12}$ deficiency alone	• *sallow complexion,* • *posterior column disease:* * decreased vibratory sensation, * loss of proprioception, • *lateral corticospinal tract disease:* UMN problems, • *dementia:* neurologic problems may occur without anemia or MCV alteration
S/S of PA alone	• *achlorhydria,* • *stomach cancer,* • *autoantibodies against parietal cells and IF,* • *correction of B$_{12}$ absorption after giving IF*
PB findings in B$_{12}$/folate deficiency	• *pancytopenia:* BM macrophage destruction of megaloblastic cells, • *macroovalocytes:* egg-shaped RBCs unique to B$_{12}$/folate deficiency, • *hypersegmented neutrophils:* >5 nuclear lobes, • *tear drop RBCs*
lab findings in folate deficiency	• *low serum folate/RBC folate* (better test), • *high plasma homocysteine,* • *increased urine FIGLu,* • *high serum LDH,* • *slightly high UCB:* BM macrophage RBC destruction
lab findings in PA	• *low serum B$_{12}$,* • *high plasma homocysteine,* • *high urine methylmalonic acid:* most sensitive test, • *high LDH,* • *high UCB,* • *Schilling's test:* * correction B$_{12}$ reabsorption with addition of IF, * see Table 8–2, • *high serum folate:* absence of B$_{12}$ causes methyl-FH$_4$ in cells to leak back into blood

Table continued on following page

Table 8–5. MACROCYTIC ANEMIAS *Continued*

Most Common...	Answer and Explanation
Rx of folate/B_{12} deficiency	• *folic acid for folate deficiency:* corrects hematologic problems in B_{12} deficiency, but not neurologic problems, • *IM B_{12} for B_{12} deficiency,* • *iron:* erythropoiesis uses up iron

Question: Which of the following distinguish PA from other causes of B_{12} deficiency and folate deficiency? **SELECT 4**
- (A) Urine methylmalonic acid
- (B) Schilling's test
- (C) Plasma homocysteine
- (D) Anti-parietal cell antibodies
- (E) Hypersegmented neutrophils
- (F) Neurologic exam
- (G) Achlorhydria
- (H) Urine FIGLu
- (I) Serum LDH
- (J) Serum gastrin levels

Answers: (B), (D), (G), (J): There is an increase in urine methylmalonic acid in any cause of B_{12} deficiency (normal in folate deficiency, **choice A is incorrect**). Correction of Schilling's test **(choice B)** with the addition of IF along with radioactive B_{12} separates PA from other causes of B_{12} deficiency and folate deficiency. Homocysteine levels are increased in both B_{12} and folate deficiency **(choice C is incorrect)**. Anti-parietal cell antibodies **(choice D)**, achlorhydria **(choice G)**, and increased serum gastrin levels **(choice J**; no negative feedback of acid on gastrin release) are present only in PA. Hypersegmented neutrophils and an increase in serum LDH are present in both B_{12} and folate deficiency **(choices E and I are incorrect)**. Urine FIGLu is increased in folate deficiency **(choice H is incorrect)**. The neurologic exam is abnormal in any cause of B_{12} deficiency and is normal in folate deficiency **(choice F is incorrect)**.

BCPs = birth control pills, BM = bone marrow, CoA = coenzyme A, EPO = erythropoietin, FH_4 = tetrahydrofolate, FIGLu = formiminoglutamic acid, IF = intrinsic factor, LDH = lactate dehydrogenase, MCC = most common cause, MCV = mean corpuscular volume, PA = pernicious anemia, PB = peripheral blood, RBC = red blood cell, Rx = treatment, S/S = signs and symptoms, UCB = unconjugated bilirubin, UMN = upper motor neuron.

Table 8–6. NORMOCYTIC ANEMIAS AND INFECTIONS OF THE BLOOD

Most Common...	Answer and Explanation
initial effect of acute blood loss on Hb concentration	*no effect:* * equal amount of RBCs and plasma are lost, * plasma initially replaced and uncovers RBC deficit in few hours to few days
effect of IV normal saline in a patient with acute blood loss on the Hb concentration	*uncovers RBC deficit:* normal saline remains in ECF compartment
cause of acute blood loss	*GI bleed:* most commonly from PUD (e.g., duodenal ulcer)
cause of aplastic anemia	• **idiopathic,** • **drugs:** * MC known cause, * e.g., busulfan, chloramphenicol, gold salts, phenylbutazone, sulfonamides, • *infection:* * **NANBH,** * EBV, * CMV, * parvovirus, • *chemicals:* * benzene, * insecticides, • *genetic:* Fanconi's anemia (AR disease with risk for acute leukemia), • *radiation,* • *other anemias:* * aplastic crisis in HbSS (relation to parvovirus), * PNH
S/S in aplastic anemia	• **bleeding/petechia/ecchymoses:** thrombocytopenia, • *fever:* infection from neutropenia, • *fatigue:* anemia
lab findings in aplastic anemia	• *normocytic anemia with corrected retic count <2%,* • *pancytopenia,* • *hypocellular bone marrow*
Rx for aplastic anemia	• **bone marrow transplantation for patients <50 y old,** • *antithymocyte/antilymphocyte globulins,* • *cyclosporine,* • *corticosteroids,* • *growth factors:* e.g., * EPO, * CSF-GM and G, * thrombopoietin
causes of pure RBC aplasia	• **severe hemolytic anemias in association with parvovirus infections:** * sickle cell anemia, * congenital spherocytosis, • *Blackfan-Diamond syndrome:* AR disease, • *thymoma*
lab findings in pure RBC aplasia	• *severe anemia,* • *absent PB retics,* • *no RBC precursors in BM*
cause of anemia in renal disease	• **EPO deficiency,** • *dialysis-related iron/folate deficiency,* • *microangiopathic hemolytic anemia*

Table continued on following page

Table 8–6. NORMOCYTIC ANEMIAS AND INFECTIONS OF THE BLOOD Continued

Most Common...	Answer and Explanation
hematologic findings in renal disease	• *normocytic anemia with corrected retic count <2%,* • *burr cells:* * undulating RBC membrane, * correctable with dialysis, • *prolonged BT:* * qualitative platelet defect, * reversible with dialysis
Rx of anemia in renal disease	*EPO*
anemia in malignancy	• **ACD:** ~50%, • *iron deficiency:* usually GI blood loss, • *marrow invasion by tumor:* called myelophthisis, • *chemotherapy suppression of BM,* • *hemolytic anemia:* * HUS triggered by mitomycin C, * AIHA, * folate deficiency
general mechanisms of hemolysis in hemolytic anemias	**extravascular:** macrophage-induced, • *intravascular*
types of intrinsic (RBC defect) hemolytic anemias	• *membrane defects:* * **congenital spherocytosis,** * hereditary elliptocytosis, * PNH, • *abnormal Hb:* * **sickle cell disease** and its variants, * HbC disease, • *deficient enzymes:* * **G6PD deficiency,** * PK deficiency
types of extrinsic (defect outside the RBC) hemolytic anemias	• **AIHA:** * **SLE,** * drugs, • *microangiopathic:* * **DIC,** * TTP, * HUS, * HELLP syndrome, • *macroangiopathic:* * **calcific aortic stenosis,** * prosthetic heart valves
lab finding in hemolytic anemias	• **corrected reticulocyte count >3%:** corrected for anemia and the presence or absence of polychromasia, • *positive direct Coombs' test,* • *low to absent serum haptoglobin:* * primarily intravascular types, * extravascular types only if severe, • *high LDH, high UCB:* extravascular types, • *hemoglobinuria:* * primarily intravascular types, * extravascular types only if severe
hemolytic anemias with predominantly extravascular hemolysis	• *congenital spherocytosis,* • *congenital elliptocytosis,* • *sickle cell disease,* • *warm AIHA*
hemolytic anemias with predominantly intravascular hemolysis	• **microangiopathic, macroangiopathic** • *PNH,* • *G6PD deficiency:* plus lesser element of extravascular, • *cold AIHA*

Table 8–6. NORMOCYTIC ANEMIAS AND INFECTIONS
OF THE BLOOD *Continued*

Most Common...	Answer and Explanation
defect in congenital spherocytosis	*AD disease with a defect in spectrin and band 4.1 in RBC membrane:* * decreased surface to volume ratio (membrane loss), * increased glycolysis (decreased ATP, low RBC glucose)
clinical triad in congenital spherocytosis	• *splenomegaly,* • *anemia,* • *jaundice:* UCB type, • *additional:* * cholecystitis (♦ 55–75%, ♦ jet black calcium bilirubinate stones), * hemolytic crises resulting in aplastic anemia (often triggered by parvovirus)
lab findings in congenital spherocytosis	• **increased osmotic fragility of RBCs in progressively hypotonic salt solutions:** low ATP levels hamper proper functioning of ATPase pump that normally keeps Na^+ out of RBCs, • *spherocytes in PB:* no central area of pallor, • *high MCHC:* loss of RBC membrane concentrates Hb, * spherocytes MCC of high MCHC, • *corrected retic >3%*
Rx of congenital spherocytosis	*splenectomy in patients with Hb <11 g/dL and corrected reticulocyte count >6%:* * Pneumovax/Hib vaccines given prior to splenectomy, * spherocytes present after splenectomy
defect in hereditary elliptocytosis	*AD disease with defects in spectrin*
lab findings in hereditary elliptocytosis	• *elliptocytes:* * >25% of RBCs, * elliptocytes also seen in iron deficiency, • *retic >3%,* • *compensated hemolytic anemia:* * normal Hb, * marrow keeps pace with anemia
Rx of hereditary elliptocytosis	*usually none*
membrane defects in PNH	• **lack glycosylphosphatidylinositol-linked proteins** (GPI-linked proteins, e.g., CD59) **in erythroid, granulocytic, megakaryocytic stem cells,** • *lack decay accelerating factor:* see Table 8–2, • *low levels of RBC acetylcholinesterase*
S/S of PNH	• **episodic hemoglobinuria,** • *pain:* low back, esophageal, abdominal, • *vessel thrombosis:* * hepatic vein (Budd-Chiari syndrome), * portal vein, * mesenteric vein, * sagittal sinus

Table continued on following page

Table 8–6. NORMOCYTIC ANEMIAS AND INFECTIONS OF THE BLOOD *Continued*

Most Common...	Answer and Explanation
screening/ confirmatory test for PNH	• *screening test:* * sugar water test, * see Table 8–2, • *confirmatory test:* * acidified serum test (Ham's test), * see Table 8–2, • *flow cytometry for detection of GPI-linked proteins:* best confirmatory test, • *other lab findings:* * pancytopenia, * aplastic marrow, * iron deficiency (hemoglobinuria), * hemosiderinuria, * low serum haptoglobin levels, * low LAP score
Rx of PNH	• *ferrous sulfate for iron deficiency:* may exacerbate hemolysis, • *androgen therapy:* beneficial in hypocellular marrows, • *corticosteroids:* may inhibit activation of alternative complement pathway, • *marrow transplantation:* for aplastic anemia, • *antithymocyte globulin*
COD in PNH	*hepatic vein thrombosis:* * venous thrombosis accounts for ~50% of deaths, * other COD: ♦ aplastic anemia, ♦ acute nonlymphocytic leukemia (5–10%)
Hb disorder in blacks	**sickle cell trait**/*disease:* sickle cell gene in ~8% of blacks
defect in sickle cell disease	*AR disease with a point mutation* (adenine replaces thymidine) *leading to substitution of valine for glutamic acid at 6th position of the* β-*globin chain:* substitution causes polymerization of HbS → permanently altered RBC membrane proteins
cause of sickling of RBCs in HbSS	• **increased amount of sickle Hb:** >60%, • *reduced O_2 tension:* * high altitude, * renal medulla, • *high 2,3-BPG levels:* increased O_2 release from Hb, • *presence of other Hbs:* e.g., HbC, • *volume depletion,* • *acidosis:* right shifts ODC with release more O_2
Hb that inhibits sickling	*HbF:* HbF in RBCs of newborns prevents sickling for 6–9 mths
S/S of sickle cell trait	• **usually asymptomatic,** • exceptions: * microscopic/macroscopic hematuria, * potential for sudden death with vigorous exercise, * splenic infarction at altitudes >10,000 feet, * bacteriuria, * pyelonephritis in pregnancy, * isosthenuria (inability to concentrate/dilute

Table 8–6. NORMOCYTIC ANEMIAS AND INFECTIONS OF THE BLOOD *Continued*

Most Common...	Answer and Explanation
Continued	urine), * renal papillary necrosis, • *trait* (not disease) *protective against falciparum malaria*
problems in sickle cell disease (HbSS)	• **vaso-occlusive disease:** combination of sickle cells blocking microcirculation and nonsickled cells sticking to endothelium, • *chronic hemolytic anemia:* * primarily extravascular, * intravascular to lesser extent
manifestation of HbSS	*vaso-occlusive painful crises:* * occur in limbs, back, chest, * no RBC hemolysis
initial site for vaso-occlusive crisis in HbSS	• **hands/feet:** dactylitis, • *brain:* strokes, particularly in children, • *lungs:* acute chest syndrome, • *liver:* liver cell necrosis, • *bone marrow:* aplastic crisis, • *spleen:* sequestration crisis, • *penis:* priapism
clinical findings of acute chest syndrome	• **fever/chest pain,** • *pulmonary infiltrates,* • *neutrophilic leukocytosis,* • *hypoxemia,* • *children:* pneumonia precipitates sickling in lungs as secondary event, • *adults:* * sickling primary event, * no preexisting infection, • *mortality:* accounts for ~20% of deaths
hematologic crises in HbSS	• *aplastic crisis:* * precipitated by parvovirus infection, * low retic count, * marrow aplastic, • *splenic sequestration crisis:* * sudden onset of painful splenomegaly/shock due to RBC trapping, * high retic count, * BM with RBC hyperplasia
cause of priapism in HbSS	*vaso-occlusion of vessels leading to painful erection*
cause of stroke in HbSS	*vaso-occlusion of cerebral vessels leading to a cerebral infarction:* MC in children
bone complications in HbSS	• *delayed bone growth,* • *aseptic necrosis of femoral head:* bone infarction, • *osteomyelitis:* * most often *Staphylococcus aureus,* * less commonly, *Salmonella* species, • *radiograph:* * vertebra with fish-mouth appearance, * reactive bone formation in aseptic necrosis
spleen complications in HbSS	• *painful splenomegaly,* • *splenic dysfunction:* usually complete by 2–3 y of age, • *autosplenectomy:* usually in late adolescence, • *splenic sequestration:* see above

Table continued on following page

Table 8–6. NORMOCYTIC ANEMIAS AND INFECTIONS OF THE BLOOD *Continued*

Most Common...	Answer and Explanation
complications of chronic hemolysis in HbSS	• *jaundice,* • *calcium bilirubinate stones,* • *iron overload:* heavy transfusion requirement
ocular findings in HbSS	*retinal vascular lesions:* * proliferative retinopathy, * vitreous hemorrhages, * retinal detachment
effect of pregnancy in HbSS	• *increased incidence of maternal death,* • *premature delivery/fetal demise:* 20%
lab findings in sickle cell trait	• *normal CBC,* • *Hb electrophoresis:* * HbS ~40%, * HbA ~60%
lab findings in sickle cell disease	• Hb electrophoresis: * HbS 85–98%, * HbF 5–15%, * no HbA, • hematologic findings: * sickle cells (♦ reversible, ♦ irreversible), * target cells (♦ excellent hemoglobinopathy marker, ♦ increased RBC membrane with central bulge), * Howell-Jolly bodies (♦ nuclear remnant, ♦ indicate absent/dysfunctional spleen), * nucleated RBCs, * polychromasia, * retics >3%, * neutrophilic leukocytosis, * low ESR, * thrombocytosis (dysfunctional/autosplenectomized spleen), • other findings: * high serum UCB, * low haptoglobin levels, * hematuria, * isosthenuria, • *prenatal Dx:* * Southern blot technique with cleavage of fetal DNA using restriction endonuclease into fragments of DNA, * abnormal gene sites are detected with nuclear probe
Rx of painful crises in HbSS	• **hydration:** not blood transfusion, • *morphine sulfate:* analgesic of choice, • *O₂*
crises in HbSS requiring blood transfusion	• *acute chest syndrome,* • *stroke,* • *aplastic/ sequestration crises,* • *priapism*
use of hydroxyurea in HbSS	• **decreases incidence of vaso-occlusive pain episodes by increasing synthesis of HbF,** • *BM transplantation:* option in severe cases
COD in children <5 years old who have HbSS	*sepsis secondary to Streptococcus pneumoniae:* * less commonly *Haemophilus influenzae,* * underscores importance of vaccination
COD in adults with HbSS	• **acute chest syndrome,** • *stroke,* • *infection*

Table 8–6. NORMOCYTIC ANEMIAS AND INFECTIONS OF THE BLOOD *Continued*

Most Common...	Answer and Explanation
cause of sickling and low MCV	*HbS/β° or HbS/β+ thal:* * clinical severity < HbSS, * HbF 10–20%, * less HbS (70–80% in β°, 60–75% in β+), * some HbA (10–20% in β+), HbA$_2$ 3–5%, * functional spleen, * retinopathy > HbSS
defect in HbC disease	*AR disease with a substitution of lysine for glutamic acid in 6th position of β-chain*
clinical findings of HbC disease	• *splenomegaly,* • *mild to moderate anemia,* • *HbC crystals in PB:* look like Washington monument, • *numerous target cells*
S/S of HbS/C disease compared to HbSS	• *greater severity than HbSS:* * proliferative retinopathy, * renal papillary necrosis, * pulmonary infarctions, * acute chest syndrome secondary to fat emboli in late pregnancy, * aseptic necrosis, • *lesser severity than HbSS:* * degree of anemia, * number of sickle cell crises, * propensity for splenic infarctions (spleen is functional)
lab findings in HbS/C disease	• *hybrid crystals:* * cross between sickle cell and HbC Washington monument, * sickle cells rare, • *target cells:* ~50% of RBCs, • *no Howell-Jolly bodies,* • *Hb electrophoresis:* * HbS, * HbC, * HbF, * no HbA
defect in G6PD deficiency causing hemolysis	*absence of GSH:* SXR disease
precipitating factors leading to hemolysis in G6PD deficiency	• **infections,** • *oxidizing drugs:* e.g., * primaquine, * dapsone, * nitrofurantoin, * sulfa drugs, • *eating fava beans:* Mediterranean variant
defect in black variant of G6PD versus Mediterranean	black variant: * defective G6PD only in older RBCs, * hemolysis less severe, • *Mediterranean variant:* * G6PD defective or deficient in all RBCs, * hemolysis severe
PB findings in G6PD deficiency	• *bite cells:* * macrophage removes part of RBC membrane, * useful finding in acute hemolysis, • *Heinz bodies:* see Table 8–2

Table continued on following page

Table 8–6. NORMOCYTIC ANEMIAS AND INFECTIONS OF THE BLOOD *Continued*

Most Common...	Answer and Explanation
method of diagnosing G6PD deficiency in active hemolysis versus a nonhemolytic state	• *active hemolysis:* * Heinz body prep, * enzyme studies normal to increased (only RBCs with enzyme left), • *nonhemolytic state:* enzyme assays
Rx of G6PD deficiency	• *adequate hydration,* • *avoid drugs known to precipitate hemolysis,* • *splenectomy: not indicated*
mechanism of hemolysis in PK deficiency	*AR disease leading to reduction in ATP synthesis and reduced consumption of glucose:* * PK catalyzes following reaction: PEP + ADP → Pyruvate + ATP, * PK deficiency causes increase in substrates proximal to block and decrease in ATP, * low ATP alters RBC membrane with loss of K⁺ resulting in volume contraction of RBCs (echinocytes), * RBCs susceptible to macrophage removal in spleen
S/S of PK deficiency	• *splenomegaly,* • *jaundice,* • *increased incidence of calcium bilirubinate stones*
lab findings in PK deficiency	• *mild normocytic anemia,* • *retics >3%,* • *high serum UCB,* • *high RBC 2,3-BPG:* * proximal to enzyme block, * right shifts ODC: tissue hypoxia not severe, • *RBC enzyme assay:* confirmatory test
Rx of PK deficiency type of anemia	*no specific Rx:* splenectomy in severe cases
types of AIHA	• **warm AIHA:** e.g., * **SLE,** * CLL, * lymphoma, • *drug-induced AIHA:* see below, • *cold AIHA:* e.g., * *Mycoplasma pneumoniae* with anti-I-IgM antibodies, * infectious mononucleosis with anti-i-IgM antibodies, * CLL
mechanisms of hemolysis in AIHA	• *warm AIHA:* * IgG with/without C3b (SLE has both) attaches to RBC membrane → extravascular hemolysis, * antibodies directed against Rh antigens, • *drug-induced AIHA:* see below, * *cold AIHA:* * IgM/C3b attach to RBC membrane → intravascular hemolysis, * IgM activates classical complement pathway

Table 8–6. NORMOCYTIC ANEMIAS AND INFECTIONS OF THE BLOOD *Continued*

Most Common...	Answer and Explanation
S/S of AIHA	• *fever,* • *jaundice:* high UCB, • *generalized lymphadenopathy,* • *hepatosplenomegaly*
mechanism of AIHA with penicillin	• *penicillin (cephalosporin) acts as hapten and attaches to RBC membrane → IgG antibodies directed against drug,* • *type II HSR*
mechanism of AIHA with methyldopa, α-interferon	• *drugs produce IgG autoantibodies against Rh antigens,* • *type II HSR*
mechanism of AIHA with quinidine, INH	• *IgM antibodies combine with drug and attach to RBCs → IgM activates complement system → intravascular hemolysis,* • *type III HSR*
tests used to identify an AIHA	**direct**/*indirect Coombs' test:* see Table 8–2
PB findings in AIHA	• *spherocytes:* macrophages remove part of RBC membrane with IgG, • *polychromasia,* • *NRBC*
Rx of warm AIHAs	• **corticosteroids:** * first step, * avoid transfusion if possible (RBCs hemolyzed), • *splenectomy:* second step, if steroids unsuccessful, • *alkylating agents:* last resort
Rx of cold AIHA	*alkylating agents*
Rx of drug-induced AIHA	*withdraw drug*
Rx of life-threatening AIHA unresponsive to the above treatments	*IV gamma globulin:* * IgG binds to Fc receptors on macrophages and prevents them from phagocytosing sensitized RBCs, * temporary Rx
mechanism of hemolysis in PCH	*bithermal IgG antibody* (Donath-Landsteiner antibody): * see Table 8–2, * direct Coombs' test negative at body temperature but positive in cold temperatures
causes of PCH	• **syphilis,** • *infectious mononucleosis,* • *mumps,* • *measles*
PB finding in micro- and macroangiopathic hemolytic anemias	*schistocytes:* fragmented RBCs

Table continued on following page

Table 8–6. NORMOCYTIC ANEMIAS AND INFECTIONS OF THE BLOOD *Continued*

Most Common...	Answer and Explanation
lab findings in micro- and macroangiopathic hemolytic anemias	• *low to absent serum haptoglobin,* • *hemoglobinuria,* • *hemosiderinuria,* • *possibility of iron deficiency: loss of iron in urine*
lab findings in HELLP syndrome	• *H = hemolysis,* • *EL = elevated transaminases,* • *LP = low platelets,* • schistocytes in PB, • *~40% associated with DIC,* [HELLP is associated with pre-eclampsia. Rx is prompt delivery of the baby.]
infectious causes of hemolysis	• **malaria:** *Plasmodium falciparum* most severe type, • *babesiosis:* * *Babesia microti,* * carried by Iodides tick, • *bartonellosis*
anemias in alcoholics	• **ACD:** 80%, • *folate deficiency:* 30%, • *acute blood loss:* 25%, • *sideroblastic anemia:* 25%, • *iron deficiency:* 13%, • *hemolytic anemias:* uncommon, • *~50% have single cause for anemia, 30% two causes, 20% ≥three causes*
anemias in AIDS	• **ACD,** • *MDS:* see below, *hemolytic:* immune mechanisms, • *microangiopathic:* from disseminated cancer or DIC
types of blood cultures	• *aerobic,* • *anaerobic* [Volume of blood drawn is more important than timing. 10 mL into each culture container (aerobic/anaerobic) is minimum amount. One mL in children is minimal amount.]
contaminants in blood culture	• ***Staphylococcus epidermidis:*** coagulase negative, • *Bacillus species,* • *Corynebacterium species* [Suspect contamination if blood culture drawn in other arm is negative.]
findings in systemic inflammatory response syndrome (SIRS)	• **fever >38°C or <36°C,** • *heart rate >90/min:* exception is sinus bradycardia in typhoid fever, • *respiratory rate >20/min,* • *hypoxemia,* • *lethargy,* • *increased/decreased WBC count:* e.g., * high in *Staphylococcus aureus* septicemia, * low in *Escherichia coli* septicemia, • *left-shifted smear:* left-shifted even with low WBC counts, particularly in the elderly
cause of pneumonia/sepsis in ICU	*Pseudomonas aeruginosa:* respirator is the source
hospital risk factor for sepsis	• **indwelling urinary catheter:** *E. coli* sepsis, • *indwelling line in place >48 h: S. aureus* sepsis

Table 8–6. NORMOCYTIC ANEMIAS AND INFECTIONS OF THE BLOOD *Continued*

Most Common...	Answer and Explanation
patient risk factors for sepsis	• **immunosuppression from cancer Rx:** usually gram-negative sepsis, • *chronic illness,* • *DM,* • *therapeutic procedure:* e.g., * indwelling urinary catheter, * respirator, • *angiography*
diseases predisposing to sepsis	• **pneumonia:** *Streptococcus pneumoniae,* • *AIDS,* • *pyelonephritis: E. coli,* • *burns:* * ***Pseudomonas aeruginosa,*** * *Staphylococcus aureus,* • *trauma,* • *pancreatitis,* • *biliary tract infection: E. coli,* • *sickle cell disease: S. pneumoniae,* • *splenectomy: S. pneumoniae,* • *peritonitis:* * *E. coli,* * *Bacteroides fragilis,* • *ascites:* spontaneous peritonitis due to *E. coli,* • *absolute neutropenia with WBC count <500 cells/μL:* usually *P. aeruginosa* sepsis
clinical findings in candidemia	• *predisposing causes:* * indwelling catheters for TPN, * broad-spectrum antibiotics, * neutropenia, • *clinical:* * 5–10% nosocomial septicemias, * nodular skin lesions (metastatic abscess), * fluffy white chorioretinal exudates (endophthalmitis), * fever unresponsive to empirical antibacterial agents, • *Rx:* * replace indwelling catheter, * amphotericin B or high-dose fluconazole
clinical findings in relapsing fever	• *pathogen:* * *Borrelia recurrentis,* * tick/louse transmitted, • *clinical:* * relapses of high fever, * hepatosplenomegaly, • *lab:* * spirochetes in PB, • *Rx:* doxycycline
clinical findings in leptospirosis	• *pathogen:* * *Leptospira interrogans* (cause of Weil's disease), * rodents/domesticated animals (particularly dogs) are reservoirs for the disease (shed organisms in urine into soil/ponds), * tightly wound spirochete, * contracted from swimming in infected ponds, • *clinical:* * initial septicemic phase: ♦ anicteric hepatitis, ♦ flu-like syndrome, ♦ conjunctivitis, ♦ tubulointerstitial disease (oliguria, potential for renal failure), ♦ meningitis, * immune phase: ♦ antibodies develop, ♦ numerous organisms in urine, • *lab:* * spirochetes noted in urine (best body fluid to examine) by phase contrast or darkfield microscopy, * serologic tests, • *Rx:* doxycycline or penicillin G

Table continued on following page

Table 8–6. NORMOCYTIC ANEMIAS AND INFECTIONS OF THE BLOOD *Continued*

Most Common...	Answer and Explanation
organism transmitted along with *Borrelia burgdorferi*	*Babesia microti:* intra-erythrocytic sporozoan
clinical findings of babesiosis	• *pathogen:* * *Babesia microti*, * transmitted by tick *Ixodes dammini*, * parasitizes RBCs, • *clinical:* self-limited hemolytic anemia, • *lab:* * examine peripheral blood for organisms, • *Rx:* clindamycin + quinine
types of malaria worldwide	• ***Plasmodium vivax:*** 55%, • *P. falciparum:* 40%, • *P. malariae:* 5%, • *P. ovale:* <1%
malaria with fever spikes q 48-h	*P. viva:* * tertian malaria, * fever corresponds with RBC hemolysis and parasite release
malaria with fever spikes q 72-h	*P. malariae:* quartan malaria
malaria with intermittent fever spikes	*P. falciparum:* * quotidian malaria, * most dangerous malaria
mechanisms of hemolysis in malaria	• **intravascular,** • *extravascular*
method of transmission of malaria	• **mosquito bite:** female *Anopheles* mosquito, • *blood transfusion*, • *mosquito transmits infected blood from one patient to the next*
types of malaria with no relapses	• *P. vivax*, • *P. malariae* [Absence of relapses indicates that there is no hepatocyte reinfection. *P. malariae/P. ovale* have relapses.]
clinical findings in malaria	• **spiking fever,** • *splenomegaly:* * massive splenomegaly may occur, * spontaneous splenic rupture may occur, • *hemolytic anemia*, • *IC disease:* membranous GN with nephrotic syndrome in *P. malariae*, • *cerebral malaria: P. falciparum*, • *ARDS: P. falciparum*, • *hemoglobinuria: P. falciparum*
lab Dx of malaria	• **examination of thick/thin PB smears,** • *serologic tests*, • *DNA probes*
prophylaxis for malaria	*chloroquine*
prophylaxis for malaria in chloroquine-resistant areas	• **mefloquine,** • *doxycycline*

Table 8–6. NORMOCYTIC ANEMIAS AND INFECTIONS OF THE BLOOD Continued

Most Common...	Answer and Explanation
Rx of infection due to *P. vivax, P. malariae,* susceptible *P. falciparum*	*chloroquine:* * blood schizonticide, * may produce irreversible retinopathy/myopathy (check vision/muscle strength periodically)
Rx of infection of malaria with chloroquine-resistant strains	*quinine or mefloquine and doxycycline*
use of primaquine in Rx of malaria	*Rx liver infestation by P. malariae, P. ovale:* * primaquine is a tissue schizonticide to above types, * gametocidal to all types of malaria, * can produce hemolytic anemia in patients with G6PD deficiency.
blood group that offers protection against *P. vivax*	*absence of Duffy blood group:* common in blacks
conditions that offer protection against *P. falciparum*	• *sickle cell trait:* sickle cell disease as well to a less extent, • *G6PD deficiency,* • α/β-*thal*

Question: Which of the following normocytic anemias are likely to have a UCB hyperbilirubinemia and an increased corrected reticulocyte count? **SELECT 3**
- (A) PK deficiency
- (B) Sickle cell trait
- (C) Anemia in chronic renal disease
- (D) Congenital spherocytosis
- (E) Aplastic anemia
- (F) Warm AIHA
- (G) Cold AIHA
- (H) PCH
- (I) Microangiopathic hemolytic anemia
- (J) PNH

Answers: (A), (D), (F): In most instances, extravascular hemolytic anemias are those most commonly associated with UCB-related jaundice and an increased corrected reticulocyte count **(choices A, D, F).** Sickle cell trait is not associated with anemia **(choice B is incorrect).** Anemia in chronic renal disease is most commonly due to low levels of EPO **(choice C is incorrect).** Aplastic anemia is not a hemolytic anemia **(choice E is incorrect).** Cold AIHA, PCH, microangiopathic hemolytic anemia, and PNH are primarily intravascular hemolytic anemias **(choices G, H, I, and J are incorrect).** Only in very severe intravascular hemolysis is jaundice a possibility owing to increased phagocytosis of the haptoglobin-Hb complex by macrophages and the breakdown of Hb.

ACD = anemia of chronic disease, AD = autosomal dominant, ADP = adenosine diphosphate, AIDS = acquired immunodeficiency syndrome, AIHA = autoimmune hemolytic anemia, AR = autosomal recessive, ARDS = adult respiratory distress syndrome, ATP = adenosine triphosphate, BM = bone marrow, 2,3-BPG = 2,3 bisphosphoglycerate, BT = bleeding time, CBC = complete blood count, CLL = chronic lymphocytic leukemia, CMV = cytomegalovirus, COD = cause of death, CSF-G = colony-stimulating factor–granulocytes, CSF-GM = colony stimulating-factor–granulocytes/macrophage, DIC = disseminated intravascular coagulation, DM = diabetes mellitus, Dx = diagnosis, EBV = Epstein-Barr virus, ECF = extracellular fluid, EPO = erythropoietin, ESR = erythrocyte sedimentation rate, G6PD = glucose 6-phosphate dehydrogenase, GI = gastrointestinal, GN = glomerulonephritis, GPI = glycosylphosphatidylinositol-linked proteins, GSH = glutathione, Hb = hemoglobin, Hib = *Haemophilus influenzae* type B, HbSS = sickle cell anemia, HELLP = Hemolysis, ELevated transaminases, Low Platelets, HSR = hypersensitivity reaction, HUS = hemolytic uremic syndrome, IC = immunocomplex, ICU = intensive care unit, Ig = immunoglobulin, INH = isoniazid, IV = intravenous, LDH = lactate dehydrogenase, MC = most common, MCHC = mean corpuscular hemoglobin concentration, MDS = myelodysplastic syndrome, NANBH = non-A non-B hepatitis, NRBC = nucleated RBC, ODC = oxygen dissociation curve, PB = peripheral blood, PCH = paroxysmal cold hemoglobinuria, PEP = phosphoenolpyruvate, PK = pyruvate kinase, PNH = paroxysmal nocturnal hemoglobinuria, PUD = peptic ulcer disease, RBC = red blood cell, Rx = treatment, S/S = signs and symptoms, SLE = systemic lupus erythematosus, SXR = sex-linked recessive, TPN = total parenteral nutrition, UCB = unconjugated bilirubin, WBC = white blood cell.

Table 8–7. BENIGN WHITE BLOOD CELL DISORDERS

Most Common...	Answer and Explanation
cause of absolute neutrophilic leukocytosis (>7000 cells/μL)	• **bacterial infection:** e.g., * acute appendicitis, * cellulitis, • *decreased adhesion molecule synthesis:* e.g., * corticosteroids, * lithium, * catecholamines, • *sterile inflammation:* e.g., * AMI, * blood in peritoneal cavity, * smoking, • *uremia,* • *DKA,* • *stress,* • *MPD*
medically significant absolute neutrophil count	*absolute neutrophil count >14,000 cells/μL*
PB findings in acute bacterial infections	• **absolute neutrophilic leukocytosis,** • *toxic granulation:* prominence of azurophilic granules containing MPO, • *left shift,* • *Dohle bodies:* dull gray cytoplasmic inclusions representing parallel strands of RER
causes of leukemoid reaction (benign increase in WBCs >30,000 cells/μL)	• **infection:** e.g., * TB, * whooping cough, • *malignancy:* e.g., renal adenocarcinoma [Differential count in these reactions should not include myeloblasts/lymphoblasts.]

Table 8–7. BENIGN WHITE BLOOD CELL
DISORDERS *Continued*

Most Common...	Answer and Explanation
cause of leukoerythroblastic reaction	• *metastasis to bone:* e.g., breast cancer, • *myelofibrosis,* • *excess bone replacing BM:* osteopetrosis [PB contains "blasts" and NRBCs.]
cause of absolute neutropenia (<1500 cells/μL)	• **decreased production due to drugs:** e.g., * chemotherapy agents, * see aplastic anemia under Table 8–6, • *chemicals:* e.g., benzene, • *increased margination:* e.g., * normal finding in blacks, * endotoxins, • *infection:* e.g., typhoid, • *destruction:* e.g., Felty's syndrome (autoimmune neutropenia + splenomegaly + RA), * AIDS, • *cyclic neutropenia:* see below
WBC count for antibiotic prophylaxis in neutropenia	≤*500 cells/μL*
empiric Rx for neutropenic patients with fever	*monotherapy with ceftazidime or imipenem:* gram negatives like *Pseudomonas aeruginosa* are of most concern
S/S of cyclic neutropenia	• *fever,* • *aphthous ulcers,* • *furuncles,* • *neutropenia occurs q 19–23 d:* neutrophil production disorder at regulation phase
cause of absolute lymphocytosis (>4,000 cells/μL)	• **viral infections:** e.g., * HIV, * IM, * infectious lymphocytosis, • *bacterial infections:* e.g., * *Bordetella pertussis,* * TB, • *Graves' disease,* • *drugs:* e.g., phenytoin
infections with lymphocytosis and normal lymphocytes	• *whooping cough,* • *infectious lymphocytosis:* probable coxsackievirus infection
cause of atypical lymphocytosis (>10% cells)	• **infectious mononucleosis,** • *viral hepatitis,* • *CMV,* • *toxoplasmosis,* • *HIV,* • *phenytoin*
method of transmission of IM	• **deep kissing:** * virus in saliva, * initially replicates in oropharynx, • *blood transfusion,* • *sexual transmission* [EBV attaches to CD_{21} receptors on B cells. T cells react against infected B cells and represent the atypical lymphocyes in PB. EBV remains in B cells throughout life.]
S/S of IM	• **fever:** >90%, • *pharyngitis:* * often exudative, * palatal petechia, • *generalized lymphadenopathy:* 80–90%, • *rash with ampicil-*

Table continued on following page

Table 8–7. BENIGN WHITE BLOOD CELL
DISORDERS *Continued*

Most Common...	Answer and Explanation
Continued	lin, • *hepatomegaly:* 10–15%, • *spleno-megaly:* * 50–60%, * spontaneous rupture rare * rupture MC with contact sports
lab findings of IM	• **atypical lymphocytosis,** • *positive heterophile antibody test:* see Table 8–2, • *elevated transaminases:* * 80–90%, * anicteric hepatitis, * self-limited, • *increased antiviral capsid antigen IgM:* most sensitive antibody test, • *cold autoimmune hemolytic anemia:* anti-i-IgM antibodies
cause of absolute lymphopenia (<1500 cells/μL)	• **viral infection:** initial phase, • *drugs:* e.g., corticosteroids, • *immunodeficiency syndromes:* e.g., AIDS
cause of eosinophilia (>700 cells/μL)	• **type I HSR:** e.g., * drug reaction, * hay fever, * asthma, • *invasive helminthic diseases:* no protozoal diseases or noninvasive helminths like *Enterobius vermicularis* or adult *Ascaris lumbricoides* infections, • *Addison's disease:* low cortisol has opposite effect as increase in cortisol on eosinophil count, • *Hodgkin's disease,* • *PAN,* • *MPD*
cause of eosinopenia	• **corticosteroids,** • *Cushing's syndrome*
cause of basophilia (>110 cells/μL)	• **MPDs:** e.g., * PRV, * CML, • *CD,* • *myxedema*
cause of monocytosis (>800 cells/μL)	• **chronic inflammation,** • *autoimmune disease,* • *malignancy*
PB findings in corticosteroid Rx	• **absolute neutrophilic leukocytosis,** • *lymphopenia,* • *eosinopenia*
clues suggesting a phagocytic disorder	• *delayed separation of umbilical cord:* * β_2-integrin (CD11/CD18 glycoprotein) adhesion molecule defect, * no marginating neutrophils, * no neutrophils in umbilical cord tissue, • *unusual pathogens:* e.g., * *Serratia marcescens,* * *Staphylococcus epidermidis,* • *child always sick,* • *chronic periodontitis and loss of teeth,* • *"cold" soft tissue abscesses:* * no inflammatory response, * chemotaxis problem

Table 8–7. BENIGN WHITE BLOOD CELL
DISORDERS Continued

Most Common...	Answer and Explanation
S/S of Job's syndrome	• *chronic eczema*, • *red hair*, • *leonine face*, • *"cold" soft tissue abscesses due to Staphylococcus aureus*, • *increased IgE*: hyperimmune E syndrome, • *primarily chemotaxis defect*
cause of hemolytic anemia precipitated by infection	*G6PD deficiency*
phagocytic defects in diabetics	• impaired— • chemotaxis, • phagocytosis, • intracellular killing of bacteria [Hyperglycemia is responsible for defects, hence importance of good glycemic control.]
phagocytic defects in HIV-positive patients	*defective neutrophil and monocyte chemotaxis*
PB WBC findings in AIDS	• **lymphopenia:** * 70–95%, * direct HIV lymphocytotoxic effect on CD$_4$ T helper cells, • *neutropenia:* * 45–75%, * immune mediated, • *pancytopenia:* 35–40%
BM findings in AIDS	• **hypercellular,** • *normocellular,* • *hypocellular,* • *reactive plasmacytosis,* • *increased iron stores* [MDS findings (see below) with ringed sideroblasts and increased myeloblasts are common.]

Question: In which conditions is atypical lymphocytosis expected? **SELECT 5**
  (A) Whooping cough
  (B) Phenytoin therapy
  (C) Viral hepatitis
  (D) Infectious lymphocytosis
  (E) Corticosteroid therapy
  (F) CMV infections
  (G) Rheumatoid arthritis
  (H) Infectious mononucleosis
  (I) Drug allergies
  (J) Toxoplasmosis

Answers: (B), (C), (F), (H), (J): Viral hepatitis **(choice B)**, phenytoin **(choice C)**, CMV **(choice F)**, infectious mononucleosis **(choice H)**, and toxoplasmosis **(choice J)** are all associated with atypical lymphocytosis. The lymphocytosis of whooping cough and infectious lymphocytosis involves mature lymphocytes **(choices A and D are incorrect)**. Corticosteroids produce lymphopenia, rheumatoid arthritis monocytosis, and drug allergies eosinophilia **(choices E, G, and I are incorrect)**.

AMI = acute myocardial infarction, BM = bone marrow, CD = Crohn's disease, CML = chronic myelogenous leukemia, CMV = cytomegalovirus, DKA = diabetic ketoacidosis, EBV = Epstein-Barr virus, G6PD = glucose 6-phosphate dehydrogenase, HIV = human immunodeficiency virus, HMP = hexose monophosphate shunt, HSR = hypersensitivity reaction, Ig = immunoglobulin, IM = infectious mononucleosis, MC = most common, MDS = myelodysplastic syndrome, MPD = myeloproliferative disease, MPO = myeloperoxidase, NRBC = nucleated RBC, PAN = polyarteritis nodosa, PB = peripheral blood, PRV = polycythemia rubra vera, RA = rheumatoid arthritis, RER = rough endoplasmic reticulum, Rx = treatment, S/S = signs and symptoms, TB = tuberculosis, WBC = white blood cell.

Table 8–8. NEOPLASTIC WHITE BLOOD CELL DISORDERS

Most Common...	Answer and Explanation
cause of MPDs	*acquired, neoplastic clonal stem cell disorders with unregulated proliferation of specific cell lines*
MPDs	• **PRV,** • *CML,* • *AMM,* • *ET*
clinical findings in all MPDs	• *myelofibrosis,* • *leukemic transformation:* usually AML, • *splenomegaly*
MPD with a chromosome abnormality	*CML:* t(9;22) with fusion of abl proto-oncogene on chromosome 9 with bcr on chromosome 22 (Philadelphia chromosome)
cause of polycythemia	*relative polycythemia:* see Table 8–2
appropriate absolute polycythemia	*hypoxemia-induced secondary polycythemia:* e.g., * **smoker's polycythemia** (CO-induced), * COPD, * high altitude, * right-to-left shunt in the heart, * see Table 8–2
inappropriate absolute polycythemia	• **PRV,** • *EPO production in renal disease* • *hepatocellular carcinoma* [See Table 8–2.]
mechanism of polycythemia in pheochromocytoma	• *catecholamines increase RBC mass,* • *vasoconstriction reduces plasma volume*
cause of PRV	*clonal expansion of multipotential myeloid stem cell:* increased production of RBCs, WBCs (not lymphocytes), platelets

Table 8–8. NEOPLASTIC WHITE BLOOD CELL
DISORDERS *Continued*

Most Common...	Answer and Explanation
clinical findings of PRV	• **hyperviscosity signs:** predisposes to thrombosis leading to AMI, stroke, bowel infarction, • *hypervolemia:* only MPD with increased plasma volume, • *hyperuricemia:* increased turnover of nucleated cells may lead to gout, • *histaminemia:* * histamine released from mast cells/basophils, * causes vasodilatation (plethoric face, headache), * pruritus after bathing
lab findings of PRV	• **category A:** * high RBC mass, * SaO_2 ≥92%, * splenomegaly, • **category B:** * platelet count >400,000 cells/µL, * leukocytosis >12,000 cells/µL, * LAP score >100 (see Table 8–2), * serum B_{12} >900 pg/mL (WBCs carry transcobalamin I), • *PRV Dx:* * all three category A are present, * high RBC mass along with any other category A criteria plus two out of four category B criteria, • *other lab findings:* * normal/high plasma volume, * low EPO (elevated O_2 content), * high uric acid, * low MCV (secondary to iron deficiency from bleeding or phlebotomy), * Hct >58% in males and >52% in females
Rx of PRV in asymptomatic/ symptomatic patients	• *asymptomatic:* * phlebotomy, * reduce RBC mass, * produce iron deficiency (decreases RBC production), • *symptomatic:* * **hydroxyurea,** * anagrelide, * ^{32}P, * alkylating agents and radioactive phosphorus increase risk for leukemic transformation
lab findings of absolute polycythemia associated with tissue hypoxia	• *high RBC mass,* • *normal plasma volume,* • SaO_2 ≤88%, • *high EPO,* • *examples:* * COPD, * high altitude, * hypoventilation syndromes (obstructive sleep apnea), * cyanotic CHD, * methemoglobinemia, * CO poisoning
lab findings of absolute polycythemia with SaO_2 ≥92%	• *high RBC mass,* • *normal plasma volume,* • SaO_2 ≥92%, • *high EPO,* • *examples:* * renal disorders (♦ renal adenocarcinoma: includes von Hippel-Lindau disease, ♦ Wilms' tumor, ♦ cysts, ♦ hydronephrosis: includes uterine leiomyoma pressing on ureter), * HCC
lab findings of smoker's polycythemia	• *high RBC mass:* CO effect, • *low plasma volume:* vasoconstrictive effects of catecholamines, • *variable SaO_2,* • *variable EPO*

Table continued on following page

Table 8–8. NEOPLASTIC WHITE BLOOD CELL DISORDERS *Continued*

Most Common...	Answer and Explanation
differentiating lab features of PRV versus COPD	• **Sao₂:** * ≥92% PRV, * ≤88% COPD, • *plasma volume:* * high in PRV, * normal in COPD, • *EPO:* * low in PRV, * high in COPD, • *BM exam:* * all cell lines increased in PRV, * only RBC hyperplasia in COPD
differentiating lab features of PRV versus renal disease	• **EPO:** * low in PRV, * high in renal, • *plasma volume:* * high in PRV, * normal in renal, • *BM exam:* * all cell lines increased in PRV, * only RBC hyperplasia in renal disease
cause of CML	*neoplastic clonal expansion of PPSC prompted by a translocation of abl proto-oncogene from chromosome 9 to chromosome 22 with fusion with bcr to form a fusion gene* (Philadelphia chromosome) *that enhances tyrosine kinase activity:* CML accounts for ~20% of all leukemias
S/S of CML	• *hypermetabolic state:* * fever, * weight loss, * sweating, • *hepatosplenomegaly:* metastasis, • *generalized lymphadenopathy:* metastasis, • *chloromas:* * soft tissue collection neoplastic cells, * orbit common site, • *myeloblast or lymphoblast crisis after ~2–3 y*
lab findings of CML	• *leukoerythroblastic smear:* 50,000–150,000 cells/μL, • *normocytic anemia,* • *basophilia,* • *thrombocytosis:* * 40–50%, * only leukemia with thrombocytosis, • *myeloblasts: <10% in BM,* • *low LAP score:* see Table 8–2, • *Philadelphia chromosome:* * 95%, * poor prognosis if absent, • *positive bcr-fusion gene study:* 100%, • *high serum B₁₂:* * high transcobalamin I in WBCs, • *high serum acid phosphatase:* present in WBCs
Rx for CML	• **hydroxyurea:** most frequently used drug, • *α-interferon or busulfan* [Blast crisis in 2–3 y • AML blast crisis Rx like AML. Lymphoid blast crisis Rx like ALL. BM transplant only curative Rx. Philadelphia chromosome remains after hydroxyurea Rx but disappears with α-interferon.]
cause of AMM	*proliferation of neoplastic stem cells that begin in marrow and move to the spleen, where extramedullary hematopoiesis continues:*

Table 8–8. NEOPLASTIC WHITE BLOOD CELL DISORDERS *Continued*

Most Common...	Answer and Explanation
Continued	megakaryocytes in BM secrete growth factors that stimulate collagen synthesis
S/S of AMM	• *massive splenomegaly:* hallmark of AMM, • *abdominal pain:* * splenic infarctions, * stretching of capsule, • *left-sided friction rubs:* splenic infarctions, • *left-sided pleural effusions:* splenic infarctions, • *PH*
lab findings in AMM	• **leukoerythroblastic smear:** hematopoietic cells in spleen directly released into blood through sinusoids, • *normocytic anemia,* • *thrombocytosis,* • *marrow fibrosis:* dry BM aspirate, • *teardrop RBCs in PB:* derive from damaged RBCs remaining in fibrosed BM, • *increased LAP score,* • *absent Philadelphia chromosome*
Rx of AMM	• *androgens:* stimulate erythropoiesis, • *splenic irradiation:* Rx for infarcts
differentiating features of AMM versus CML	• *LAP score:* * high in AMM, * low in CML, • *Philadelphia chromosome:* * absent in AMM, * present in CML
cause of ET	*clonal stem cell disorder primarily involving megakaryocytes*
S/S of ET	• **venous thrombosis,** • *bleeding:* * usually GI, * platelets defective, • *TIAs,* • *splenomegaly*
lab findings of ET	• *thrombocytosis:* >600,000 cells/μL, • *iron deficiency anemia:* GI bleeding, • *neutrophilic leukocytosis,* • *abnormal megakaryocytes in BM* [Difficult to distinguish iron deficiency with thrombocytosis from ET leading to iron deficiency.]
Rx of ET	• *platelet pheresis,* • *hydroxyurea*
cause of MDS	*clonal stem cell disorder with defects in maturation involving all hematopoietic cell lines:* * chromosomal defects common (e.g., ♦ 5q⁻, ♦ trisomy 8), * may be induced by ♦ radiation, ♦ chemotherapy, ♦ toxin exposure
FAB types of MDS	• **refractory anemia:** 24%, • **refractory anemia with ringed sideroblasts:** * 24%, * lowest rate of leukemic transformation, • *refractory*

Table continued on following page

Table 8–8. **NEOPLASTIC WHITE BLOOD CELL DISORDERS** *Continued*

Most Common...	Answer and Explanation
Continued	*anemia with excess blasts:* 23%, • *refractory anemia with excess blasts in transformation:* * 9%, * highest rate leukemic transformation, • *chronic myelomonocytic leukemia:* 16%
clinical presentation of MDS	*elderly patient with severe anemia requiring constant transfusions:* 10–40% progress into acute leukemia
lab findings of MDS	• **dimorphic RBC population:** micro-, macrocytic, • *pancytopenia,* • *megaloblastic marrow:* some use term megaloblast**oid** to differentiate it from folate B_{12} deficiency, • *increased myeloblasts:* <30%, • *ringed sideroblasts*
Rx of MDS	*supportive with blood transfusions:* BM transplantation option in patients <55 y
overall leukemia	*CLL*
leukemia in newborns to 14 y old	*ALL:* * MC overall cancer/leukemia in children, * uncommon in adults
leukemia in 15–39 y old age bracket	*AML*
leukemia in 40–60 y old age bracket	• **AML,** • *CML*
leukemia in >60 y old age bracket	*CLL:* MC cause of generalized lymphadenopathy in patients >60 y old
method of distinguishing acute from chronic leukemia	• *acute leukemia:* * BM blast count >30% (e.g., myeloblasts, lymphoblasts, monoblasts, erythroblasts), * thrombocytopenia, circulating blasts, * normocytic/slightly macrocytic anemia (folate deficiency), • *chronic leukemia:* * BM blast count <30%, * greater degree of WBC maturation in PB, * thrombocytopenia, * normocytic/macrocytic anemia
causes of leukemia	• *chromosomal abnormalities:* * Down syndrome, * chromosome instability syndromes (♦ Fanconi syndrome, ♦ ataxia telangiectasia), • *radiation,* • *alkylating agents:* * **melphalan,**

Table 8–8. NEOPLASTIC WHITE BLOOD CELL
DISORDERS *Continued*

Most Common...	Answer and Explanation
Continued	* cyclophosphamide, * chlorambucil, • *benzene*, • *immunodeficiency syndromes:* e.g., Wiskott-Aldrich syndrome, • *viruses:* HTLV-1
S/S of leukemia	• *fever:* * gram-negative infections, * hypermetabolic state, • *hepatosplenomegaly:* metastasis, • *petechiae/ecchymoses:* thrombocytopenia, • *generalized lymphadenopathy:* metastasis, • *bleeding:* * thrombocytopenia, * DIC (particularly acute progranulocytic leukemia), • *bone pain:* BM infiltration, • *gum infiltration:* acute monocytic type
initial step in leukemia work-up	*BM aspirate and Bx*
ancillary lab findings in leukemia	• *hyperuricemia:* * increased cell turnover, * danger of urate nephropathy, • *high LDH:* nonspecific tumor marker, • *macrocytic anemia:* folate deficiency from overutilization, • *pseudohyperkalemia:* K^+ leaks out of WBCs in collection tube when WBC count >50,000 cells/μL
stains used in Dx of leukemias	*see Table 8–2*
type of ALL	Pre B cell ALL that is CALLA positive, TdT positive [ALL type most important prognostic factor. Most adult ALLs are B cell origin. Mature B cell ALL has worst prognosis. T cell ALL has intermediate prognosis.]
Rx for ALL	• *remission/induction:* * prednisone, * vincristine, * asparaginase, • *consolidation:* same drugs at lower doses, • *maintenance:* * 6-mercaptopurine, * methotrexate, • prognosis: * best prognosis between ages of 3 and 10 y, * CALLA positive, * 60–70% long-term disease-free interval in children versus only 10–40% in adults
sites for residual blasts after remission/induction Rx in ALL	• **bone marrow,** • *CNS,* • *testes* [Intrathecal administration of methotrexate and radiation of neuraxis obliterate blast cells in CNS.]

Table continued on following page

Table 8–8. NEOPLASTIC WHITE BLOOD CELL
DISORDERS *Continued*

Most Common...	Answer and Explanation
cell type of CLL	*virgin B cells:* * unable to produce plasma cells, * hypogammaglobulinemia, * rare in Asians
complication associated with CLL	• **hypogammaglobulinemia:** * 50%, * infections MC COD, • *warm/cold AIHA,* • *second malignancies:* * lung, * skin (BCE, squamous), • *transformation into malignant lymphoma:* Richter's syndrome
lab findings in CLL	• *normocytic anemia,* • *lymphocytosis:* 15,000–200,000 cells/μL, * "smudge" cells (fragile neoplastic B cells), * <55% of cells are prolymphocytes (most cells look "normal"), • *thrombocytopenia,* • *diffuse BM infiltration,* • *monoclonal IgM spike,* • *trisomy 12:* MC chromosome abnormality, • *hypogammaglobulinemia*
Rx of CLL	**chlorambucil** *with or without prednisone or fludarabine:* * fludarabine Rx of choice if relapses occur with chlorambucil, * IV γ-globulin given if γ-globulin levels <0.3 g/dL
cause of adult T cell leukemia	*HTLV-1 retrovirus:* more common in Japan than in United States
complications associated with adult T cell leukemia	• *hypercalcemia:* lytic bone lesions, • *skin infiltration:* feature of all T cell malignancies, • *prognosis:* majority die within 1 y
cause of HCL	*stem cell disorder involving B cells:* * cells have cytoplasmic projections, * splenic red pulp primary site for neoplastic proliferation
S/S of HCL	• **splenomegaly,** • *hepatomegaly,* • *absence of generalized lymphadenopathy:* unusual for leukemia, • *autoimmune vasculitis,* • *arthritis,* • *disseminated MAI infections*
Rx of HCL	*2-chlorodeoxyadenosine:* * ~90% response rate, * splenectomy no longer routine Rx, * α-interferon used in some cases
COD in HCL	*infection*
acute nonlymphocytic leukemia	*FAB classification:* * M2 (AML with maturation)

Table 8–8. NEOPLASTIC WHITE BLOOD CELL
DISORDERS *Continued*

Most Common...	Answer and Explanation
cytoplasmic abnormality in AML	*Auer rods:* * only in acute leukemias arising from neutrophils (missing in monocytic leukemias, CML, CML in AML blast crisis), * Auer rods are a fusion of cytoplasmic granules
leukemia associated with DIC	*FAB classification:* * M3 (acute progranulocytic leukemia), * hypergranular blasts, * t(15;17) characteristic, * high doses of transretinoic acid produce remissions
leukemia associated with gum infiltration	*FAB classification:* M5 (acute monocytic leukemia)
leukemia with bizarre, multinucleated erythroblasts	*FAB classification:* * M6 (Diguglielmo's disease), * blasts PAS positive, * may occur in Down syndrome
Rx of AML	• **cytosine arabinoside:** ara-C, • *daunorubicin* or *idarubicin,* • *BM transplantation:* only curative Rx
COD in leukemia	• **infections:** usually gram-negatives, • *bleeding*

Question: Which of the following differentiate PRV from all other causes of polycythemia? **SELECT 4**
    (A) Hypercellular bone marrow
    (B) SaO$_2$ ≤88%
    (C) High plasma volume
    (D) Low EPO
    (E) Basophilia/eosinophilia
    (F) Neoplastic stem cell disorder
    (G) High RBC count and RBC mass
    (H) Low LAP score

Answers: (C), (D), (E), (F): High plasma volume (**choice C**), low EPO (**choice D**), basophilia/eosinophilia (**choice E**), and neoplastic transformation of a stem cell (**choice F**) are unique to PRV. Hypercellular marrows and a high RBC count and RBC mass are noted in all the absolute polycythemias owing to RBC hyperplasia (**choices A and F are incorrect**). PRV has a SaO$_2$ ≥92% and a LAP score >100 (**choices B, H are incorrect**).

ALL = acute lymphoblastic leukemia, AMI = acute myocardial infarction, AML = acute myelogenous leukemia, AMM = agnogenic myeloid metaplasia, BCE = basal cell epithelioma, bcr = break cluster region, BM = bone marrow, Bx = biopsy, CALLA = common acute lymphoblastic leukemia antigen, CHD = congenital heart disease, CLL

= chronic lymphocytic leukemia, CML = chronic myelogenous leukemia, CNS = central nervous system, CO = carbon monoxide, COD = cause of death, COPD = chronic obstructive pulmonary disease, DIC = disseminated intravascular coagulation, Dx = diagnosis, EPO = erythropoietin, ET = essential thrombocythemia, FAB = French-American-British, GI = gastrointestinal, HCC = hepatocellular carcinoma, HCL = hairy cell leukemia, HTLV-1 = human T cell lymphotropic virus, IV = intravenous, LAP = leukocyte alkaline phosphatase, LDH = lactate dehydrogenase, MAI = *Mycobacterium avium intracellulare,* MC = most common, MDS = myelodysplastic syndrome, MPD = myeloproliferative disease, PAS = periodic acid–Schiff, PB = peripheral blood, PH = portal hypertension, PPSC = pluripotential stem cell, PRV = polycythemia rubra vera, RBC = red blood cell, Rx = treatment, Sao₂ = oxygen saturation of arterial blood, S/S = signs and symptoms, TdT = terminal deoxynucleotidyl transferase, TIAs = transient ischemic attacks, WBC = white blood cell.

Table 8–9. LYMPH NODE DISORDERS

Most Common...	Answer and Explanation
roles of IL-2, -4, -5 in B cell differentiation in lymph node	• *IL-2:* activates B cells, • *IL-4:* stimulates B cell growth and enhances isotype switching from synthesis of IgM to IgG, • *IL-5:* stimulates B cell differentiation [All of these interleukins are secreted by CD₄ helper T cells.]
causes of generalized tender lymphadenopathy	• **infections:** e.g., * HIV, * IM, * CMV, * secondary syphilis, • *drugs:* e.g., phenytoin, • *autoimmune disease:* e.g., * SLE, * RA
benign nodal disorder confused with metastatic malignant melanoma	*dermatopathic lymphadenopathy:* * lymph nodes draining skin lesions with excessive squamous proliferation (e.g., psoriasis), * macrophages phagocytose melanin pigment
cause of cat-scratch disease	*Bartonella henselae:* * isolated skin lesion, usually on hands, followed by regional, painful lymphadenopathy, * granulomatous microabscesses, * organisms identified with silver stains, * S/S usually resolve without Rx in 2–6 mths
Rx of cat-scratch disease	• *antibiotics are controversial,* • *in severe disease, rifampin, ciprofloxacin, or TMP/SMX may be used*
benign nodal disorder mistaken for HD	*lymph nodes in IM:* infected B cells transform into plasmacytoid immunoblasts that resemble Reed-Sternberg cells

Table 8–9. LYMPH NODE DISORDERS *Continued*

Most Common...	Answer and Explanation
drug producing generalized lymphadenopathy/ and atypical lymphocytosis	*phenytoin:* * fever, * skin rash, * eosinophilia also noted
benign nodal disorder associated with malignancy	*sinus histiocytosis:* favorable sign in breast cancer
malignancy associated with Virchow's node	*stomach adenocarcinoma:* left supraclavicular nodes, which drain abdominal cavity
malignancies associated with para-aortic lymph node enlargement	• **primary malignant lymphomas,** • *metastatic testicular cancers*
causes of hilar lymph node enlargement	• **primary lung cancer:** MC initial site of metastasis, • *sarcoidosis,* • *TB,* • *systemic fungal infections*
cause of nontender unilateral epitrochlear node	*NHL*
causes of generalized nontender lymphadenopathy	• **acute/chronic leukemias,** • *NHL*
cause of lymphadenopathy in patient <30 y old	*benign disease in ~80%:* e.g., infection
cause of lymphadenopathy in patient >30 y old	*malignancy:* most often metastatic disease
types of lymphoma	• **NHL,** • HD
extranodal site for a primary lymphoma	*stomach:* * majority arise in mucosa-associated lymphoid tissue and are high grade, * *Helicobacter pylori* causes low-grade B cell lymphoma
primary site for HIV-induced lymphoma	*CNS:* AIDS is MC cause for increase in primary CNS lymphomas in United States

Table continued on following page

Table 8–9. LYMPH NODE DISORDERS *Continued*

Most Common...	Answer and Explanation
malignancy of lymph nodes	*metastasis:* e.g., * breast cancer, * primary lung cancer
organ metastasized to	*lymph nodes*
CD antigen marker for lymphomas	CD_{45}: identifies ~90% of lymphomas
translocations associated with lymphoma	• **t(14;18) in B cell follicular lymphomas** • t(8;14) in Burkitt's lymphoma
cause for increase in NHL in United States	• **increase in HIV-positive patients,** • *immunosuppressive Rx:* alkylating agents, • *congenital immunodeficiencies:* e.g., Wiskott-Aldrich syndrome, • *autoimmune disease:* e.g., Sjögren's syndrome, • *EBV infections*
location for Burkitt's lymphoma	*equatorial Africa:* strong relationship with EBV and jaw involvement
classification scheme for NHL that utilizes pattern and size of the cells	*Rappaport classification:* * patterns are nodular/diffuse, * size based on comparison of lymphoma cells with endothelial cells, * nodular more favorable than diffuse
classification scheme based on marker studies	*Lukes-Collins classification:* * more accurate than Rappaport system, * more expensive and complicated
classification scheme that groups NHL by natural history and response to Rx	*The Working Formulation for Clinical Usage:* * NHL is subdivided low, intermediate, and high grades [Revised European-American Classification of Lymphoid Neoplasms (REAL) is now in vogue. Based on immunophenotyping-mature/immature B cell and T cell neoplasms, NK neoplasms.]
low grade NHL using the Working Formulation	*malignant lymphoma: follicular, small cleaved type:* * translocation of B cell Ig heavy chain gene site located on chromosome 14 to a location in proximity to bcl 2 oncogene site on chromosome 18, * causes overexpression of bcl 2 gene protein product, which inactivates apoptosis gene (cells immortal)
features of low-grade NHL	• *usually incurable,* • *occur in older patients,* • *present as stage III or IV disease:* BM involvement common, • *respond well to chemotherapy,* • *have a long survival, even after relapse:* median survival ~8 y

Table 8–9. LYMPH NODE DISORDERS *Continued*

Most Common...	Answer and Explanation
features of high-grade NHL	• *potentially curable,* • *may progress to more aggressive lymphoma,* • *length of survival is short in those who do not go into remission*
S/S of low grade NHL	*painless lymphadenopathy*
S/S of high-grade NHL	• *fever,* • *drenching night sweats,* • *weight loss,* • *abdominal pain:* typical for American Burkitt's lymphoma
B cell NHL confused with CLL involving lymph nodes	*malignant lymphoma: small lymphocytic:* * low-grade lymphoma, * involves BM and has leukemic phase
NHL in children	*Burkitt's lymphoma:* * malignant lymphoma: small noncleaved cell, * high-grade B-cell lymphoma
site for Burkitt's lymphoma	*abdominal cavity:* * in boys, it most often occurs in small intestine, * in girls, it favors pelvic organs, * African type more common in jaws and has greater EBV relationship
NHL associated with immunosuppression	*malignant lymphoma: large cell immunoblastic:* high-grade lymphoma
T cell lymphoma with skin/PB involvement	*mycosis fungoides:* * neoplastic T cells (CD_4 T helper cells) involve skin, lymph nodes, other organs, * called *Sezary syndrome* when neoplastic cells (characteristic nuclear cleft) enter PB
T cell lymphoma in children with leukemic phase resembling ALL	*malignant lymphoma: lymphoblastic:* * high-grade tumor, * involves anterior mediastinum and PB
work-up of NHL	• *chest radiograph,* • *CT abdomen/pelvis,* • *bilateral BM aspirates/Bx:* BM involved more commonly in low than high-grade NHL (stage IV disease)
Rx of low-grade lymphomas	*observation in most cases until patients become more symptomatic:* * chlorambucil or * CVP (cyclophosphamide, vincristine, prednisone) MC Rx regimens
Rx of intermediate to high-grade lymphomas	• **CHOP therapy:** * cyclophosphamide, * doxorubicin, * vincristine, * prednisone, • *autologous BM transplantation when in relapse*

Table continued on following page

Table 8–9. LYMPH NODE DISORDERS *Continued*

Most Common...	Answer and Explanation
diseases encompassed by term histiocytosis X	• *eosinophilic granuloma:* benign, • *Hand-Schuller-Christian disease:* malignant, • *Letterer-Siwe disease:* malignant [Histiocytes are CD_1 positive]
S/S of an eosinophilic granuloma	*unifocal lytic lesion in bone in adolescent or adult:* bone pain/pathologic fractures
features more often associated with HD than with NHL	• *younger people,* • *fever,* • *rarely involves Waldeyer's ring:* tonsils, adenoids, • *rarely involves skin/GI tract,* • *localized lymphadenopathy,* • *pain in an involved lymph node following ingestion of alcohol*
subtypes of HD in order of increasing number of RS cells, decreasing survival, increasing age	• *LP:* * 5%, * male dominant, • *NS:* * 40–70%, * female dominant, * MC type, • *mixed cellularity:* * 20–40%, * male dominant, • *LD:* * rare, * male dominant
neoplastic cell in HD	*RS cells:* * B or T cells, * essential for Dx of HD, * single cell with two or more nuclei or nuclear lobes, * large red nucleolus surrounded by clear halo ("owl-eye")
viral association with HD	*PCR detects EBV in 60–80%*
HD subtype with mediastinal involvement	*NS*
factors determining prognosis in HD	• **clinical stage,** • *type of HD:* * LP best, * LD worst
initial work-up of HD	• *complete history/physical exam,* • *chest radiograph,* • *CT:* * thorax, * abdomen, * pelvis, • *bipedal lymphangiography,* • *CBC with differential,* • *bilateral BM aspiration/Bx,* • *serum albumin,* • *serum calcium,* • *serum LDH,* • *liver function tests:* * bilirubin, * AST, * ALT, * ALP, * GGT
stage at initial presentation of HD	• *stage IIA:* * ≥ two lymph node regions on same side of diaphragm, * large case letter **A** indicates absence of fever >38°C, drenching night sweats, weight loss >10% of body weight within preceding 6 mths, * B indicates presence of above S/S

Table 8–9. LYMPH NODE DISORDERS Continued

Most Common...	Answer and Explanation
criteria for other stages of HD	• **stage I:** single lymph node region, • *stage III:* nodal involvement above and below diaphragm, • *stage IV:* disseminated disease involving liver or BM
Rx of HD	• *localized disease* (stage IA, IIA): radiation, • *intermediate disease* (stage IIB, IIIA): combination chemotherapy (♦ doxorubicin, ♦ bleomycin, ♦ vincristine, ♦ dacarbazine), • *disseminated disease* (stage IIIB, IV): intensive chemotherapy with high doses of ♦ doxorubicin, ♦ bleomycin, ♦ vincristine, ♦ dacarbazine
Rx complications in HD	• **second malignancies related to alkylating agents:** e.g., * acute nonlymphocytic leukemia, * B cell NHL, * MDS, • *solid tumors related to radiation:* cancers of * thyroid, * breast, * skin, * stomach, * head/neck, • *infertility*, • *hypothyroidism:* radiation effect, • sepsis: *Streptococcus pneumoniae* in splenectomized patients, • *congestive cardiomyopathy:* doxorubicin effect

Question: Which of the following lymph node enlargements **MOST LIKELY** represent a malignant lymph node disorder? **SELECT 4**

    (A) Submental lymph node enlargement in a smoker
    (B) Axillary lymph node enlargement in a cat lover
    (C) Left supraclavicular lymph node enlargement in a patient with weight loss
    (D) Para-aortic lymph enlargement in a 22-year-old man with a painless testicular mass
    (E) Generalized lymphadenopathy in an HIV-positive patient
    (F) Generalized lymphadenopathy in a patient with SLE
    (G) Axillary lymph node enlargement in a 55-year-old woman with a normal mammogram

Answers: (A), (C), (D), (G): A smoker with a submental lymph node **(choice A)** most likely has metastatic squamous cancer from the lateral border of the tongue. Cat-scratch disease is the most likely cause of axillary adenopathy in a cat-lover **(choice B is incorrect)**. Involvement of Virchow's node **(choice C)** is most likely in a patient with metastatic adenocarcinoma of the stomach. A testicular mass in a young man with para-aortic nodal involvement **(choice D)** is most likely metastatic seminoma. Generalized lymphadenopathy is a common benign finding in HIV-positive patients **(choice E is incorrect)**. Patients with SLE commonly have generalized lymphadenopathy **(choice F is incorrect)**. Axillary nodes in a woman over 50 years old is metastatic breast cancer regardless of the mammogram results **(choice G)**. It must be excised.

ALL = acute lymphoblastic leukemia, ALP = alkaline phosphatase, ALT = alanine aminotransferase, AST = aspartate aminotransferase, BM = bone marrow, Bx = biopsy, CBC = complete blood count, CD = cluster designation, CHOP = cyclophosphamide, doxorubicin, vincristine, prednisone, CLL = chronic lymphocytic lymphoma, CMV = cytomegalovirus, CNS = central nervous system, CT = computed tomography, CVP = cyclophosphamide, vincristine, prednisone, Dx = diagnosis, EBV = Epstein-Barr virus, GI = gastrointestinal, GGT = γ-glutamyltransferase, HD = Hodgkin's disease, HIV = human immunodeficiency virus, Ig = immunoglobulin, IL = interleukin, IM = infectious mononucleosis, LD = lymphocyte depleted, LDH = lactate dehydrogenase, LP = lymphocyte predominant, MC = most common, MDS = myelodysplastic syndrome, NHL = non-Hodgkin's lymphoma, NK = natural killer, NS = nodular sclerosis, PB = peripheral blood, PCR = polymerase chain reaction, RA = rheumatoid arthritis, RS = Reed-Sternberg cells, Rx = treatment, SLE = systemic lupus erythematosus, S/S = signs and symptoms, TB = tuberculosis, TMP/SMX = trimethoprim/sulfamethoxazole.

Table 8–10. PLASMA CELL DISORDERS AND AMYLOIDOSIS

Most Common...	Answer and Explanation
monoclonal gammopathy (MG)	*MGUS:* * 56%, * MC in patients >65 y old
clinical findings in MGUS	• M protein <3 g/dL, • BM plasma cell count <10%, • no anemia, osteolytic bone lesions, hypercalcemia, • ~24% develop MM/related disorder over next 20 y
location for MG on an SPE	*γ-globulin region:* * ~90%, * majority MGs are IgG (60%) followed by IgM and IgA
primary malignancy of bone	*MM:* * ~20% of MG, * median age ~60 y old, * women > men, * black > white
S/S of MM	• **bone pain:** * ~65%, * back/ribs, * BM infiltration/osteolytic lesions, • *pathologic fractures:* * osteolytic lesions in axial skeleton (♦ skull, ♦ spine, ♦ ribs, ♦ proximal long bones), * osteoporosis, • *renal failure:* * ~50%, * see Table 10–4, • *fatigue:* anemia, • *recurrent infections:* MC COD, particularly *Streptococcus pneumoniae,* • *spinal cord compression*
lab findings of MM	• **IgG M spike:** * IgA or light chain types less common, • *M protein ≥3 g/dL,* • *sheets of malignant plasma cells* (>10%) *in BM,* • *BJ proteinuria:* see Table 10–1, • *hypercalcemia:* 30%, • *high ESR,* • *prolonged bleeding time:* qualitative platelet defect, • *low anion gap:*

Table 8–10. PLASMA CELL DISORDERS AND AMYLOIDOSIS *Continued*

Most Common...	Answer and Explanation
Continued	IgG has positive charge and lowers AG (AG = unmeasured anions − unmeasured cations), • *pseudohyponatremia:* see Table 10–2, • *high β_2-microglobulins:* >2.7 µg/mL indicate poor prognosis, • *radionuclide bone scans:* not useful since lesions are lytic and have no osteoblastic response
Rx of MM	• **melphalan and prednisone:** * vincristine, doxorubicin, dexamethasone may be replacing the above Rx owing to less BM toxicity, • *EPO/α-interferon:* useful adjuncts, • *local radiation/bisphosphonates:* useful for palliation of bone pain, • *BM transplant:* some survival benefit
MG associated with hyperviscosity	*Waldenstrom's macroglobulinemia* (WMG): * IgM ≥3 g/dL, * median age 60 y, * male dominant
S/S of WMG	• **hyperviscosity syndrome:** * dizziness, * retinal hemorrhages, * blurry vision, * mucous membrane bleeding (qualitative platelet defect), * papilledema, * Raynaud's phenomenon, • *hepatosplenomegaly,* • *lymphadenopathy*
lab findings in WMG	• **anemia,** • *qualitative platelet defects,* • *BM with plasmacytoid lymphocytes,* • *increased serum viscosity,* • *IgM M spike on SPE,* • *BJ protein in 55%*
differences between MM and WMG	• *lytic bone lesions:* * present in MM, * absent in WMG, • *monoclonal spike:* * IgG, IgA, light chains in MM, * IgM in WMG, • *lymphadenopathy:* * absent in MM, * present in WMG, • *splenomegaly:* * absent in MM, * present in WMG, • *cell type:* * plasmablasts in MM, * lymphoplasmacytoid lymphocytes in WMG
Rx of WMG	• **plasmapheresis:** >80% of IgM in vascular compartment, • *chlorambucil plus prednisone,* • *prognosis:* 60% median 5 y survival
heavy chain diseases	• **α-heavy chain disease:** * small bowel lymphoma with malabsorption, * localized disease in upper respiratory tract less common, • *μ-heavy chain disease:* resembles CLL

Table continued on following page

Table 8–10. PLASMA CELL DISORDERS AND
AMYLOIDOSIS *Continued*

Most Common...	Answer and Explanation
characteristics of heavy chains in heavy chain disease	• *MG protein part of heavy chain without light chains,* • *BJ proteinuria uncommon*
locations for solitary plasmacytomas of bone	*vertebra, ribs, pelvis* [MM must be excluded before Dx confirmed. ~75% progress into MM. Rx is radiation.]
location for extramedullary plasmacytoma	*upper respiratory tract:* * 85%, * nasopharynx, larynx, sinuses [Exclude MM. Unlike solitary plasmacytoma of bone, most do not progress into MM. Potentially curable with radiation.]
types of amyloidosis and their protein derivation	• **systemic amyloidosis:** * *primary:* ♦ 90%, ♦ γ light chains, * *secondary:* ♦ chronic disease (e.g., RA), ♦ SAA protein, * *familial Mediterranean fever:* SAA protein, * *familial amyloidosis neuropathies:* prealbumin, * *hemodialysis-associated:* β₂-microglobulins, • *localized amyloidosis:* * *senile cardiac:* prealbumin, * *senile cerebral:* ♦ Alzheimer's disease, ♦ β₂: amyloid protein coded for on chromosome 21, ♦ Down syndrome relationship, * *medullary carcinoma of thyroid:* ♦ calcitonin, * *β-islet cells:* ♦ type II DM, ♦ islet amyloid peptide
staining/EM appearance of amyloid	• *staining:* * pink with routine H/E stain, * after Congo red staining → apple-green birefringence under polarized light, • *EM:* linear, nonbranching fibrils, • *amyloid:* * fibrillary protein deposited in interstitial tissue, * twisted β-pleated sheet (β-fibrilloses)
sites/clinical S/S of amyloid disease	• **kidneys:** * MC site for primary type, * nephrotic syndrome, • *heart:* * restrictive cardiomyopathy with heart failure, * low voltage ECG, * conduction defects, * ECHO abnormal in 60%, • *peripheral nerves:* * sensory neuropathy, * carpal tunnel syndrome (50%), * *autonomic dysfunction:* * orthostatic hypotension, * diarrhea, • *spleen:* splenomegaly, • *liver:* * high serum ALP, * hepatomegaly, • *tongue:* macroglossia, • *neurons:* Alzheimer's disease

Table 8–10. PLASMA CELL DISORDERS AND
AMYLOIDOSIS *Continued*

Most Common...	Answer and Explanation
method of diagnosing amyloidosis	• **SIEP/UIEP to document a MG:** most important screening test, since >90% have primary amyloidosis, • *fat aspiration of abdominal wall:* 80% sensitivity, • *rectal Bx:* 75% sensitivity, • *BM Bx:* ~55% sensitivity
Rx of amyloidosis	• *colchicine for familial Mediterranean fever,* • *melphalan plus prednisone:* ~20% response for systemic disease, • *survival:* 2 y survival for systemic disease

Question: In which of the following disorders would you expect an abnormality on an SPE? **SELECT 3**
  (A) Primary amyloidosis
  (B) Secondary amyloidosis
  (C) Medullary carcinoma of thyroid
  (D) CLL
  (E) Eosinophilic granuloma
  (F) Waldenstrom's macroglobulinemia

Answers: (A), (D), (F): Primary amyloidosis **(choice A)** is the most common cause of amyloidosis in the United States and is associated with MGs. Secondary amyloidosis is associated with chronic inflammatory states and not MGs **(choice B is incorrect).** Medullary thyroid cancer is a localized type of amyloidosis and is not associated with an MG **(choice C is incorrect).** CLL **(choice D)** is commonly associated with hypergammaglobulinemia and may have an IgM MG. Eosinophilic granuloma is a benign histiocytosis involving bone **(choice E is incorrect).** WMG **(choice F)** is an IgM MG.

AG = anion gap, ALP = alkaline phosphatase, BJ = Bence-Jones protein, BM = bone marrow, Bx = biopsy, CLL = chronic lymphocytic lymphoma, COD = cause of death, DM = diabetes mellitus, Dx = diagnosis, ECG = electrocardiogram, ECHO = echocardiogram, EM = electron microscope, EPO = erythropoietin, ESR = erythrocyte sedimentation rate, H/E = hematoxylin/eosin, Ig = immunoglobulin, M = monoclonal, MC = most common, MG = monoclonal gammopathy, MGUS = monoclonal gammopathy of undetermined significance, MM = multiple myeloma, RA = rheumatoid arthritis, Rx = treatment, SAA = serum associated amyloid, SIEP = serum immunoelectrophoresis, SPE = serum protein electrophoresis, S/S = signs and symptoms, UIEP = urine immunoelectrophoresis, WMG = Waldenstrom's macroglobulinemia.

Table 8–11. GENERAL CONCEPTS OF HEMOSTASIS

Most Common...	Answer and Explanation
components of hemostasis system	• *blood vessels,* • *platelets,* • *coagulation system,* • *fibrinolytic system*
endothelial cell–derived anticoagulants	• *tissue plasminogen activator:* * tPA, * activates plasminogen to produce plasmin, • *heparin-like products:* enhance ATIII activity, • *prostacyclin:* * PGI_2, * prevents platelet aggregation/vasodilator, * endothelial cell prostacyclin synthetase converts PGH_2 into PGI_2
liver-derived anticoagulants	• *antithrombin III:* inhibits serine proteases (e.g., ♦ thrombin, ♦ factor X), • *proteins C and S:* * enhance fibrinolytic activity, * inactivate factors V/VIII
endothelial cell–derived procoagulants (enhance vessel thrombosis)	• *VII:Ag:* antigenic determinant of VIII:C, • *VIII:VWF:* initial adhesion agent for platelets in endothelial injury, • *VIII:RCo:* activity necessary for platelet aggregation due to ristocetin, • *tissue thromboplastin:* activates factor VII in extrinsic coagulation system
platelet-derived procoagulants	• *thromboxane A_2 (TXA$_2$):* * platelet aggregator, * vasoconstrictor, * bronchoconstrictor, * thromboxane synthetase converts PGH_2 into TXA_2, • *VIII:VWF:* * synthesized by megakaryocytes, * stored in α-granules within platelets, * circulates as multimers, • *ADP:* platelet aggregator located in platelet dense bodies
liver-derived procoagulants	*all coagulation factors except VIII:VWF and VIIIC:Ag*
site of platelet production	*BM:* * cytoplasmic fragmentation of megakaryocytes ($\sim$1000–3000 platelets per meg), * live $\sim$10 d, * $\sim$one-third stored in spleen
platelet enzyme blocked by aspirin and NSAIDs	*platelet cyclooxygenase:* * converts arachidonic acid $\rightarrow PGG_2 \rightarrow PGH_2$ + thromboxane synthetase $\rightarrow TXA_2$, • *endothelial cell cyclooxygenase less affected by these drugs*
binding agent for vitamin K–dependent factors (factors II prothrombin), VII, IX, X, protein C/S	*calcium:* * binds vitamin K–dependent factors to platelet factor 3 (PF_3), the phospholipid substrate upon which coagulation occurs, * factors γ-carboxylated by vitamin K can bind to calcium and PF_3

Table 8–11. GENERAL CONCEPTS OF HEMOSTASIS
Continued

Most Common...	Answer and Explanation
sequence of reactions in extrinsic coagulation system down to final common pathway	• *factor VII:* activated by tissue thromboplastin → • *activates factor X in final common pathway:* * see below, * VIIa also activates factor IX in intrinsic pathway
sequence of reactions in intrinsic coagulation system down to final common pathway	• *factor XII:* * Hageman's factor, * activated by exposed subendothelial collagen and kallikrein, * kininogen cascade system between factor XII and XI (activated by XIIa) →• *factor XI →* • *factor IX →* • *IXa, VIII:C, PF_3 Ca^{++}:* four-component system → • *activates factor X in final common pathway*
sequence of reactions in final common pathway	• *VIIa* (extrinsic system) or *IXa, VIII, PF_3, Ca^{++}* (intrinsic system) *activate factor X →* • *Xa, factor V, PF_3, Ca^{++}* complex) *activates factor II* (prothrombin) *to produce thrombin →* • *thrombin activates factor I:* fibrinogen → • *thrombin cleaves fibrinogen into a fibrin monomer + fibrinopeptides A and B →* • *fibrin monomers form fibrin aggregates →* • *fibrin aggregates form soluble fibrin:* urea soluble → • *soluble fibrin converted into insoluble fibrin* (urea insoluble clot) *by factor XIII, which produces strong covalent cross-links necessary to form stable clot*
site for synthesis of the vitamin K–dependent factors	*liver:* * produces nonfunctional precursors, * functional (able to bind with calcium) when vitamin K_1 γ-carboxylates their terminal glutamic acid residues
coagulation factors consumed in forming a fibrin clot	• *factors I:* fibrinogen, • *II:* prothrombin, • *V,* • *VIII* [Above factors absent in serum and present in plasma.]
activators of plasminogen in fibrinolytic pathway	• *tPA,* • *XII,* • *streptokinase,* • *urokinase* [tPA, streptokinase, urokinase are clinically used to activate fibrinolytic system to dissolve clots.]
vessel response in small vessel injury	*vasoconstriction:* reduces blood flow to facilitate platelet adhesion
platelet response in small vessel injury	*see Table 8–2 under bleeding time*

Table continued on following page

Table 8–11. GENERAL CONCEPTS OF HEMOSTASIS
Continued

Most Common...	Answer and Explanation
coagulation system response in small vessel injury	• *release of tissue thromboplastin:* activates extrinsic pathway, • *activation of factor XII in intrinsic system* [Both systems produce thrombin. Thrombin converts platelet-associated fibrinogen into fibrin with formation of a stable platelet plug.]
fibrinolytic system response in small vessel injury	*plasminogen activated by tPA and activated factor XII:* * plasmin released, * dissolves stable platelet plug by breaking up fibrin strands
tests evaluating hemostasis	*see Table 8–2*

Question: Which of the following disorders prolong the BT? **SELECT 4**
- (A) Hemophilia A
- (B) Factor XIII deficiency
- (C) DIC
- (D) Thrombocytopenia
- (E) Aspirin
- (F) Heparin
- (G) Warfarin
- (H) Multiple myeloma

Answers: (C), (D), (E), (H): The BT is a test of vessel and platelet function and is not affected by coagulation disorders **(choices A and B are incorrect)** or drugs that inhibit coagulation, like heparin and warfarin **(choices F and G are incorrect).** DIC **(choice C**, produces thrombocytopenia, FDPs inhibit platelet aggregation), platelet counts <90,000 cells/μL **(choice D**, not enough platelets to adhere), aspirin **(choice E**, inhibits platelet aggregation), and multiple myeloma **(choice H**, increased γ-globulins interfere with platelet aggregation) all affect the mechanics of the BT.

ADP = adenosine diphosphate, ATIII = antithrombin III, BM = bone marrow, BT = bleeding time, DIC = disseminated intravascular coagulation, FDPs = fibrin(ogen) degradation products, NSAIDs = nonsteroidal anti-inflammatory drugs, PF$_3$ = platelet factor 3, PG = prostaglandin, PGI$_2$ = prostacyclin, tPA = tissue plasminogen activator, TXA$_2$ = thromboxane A$_2$, VIII:Ag = antigenic determinant of VIII:C, VIII:C = VIII coagulant, VIII:VWF = von Willebrand factor, VIII:RCo = von Willebrand factor activity with ristocetin.

Table 8–12. SELECTED VASCULAR AND PLATELET DISORDERS

Most Common...	Answer and Explanation
S/S associated with vessel/platelet disorders	• **epistaxis:** nosebleeds, • *petechiae:* 13 mm, red, nonblanching, nonpalpable hemorrhages on skin/mucous membranes, • *ecchymoses:* purpuric lesions about size of quarter, • *easy/spontaneous bruising,* • *bleeding from superficial scratches:* no primary hemostatic plug, • *spontaneous mucous membrane bleeding*
genetic vascular disorders	• *hereditary hemorrhagic telangiectasia:* see Table 5–3, • *Marfan syndrome:* AD defect in fibrillin, • *Ehlers-Danlos syndrome:* defect in collagen
age-dependent vessel disease in elderly	*senile purpura:* due to atrophy of perivascular support leading to purpura (ecchymoses) on extensor surfaces of hands/forearms
nutritional vascular disease	*scurvy:* see Table 9–11
metabolic vascular disease	*excess glucocorticoids:* e.g., patient on * steroids, * Cushing's syndrome, * steroids interfere with collagen synthesis
infectious vascular diseases	• **viral infections:** e.g., * rubella, * rubeola, • *RMSF:* rickettsial vasculitis, • *scarlet fever:* erythrogenic toxin
causes of giant platelets in the PB	• **recovery phase of thrombocytopenia,** • *MPDs:* e.g., * PRV, * CML, • *Bernard-Soulier syndrome:* see below, • *May-Hegglin anomaly:* * AD disease, * thrombocytopenia, * giant platelets, * Döhle bodies
cause of small platelets in PB	• **aspirin,** • *Wiskott-Aldrich syndrome:* * SXR disease, * thrombocytopenia, * chronic eczema, * B/T deficiencies, * increased IgE
causes of falsely low platelet count	• **satellitosis of platelets around WBCs,** • *EDTA-induced platelet clumping in a purple top tube:* antibody-mediated phenomenon
causes of thrombocytopenia	• **increased destruction:** e.g. * **immune,** * DIC, * TTP, * HUS, • *decreased production:* e.g., * BM suppression, * marrow infiltration, • *abnormal sequestration:* splenomegaly

Table continued on following page

Table 8–12. SELECTED VASCULAR AND PLATELET DISORDERS *Continued*

Most Common...	Answer and Explanation
cause of thrombocytopenia in children	*idiopathic thrombocytopenic purpura* (ITP): * IgG antibodies develop against platelet GPIIb/IIIa receptor, * type II HSR, * recovery the rule, * corticosteroids used if symptomatic
clinical findings of ITP	• *S/S:* * epistaxis, * petechiae/ecchymoses, * mucous membrane bleeding, * no splenomegaly (significant negative finding), * follows an URI (85%), • *lab:* * platelets <50,000 cells/μL, * normal WBC count, * normal Hb/Hct, * megakaryocytes present in BM
Rx of ITP	• ≥*50,000 cells/μL:* observe, • *<30,000 cells/μL:* corticosteroids, • *30,000–50,000 cells/μL:* Rx if symptomatic [Steroids decrease antibody production and reduce macrophage clearance of platelets.]
cause of thrombocytopenia in adults	*immune thrombocytopenia:* * IgG antibodies against platelets with extravascular removal by macrophages, * type II HSR
clinical findings in adult immune thrombocytopenia	• *S/S:* * insidious, * often becomes chronic, * less responsive to Rx than in children, * splenomegaly, * SLE is common cause, • *lab:* BM exam required in adults >60 y old to R/O underproduction of platelets
Rx of immune thrombocytopenia in adults	• **initially corticosteroids:** * 70% response, * if no response → • *splenectomy:* 75% response, * definitive Rx, * if no response → • *danazol:* * blocks macrophage Fc receptors sites, * if no response → • *immunosuppressive agents:* vincristine, vinblastine, azathioprine, cyclophosphamide, cyclosporine, * if life-threatening → • *IV γ-globulin plus platelet transfusions:* IV γ-globulin blocks IgG Fc receptor sites on macrophages
causes of thrombocytopenia in pregnancy	• **incidental thrombocytopenia:** * 75%, * self-limited, * not necessary to Rx, • *immune,* • *pre-eclampsia:* 50% have low platelets, • *HELLP syndrome:* see Table 8–6, • *HIV,* • *drugs:* heparin, • *folate deficiency*
Rx of immune thrombocytopenia in pregnancy	• *IV γ-globulin,* • *corticosteroids:* possibility of developing * GDM, * HTN

Table 8–12. SELECTED VASCULAR AND PLATELET
DISORDERS *Continued*

Most Common...	Answer and Explanation
mechanisms for drug-induced thrombocytopenia	• **drug + carrier protein in plasma elicits synthesis of IgG antibody, which forms IC that adheres to platelet leading to its destruction:** type III HSR, • *drug attaches to GPIb or GIIb/IIIa and IgG antibody develops against complex leading to hemolysis:* type III localized HSR, • *common drugs:* * heparin, * quinidine, * quinine, * gold salts, * sulfonamides, * thiazides, • *Rx:* * drug withdrawal, * reverses disease in 4–14 d except for gold salts, which may take longer
drug associated with immune thrombocytopenia in hospitalized patient	*heparin:* * type I variant: ♦ occurs early, ♦ transient, ♦ not immune-mediated, * type II variant: ♦ immune-mediated (heparin-specific antibody against platelet heparin complex on platelet) leading to non-dose-related platelet destruction (median time 10 d post Rx), ♦ platelet release reaction of thrombogenic agents may produce venous (more common) or arterial thromboses
virus-associated immune thrombocytopenias	• **HIV:** * MC coagulation abnormality in AIDS, * 30–45% of patients, • *CMV,* • *EBV*
cause of TTP	*unknown circulating platelet-agglutinating factor:* * occlusive platelet thrombi develop in terminal arterioles/capillaries, * relationship with pregnancy/birth control pills, * VIII:VWF involved in platelet thrombus development
S/S of TTP	*pentad of* • *fever,* • *thrombocytopenia:* * ~95%, * petechia/purpura, * CNS/retinal bleeding, * GI bleeding, * hematuria, • *microangiopathic hemolytic anemia with schistocytes:* fragmented RBCs must be present for Dx, • *neurologic abnormalities,* • *renal failure:* 20%
lab findings in TTP	• *normocytic anemia with retics >3%,* • *low serum haptoglobin,* • *thrombocytopenia,* • *prolonged BT,* • *normal PT/PTT:* * not DIC, * no intravascular consumption of clotting factors, • *BM Bx:* platelet thrombi present, • *high serum creatinine:* <20%

Table continued on following page

Table 8–12. SELECTED VASCULAR AND PLATELET
DISORDERS *Continued*

Most Common...	Answer and Explanation
Rx of TTP	• **plasmapheresis/replacement with FFP,** • *aspirin,* • *dipyridamole,* • *prednisone,* • prognosis: * multiorgan failure, * >90% mortality if left untreated, * 70–80% survival with Rx
causes of adult HUS	• *complication of pregnancy,* • *estrogen use,* • *malignant HTN,* • *toxin-induced endothelial damage by E. coli serotype O157:H7:* eating undercooked hamburger meat, • *drugs:* e.g., * mitomycin, * cyclosporine, * cisplatin
S/S of adult HUS	*similar to TTP* (see above) *except pathologic changes target kidneys:* * renal disease worse in HUS than in TTP, * thrombocytopenia milder than TTP, * neurologic disease absent
lab findings in HUS	*similar to TTP* (see above) *except serum creatinine more likely to be >3 mg/dL*
Rx of adult HUS	*similar to TTP:* left untreated, mortality is high and 80% develop CRF
mechanism of post-transfusion purpura	*PL^A1 negative patient with previous exposure to PL^A1 positive platelets develops IgG antibodies and on re-exposure to PL^A1 positive platelets develops severe thrombocytopenia ~5–7 d after transfusion:* * donor and patient platelets destroyed, * mortality 10–15%
cause of sequestration of platelets leading to thrombocytopenia	*congestive splenomegaly:* * MC in PH due to cirrhosis, * splenic destruction of cells is called hypersplenism
cause of primary thrombocytosis	*myeloproliferative disease:* * e.g., ♦ PRV, ♦ ET, * thrombosis/bleeding
causes of secondary thrombocytosis	• **malignancy:** * 35%, * IL-6 stimulation of platelet production, * hypercoagulability in paraneoplastic syndrome, • *infection:* e.g., TB, • *rebound after thrombocytopenia,* • *chronic iron deficiency,* • *splenectomy*
acquired cause of qualitative platelet defect with normal platelet count and prolonged BT	*patient taking aspirin/NSAIDs:* * irreversible effect of aspirin on platelet cyclooxygenase, * reversible with NSAIDs after 48 h

Table 8–12. SELECTED VASCULAR AND PLATELET
DISORDERS *Continued*

Most Common...	Answer and Explanation
genetic cause of a qualitative platelet defect	*VWD:* classical type is associated with absence of VIII:VWF (see below)
platelet abnormality in uremia	*platelet dysfunction secondary to guanidino-succinic acid inhibiting platelet PF₃ and interfering with platelet adhesion and aggregation:* reversed with * dialysis, * desmopressin (ADH), * combined estrogen/progestin pills
defects in Glanzmann's thrombasthenia	• *AR disease,* • *deficiency of platelet GPIIb/IIIa fibrinogen receptor,* • *absence of thrombosthenin:* contractile protein
S/S of Glanzmann's thrombasthenia	• *early onset of petechiae/ecchymoses,* • *epistaxis,* • *poor wound healing*
lab findings in Glanzmann's thrombasthenia	• *normal platelet count,* • *prolonged BT,* • *no first phase aggregation of platelets with addition of aggregating agents like ADP:* no GPIIb/IIIa receptors to aggregate platelets, • *poor clot retraction:* no thrombosthenin, • *normal ristocetin cofactor assay:* no problems with VIII:VWF or its receptor
defects in Bernard-Soulier syndrome	• *AR disease,* • *absence of GPIb:* receptor for VWF and ristocetin-induced VIII:VWF-dependent platelet aggregation, • *thrombocytopenia,* • *giant platelets*
S/S of Bernard-Soulier syndrome	• *menorrhagia,* • *bleeding problems with surgery*
lab findings in Bernard-Soulier syndrome	• *prolonged BT,* • *thrombocytopenia,* • *giant platelets,* • *normal first phase aggregation with ADP,* • *abnormal second phase of aggregation:* platelet's own ability to aggregate is abnormal because of missing receptor, • *abnormal ristocetin cofactor assay,* • *normal clot retraction*
genetic platelet storage pool diseases	• *Hermansky-Pudlak syndrome:* lack of ADP in dense bodies of platelets, • *gray platelet syndrome:* absence of α-granules in platelets

Table continued on following page

Table 8–12. SELECTED VASCULAR AND PLATELET DISORDERS *Continued*

Question: Immune mechanisms are involved in the pathogenesis of which of the following causes of thrombocytopenia? **SELECT 4**
- (A) Hypersplenism
- (B) HIV
- (C) Adult HUS
- (D) DIC
- (E) Heparin
- (F) Idiopathic thrombocytopenic purpura
- (G) Post-transfusion thrombocytopenia
- (H) TTP

Answers: (B), (E), (F), (G): Hypersplenism is most often secondary to congestive splenomegaly in patients with portal hypertension from cirrhosis (choice A is incorrect). Thrombocytopenia associated with HIV (choice B), heparin (choice E), ITP (choice F), and post-transfusion (choice G) are all immune-mediated. Adult HUS and TTP are due to platelet thrombi developing in small vessels with consumption of the platelets (choices C and H are incorrect). DIC consumes platelets in the formation of fibrin clots (choice D is incorrect).

AD = autosomal dominant, ADH = antidiuretic hormone, ADP = adenosine diphosphate, AIDS = acquired immunodeficiency syndrome, AR = autosomal recessive, BM = bone marrow, BT = bleeding time, Bx = biopsy, CRF = chronic renal failure, CML = chronic myelogenous leukemia, CMV = cytomegalovirus, CNS = central nervous system, DIC = disseminated intravascular coagulation, Dx = diagnosis, EBV = Epstein-Barr virus, EDTA = ethylenediaminetetraacetic acid, ET = essential thrombocytopenia, FFP = fresh frozen plasma, GDM = gestational diabetes mellitus, GI = gastrointestinal, GP = glycoprotein, Hb = hemoglobin, Hct = hematocrit, HELLP = *h*emolysis, *e*levated transaminases, *l*ow *p*latelets, HIV = human immunodeficiency virus, HSR = hypersensitivity reaction, HTN = hypertension, HUS = hemolytic uremic syndrome, IC = immunocomplex, Ig = immunoglobulin, IL = interleukin, ITP = idiopathic thrombocytopenic purpura, IV = intravenous, MC = most common, NSAIDs = nonsteroidal antiinflammatory drugs, PB = peripheral blood, PF$_3$ = platelet factor 3, PH = portal hypertension, PRV = polycythemia rubra vera, PT = prothrombin time, PTT = activated partial thromboplastin time, RBC = red blood cell, RMSF = Rocky Mountain spotted fever, R/O = rule out, Rx = treatment, SLE = systemic lupus erythematosus, S/S = signs and symptoms, SXR = sex-linked recessive, TB = tuberculosis, TTP = thrombotic thrombocytopenic purpura, URI = upper respiratory infection, VIII:VWF = von Willebrand factor, VWD = von Willebrand disease, WBC = white blood cell.

Table 8–13. COAGULATION AND FIBRINOLYTIC DISORDERS

Most Common...	Answer and Explanation
signs of a coagulation disorder	• *delayed bleeding:* e.g., * after molar dental extraction, * primary hemostatic plug present but not a stable platelet plug, • *hemarthroses:* only severe hemophilia A/B, • *bleeding into spaces: only severe hemophilia A/B,* • *hematuria,* • *GI bleeds,* • *deep ecchymoses*
causes of coagulation deficiency	• **defective production:** e.g., hereditary, • **acquired:** e.g., * liver disease, * vitamin K deficiency, • *increased consumption:* e.g., DIC, • *increased destruction:* e.g., circulating anticoagulants (♦ antibodies, ♦ inhibitors), • *combinations of above*
SXR hereditary coagulation disorders	• **hemophilia A:** * SXR (85%), * spontaneous mutations in remainder, * deficiency of VIII:C, * asymptomatic female carrier transmits disease to 50% of her sons, • *hemophilia B:* * SXR, * factor IX deficiency
method of detecting asymptomatic female carriers of hemophilia A or B	• **DNA techniques:** identification of abnormal locus on X chromosome, • *ratio of VIII:C/ VIII:Ag <0.75,* * VIII:Ag normal in hemophilia A
factor determining severity of hemophilia A	*factor VIII:C concentration:* e.g., * severe if factor VIII:C <1% of normal (♦ spontaneous hemarthroses, ♦ subcutaneous hematomas, ♦ atrophied muscles, ♦ hematomas in GI/GU tract), * moderately severe if VIII:C 1–5%, * mild if VIII:C level 6–25%, * asymptomatic if VIII:C 25–50% (unless hemodynamically stressed by major surgery or trauma)
bleeding sites in severe hemophilia A	• **joints,** • *muscle,* • *GI tract* [Severe hemophiliacs bleed spontaneously and do not require trauma or a surgical insult to bleed. 50% of male newborns bleed at circumcision.]
lab findings in hemophilia A	• *prolonged PTT,* • *normal PT,* • *normal platelet count,* • *normal BT,* • *low factor VIII:C,* • *normal VIII:Ag,* • *normal VIII:VWF,* • *infusion of products containing factor VIII:C:* immediate, non-sustained increase in de novo synthesis of factor VIII:C not in excess of amount infused

Table continued on following page

Table 8–13. **COAGULATION AND FIBRINOLYTIC DISORDERS** *Continued*

Most Common...	Answer and Explanation
Rx of hemophilia A	• *mild hemophilia:* desmopressin acetate (increases synthesis of all factor VIII components), • *moderate/severe:* * trial of desmopressin initially for moderate hemophilia, * most require factor VIII infusion (produced by monoclonal antibodies or recombinant DNA techniques, no risk for HIV, HBV, HCV) [~75% of hemophilia A patients Rx with factor VIII concentrates (pooled VIII:C from multiple donors) before 1985 (before screening was available) became infected with HIV.]
Rx of factor VIII inhibitors secondary to therapy with factor VIII infusions	• **porcine factor VIII:** best initial step, • *bypass with activated factor IX complexes:* danger of venous thrombosis, • *larger infusions of factor VIII* [Titers of antibody are expressed in Bethesda units. 1 Bethesda unit/mL is an activity sufficient to lower the factor VIII level by 50% after a 2-h incubation in vitro. ~5–20% of hemophiliacs develop inhibitors.]
hereditary coagulation disorder	*classical VWD:* * AD disorder, * 70–80% of all cases of VWD
differences among VWD variants	• *inheritance patterns,* • *BT results,* • *platelet response to ristocetin,* • *multimeric patterns on agar gel electrophoresis,* • *concentration of different factor VIII components*
S/S of VWD	*signs of platelet and coagulation defects:* * epistaxis, * menorrhagia (main complaint in women), * ecchymoses, * bleeding from superficial scratches, * bleeding from tooth extractions, * GI bleeding, * easy bruiseability, * bleeding exacerbated by aspirin
GI association with VWD	*angiodysplasia:* see Table 9–5
lab findings in classical VWD	• **low VIII:RCo:** * best overall test, * no platelet aggregation with ristocetin, • *low VIII:Ag:* antigenic determinant of VIII:C, • *low VIII:VWF:* adhesion agent, • *low VIII:C:* intrinsic system factor, • *prolonged BT,* • *prolonged PTT,* • *normal PT,* • *infusion of products containing factor VIII:* slow but sustained increase in de novo synthesized factor VIII:C in excess of amount infused

Table 8–13. COAGULATION AND FIBRINOLYTIC DISORDERS *Continued*

Most Common...	Answer and Explanation
Rx for mild VWD	*minor bleeding problems:* * demopressin acetate, * oral contraceptives for women with menorrhagia (estrogen increases the synthesis of all factor VIII components), • *moderate bleeding problems:* intermediate purity factor VIII concentrate (Humate P) that are rich in high molecular weight multimers of VIII:VWF (most important for platelet adhesion), • *minor surgery:* desmopressin 1 h preoperatively and daily for 23 d postoperatively, • *major surgery:* * monitoring of VIII:C and VIII:RCo levels, * more frequent intervals of infusion of desmopressin, • *cryoprecipitate:* previous gold standard of Rx of VWD, * blood product limits its usefulness (potential for HIV, HBV, HCV)
clinical features of factor XII deficiency	• *AR disease,* • *increased predisposition to venous/arterial thromboses:* factor XII normally activates plasminogen, • *no evidence of bleeding,* • *markedly prolonged PTT:* >150 sec
clinical features of factor XI deficiency (hemophilia C)	• *AR disease,* • *increased incidence in Ashkenazi Jews,* • *mildest coagulation bleeding disorder,* • *prolonged PTT,* • *normal PT*
clinical features of factor IX deficiency (hemophilia B, Christmas disease)	• *SXR disease,* • *similar in S/S as hemophilia A,* • *risk for venous thrombosis when infused with purified factor IX complex:* * presence of activated factors VII and X, * also contains factors IX and II, • *prolonged PTT,* • *normal PT*
clinical features of factor VII deficiency	• *AR disease,* • *S/S similar to platelet abnormality:* * epistaxis, * gingival bleeding, * bleeding after trauma, • *menorrhagia,* • *hemarthroses,* • *paradoxical increase in venous thrombosis,* • *prolonged PT,* • *normal PTT,* • *normal Russell viper venom test:* * see Table 8–2, * Stypven time
clinical features of factor X deficiency	• *AR disease,* • *acquired deficiency associated with amyloidosis:* binds the factor, • *bleeding similar to factor VII deficiency,* • *prolonged PTT and PT,* • *abnormal Russell viper venom test* (Stypven time)

Table continued on following page

Table 8–13. COAGULATION AND FIBRINOLYTIC DISORDERS *Continued*

Most Common...	Answer and Explanation
clinical features of factor V deficiency	• *AR disease,* • *acquired deficiency in some MPDs,* • *acquired inhibitors with drugs:* * aminoglycosides, * streptomycin, • *prolonged PTT/PT*
clinical features of prothrombin deficiency	• *AR disease,* • *associated with LA,* • *prolonged PTT/PT*
clinical features of fibrinogen deficiency	• *AR disease,* • *umbilical cord bleeding,* • *poor wound healing,* • *low fibrinogen:* functional and immunologic assays, • *prolonged reptilase time:* see Table 8–2, • *prolonged TT:* see Table 8–2, • *prolonged BT*
clinical features of dysfibrinogenemia	• *MCC is liver disease,* • *predisposes to bleeding problems/thrombosis,* • *prolonged functional fibrinogen assay but normal immunologic,* • *prolonged reptilase time,* • *normal BT,* • *prolonged TT*
clinical features of factor XIII deficiency	• *AR disease,* • *poor wound healing,* • *umbilical cord bleeding,* • *prolonged hemorrhage from cuts,* • *normal PTT/PT,* • *abnormal 5-molar urea clot solubility test:* see Table 8–2
circulating anticoagulant	*antibodies against factor VIII*
clinical findings in factor VIII anticoagulant	• *causes:* * **Rx of hemophilia A,** * postpartum, * chlorpromazine, • *lab:* prolonged PTT does not correct with addition of normal plasma (see Table 8–2)
circulating anticoagulant against platelet PF$_3$	*lupus anticoagulant* (LA): * prolongs PTT (90%), * less commonly prolongs PT (20%), * addition of phospholipid to test system corrects PTT, * antibodies may be IgG, IgM, or, less commonly, IgA
circulating anticoagulant producing false positive RPR/VDRL	*anticardiolipin antibody* (ACA): * test substrate in RPR/VDRL is beef cardiolipin, * anticardiolipin antibodies react against substrate causing FP test
syndrome associated with LA and/or ACA	*antiphospholipid* (APL) *syndrome:* * both antibodies present in 60%, * one of two antibodies in 40%

Table 8–13. COAGULATION AND FIBRINOLYTIC
DISORDERS *Continued*

Most Common...	Answer and Explanation
mechanism of thrombosis in LA/ACA	*antibodies react against phospholipids in endothelial cells resulting in damage and thrombosis*
coagulation abnormalities associated with APLs	• **venous thrombosis:** * placental bed, * hepatic vein (Budd-Chiari syndrome), * DVTs, cutaneous (skin necrosis), * renal vein, • *arterial thrombosis:* * CNS, * coronary arteries, * renal artery, • *recurrent spontaneous abortions:* thrombosis of placental bed, • *premature delivery,* • *livedo reticularis,* • *multiinfarct dementia*
Rx/prevention of thrombosis in APL syndrome	• **heparin followed by warfarin:** INR >3, • *prednisone:* rapidly eliminates LA, • *pregnancy:* low doses of aspirin and heparin
fat-soluble vitamin deficiency resulting in a coagulation disorder	*vitamin K deficiency:* see Table 9–11
adult causes of vitamin K deficiency	*see Table 9–1:* common scenario for vitamin K deficiency is postoperative patient who is not eating properly and is on antibiotics
mechanism of DIC	*thrombohemorrhagic disorder:* intravascular clotting leads to consumption of clotting factors with secondary fibrinolysis
causes of DIC	• **malignancy:** * leukemia (particularly acute progranulocytic), * prostate cancer, * lung cancer, • *septicemia:* particularly gram-negatives, • *surgery/trauma,* • *obstetric problems:* e.g., amniotic fluid embolism, retained dead fetus, • *hemolytic transfusion reaction,* • *snake envenomation*
factors consumed in DIC	• *fibrinogen,* • *II,* • *V,* • *VIII,* • *platelets,* • *ATIII:* used up in neutralizing serine proteases
S/S of acute DIC	• **oozing of blood from wounds and venipuncture sites,** • *hypovolemic shock:* * activation of complement system by plasmin with release of anaphylatoxins, * blood loss, • *widespread ecchymoses:* * platelet dysfunction from FDPs, * thrombocytopenia, • *wide-*

Table continued on following page

Table 8–13. COAGULATION AND FIBRINOLYTIC DISORDERS *Continued*

Most Common...	Answer and Explanation
Continued	spread organ dysfunction: e.g., * renal failure, * intracranial hemorrhage, • *chronic DIC:* more likely to present with thrombosis than with bleeding
lab findings in DIC	• *screening tests commonly available:* * platelet count: ♦ thrombocytopenia, ♦ sensitivity 90%, * PT: ♦ prolonged, ♦ sensitivity 90%, * fibrinogen: ♦ low, ♦ sensitivity 70% (particularly if serial assays obtained and progressive drop in concentration is noted), • *confirmatory tests commonly available:* * D-dimers: ♦ best all-around test, dimers present, ♦ see Table 8–2, * FDPs (see Table 8–2), • *other lab findings:* * normocytic anemia, * prolonged PTT, * schistocytes, • *sensitive tests not commonly available:* * AT III: ♦ low, * fibrinopeptide A: ♦ increased, ♦ cleavage product of fibrinogen, * PF_4: ♦ increased, ♦ indicates platelet activation
Rx of DIC	• **Rx underlying cause of DIC,** • *packed RBCs,* • *FFP,* • *platelet concentrates,* • *cryoprecipitate:* contains fibrinogen and factor VIII, • *full dose and subcutaneous heparin:* prevent clot formation (cause of factor consumption)
mechanisms of coagulation deficiency in liver disease	• **multiple factor deficiencies:** * decreased production, * malabsorption vitamin K due to bile salt deficiency, * factor VII first to decrease in liver disease, • *increased fibrinolysis:* less clearing of plasminogen activator (decreased production of α_2-antiplasmin), • *dysfibrinogenemia:* see above, • *platelet dysfunction:* * FDPs increased (less clearing by macrophages), * FDPs interfere with platelet aggregation, • *thrombocytopenia:* decreased production in BM
causes of multiple factor deficiencies	• **severe liver disease,** • *DIC,* • *vitamin K deficiency,* • *anticoagulation with heparin/warfarin*
cause of secondary fibrinolysis	*DIC:* activation of factor XII leads to concomitant activation of plasminogen → plasmin release

Table 8–13. COAGULATION AND FIBRINOLYTIC
DISORDERS *Continued*

Most Common...	Answer and Explanation
causes of primary fibrinolysis	• **radical prostatectomy:** urokinase release, • *metastatic prostate cancer,* • *open heart surgery* [Serious bleeding is likely to occur once α_2-plasmin inhibitor is used up in neutralizing excess plasmin.]
lab findings in primary fibrinolysis	• *increased FDPs,* • *absent D-dimers,* • *low fibrinogen,* • *prolonged PTT/PT:* * coagulation factors degraded by plasmin, * FDPs interfere with clotting, • *normal platelet count*
lab findings that differentiate primary from secondary fibrinolysis	• **D-dimer assay:** * absent in primary, * increased in secondary, • *platelet count:* * normal in primary, * low in secondary
Rx of primary fibrinolysis	ε-*aminocaproic acid:* * binds to plasminogen and plasmin, * prevents plasmin from degrading fibrinogen/other clotting factors
mechanism of heparin as an anticoagulant	*enhances ATIII activity:* * ATIII 1000 times faster, * heparin binds ATIII and forms a complex and is then reused, * ATIII primarily inactivates thrombin, Xa, and IXa (not VIIa even though it is a serine protease), * ATIII-serine protease complex cleared by macrophages (lowers ATIII levels), * in thrombosis, ATIII levels are significantly reduced (reduces effectiveness of heparin), * ATIII synthesized in liver
mechanism of clearance of heparin	*macrophage uptake in liver with subsequent degradation into inactive products which are excreted in urine:* * heparin half-life is ~90 min, * liver/renal disease alter its metabolism, * it does not cross the placenta (useful in pregnancy)
complications of heparin Rx	• **bleeding:** 5–10%, • *hypersensitivity reactions:* * chills, * fever, * urticaria, * shock, • *thrombocytopenia:* see Table 8–12, • *osteoporosis,* • *paradoxical venous/arterial thrombosis:* * release of PF_4 (heparin neutralizing agent) and serotonin from platelets, * causes platelet aggregation and potential for a thrombosis of aorta, iliac artery, skin necrosis

Table continued on following page

Table 8–13. COAGULATION AND FIBRINOLYTIC DISORDERS *Continued*

Most Common...	Answer and Explanation
cause of heparin resistance	• **low ATIII levels:** acquired or hereditary, • *high levels of factor VIII,* • *high levels of heparin-binding proteins:* e.g., PF$_4$
Rx of significant bleeding due to heparin	*protamine sulfate*
clinical uses of heparin	• **anticoagulation in DVT,** • *pulmonary embolus,* • *post-thrombolytic Rx,* • *prevent mural thrombosis in AMI,* • *Rx of DIC,* • *venous thrombi and pulmonary emboli in pregnancy,* • *prevention of DVTs prior to orthopedic procedures*
method of monitoring heparin therapy	*PTT:* should be maintained between 1.5 and 2.5 times normal
mechanism of low molecular weight (fractionated) heparin	*primarily inactivates factor Xa:* * longer half-life than unfragmented heparin, * more predictable acting, * does not require lab monitoring (does not prolong PTT or TT), * less risk for heparin-induced thrombocytopenia
mechanism of warfarin as an anticoagulant	*inhibits epoxide reductase:* see above
complications of warfarin therapy	• **bleeding:** * 10–20%, * INR >5 at increased risk, • *drug interactions:* see below, • *hemorrhagic skin necrosis:* see Table 8–14, • *urticaria,* • *alopecia,* • *teratogenic:* * nasal hypoplasia, * CNS abnormalities, * contraindicated in first trimester
conditions potentiating warfarin activity (need less warfarin, prolongs the PT)	• *drugs leading to vitamin K deficiency:* broad-spectrum antibiotics, • *drugs displacing plasma-bound warfarin:* * phenylbutazone, * clofibrate, • *competitive inhibition for hepatic degradation:* * phenytoin, * tolbutamide, • *enhanced affinity for hepatic receptor sites:* * high-dose salicylates, * quinidine, • *drugs inhibiting platelet function:* aspirin, • *liver disease,* • *CHF,* • vitamin E toxicity

Table 8–13. COAGULATION AND FIBRINOLYTIC
DISORDERS *Continued*

Most Common...	Answer and Explanation
conditions antagonizing warfarin activity (need more warfarin, lowers PT)	• *drugs inducing hepatic cytochrome system:* e.g., * alcohol, * barbiturates, * rifampin, * griseofulvin, • *diuretics:* thiazides, • *decrease GI absorption:* cholestyramine, • *oral contraceptives,* • *administration of vitamin K*
clinical uses of warfarin	• **Rx and prophylaxis for DVT and PE,** • *prevention of thrombi on mechanical valves,* • *prevention of thrombi in cardiac conditions:* * AMI, * ventricular aneurysm, * left atrial enlargement in MS, • *prevention/Rx of thrombi in hereditary thrombotic conditions:* * ATIII deficiency, * protein C/S deficiency
method of monitoring warfarin therapy	*INR:* * see Table 8–2, * INR usually kept at 2–3, * kept at higher value for mechanical valves (2.5–3.5)
reason heparin and warfarin anticoagulation are started simultaneously in Rx of venous thrombosis	*heparin immediately anticoagulates the patient, while warfarin requires 4–5 days for full anticoagulation owing to the different half-lives of vitamin K–dependent factors that have already been γ-carboxylated:* * protein C/factor VII have shortest half-lives (4–6 h), * factor II has longest half-life (72 h)
Rx of life-threatening hemorrhage in a patient on warfarin	*infusion fresh frozen plasma (FFP):* * contains functional coagulation factors, * oral or intramuscular vitamin K recommended for less serious bleeds
cause of normal platelet count, prolonged BT, normal PTT and PT	*aspirin or NSAIDs*
cause of low platelet count, prolonged BT, normal PTT and PT in child	*ITP*
cause of low platelet count, prolonged BT, normal PTT and PT in woman with schistocytes in PB	*TTP*

Table continued on following page

Table 8–13. COAGULATION AND FIBRINOLYTIC DISORDERS *Continued*

Most Common...	Answer and Explanation
cause of low platelet count, prolonged BT, normal PTT and PT in child with renal failure and schistocytes in PB	*HUS*
cause of normal platelet count, prolonged BT, prolonged PTT, normal PT	*classical VWD*
cause of normal platelet count, normal BT, normal PTT, prolonged PT	*factor VII deficiency*
cause of normal platelet count, normal BT, prolonged PTT, normal PT	*hemophilia A*
cause of normal platelet count, normal BT, prolonged PTT, normal PT not corrected by mixing studies	*circulating inhibitor against factor VIII*
coagulation lab findings in patients on warfarin or heparin	• *normal platelet count,* • *normal BT,* • *prolonged PTT:PT* [The PT has most of the vitamin K–dependent factors (II, VII, X, not IX) and provides a better monitor for warfarin therapy than PTT. The PTT has most of the serine proteases inhibited by ATIII (XII, XI, IX, X, II, thrombin) and provides a better monitor for monitoring heparin than does warfarin.]
coagulation lab findings in a patient with uncompensated acute DIC	• *low platelet count,* • *prolonged BT,* • *prolonged PTT,* • *prolonged PT* [This rarely occurs since coagulation factors are often 2–3 times normal (VIII, V, fibrinogen). Factors must be below 30–40% of normal before PT and PTT are prolonged.]

Table 8–13. COAGULATION AND FIBRINOLYTIC DISORDERS Continued

Question: Which of the following hemostasis disorders have a prolonged BT and a prolonged PTT and PT? **SELECT 3**
- (A) DIC
- (B) TTP
- (C) Classical VWD
- (D) Chronic liver disease
- (E) Hemophilia A
- (F) Afibrinogenemia
- (G) Vitamin K deficiency
- (H) Patient on heparin

Answers: (A), (D), (F): In DIC (choice A), there is thrombocytopenia (prolongs BT) and production of FDPs (prolong BT), and consumption of fibrinogen V, VIII, and II, hence both the PTT and PT are prolonged. TTP is associated with the consumption of platelets (prolongs the BT); however, there is no consumption of coagulation factors as in DIC (choice B is incorrect). Classic VWD produces a prolonged BT (low VWF), prolonged PTT (low VIII:C), but a normal PT (choice C is incorrect). Chronic liver disease (choice D) produces a prolonged BT (low fibrinogen, dysfibrinogenemia, increased FDPs prevent platelet aggregation) and multiple coagulation deficiencies, hence both the PT and PTT are prolonged. Hemophilia A only prolongs the PTT (low VIII:C, choice E is incorrect). Afibrinogenemia (choice F) prolongs the BT (no fibrinogen to hold the primary platelet plug together) and prolongs the PT and PTT, since the end-stage of the tests is the formation of a clot. Vitamin K deficiency results in a deficiency of factors II, VII, IX, and X, hence the BT is normal in the presence of a prolonged PT and PTT (choice G is incorrect). A patient on heparin with enhancement of ATIII activity leads to the neutralization of factors XII, XI, IX, X, II, and thrombin, hence the BT is normal, while the PT and PTT are both prolonged (choice H is incorrect).

ACA = anticardiolipin antibody, AD = autosomal dominant, AMI = acute myocardial infarction, APL = antiphospholipid, PTT = partial thromboplastin time, AR = autosomal recessive, ATIII = antithrombin III, BM = bone marrow, BT = bleeding time, CHF = congestive heart failure, CNS = central nervous system, DIC = disseminated intravascular coagulation, DVT = deep venous thrombosis, FDPs = fibrin(ogen) degradation products, FFP = fresh frozen plasma, FP = false-positive, GI = gastrointestinal, GU = genitourinary, HBV = hepatitis B, HCV = hepatitis C, HIV = human immunodeficiency virus, HUS = hemolytic uremic syndrome, Ig = immunoglobulin, INR = International Normalized Ratio, ITP = idiopathic thrombocytopenic purpura, LA = lupus anticoagulant, MCC = most common cause, MPD = myeloproliferative disease, MS = mitral stenosis, NSAIDs = nonsteroidal anti-inflammatory drugs, PB = peripheral blood, PE = pulmonary embolus, PF_4 = platelet factor 4, PT = prothrombin time, PTT = partial thromboplastin time, RBC = red blood cell, RPR = rapid plasma reagin, Rx = treatment, S/S = signs and symptoms, SXR = sex-linked recessive, TT = thrombin time, TTP = thrombotic thrombocytopenic purpura, VIII:Ag = antigenic determinant of VIII:C, VIII:C = factor VIII coagulant, VIII:RCo = von Willebrand factor activity with ristocetin, VIII:VWF = von Willebrand factor, VDRL = Veneral Disease Research Laboratory, VWD = von Willebrand disease.

Table 8–14. THROMBOEMBOLIC DISORDERS

Most Common...	Answer and Explanation
blood components in an arterial thrombus	*platelets held together by fibrin strands* [They develop in areas of rapid arterial blood flow where there is endothelial damage (e.g., TTP, cigarette smoke) or turbulence (e.g., **atherosclerotic plaque,** branching points in arteries).]
blood components in a venous thrombus	• *coagulation factors:* * fibrinogen, * V, * VIII, * II, • *fibrin,* • *platelets,* • *entrapped RBCs* [They develop in areas of stasis (e.g., venous system) or in hypercoagulable states (e.g., ATIII deficiency).]
risk factors for venous thrombosis	• **stasis:** e.g., **postoperative state,** • *CHF:* decreased venous return to heart, • *obesity,* • *oral contraceptives:* decreased ATIII levels, • *smoking,* • *orthopedic surgery:* hip, • *malignancy,* • *nephrotic syndrome:* ATIII loss in urine, • *sepsis,* • *varicose veins*
risk factors for arterial thrombosis	• **age:** * >45 in man, * >55 in woman, • *LDL >160 mg/dL,* • *HDL <35 mg/dL,* • *DM,* • HTN, • *smoking,* • *family Hx of premature CAD/stroke,* • *high plasma homocysteine levels:* damage vessel endothelium, • *oral contraceptives,* • *malignancy,* • *PRV*
Rx of venous thrombi	*see Table 5–3*
Rx of arterial thrombosis	• *low dose aspirin:* * see Table 5–8, • ticlopidine used if patients are allergic to aspirin, • *fibrinolytic agents:* e.g., * tPA, * streptokinase, * dissolve large clots (e.g., CA thrombosis)
hereditary causes of a hypercoagulable state	• **factor V Leiden mutation:** * AD, * resistant to degradation by activated protein C, • *protein C deficiency:* AD disease, • *protein S deficiency:* AD disease, • *ATIII deficiency:* AD disease

Table 8–14. THROMBOEMBOLIC DISORDERS *Continued*

Most Common...	Answer and Explanation
clues favoring a hereditary hypercoagulable state	• *recurrent DVT with/without PE,* • *family Hx,* • *DVT/PE at early age,* • *unusual sites for venous thrombosis:* e.g., * axilla, * dural sinuses
clinical findings in factor V Leiden mutation	*recurrent venous thrombosis:* * heterozygotes have 30-fold risk for venous thrombosis, * homozygotes have 80-fold risk, * managed with heparin/warfarin
acquired causes of protein C deficiency	• **warfarin Rx:** vitamin K-dependent factor, • *DIC,* • *L-asparaginase,* • *liver disease:* synthesized in liver, • *malignancy*
clinical findings in protein C deficiency	• *homozygotes die in infancy of neonatal purpura fulminans,* • *S/S in heterozygotes occur in mid to late teens,* • *recurrent DVTs:* ~65%, • *PE:* ~40%, • *hemorrhagic skin necrosis:* see below, • *recurrent superficial thrombophlebitis,* • *low protein C by functional and immunologic tests,* • *normal BT,* • *normal PTT/PT*
cause of hemorrhagic skin necrosis in a patient placed on warfarin	*heterozygote carrier with protein C deficiency:* patients have 30–60% protein C, * become "homozygous" when placed on warfarin (protein C nonfunctional in ~7 h), * patients thrombose in ~48 h, * thrombosis mainly occurs in skin vessels, * same disorder may occur with protein S deficiency
Rx of DVTs due to protein C deficiency	*heparin followed by warfarin:* * warfarin at much lower doses than normal to prevent skin necrosis, * patients remain on warfarin for life
causes of acquired protein S deficiency	*similar to causes listed for acquired protein C deficiency*
clinical findings in protein S deficiency	• *homozygotes more likely to die in utero or very early infancy,* • *S/S similar to protein C deficiency,* • *low protein S by functional and immunologic assays,* • *Rx:* similar to protein C

Table continued on following page

Table 8–14. THROMBOEMBOLIC DISORDERS *Continued*

Most Common...	Answer and Explanation
causes of acquired ATIII deficiency	• **oral contraceptives**, • *DIC*, • *severe liver disease*, • *nephrotic syndrome*, • *heparin Rx*
clinical findings in ATIII deficiency	• *recurrent DVTs*, • *PE*, • *mesenteric thrombosis*, • *no prolongation of PTT at standard doses of heparin:* first clue for Dx, • *low ATIII levels for both the immunologic and functional assays*
Rx of ATIII deficiency	*much higher doses of heparin must be given than normal:* * patients sent home on warfarin, * ATIII concentrates are available
origin of emboli to the lungs in the venous system	*femoral veins in upper thigh:* femoral/iliac vein thrombosis usually result of propagation from deep vein thrombosis in calf
origin of emboli in the arterial system	*clots dislodged from the left side of heart:* e.g., * mural thrombus, * vegetations
cause of paradoxical embolization	*thromboembolism from venous system through a patient foramen ovale into systemic circulation:* associated with ASD
cause of fat embolization	*fractures of lung bones or pelvis:* fat enters circulation from disrupted marrow and fat surrounding fractures
clinical findings in fat embolism	• *S/S:* * occur within 3 d, * mental status alterations, * dyspnea, * petechia limited to upper half of torso, • *lab findings:* * hypoxemia <60 mm Hg, * thrombocytopenia <15,000 cells/μL (platelets adhere to fat globules), * high serum lipase, * lipiduria
Rx of fat embolism	• *O$_2$ delivered with PEEP*, • *corticosteroids*, • *mortality:* ~10%
COD in amniotic fluid embolization	*DIC:* * AF rich in thromboplastin (initiates DIC), * lanugo hair/fetal squamous cells in lungs of women who die, * >80% mortality

Table 8–14. THROMBOEMBOLIC DISORDERS *Continued*

Question: A 22-year-old man with a history of recurrent DVTs and one episode of a PE to the left lower lobe presents with swelling and pain of the left lower leg consistent with a DVT. The platelet count, BT, PTT, and PT are all normal. Heparin is initiated and the PTT returns to normal. What condition does the patient **MOST LIKELY** have? **SELECT 1**

  (A) Protein C deficiency
  (B) Protein S deficiency
  (C) ATIII deficiency
  (D) Factor V Leiden mutation
  (E) Lupus anticoagulant

Answers: (C): Heparin must enhance the activity of ATIII to neutralize the serine proteases for anticoagulation to occur. At standard doses of heparin for DVTs, a patient with ATIII deficiency **(choice c)** will not have prolongation of the PTT; much greater doses will eventually cause prolongation of the PTT. Protein C, protein S, and factor V Leiden mutations will respond appropriately to heparin with prolongation of the PTT **(choices A, B, D are incorrect).** Patients with a LA usually have prolongation of the PTT **(choice E is incorrect).**

AD = autosomal dominant, AF = amniotic fluid, APL = antiphospholipid, ASD = atrial septal defect, ATIII = antithrombin III, BT = bleeding time, CA = coronary artery, CAD = coronary artery disease, CHF = congestive heart failure, COD = cause of death, DIC = disseminated intravascular coagulation, DM = diabetes mellitus, DVT = deep venous thrombosis, Dx = diagnosis, HDL = high density lipoproteins, HTN = hypertension, LDL = low density lipoproteins, PE = pulmonary embolus, PEEP = positive end-expiratory pressure, PRV = polycythemia rubra vera, PT = prothrombin time, PTT = activated partial thromboplastin time, RBC = red blood cell, Rx = treatment, S/S = signs and symptoms, tPA = tissue plasminogen activator, TTP = thrombotic thrombocytopenic purpura.

Table 8–15. IMMUNOHEMATOLOGY

Most Common...	Answer and Explanation
ABO blood group	*blood group O:* * O gene is inactive, * neither A or B antigens are present
universal recipient	*blood group AB:* no isohemagglutinins (anti-A or anti-B) in plasma to attack A or B antigens on other RBCs
blood group that can be transfused only with blood group O	*blood group O:* * O patients have anti-A-IgM, anti-B-IgM, and anti A,B-IgG, * can only receive blood negative for both A/B antigens

Table continued on following page

Table 8–15. **IMMUNOHEMATOLOGY** *Continued*

Most Common...	Answer and Explanation
universal donor	*blood group O:* ∗ anti-A-IgM from B patients and anti-B-IgM from A patients cannot destroy O RBCs, since they lack A and B antigens
maternal blood group involved in ABO incompatibility	*blood group O:* ∗ O mothers have anti A,B-IgG (normal antibody, not from previous sensitization), ∗ IgG antibody crosses placenta and attaches to fetal RBCs with A or B antigen, ∗ fetal RBCs undergo extravascular destruction in splenic macrophages in fetal spleen, ∗ mild hemolytic anemia
blood groups with high incidence of duodenal ulcer/ gastric cancer	*blood group O, blood group A, respectively*
Rh antigen	*D antigen:* 85% of the population are positive; designated Rh positive [Other Rh antigens include C, c, E, e (there is no d antigen).]
clinically significant antibody in clinical medicine	*anti-D antibodies:* ∗ strong IgG antibodies, ∗ produce brisk hemolytic anemia
blood group antigen that protects blacks from *Plasmodium vivax*	*Duffy antigen:* ∗ antigen is receptor for *P. vivax,* ∗ blacks lack this antigen
cold (IgM) antibodies of clinical significance	• *anti-I:* hemolytic anemia in *Mycoplasma pneumoniae* infections, • *anti-i:* hemolytic anemia in infectious mononucleosis, • *anti-P antibodies*
naturally occurring antibody	*anti-Lewis-IgM antibodies:* ∗ weak antibodies, ∗ no clinical significance
tests performed on donor blood in blood bank	• *ABO,* • *Rh,* • *ABS:* indirect Coombs', • *RPR or VDRL,* • *HBsAg,* • *anti-HCV antibodies,* • *anti-HIV1/HIV-2 antibodies,* • *anti-HTLVI/II antibodies*
antibody in United States	*anti-CMV antibodies*
infection transmitted by blood transfusion	*CMV:* present in donor lymphocytes

Table 8–15. IMMUNOHEMATOLOGY *Continued*

Most Common...	Answer and Explanation
infection rates post-transfusion for HBV, HCV, HTLV I/II, and HIV	• *HBV = 1:200,000 per unit*, • *HCV = 1:3300 per unit*, • *HTLVI/II = 1:200,000 per unit*, • *HIV = 1:676,000 per unit*
cause of post-transfusion hepatitis	*HCV:* 90%
preservative used in the blood bank	*CPDA1:* * *c*itrate: ♦ anticoagulant, ♦ binds calcium, * *p*hosphate: ♦ maintain 2,3 BPG levels (100% for 1 wk), * *d*extrose: ♦ fuel for RBCs, * *a*denine: ♦ substrate for ATP, * shelf life: ~35 d
pretransfusion tests performed on a patient	• *ABO*, • *Rh*, • *ABS:* detects atypical antibodies, • *direct Coombs':* detects antibodies on patient RBCs, • *major crossmatch:* * patient serum reacted against donor RBCs, * goal is to not have patient antibodies attacking donor RBC antigens
use of type and screen	*conserve blood/decrease patient cost:* all standard tests performed except the major crossmatch with donor unit
method of preventing GVH and CMV infection in recipient of a blood transfusion	*irradiation of unit:* * kills donor lymphocytes that cause GVH, * also kills lymphocytes containing CMV, * using leukocyte-depleting filters is less expensive way of eliminating WBCs that could transmit CMV
risks when transfusing blood	• **development of antibodies against foreign antigens**, • *transmitting infection:* e.g., * CMV, * HBV, * HCV, * HIV, * HTLV I/II, * *Yersinia enterocolitica*, • *transfusion reactions:* see below, • *volume overload*, • *noncardiogenic pulmonary edema:* * related to anti-HLA antibodies against donor leukocytes, * see below, • *GVH reaction*
type of RBC transfusion that eliminates all risks	*autologous transfusion:* process of collecting, storing, reinfusing the patient's own blood
time frame for transfusing RBCs	*within 4 h*

Table continued on following page

Table 8–15. IMMUNOHEMATOLOGY *Continued*

Most Common...	Answer and Explanation
indication for washed RBCs	• **patient with a previous febrile reaction,** • *patient with IgA deficiency:* anaphylactic reactions (1:100,000 risk) may occur if IgA deficient patients with anti-IgA antibodies are infused plasma products with IgA
indication for transfusing packed RBCs	*symptomatic anemia that cannot be adequately corrected by medical therapy:* * 1 unit of packed RBCs raises patient Hb by 1 g/dL and Hct by 3%, * patients with a Hb <7 g/dL should be transfused (O_2-carrying capacity compromised)
indication for transfusion of whole blood	*loss of massive amounts of whole blood*
indication for transfusing platelet concentrates	*see Table 8–12*
indication for transfusing granulocytes	• *patients with severe sepsis,* • *WBC count <500 cells/μL:* plus no response to antibiotics
indication for infusion of FFP	*multiple coagulation deficiencies:* e.g., * cirrhosis, * DIC, * over-anticoagulated with warfarin [Never use FFP as volume expander.]
indication for infusion of cryoprecipitate	• **DIC,** • *afibrinogenemia* [Desmopressin acetate has replaced cryoprecipitate for Rx of mild/moderate VWD/hemophilia A owing to the latter's risk of transmitting infection.]
indication for ISG	• **prevention of HAV in patient exposed to an active HAV infection:** should be given within 10 d, • *B cell immunodeficiencies:* e.g., * CLL, • *temporary prevention of hemolysis or thrombocytopenia in AIHA/autoimmune thrombocytopenia:* IgG blocks macrophage Fc receptors for IgG, • *Rx of Kawasaki's disease*
transfusion reaction	*mild allergic reactions:* * 1:100, * patient has IgE antibodies (type I HSR) against plasma proteins, * S/S range from urticaria to fever to an anaphylactic reaction
mechanism of a febrile reaction	*anti-HLA antibodies in patient directed against donor leukocyte HLA antigens:* * type II HSR, * patients must be exposed to human blood products to develop anti-HLA

Table 8–15. IMMUNOHEMATOLOGY *Continued*

Most Common...	Answer and Explanation
Continued	antibodies, * Rx: leukocyte-depletion filters, antipyretics
types of HTRs	• **intravascular:** * ABO mismatch between recipient and donor, * e.g., blood group A patient receives B blood, * most often result of human error (~50%), • *extravascular:* * due to presence of previously undetected antibodies in recipient (FN antibody screen) that are directed against donor RBC antigen, * RBCs are removed extravascularly by macrophages (type II HSR), * some reactions delayed (1–2 wks), particularly those related to anti-Kidd or anti-Rh type antibodies, * more common in women (sensitized from previous pregnancies) [1:6000 risk of HTR per unit.]
S/S of HTR	• *pain at infusion site or in back, abdomen, or chest,* • *fever,* • *drop in Hb/Hct,* • *hypotension,* • *oliguria,* • *jaundice,* • *bleeding:* secondary to DIC
lab tests and findings in HTRs	*see Table 8–2*
Rx of HTRs	• *immediate termination of transfusion:* keep IV open with 0.9% saline, • *loop diuretic to keep urine flowing:* some use mannitol, • *alkalinize urine:* sodium bicarbonate, • *fatality rate of HTR per unit is 1:100,000*
complications of massive transfusions	• *coagulopathies:* coagulation/platelet deficiencies, • *hypothermia:* * can precipitate arrhythmias, * use a blood warmer, • *citrate toxicity:* hypocalcemia may occur, • *electrolyte abnormalities:* * hyperkalemia from old transfused RBCs, * metabolic acidosis [Massive transfusion refers to transfusion of blood that is greater than the patient's blood volume in <24 h.]
cause of transfusion-associated ARDS	*anti-HLA antibodies against donor WBCs* (granulocytes and/or lymphocytes): risk per unit is 1:10,000
S/S of post-transfusion ARDS	*within ~6 h, patient develops: fever, dyspnea, pulmonary infiltrates* (noncardiogenic pulmonary edema): PCWP <18 mm Hg (R/O circulatory overload or left heart failure)

Table continued on following page

Table 8–15. IMMUNOHEMATOLOGY *Continued*

Most Common...	Answer and Explanation
Rx of post-transfusion ARDS	• O_2, • *PEEP therapy*, • *furosemide*, • *dopamine* [Recovery usually occurs within 24–48 h.]
cause of Rh HDN	*anti-D antibodies that develop in an Rh-negative woman from a previous pregnancy*
method of antenatal protection against Rh sensitization	*infusion of RhIG at 28 weeks in anti-D negative women:* RhIG is pooled, purified IgG human anti-D (very little crosses placenta)
postnatal method of protecting Rh-negative, anti-D-negative women who deliver an Rh-positive child	*Kleihauer-Betke test* (or similar type test) *of maternal blood to identify fetal RBCs* (fetal-maternal bleed): * number of vials in RhIG are given to the mother is based on amount of fetal RBCs in her blood, * anti-D in RhIG protects mother from developing an antibody response against Rh-positive fetal cells, * RhIG is usually given within 3 d of delivery, * not indicated for women who already have anti-D antibodies

Question: A 26-year-old woman develops fever, chills, jaundice, and fatigue 2 weeks after delivering a baby boy. She received 2 units of packed RBCs post-delivery owing to a retained placenta. Her antibody screen prior to transfusion was negative and the major crossmatch was compatible for both units. At this time, which of the following would you expect the patient to have? **SELECT 2**
- (A) A negative antibody screen
- (B) UCB hyperbilirubinemia
- (C) Anti-HCV antibodies
- (D) Positive direct Coombs'
- (E) Normal Hb/Hct

Answers: (B), (D): The patient has a delayed HTR. You would expect a positive antibody screen **(choice A is incorrect)**, high UCB level **(choice B)**, negative anti-HCV **(choice C is incorrect)**, most cases of post-transfusion HCV are anicteric and would not occur in this short a time period), positive direct Coombs' **(choice D)**, and low Hb/Hct levels **(choice E is incorrect)**. The false-negative antibody screen prior to her transfusion was due to either an antibody titer too low for the antibody screen to detect or no titer at all. Memory B cells were stimulated by the antigen (e.g., Rh, Kidd) leading to a progressive increase in titers and subsequent extravascular hemolysis (type II HSR).

ABO = blood groups A, B, and O, ABS = antibody screen, AIHA = autoimmune hemolytic anemia, ARDS = adult respiratory distress syndrome, ATP = adenosine triphosphate, BPG = bisphosphoglycerate, CLL = chronic lymphocytic leukemia, CMV = cytomegalovirus, CPDA

= citrate/phosphate/dextrose/adenine, DIC = disseminated intravascular coagulation, FFP = fresh frozen plasma, FN = false-negative, GVH = graft versus host, HAV = hepatitis A, Hb = hemoglobin, HBsAg = hepatitis B surface antigen, HBV = hepatitis B, HCV = hepatitis C, Hct = hematocrit, HDN = hemolytic disease of the newborn, HIV = human immunodeficiency virus, HLA = human leukocyte antigen, HSR = hypersensitivity reaction, HTLV = human T cell lymphotropic virus, HTR = hemolytic transfusion reaction, Ig = immunoglobulin, ISG = immune serum globulin, IV = intravenous, PCWP = pulmonary capillary wedge pressure, PEEP = positive end-expiratory pressure, RBC = red blood cell, RhIG = Rh immune globulin, R/O = rule out, RPR = rapid plasma reagin, Rx = treatment, S/S = signs and symptoms, UCB = unconjugated bilirubin, VDRL = Venereal Disease Research Laboratory, VWD = von Willebrand's disease, WBC = white blood cell.

GASTROENTEROLOGY

CONTENTS

Table 9–1. SIGNS AND SYMPTOMS OF GASTROINTESTINAL DISEASE EXCLUDING HEPATOBILIARY

Most Common...	Answer and Explanation
S/S of esophageal disease	• **heartburn:** * burning sensation in the epigastrium, e.g., * GERD, • *dysphagia:* * difficulty with swallowing food, * dysphagia for solids alone: obstruction, * dysphagia for solids/liquids: motility disorder, • *odynophagia:* * painful swallowing, * e.g., esophagitis, • *regurgitation of acid:* e.g., GERD
S/S of stomach disease	• **N/V:** * not bile stained in pyloric obstruction, * bile stained if obstruction is below ampulla of Vater, • *epigastric pain:* e.g., PUD, • *hematemesis:* * vomiting of blood, * e.g., PUD, • *melenemesis:* * vomiting of blood with coffee-ground appearance, * e.g., PUD, • *melena:* * black, tarry stool, * e.g., PUD, • *early satiety:* e.g., * gastroparesis, * pyloric obstruction, • *distention:* e.g., pyloric obstruc-

Table continued on following page

Table 9–1. SIGNS AND SYMPTOMS OF
GASTROINTESTINAL DISEASE EXCLUDING
HEPATOBILIARY *Continued*

Most Common...	Answer and Explanation
Continued	tion, • *Sister Mary Joseph sign:* metastasis to umbilicus in stomach cancer, • *acanthosis nigricans:* * pigmented axillary skin lesion, * marker for stomach cancer, • *Leser-Trelat sign:* * outcroppings of seborrheic keratosis, * marker of stomach cancer, • *Virchow's node:* * left supraclavicular node, * metastatic stomach cancer, • *enlarged ovaries:* Krukenberg tumors from stomach cancer metastasis
S/S of duodenal disease	• **pain:** e.g., duodenal ulcer, • *N/V:* e.g., acute pancreatitis, • *hematemesis:* e.g., duodenal ulcer, • *diarrhea:* malabsorption from: * bacterial overgrowth, * celiac disease
S/S of jejunal/ileal disease	• **diarrhea:** e.g., carcinoid syndrome, • *pain:* * obstruction, • *anemia:* e.g., folate/B_{12} deficiency from malabsorption, • *distention:* e.g., bowel obstruction, • *bloody diarrhea:* e.g., infarction
S/S of pancreatic disease	• **pain:** e.g., acute pancreatitis, • *weight loss:* e.g., adenocarcinoma, • *N/V:* e.g., acute pancreatitis, • *diarrhea:* e.g., * ZE syndrome, • *steatorrhea:* e.g., chronic pancreatitis, • *anemia:* e.g., B_{12} deficiency (lack of enzymes to cleave off R factor), • *jaundice:* e.g., carcinoma head of pancreas, • *mass:* e.g., pancreatic pseudocyst, • *flank hemorrhage:* Grey-Turner sign in hemorrhagic pancreatitis, • *periumbilical hemorrhage:* Cullen's sign in hemorrhagic pancreatitis, • *Courvoisier's sign:* distended gallbladder in carcinoma head of pancreas, • *localized ileus:* e.g., sentinel loop of duodenum in acute pancreatitis
S/S of colon disease	• *diarrhea:* e.g., * infectious, • *constipation:* e.g., low fiber, • *pain:* e.g., ischemic/ulcerative colitis, • *distention:* e.g., * obstruction, • *anemia:* e.g., iron deficiency: colorectal cancer, • *bloody diarrhea:* e.g., ischemic colitis, • *hematochezia:* * bright red blood in stool, e.g., * diverticulosis, • *mass:* e.g., cancer, • *ileus:* e.g., obstruction (late sign), • *hyperperistalsis:* e.g., early obstruction, • *rebound tenderness:* e.g., peritonitis

Table 9–1. SIGNS AND SYMPTOMS OF GASTROINTESTINAL DISEASE EXCLUDING HEPATOBILIARY *Continued*

Most Common...	Answer and Explanation
S/S of anorectal disease	• **bleeding:** e.g., internal hemorrhoids (painless), • *pain:* e.g., anal fissure, • *tenesmus:* * pain with urge to defecate, e.g., UC, • *pruritus:* e.g., * pinworm, * *ulceration:* e.g., STDs, • *mass:* e.g., anal carcinoma, • *anal fistula:* e.g., CD, • *hematochezia:* e.g., solitary rectal ulcer
S/S of functional GI disease	• **absence of fever/weight loss,** • *alternating diarrhea/constipation:* IBS, • *daytime diarrhea:* nocturnal diarrhea has an organic cause • *normal Hb/Hct,* • *negative stool guaiac*
mechanisms for vomiting	• *afferent stimulation of the vomiting center:* * dorsal portion of the lateral reticular formation, * controls act of vomiting, • *afferent stimulation of CTZ:* * area postrema in medulla, * sends efferent impulses to the vomiting center
afferent stimuli to the vomiting center	• **vagal fibers from the GI tract:** e.g., * **infections,** * mechanical obstruction, • *vestibular system:* e.g., Meniere's syndrome, • *high brain stem/cortical centers:* e.g., increased CNS pressure, • *CTZ:* see below
stimuli of the CTZ	• **drugs:** e.g., * opiates, * digitalis, • *bacterial toxins,* • *radiation,* • *metabolites in uremia*
cause of vomiting	*viral illness*
complications of vomiting	• **electrolyte disorders:** e.g., * hypochloremic metabolic alkalosis, * hypokalemia, • *volume depletion,* • *tears:* Mallory-Weiss syndrome, • *rupture:* Boerhaave's syndrome, • *pulmonary aspiration*
causes of N/V of undigested food 4–6 h after eating	• **gastroparesis:** e.g., DM, • *pyloric obstruction:* e.g., duodenal ulcer
causes of N/V when waking in the morning	• **pregnancy,** • *uremia,* • *alcoholic gastritis*
cause of N/V associated with vertigo/tinnitus	*Meniere's disease*

Table continued on following page

Table 9–1. SIGNS AND SYMPTOMS OF GASTROINTESTINAL DISEASE EXCLUDING HEPATOBILIARY *Continued*

Most Common...	Answer and Explanation
cause of projectile vomiting associated with headache	*increased intracranial pressure*
Rx of N/V	• *serotonin antagonists:* e.g., ondansetron, • *central dopamine antagonists:* e.g., metoclopramide, • *antihistamines:* e.g., promethazine, • *anticholinergics:* e.g., scopolamine, • *drugs stimulating cholinergic nerves:* e.g., cisapride, • *drugs interacting with motilin receptors on GI smooth muscle membranes:* e.g., erythromycin
pathogenesis of hiccups	• **direct stimulation of the phrenic nerve:** e.g., diaphragmatic irritation/trauma to phrenic nerve, • *central stimulation of phrenic nerve:* e.g. * **uremia,** * cerebral atherosclerosis
cause of hiccups	*aerophagia:* swallowing air when eating
cause of chronic hiccups	• **atherosclerotic cerebrovascular disease,** • *uremia*
Rx of hiccups	*chlorpromazine*
manifestation of esophageal disease	*dyspepsia:* * heartburn, * burning sensation in retrosternal area, * bloating, * early satiety
causes of dyspepsia	• **GERD,** • *non-ulcer dyspepsia,* • *food intolerance*
cause of dysphagia for solids but not liquids	*obstructive lesions in the esophagus:* e.g., * web, * cancer [An esophageal lumen <12 mm causes mechanical obstruction.]
cause of dysphagia for solids and liquids	*motility disorders:* e.g., * PSS/CREST syndrome, * DM/PM, * MG, * achalasia, * previous stroke [Upper one-third of esophagus is skeletal muscle, middle one-third is skeletal/smooth muscle, lower one-third is smooth muscle. DM/PM, stroke, MG affect striated muscle: oropharyngeal dysphagia. PSS/CREST syndrome, and achalasia affect smooth muscle: lower esophageal dysphagia.]
causes of oropharyngeal dysphagia	• **neuromuscular disorders:** e.g., * DM/PM, * MG, * ALS, * stroke, • *structural disorders:* e.g., Zenker's diverticulum [Oropharyngeal

Table 9–1. SIGNS AND SYMPTOMS OF GASTROINTESTINAL DISEASE EXCLUDING HEPATOBILIARY *Continued*

Most Common...	Answer and Explanation
Continued	dysphagia is a faulty transfer of food from oral pharynx to esophagus.]
S/S of oropharyngeal dysphagia	• **coughing/choking,** • *nasal regurgitation,* • *pulmonary aspiration*
cause of odynophagia	*inflammation:* e.g., * **infectious esophagitis,** * GERD
cause of intermittent dysphagia for solids only	*lower esophageal ring*
cause of progressive dysphagia for solids with associated heartburn	*peptic stricture secondary to GERD*
cause of progressive dysphagia for solids in elderly patients with weight loss	*esophageal cancer* [If hoarseness is present, invasive esophageal cancer with involvement of the recurrent laryngeal nerve is likely.]
cause of intermittent dysphagia for solids/ liquids associated with noncardiac chest pain	• **GERD,** • *nutcracker esophagus:* very high pressures recorded by manometry, • *diffuse esophageal spasm:* "corkscrew" esophagus on barium studies
Rx of esophageal disorders causing noncardiac chest pain	• *nitroglycerin,* • *calcium channel blockers,* • *anticholinergics*
causes of hematemesis	• **duodenal ulcer,** • *gastric ulcer,* • *esophageal varices* [Hematemesis is the vomiting of blood.]
causes of melenemesis	• **duodenal ulcer,** • *gastric ulcer* [Melenemesis is the vomiting of coffee ground material.]
mechanism of black pigment in vomitus/ stools	*stomach acid converts Hb into a black pigment called hematin*

Table continued on following page

Table 9–1. SIGNS AND SYMPTOMS OF GASTROINTESTINAL DISEASE EXCLUDING HEPATOBILIARY *Continued*

Most Common...	Answer and Explanation
cause of bloody stools after liver trauma	*hematobilia:* blood in biliary tree
cause of melena (black tarry stools)	*duodenal ulcer* [~90% of causes of melena are proximal to the ligament of Treitz (junction of the duodenum/jejunum). ~50–100 mL of blood produces melena. Slow bleeds below the ligament of Treitz may produce melena (colonic bacteria convert Hb to hematin).]
GI location for hematochezia	*below the ligament of Treitz*
causes of hematochezia	• **diverticulosis:** diverticulitis does not produce bleeding owing to scarring of the vessels, • *angiodysplasia*
causes of chronic lower GI bleeding	• **internal hemorrhoids,** • *colorectal cancer*
cause of painful defecation with blood coating the stool	*anal fissure* [It is usually due to a tear on the posterior part of the anus. A sentinel tag marks the location of the tear.]
causes of iron deficiency due to a GI bleed	• **duodenal ulcer,** • *colorectal cancer*
lab test to identify blood in the stool	*Hemoccult slide test* [The test uses guaiac to detect peroxidase activity in Hb. Newer tests have antibodies against Hb or detect heme.]
causes of a false-positive Hemoccult slide test	• **myoglobin in meat,** • *nonheme peroxidases in vegetables:* e.g., * horseradish, * cruciferous vegetables
order to follow in evaluating the abdomen	• *inspection,* • *auscultation,* • *percussion,* • *palpation*
causes of pain in hollow viscera	• *stretching of the wall,* • *inflammation,* • *ischemia,* • *forceful contractions*
causes of pain in solid viscera	• *stretching of the capsule,* • *inflammation of the capsule:* e.g., hepatomegaly

Table 9–1. SIGNS AND SYMPTOMS OF
GASTROINTESTINAL DISEASE EXCLUDING
HEPATOBILIARY *Continued*

Most Common...	Answer and Explanation
types of pain	• **visceral,** • *parietal,* • *referred*
nerve fibers responsible for visceral pain	*unmyelinated afferent C fibers* [Visceral pain is associated with irritation of the visceral organs. It is a dull pain that is slow in onset.]
localization site for visceral pain	*midline closest to the irritated viscera*
structures referring visceral pain to the epigastrium	• *stomach,* • *duodenum,* • *liver,* • *GB*
structures referring visceral pain to the umbilical area	• *jejunum/ileum,* • *appendix,* • *cecum,* • *right colon*
structures referring visceral pain to the hypogastric/ suprapubic area	• *colon,* • *internal reproductive organs*
nerve fibers responsible for parietal pain	*C fibers and myelinated A δ-fibers:* * parietal pain is associated with irritation of parietal peritoneum, * acute in onset, * sharp pain
localization site of parietal pain	*exact location of peritoneal irritation*
secretions causing parietal pain	• **blood:** e.g., ectopic pregnancy, • *pus,* • *bile,* • *pancreatic secretions,* • *cyst fluid:* e.g., ruptured follicular cyst
S/S of parietal pain	• **rebound tenderness,** • *pain with coughing or movement*
causes of acute RUQ pain	• **acute cholecystitis,** • *cholelithiasis,* • *acute hepatitis,* • *right ureteral colic:* radiates to ipsilateral groin, • *right-sided pleurisy:* * pneumonia, * PE, • *right-sided pyelonephritis:* look for urinary signs, • *subphrenic abscess*
cause of Murphy's sign	*acute cholecystitis:* palpation of the RUQ causes inspiratory arrest secondary to pain

Table continued on following page

**Table 9–1. SIGNS AND SYMPTOMS OF
GASTROINTESTINAL DISEASE EXCLUDING
HEPATOBILIARY** *Continued*

Most Common...	Answer and Explanation
findings in Charcot's triad	• *RUQ pain,* • *fever,* • *jaundice*
disorder associated with Charcot's triad	*acute cholangitis*
causes of acute LUQ pain	• **gastroenteritis,** • *IBS,* • *splenic infarction:* friction rub/pleural effusion usually noted, • *acute pancreatitis,* • *left ureteral colic:* radiates into left groin, • *left pyelonephritis*
cause of Kehr's sign	*splenic infarction:* Kehr's sign is radiation of pain to left shoulder from diaphragm irritation
causes of acute RLQ pain	• **acute appendicitis with perforation,** • *Meckel's diverticulitis,* • *typhlitis:* cecal inflammation, • *CD:* ileitis, • *perforated duodenal ulcer:* gastric contents settle in RLQ
cause of acute LLQ pain	*colonic diverticulitis:* "left-sided" appendicitis
mechanism of referred pain at a distant site from its source	*distant site shares similar neuronal pathways as the involved organ*
route of pain migration in acute appendicitis	• *initially, periumbilical:* * due to C fibers, * inflamed appendix, • *McBurney's point in the RLQ:* * due to A fibers, * localized peritonitis
site of referred pain in acute cholecystitis	*right scapular area*
site of referred pain in a perforated peptic ulcer with air under the diaphragm	*left shoulder via irritation of the phrenic nerve*
site of referred pain in acute pancreatitis	*directly into the back or flank*
site of referred pain in ureteral colic	*ipsilateral groin*
mechanism of colicky pain	*obstruction of a viscus that has peristalsis:* e.g., * colicky pain is pain followed by a pain-free interval, e.g., * obstruction due to bowel adhesions

Table 9–1. SIGNS AND SYMPTOMS OF GASTROINTESTINAL DISEASE EXCLUDING HEPATOBILIARY *Continued*

Most Common...	Answer and Explanation
sequence of pain/ N/V in a surgical abdomen	*pain occurs first and is then followed by N/V:* ∗ N/V followed by pain is a nonsurgical abdomen, ∗ e.g., gastritis
causes of explosive (immediate) onset of abdominal pain	• **perforated peptic ulcer,** • *biliary "colic,"* • *ureteral colic,* • *ruptured aortic aneurysm,* • *dissecting aortic aneurysm,* • *bowel strangulation* [Biliary "colic" is a misnomer, since the pain is usually constant owing to the weak contractile qualities of the bile ducts.]
causes of rapid onset (few minutes) of severe, steady abdominal pain	• **acute pancreatitis:** described as knife-like, • *mesenteric thrombosis:* pain is out of proportion to physical findings, • *strangulated bowel:* e.g., volvulus, • *ruptured ectopic*
causes of gradual onset (over a few hours) of steady pain	• **acute appendicitis,** • *acute diverticulitis,* • *acute cholecystitis,* • *acute hepatitis,* • *acute salpingitis* [Infection is more likely to present with a gradual onset of pain.]
causes of intermittent colicky pain (over a few hours) with free intervals	• **mechanical small bowel obstruction,** • *CD,* • *early phase of acute appendicitis* colicky pain at first but becomes constant when localized peritonitis occurs
causes of early postprandial pain	• **gastric ulcer,** • *acute gastritis*
cause of pain at night with recumbency	*GERD*
cause of relief of pain following the ingestion of food	*duodenal ulcer*
cause of late (several hours after eating) postprandial pain	*gastric outlet obstruction*
cause of steady mid-epigastric or RUQ pain that begins in the evening	*biliary colic*

Table continued on following page

Table 9–1. SIGNS AND SYMPTOMS OF GASTROINTESTINAL DISEASE EXCLUDING HEPATOBILIARY *Continued*

Most Common...	Answer and Explanation
mechanisms of constipation	• **low-fiber diet,** • *colon motility disorder,* • *anorectal dysfunction* [Constipation is defecation <3 times/week.]
life-long cause of constipation	*Hirschsprung's disease:* see below
cause of recent onset of constipation	*obstructive lesion:* e.g., * colon cancer, * ischemic stricture
causes of disturbed colonic motility leading to constipation	• **drugs:** e.g., * opiates, * anticholinergics, * aluminum antacids, • *IBS,* • *pregnancy:* progesterone effect, • *metabolic conditions:* e.g., * hypokalemia, * hypercalcemia, * hypothyroidism, * diabetes mellitus, * pheochromocytoma (increased sympathetic stimulation, • *Hirschsprung's disease:* destruction of myenteric plexus, • *systemic disease:* e.g., PSS
Rx of constipation	• **increasing fiber,** • *osmotic laxatives:* e.g., * magnesium hydroxide, * lactulose, • *emollient laxatives:* * penetrate stool, e.g., * docusate, • *stimulant laxatives:* increase peristalsis: * cascara, * senna [Rx the underlying disease.]
cause of obstipation	*complete bowel obstruction:* * obstipation is the absence of stooling and flatus, * obstruction produces both constipation and obstipation
causes of hyperperistalsis	• **diarrhea,** • *early obstruction* [Hyperperistalsis refers to increased bowel sounds.]
cause of adynamic and dynamic ileus	• *adynamic ileus:* * intestinal obstruction due to inhibition of bowel motility, e.g., * peritonitis, • *dynamic ileus:* * mechanical intestinal obstruction, e.g., * adhesions [Ileus refers to absent bowel sounds.]
causes of tenesmus	• **IBS,** • *ulcerative colitis,* • *solitary rectal ulcer syndrome* [Tenesmus is an unproductive urge to defecate. It suggests a problem in the anal sphincter next to the rectum.]
types of diarrhea	• **osmotic,** • *secretory,* • *invasive* [Diarrhea is an increase in daily stool weight of >250 grams. See Table 9–4.]

Table 9–1. SIGNS AND SYMPTOMS OF GASTROINTESTINAL DISEASE EXCLUDING HEPATOBILIARY Continued

Question: A 35-year-old man has a 3-month history of intermittent burning epigastric pain 1–3 hours after eating and pain that wakes him up at night. He now presents with an abrupt onset of epigastric pain with radiation into the back. The stool is black, tarry, and guaiac positive. Which conditions does the patient **MOST LIKELY** have: **SELECT 2**

- (A) Esophageal varices
- (B) GERD
- (C) Duodenal ulcer
- (D) Gastric ulcer
- (E) Gastric adenocarcinoma
- (F) Acute pancreatitis

Answers: (C), (F): The history of burning epigastric pain a few hours after eating, pain that wakes him up at night, and melena is consistent with a bleeding duodenal ulcer **(choice C)**. The abrupt onset of epigastric pain with radiation into the back is consistent with an acute pancreatitis **(choice F)**. The duodenal ulcer is posteriorly located and has penetrated into the pancreas, leading to pancreatitis. Esophageal varices present with an abrupt onset of hematemesis **(choice A is incorrect)**. GERD does not have this pattern of epigastric pain, nor does it commonly produce melena, nor have a relationship with acute pancreatitis **(choice B is incorrect)**. A gastric ulcer has pain soon after eating and is not associated with acute pancreatitis **(choice D is incorrect)**. Stomach cancer does not have this pattern of epigastric pain, is associated with weight loss, does not commonly produce melena, and is not associated with pancreatitis **(choice E is incorrect)**.

ALS = amyotrophic lateral sclerosis, AMI = acute myocardial infarction, CD = Crohn's disease, CNS = central nervous system, CREST = calcinosis, Raynaud's, esophageal motility disturbance, sclerodactyly, telangiectasia, CTZ = chemoreceptor trigger zone, DM = dermatomyositis, GB = gallbladder, GERD = gastroesophageal reflux disease, GI = gastrointestinal, Hb = hemoglobin, Hct = hematocrit, IBS = irritable bowel syndrome, LLQ = left lower quadrant, LUQ = left upper quadrant, MG = myasthenia gravis, N/V = nausea and vomiting, PE = pulmonary embolus, PM = polymyositis, PSS = progressive systemic sclerosis, PUD = peptic ulcer disease, RLQ = right lower quadrant, RUQ = right upper quadrant, Rx = treatment, S/S = signs and symptoms, STD = sexually transmitted disease, UC = ulcerative colitis, ZE = Zollinger-Ellison syndrome.

Table 9–2. ORAL CAVITY AND ESOPHAGEAL DISORDERS

Most Common...	Answer and Explanation
cause of herpangina	*coxsackie A:* herpangina is associated with * fever, * pharyngitis, and * palatal ulcers/vesicles surrounded by erythema
infectious cause of gingivostomatitis	*Herpes simplex:* * primary infection: fever, cervical lymphadenopathy, * virus remains dormant in sensory ganglia, * recurrent disease: nonsystemic, vermilion border of lips
Rx of *Herpes simplex*	• *primary type:* acyclovir, • *recurrent type:* usually not treated
causes of exudative tonsillitis	• **viruses:** * >50% of cases, e.g., * EBV, * coxsackievirus, • *group A Streptococcus:* 20–35%, • *Neisseria gonorrhoeae,* • *Chlamydia trachomatis,* • *Corynebacterium diphtheriae*
lab Dx of exudative tonsillitis due to group A *Streptococcus*	• **culture,** • *direct antigen detection:* * sensitivity 80–85%, * specificity >90%: * Rx if direct antigen test is positive, * if negative, Rx based on culture results
Rx of group A streptococcal pharyngitis	• **penicillin V potassium:** 250 mg tid × 10 d, or • *single IM injection of benzathine or procaine penicillin:* noncompliant patient
cause of deviation of the uvula to the contralateral side in a patient with exudative tonsillitis	*peritonsillar abscess:* also associated with odynophagia and medial deviation of the soft palate
oral manifestation of AIDS	• **candidiasis,** • *aphthous ulcers,* • *hairy leukoplakia,* • *Kaposi's sarcoma:* palate is the most common location
causes of oral candidiasis in an adult	• *dentures,* • *diabetes mellitus,* • *debilitated patients,* • *post-antibiotic/corticosteroid Rx,* • *immunocompromised patient*
types of oral candidiasis	• **pseudomembranous:** * white patches, * rubs off, leaving a bleeding surface, • *erythematous:* flat and red, • *leukoplakic:* does not rub off, • *angular cheilitis* (perlèche): cracks at angles of the mouth
Rx of oral candidiasis	• *imidazoles:* e.g., fluconazole, • *nystatin*

Table 9–2. ORAL CAVITY AND ESOPHAGEAL DISORDERS *Continued*

Most Common...	Answer and Explanation
viral cause of leukoplakia in an HIV-positive patient	*hairy leukoplakia secondary to EBV:* * predates the onset of AIDS, * not an AIDS-defining lesion
Rx for hairy leukoplakia	*high-dose acyclovir:* it recurs when acyclovir is discontinued
cause of Hutchinson's and mulberry teeth	*congenital syphilis:* * Hutchinson's teeth are peg-shaped upper incisors, * mulberry teeth are molar teeth resembling mulberries
cause of lost teeth in patients <35 years old	*dental caries*
predisposing causes of dental caries	• *sucrose,* • *Streptococcus mutans:* acts on sucrose to produce dextran (enhances plaque formation) and acid (erodes enamel), • *reduced salivation:* e.g., Sjögren's syndrome
mechanisms of fluoride prevention of dental caries	• **changes hydroxyapatite in enamel into fluorapatite,** • *bactericidal*
infectious cause of a submandibular sinus	*Actinomyces israelii:* * gram-positive, anaerobic, filamentous bacteria best identified in sulfur granules, * secondary to dental abscesses
Rx of *Actinomyces israelii* infection	• *IV ampicillin followed by PO amoxicillin,* or • *IV penicillin G followed by PO penicillin V*
bullous lesion in the oral cavity	*pemphigus vulgaris:* IgG antibodies are directed against intercellular attachments between keratinocytes
Rx of pemphigus vulgaris	*corticosteroids*
diseases associated with aphthous ulcers	• **early symptomatic phase of AIDS,** • *Reiter's syndrome:* see Table 12–1, • *CD,* • *Behçet's syndrome:* * genital ulcerations, * conjunctivitis, * uveitis [Aphthous ulcers are painful ulcerations.]
clinical findings in Stevens-Johnson syndrome	• **extension of erythema multiforme:** see Table 14–1, • *ruptured bullae with hemorrhagic crusts in the mouth,* • *target lesions on the hands/feet*

Table continued in following page

Table 9–2. ORAL CAVITY AND ESOPHAGEAL DISORDERS *Continued*

Most Common...	Answer and Explanation
cause of Stevens-Johnson syndrome	• **drugs:** e.g., * sulfonamides, * phenytoin, NSAIDs, • *Mycoplasma pneumoniae infection*
Rx of Stevens-Johnson syndrome	*corticosteroids*
syndrome associated with mucosal pigmentation	*Peutz-Jeghers* syndrome: it is an AD polyposis syndrome
endocrine disorder associated with mucosal pigmentation	*Addison's disease:* hypocortisolism leads to an increase in ACTH, which stimulates melanin synthesis
heavy metal pigmentations of the gums	• **lead,** • *mercury,* • *bismuth*
antibiotic causing tooth discoloration	*tetracycline*
cause of chalky discoloration of the teeth	*excess fluoride:* it is called fluorosis
causes of glossitis	• **vitamin deficiencies:** e.g., * vitamin C, * niacin, * riboflavin, * folate/B_{12}, • *iron deficiency*
S/S of glossitis	• **painful tongue,** • *tongue is red, smooth, and has no filiform papillae*
cause of a black hairy tongue	*Aspergillus niger:* overgrowth post-antibiotic Rx
causes of macroglossia	• **primary hypothyroidism,** • *amyloidosis,* • *acromegaly*
causes of leukoplakia	• **chronic irritation:** e.g., * dentures, * biting the cheek, • *tobacco smoking,* • *smokeless tobacco* [Leukoplakia refers to a white to red plaque that does not scrape off.]
locations for leukoplakia	• **ventrolateral tongue,** • *floor of the mouth,* • *lower lip*
management of leukoplakia	• **Bx to R/O squamous dysplasia/cancer** (4–10%), • *erythroleukoplakia:* red/white patches: 90% chance of dysplasia/cancer

Table 9–2. ORAL CAVITY AND ESOPHAGEAL
DISORDERS *Continued*

Most Common...	Answer and Explanation
cause of Wickham's striae	*lichen planus:* * striae have a net-like appearance on buccal mucosa, * lesions with an erosive component may develop into squamous dysplasia/cancer
cancer in the oral cavity	*squamous cell carcinoma*
locations of oral squamous cancer	• **lateral border of the tongue,** • *lower lip,* • *ventral aspect of the tongue*
risk factors for oral squamous cancer	• **smoking,** • *alcohol* [They have an additive effect, which further increases the risk for cancer.]
cancer associated with smokeless tobacco	*verrucous carcinoma:* * variant of squamous cancer, * most commonly develops in the mandibular sulcus, * rarely metastasizes
cancer of the upper lip	*basal cell carcinoma:* sunlight-induced
infection of the salivary glands	*mumps*
S/S of mumps	• **parotid tenderness:** usually bilateral, • **facial swelling,** • *unilateral orchitis/oophoritis:* adolescents, • *pancreatitis:* * amylase elevated in parotitis/pancreatitis, * only lipase elevated in pancreatitis
extrasalivary complication of mumps	*meningoencephalitis:* * CSF has a mixed infiltrate of cells, increased protein, and low glucose, * self-limited
site for benign/ malignant salivary gland tumors	*parotid glands:* * most parotid tumors are benign, * greater percentage of minor salivary gland tumors are malignant
overall benign salivary gland tumor in major/minor salivary glands	*mixed tumor* (pleomorphic adenoma): * most commonly located in the parotid, * rarely develop into a carcinoma (facial nerve dysfunction likely)
malignant tumor in major/minor salivary glands	*mucoepidermoid carcinoma:* most commonly located in the parotid
cause of Plummer-Vinson syndrome	*chronic iron deficiency:* more common in middle-aged women

Table continued in following page

Table 9–2. ORAL CAVITY AND ESOPHAGEAL DISORDERS *Continued*

Most Common...	Answer and Explanation
clinical findings in Plummer-Vinson syndrome	• **upper esophageal web:** dysphagia for solids, • *koilonychia,* • *achlorhydria,* • *glossitis,* • *increased risk for squamous cancers* (10–20%) *of upper esophagus*
esophageal diverticulum	*Zenker's diverticulum:* * upper esophagus, * defect in the cricopharyngeus muscle
S/S of a Zenker's diverticulum	• **oropharyngeal dysphagia,** • *halitosis,* • *diverticulitis*
systemic collagen vascular disease of the esophagus	*PSS:* CREST syndrome is a localized variant of PSS
pathophysiologic findings of PSS involving the esophagus	• *smooth muscle in lower one-third of esophagus is replaced by fibrosis,* • *mid-esophagus undergoes muscle atrophy,* • *motility dysfunction:* * aperistalsis, * proximal esophageal dilatation, * relaxed LES
clinical findings of PSS involving the esophagus	• **progressive dysphagia for solids/liquids,** • *reflux esophagitis,* • *esophagography:* * aperistalsis, * dilatation, • *esophageal manometry:* * absent to low peristaltic amplitude, * low to absent LES pressure
systemic collagen vascular diseases involving upper esophagus	*dermatomyositis/polymyositis:* involve the striated muscle of upper one-third of esophagus in ~50% of cases
S/S of DM/PM of the upper esophagus	• **oropharyngeal dysphagia,** • *regurgitation,* • *cough*
neuromuscular disorder of the esophagus	*achalasia*
pathophysiologic findings of achalasia	• **absence of ganglion cells in the myenteric plexus and Auerbach's ganglion cells of the LES,** • *loss of the vasodilator, vasointestinal peptide:* leads to sustained contraction of the LES, • *aperistalsis,* • *dilatation of proximal esophagus*
clinical findings in achalasia	• **older patient with progressive dysphagia for solids/liquids,** • *nocturnal symptoms:* * regurgitation of undigested food, * cough, • *weight loss,* • *chest radiograph showing air/*

Table 9–2. ORAL CAVITY AND ESOPHAGEAL DISORDERS *Continued*

Most Common...	Answer and Explanation
Continued	fluid level in esophagus, • *abnormal barium swallow:* * dilated, aperistaltic esophagus, * beak-like tapering at the distal end, • *abnormal esophageal manometry:* * key test, * aperistalsis, * failure of relaxation of LES
Rx of achalasia	*pneumatic dilatation*
infectious disease producing achalasia and Hirschsprung's disease	*Chagas' disease due to Trypanosoma cruzi:* neurotoxins from leishmania destroy ganglion cells of the distal esophagus/rectum
clinical findings in diffuse esophageal spasm	• **intermittent dysphagia for solids/liquids,** • *noncardiac chest pain:* closely simulates angina pectoris, • *barium study:* "corkscrew" esophagus, • *esophageal manometry:* * intermittent, simultaneous contractions, * normal peristalsis between contractions
Rx of diffuse esophageal spasm	• *calcium channel blockers,* • *nitrates*
hiatal hernia	*sliding hiatal hernia:* * herniation of the proximal stomach through a widened diaphragmatic hiatus, * GERD occurs at night
cause of heartburn	*GERD:* * transient relaxation of LES after eating, * reflux of acid/bile into the distal esophagus
factors determining reflux esophagitis	• **frequency of LES relaxations,** • *rate of gastric emptying,* • *potency of refluxate:* * acid, * bile, * pepsin, • *efficiency of esophageal clearance:* * motility, * contribution of HCO_3^- from salivary glands (neutralizes acid)
predisposing causes of GERD	• **factors lowering LES tone:** e.g., * smoking, * alcohol, * caffeine, * fatty foods, • *sliding hiatal hernia,* • *PUD,* • *pyloric obstruction*
S/S of GERD	• **heartburn 30–60 minutes after eating/reclining:** relieved by antacids, • *dysphagia:* due to acid injury, • *noncardiac chest pain:* GERD MCC, • *nocturnal cough:* GERD MCC, • *chronic cough,* • *nocturnal asthma:* GERD MCC, • *laryngitis in AM:* acid injury of vocal cords, • *water-brash:* acidic taste in the mouth in AM

Table continued in following page

Table 9–2. ORAL CAVITY AND ESOPHAGEAL
DISORDERS *Continued*

Most Common...	Answer and Explanation
complications associated with GERD	• **Barrett's esophagus:** esophageal ulceration leads to glandular metaplasia, • *increased risk for adenocarcinoma,* • *stricture:* ~10%
lab test used to document GERD	*pH electrode left in the distal esophagus overnight*
test used to document extent/ severity of GERD	*endoscopy* with Bx
test used to define whether GERD is the cause of chest pain	*acid perfusion:* * Bernstein test, * reproduction of chest pain indicates GERD is responsible
Rx of GERD	• *Step 1 Rx:* * raise head of bed, * lose weight, * stop smoking/drinking, * avoid foods/drugs that lower LES tone, * use antacids or alginic acid after meals and at bedtime, • *Step 2 Rx:* proton blockers most effective agents, • *Step 3 Rx:* surgery (Nissen fundoplication)
cause of infectious esophagitis	• **HSV,** • *CMV,* • *Candida*
clinical findings of HSV esophagitis	• **punctate ulcers without plaques,** • *multinucleated squamous cells with intranuclear inclusions*
clinical findings of CMV esophagitis	• *large ulcers,* • *intranuclear inclusions in endothelial cells/fibroblasts*
clinical findings of *Candida* esophagitis	• *nodular masses,* • *cottage cheese–like membranes*
cause of infectious esophagitis in AIDS	*Candida albicans:* esophagitis is an AIDS-defining lesion (not oral candidiasis)
Rx of *Herpes* esophagitis	*acyclovir*
Rx of CMV esophagitis	*ganciclovir:* foscarnet is used in cases that are resistant to ganciclovir
Rx of *Candida* esophagitis	• *ketoconazole or* • *fluconazole*

Table 9–2. ORAL CAVITY AND ESOPHAGEAL
DISORDERS *Continued*

Most Common...	Answer and Explanation
causes of corrosive esophagitis	• **ingestion of strong alkali:** * ammonia/lye, * cause liquefactive necrosis (greater penetration and scar), • *ingestion of acid:* * hydrochloric/sulfuric acid, * cause coagulation necrosis (more superficial damage)
initial management of corrosive esophagitis	*early endoscopy within 24-hours to evaluate the extent of damage*
complications associated with corrosive esophagitis	• **stricture,** • *perforation,* • *esophageal cancer*
drugs associated with esophagitis	• *tetracycline/doxycycline,* • *NSAIDs,* • *vitamin C,* • *ferrous sulfate,* • *potassium chloride,* • *quinidine*
age group/site of esophagitis related to drugs	• *elderly,* • *mid-esophagus*
cause of esophageal varices	*portal hypertension secondary to alcoholic cirrhosis*
COD in cirrhosis	*rupture of esophageal varices*
presentations of an upper GI bleed	• *hematemesis* and/or • *melena* [See Table 9–1.]
initial steps in management of an acute upper GI bleed	• **assess/maintain intravascular volume,** • *insert NG tube for gastric aspirate/lavage:* documents upper GI source of bleeding, • *endoscopy:* * most important diagnostic test, * value in Rx as well
Rx for acute variceal bleed	*endoscopy with variceal ligation or banding:* fewer rebleeds than sclerotherapy
pharmacologic agents used to control upper GI bleed	• **octreotide:** * somatostatin analogue given IV, * reduces splanchnic blood flow and portal vein pressure, • *vasopressin* IV: too many side effects, • *IV H_2 blockers:* ? useful in lowering the risk for rebleeding in PUD

Table continued in following page

Table 9–2. **ORAL CAVITY AND ESOPHAGEAL DISORDERS** *Continued*

Most Common...	Answer and Explanation
Rx for variceal bleed if endoscopy/drugs are not working	• *balloon tamponade:* e.g., * Sengstaken-Blakemore tube, * many complications, • *caval shunting,* • *TIPS:* * transjugular intrahepatic portosystemic shunt, * metal stent connects hepatic vein with portal vein, * reduces portal pressure but increases risk of encephalopathy, • β-*blockers/nitrates:* * reduce portal pressure, * prevent rebleeding
cause of a tear or rupture of the distal esophagus/proximal stomach	*severe vomiting/retching in an alcoholic or patient with bulimia nervosa* [A tear is called Mallory-Weiss syndrome and a rupture, Boerhaave's syndrome.]
benign tumor of the GI tract, including esophagus	*leiomyoma:* it is usually asymptomatic in the esophagus
malignant tumor of the mid-esophagus	*squamous carcinoma* [adenocarcinoma is the most common esophageal cancer.]
risk factors for squamous carcinoma of esophagus	• **smoking/alcohol,** • *nitrosamines,* • *lye strictures,* • *Plummer-Vinson syndrome,* • *achalasia,* • *HPV* [There is a 3:1 male/female ratio for esophageal cancer. It is more common in blacks than whites.]
clinical findings in esophageal cancer	• **dysphagia for solids,** • *weight loss,* • *hoarseness:* involves recurrent laryngeal nerve, • *squamous cancers can ectopically produce PTH-like peptide:* hypercalcemia, • *spread locally first and then metastasize to the lungs, liver,* • *5-year survival* <15%
cause of adenocarcinoma of the distal esophagus	*Barrett's esophagus due to GERD:* * see above, * most common esophageal cancer

Gastroenterology **377**

Table 9–2. ORAL CAVITY AND ESOPHAGEAL DISORDERS *Continued*

Question: A 45-year-old woman has dysphagia for solids and liquids. What disorders should be included in your differential? **SELECT 4**
- (A) Plummer-Vinson syndrome
- (B) Myasthenia gravis
- (C) GERD
- (D) Achalasia
- (E) PSS
- (F) Lower esophageal ring

Answers: (B), (D), (E), (F): Dysphagia for solids and liquids connotes a motility problem in the esophagus. The differential should include myasthenia gravis **(choice B)**, which involves the upper esophagus, achalasia **(choice D)**, which involves the lower esophagus, PSS **(choice E)**, which involves the lower esophagus, and a lower esophageal ring **(choice F)**, which produces intermittent obstruction at the gastroesophageal junction. The esophageal web of Plummer-Vinson syndrome, and peptic ulceration and stricture formation associated with GERD are associated with dysphagia for solids and not liquids **(choices A and C are incorrect)**.

ACTH = adrenocorticotropic hormone, AD = autosomal dominant, AIDS = acquired immunodeficiency syndrome, Bx = biopsy, CD = Crohn's disease, COD = cause of death, CMV = cytomegalovirus, CREST = calcinosis, Raynaud's phenomenon, esophageal dysfunction, sclerodactyly, telangiectasia, CSF = cerebrospinal fluid, DM = dermatomyositis, EBV = Epstein-Barr virus, GE = gastroesophageal, GERD = gastroesophageal reflux disease, GI = gastrointestinal, HIV = human immunodeficiency virus, HPV = human papilloma virus, HSV = Herpes simplex virus, Ig = immunoglobulin, IM = intramuscular, IV = intravenous, LES = lower esophageal sphincter, MCC = most common cause, NG = nasogastric, NSAIDs = nonsteroidal anti-inflammatory drugs, PM = polymyositis, PO = oral, PSS = progressive systemic sclerosis, PTH = parathormone, PUD = peptic ulcer disease, R/O = rule out, Rx = treatment, S/S = signs and symptoms, TIPS = transjugular intrahepatic portosystemic shunt.

Table 9–3. STOMACH DISORDERS

Most Common...	Answer and Explanation
gastric causes of hypergastrinemia	• **patient on an H_2 blocker:** acid has a negative feedback on the release of gastrin from the G cells in the antrum, • *gastric distention,* • *PA,* • *ZE syndrome*
cause of increased BAO and MAO in a gastric analysis	*duodenal ulcer disease* [A BAO (normal <5 mEq/h) is collected over a 1-hour period on an empty stomach. The MAO (normal 5–20 mEq/h) is collected over 1 hour after penta-

Table continued on following page

Table 9–3. STOMACH DISORDERS *Continued*

Most Common...	Answer and Explanation
Continued	gastrin stimulation. The BAO:MAO ratio is normally 0.20:1. Duodenal ulcers have an increase in BAO (5–15 mEq/h), MAO (20–60 mEq/h), and BAO:MAO ratio (0.40–0.60:1) owing to an increase in parietal cell mass and increased response to stimuli. Gastric ulcers have a normal or slightly low BAO and MAO. ZE syndrome has an extremely high BAO (>20 mEq/h), MAO (>60 mEq/h), and BAO:MAO ratio (>0.60:1.)]
complications of achlorhydria	• **protein maldigestion,** • *decreased release of B_{12} from meat products,* • *gastric polyps,* • *adenocarcinoma of the stomach* [Achlorhydria is where gastric pH never falls below 6 after pentagastrin stimulation.]
factors regulating stomach emptying	• *distention:* activates a reflex involving the vagus nerve, • *hormones:* e.g., * gastrin (stimulates), * secretin (inhibits), * gastric inhibitory peptide (inhibits), motilin (stimulates), • *composition of the gastric meal:* fats inhibit motility
causes of gastroparesis	• **autonomic neuropathy: diabetes mellitus MCC,** • *muscle disorders:* e.g., PSS, • *infiltrative disorders:* e.g., amyloidosis, • *anorexia nervosa:* gastric dysrhythmias, • *vagotomy,* • *metabolic:* e.g., * hyperglycemia (releases GIP), * hypokalemia, • *drugs:* e.g., anticholinergics, • *pyloric obstruction:* e.g., chronic duodenal ulcer
S/S of gastroparesis	• **early satiety,** • *bloating,* • *N/V:* undigested food, • *weight loss*
lab tests to confirm gastroparesis	• **ingest radiolabeled meal and measure transit time for emptying,** • *endoscopy:* R/O gastric obstruction
Rx of gastroparesis	• **prokinetic agents:** e.g., * cisapride, * metoclopramide, • *dietary changes:* e.g., * avoid fatty foods, * high-fiber diets
clinical findings in nonulcer dyspepsia	• **persistent ulcer-like symptoms but no radiographic or endoscopic abnormalities,** • *affects ~20% of people in United States,* • *Bx may reveal inflammation and Helicobacter pylori:* Rx for H. pylori does not remove the symptoms

Table 9–3. STOMACH DISORDERS *Continued*

Most Common...	Answer and Explanation
cause of acute erosive gastritis	• **NSAIDs,** • *CMV:* AIDS patients, • *smoking,* • *alcohol,* • *burns:* Curling's ulcers, • *CNS injury:* Cushing's ulcers, • *uremia*
location for NSAID-induced erosions/ ulcers	• *prepyloric area,* • *antrum* [Erosions/ulcers are dose-dependent.]
S/S of erosive gastritis	*upper GI bleed:* * hematemesis, * melena, * melenemesis
Rx of NSAID-induced erosions/ ulcers	• **reduce dose of NSAIDs,** • *D/C NSAID:* replace with acetaminophen, • *misoprostol:* * synthetic prostaglandin, * expensive, * produces diarrhea [H_2-blockers and sucralfate are not effective in preventing NSAID-induced ulcers.]
cause of type A (body/fundus) chronic gastritis	*PA:* autoimmune destruction of parietal cells in the body/fundus
antibodies found in type A chronic gastritis	• **antiparietal antibodies:** 90%, • *anti-IF antibodies:* * 50%, * less sensitive but more specific for PA
complications in type A chronic gastritis	• **achlorhydria,** • *hypergastrinemia,* • *G cell hyperplasia:* potential for gastric carcinoid tumor, • *gastric polyps,* • *increased risk for adenocarcinoma,* • *macrocytic anemia*
cause of type B (antrum/pylorus) chronic gastritis	*Helicobacter pylori*
microbiologic features of *H. pylori*	• *gram-negative, curved rod,* • *produces urease and mucolytic proteases,* • *present in 40–50% of the general population,* • *transmitted by fecal-oral route,* • *found in the mucus layer lining the antrum,* • *urease converts urea into ammonia:* ammonia destroys the bicarbonate-rich mucus layer leading to gastritis and PUD, • *gastrin levels are normal*
tests used to identify *H. pylori*	• **CLO-test:** * detects urease in gastric Bx obtained by endoscopy, * 95% sensitivity and specificity, • *serologic tests:* * most cost-effective test, * remain positive (limits usefulness for follow-up), * 95% sensitivity, * 90–95% specificity, • *radiolabeled urea breath test:* * *Table continued on following page*

Table 9–3. STOMACH DISORDERS *Continued*

Most Common...	Answer and Explanation
Continued	currently too expensive, * likely to become the test of choice in the near future, * 95–98% sensitivity and specificity
diseases caused by *H. pylori*	• **duodenal ulcer:** * 90–95%, * usually in association with gastric metaplasia, • *gastric ulcer:* ~80%, • *type B chronic atrophic gastritis,* • *gastric adenocarcinoma:* an association more so than a cause at the present time, • *low-grade B cell malignant lymphoma*
cause of type AB (environmental) chronic atrophic gastritis	*H. pylori in concert with vitamin C deficiency:* * vitamin C prevents nitrosamination, * nitrosamines produce gastritis and adenocarcinoma
cause of protein-losing enteropathy	*Ménétrier's disease:* * giant rugal folds, * glands that secrete an excessive amount of protein-rich mucus
cause of PUD	*H. pylori*
arteries responsible for bleeds in PUD	*gastric ulcer:* left gastric artery, • *duodenal ulcer:* gastroduodenal artery
clinical findings noted in duodenal versus gastric ulcers	• *most common PUD,* • *more commonly associated with H. pylori,* • *greater male to female ratio,* • *more likely to bleed/perforate,* • *located on the anterior portion of the first part of the duodenum,* • *blood group O relationship,* • *greater BAO and MAO,* • *MEN I relationship,* • *never malignant,* • *more likely to wake the patient up late at night*
clinical findings noted in gastric versus duodenal ulcers	• *ulcer located on the lesser curvature of the antrum:* type B chronic atrophic gastritis, • *1–3% chance of representing cancer,* • *pain after eating:* aggravated by food but improved with antacids, • *BAO and MAO normal to decreased*
aggravating causes of gastric ulcers	• **smoking,** • *bile reflux,* • *COPD,* • *renal failure*
aggravating causes of duodenal ulcers	• **smoking,** • *COPD,* • *renal failure,* • *cirrhosis*
Rx of *H. pylori*	• *tetracycline or amoxicillin* + • *metronidazole* + • *bismuth subsalicylate* [The above is prescribed for 2 wks.]

Table 9–3. STOMACH DISORDERS *Continued*

Most Common...	Answer and Explanation
goal of Rx of *H. pylori*	• *heal the ulcer,* • *eradicate the bacteria*
Rx of PUD	• **Rx *H. pylori:*** see above, • *antacids:* heal duodenal > gastric ulcers, • *H₂-blockers:* e.g., cimetidine/ranitidine: effective in both gastric and duodenal ulcers (reduce acid, pain, recurrences), • *hydrogen pump inhibitors:* e.g., omeprazole/lansoprazole: fastest in relieving pain and in healing duodenal > gastric ulcers, • *coating agents:* e.g., sucralfate: * binds to ulcer bed, * neutralizes pepsin, * stimulates prostaglandin production
complications of PUD	• **bleeding:** duodenal > gastric, • *perforation:* duodenal (free anterior wall, 5–10%) > gastric, • *gastric outlet obstruction:* * duodenal > gastric, * aspiration of >300 mL of fluid is diagnostic, • *pancreatitis:* duodenal > gastric
S/S of perforated PUD	• **sudden onset of epigastric pain,** • *left shoulder pain:* air under the diaphragm in 85%
Rx of perforated PUD	*surgery*
cause of dumping syndrome	*Billroth II gastrojejunostomy:* operation for intractable duodenal ulcer disease
S/S of dumping syndrome	• *early* (10–30 minutes after eating): * explosive diarrhea, * vasomotor symptoms: ♦ weakness, ♦ dizziness, ♦ flushing, ♦ palpitations, * due to rapid exit of a hyperosmolar meal into small intestine with release of vasoactive hormones, • *late* (2–4 h later): * only vasomotor symptoms, * hypoglycemia is secondary to increased glucose reabsorption and excessive release of insulin
cause of a duodenal ulcer without *H. pylori*	*ZE*
cause of ZE syndrome	*pancreatic islet cell tumor secreting excessive gastrin:* * malignant (~70%), * located in the pancreas (85%), * association with MEN I syndrome (25%)

Table continued on following page

Table 9–3. STOMACH DISORDERS *Continued*

Most Common...	Answer and Explanation
S/S of ZE	• **triad:** * peptic ulceration, * diarrhea, * acid hypersecretion, • *ulcers:* * usually a solitary duodenal ulcer, * multiple ulcers in unusual places (e.g., jejunum, duodenum) are uncommon, • *associated with MEN I syndrome*
screening and confirmatory test for ZE	• *screening:* * BAO markedly increased (see above), * MAO maximally increased, * BAO:MAO ratio >0.60:1, * serum gastrin >1000 pg/mL: diagnostic, • *confirmatory:* IV secretin test: paradoxical increase in an already high serum gastrin level
Rx of ZE	• **surgical removal:** 20–25% chance of complete removal, • *parietal cell vagotomy,* • *H_2-blockers/proton blockers:* most effective, • *chemotherapy for metastatic disease:* streptozocin and 5-fluorouracil
gastric polyps	• **hyperplastic polyp:** * most common type (~75%), * hamartomas, * rarely malignant, • *adenomatous polyp:* * neoplastic, * potential for malignant transformation if >2 cm, • *Peutz-Jeghers polyp:* * AD, * hamartomas, * rarely malignant
benign soft tissue tumor	*leiomyoma:* * most common location is the stomach, * ulcerate or bleed
malignancy	• **intestinal type of adenocarcinoma:** * *H. pylori*-related, * decreasing incidence, • *diffuse type:* * not *H. pylori*-related, * increasing incidence
causes of gastric adenocarcinoma	• ***H. pylori:*** an association more than a causal relationship at the moment, • *adenomatous polyps,* • *nitrosamines,* • *smoked foods,* • *blood group A,* • *all types of chronic atrophic gastritis,* • *smoking,* • *alcohol,* • *previous gastric surgery*
locations of gastric adenocarcinoma	• **lesser curvature of pyloroantrum:** * 50%, * same site as gastric ulcers, • *cardia:* * 25%, * rapidly increasing, • *body and fundus:* 25%
S/S of gastric cancer	• **weight loss,** • *epigastric pain,* • *early satiety,* • *vomiting,* • *epigastric mass*

Table 9–3. STOMACH DISORDERS *Continued*

Most Common...	Answer and Explanation
sites of metastasis of gastric cancer	• **regional lymph nodes,** • *liver,* • *lung,* • *ovaries:* * Krukenberg tumor, * bilateral, • *Virchow's left supraclavicular node,* • *umbilicus:* Sister Mary Joseph sign
paraneoplastic syndromes associated with gastric cancer	• *acanthosis nigricans:* dark, papillomatous plaques in intertriginous areas, • *Leser-Trelat sign:* multiple outcroppings of seborrheic keratoses
Rx and prognosis of gastric adenocarcinoma	• *surgery:* total gastrectomy, if confined to the stomach/regional nodes, • *chemotherapy:* not generally useful, • *postoperative radiation:* decreases local recurrence, • *prognosis:* * localized to mucosa/submucosa: 90% 5-year survival, * extends through the serosa/no nodes: 50% 5-year survival, * lymph node involvement: <10% 5-year survival
extranodal site for malignant lymphoma	*stomach:* * usually a high-grade, B cell immunoblastic lymphoma, * low-grade B cell lymphomas are *H. pylori*-related

Question: Which of the following characterize a duodenal ulcer rather than a gastric ulcer? **SELECT 3**
  (A) Perforation
  (B) Hematemesis
  (C) Less association with *H. pylori*
  (D) Increased risk in smokers
  (E) MEN I relationship
  (F) More often associated with ZE syndrome
  (G) Pain aggravated by eating

Answers: (A), (E), (F): Duodenal ulcers are more likely to perforate (choice A), are more often associated with *H. pylori* (choice C), are associated with MEN I (choice E) and ZE (choice F), and are more likely to have pain relieved by eating (choice G is incorrect). Both duodenal and gastric ulcers are associated with hematemesis and smoking (choices B and D are incorrect).

AD = autosomal dominant, AIDS = acquired immunodeficiency syndrome, BAO = basal acid output, Bx = biopsy, CMV = cytomegalovirus, CNS = central nervous system, COPD = chronic obstructive pulmonary disease, D/C = discontinue, G = gastrin, GI = gastrointestinal, GIP = gastric inhibitory peptide, H_2 = histamine, IF = intrinsic factor, IV = intravenous, MAO = maximal acid output, MCC = most common cause, MEN = multiple endocrine neoplasia, NSAIDs = nonsteroidal anti-inflammatory drugs, N/V = nausea and vomiting, PA = pernicious anemia, PSS = progressive systemic sclerosis, PUD = peptic ulcer disease, R/O = rule out, Rx = treatment, S/S = signs and symptoms, ZE = Zollinger-Ellison.

Table 9–4. ACUTE AND CHRONIC DIARRHEA

Most Common...	Answer and Explanation
nutrients absorbed in duodenum, jejunum, ileum	• *duodenum:* * iron, * calcium, * magnesium, * water-soluble vitamins, * monosaccharides • *jejunum:* * folate, * fatty acids, * amino acids, * monosaccharides, * water soluble vitamins, • *ileum:* * B_{12}, * conjugated bile acids, * fat-soluble vitamins, * fatty acids, * monosaccharides, * amino acids, * terminal ileum can adapt to absorbing all nutrients
functions of large bowel	• **forming stool,** • *producing mucin*
definition of diarrhea	*>250 g of stool per day*
time distinction between acute and chronic diarrhea	• *acute diarrhea <3 weeks* • *chronic diarrhea >4 weeks*
types of acute diarrhea	• **inflammatory,** • *noninflammatory*
differences between right- and left-sided diarrhea	• *right-sided small bowel:* * large volume (>1 liter), * modest increase in frequency of stooling, * no blood/mucus, * no tenesmus/urgency, * e.g., osmotic/secretory diarrheas, • *left-sided colon:* * small volume (<1 liter), * greater frequency, * blood/mucus, * tenesmus/urgency, * e.g., infectious diarrheas
mechanisms of infectious diarrhea	• *toxigenic,* • *invasive:* * enterocyte invasion, * mucosal penetration
cause of acute infectious diarrhea in adults	*viral gastroenteritis:* e.g., **Norwalk,** * Rotavirus [Most infectious diarrheas are self-limited and do not require antibiotics.]
tests used to evaluate infectious diarrheas	• **fecal smear for leukocytes:** presence of leukocytes distinguishes an invasive diarrhea (e.g., shigellosis) versus an osmotic/secretory diarrhea, • *stool cultures,* • *stools for O/P,* • *stool guaiac:* * blood plus leukocytes indicate invasive bacteria, * exceptions: ♦ UC, ♦ ischemic colitis, • *toxin assay of stool:* R/O pseudomembranous colitis due to *Clostridium difficile,* • *proctosigmoidoscopy:* R/O * pseudomembranous colitis, * UC, * cancer

Table 9–4. ACUTE AND CHRONIC DIARRHEA *Continued*

Most Common...	Answer and Explanation
causes of acute, infectious diarrhea with a negative stool for leukocytes	• **viruses:** * Rotavirus, * Norwalk, • *protozoa:* * *Giardia lamblia,* * *Cryptosporidium,* • *bacteria with preformed toxin:* * Staphylococcus aureus, * Bacillus cereus, * Clostridium perfringens,* • *bacteria with enterotoxin production and stimulation of cAMP:* * enterotoxigenic *Escherichia coli* (traveler's diarrhea), * Vibrio cholerae*
causes of acute infectious diarrhea with a positive fecal smear for leukocytes	• **bacteria with mucosal invasion:** * ***Campylobacter jejuni,*** * *Salmonella typhimurium,* * *Shigella sonnei,* * *Yersinia enterocolitica,* * *Vibrio vulnificus,* * *Staphylococcus aureus* (enterocolitis), • *bacteria with cytotoxin production:* * *Clostridium difficile,* * enterohemorrhagic *E. coli* (♦ serotype O157:H7, ♦ cause of HUS), * *Vibrio parahaemolyticus,* • *protozoa: Entamoeba histolytica,* • *virus:* CMV
causes of acute bloody diarrhea	• **invasive diarrhea:** the term dysentery is applied to infectious diarrheas with blood and leukocytes, • *ischemic colitis,* • *IBD*
cause of food poisoning in the United States	*Salmonella enteritidis:* see below
clinical findings in *Staphylococcus aureus* food poisoning	• *preformed toxin:* * egg products, * cream, * mayonnaise, • *cAMP-mediated,* • *incubation:* 1–6 hours, • *clinical:* * afebrile, * vomiting, * self-limited in 12–24 hours, • *lab Dx:* food immunoassay or culture, • *Rx:* none
clinical findings in *Clostridium perfringens* food poisoning	• *preformed toxin:* * precooked beef/turkey, * "church picnic" diarrhea, • *incubation:* 8–12 hours, • *clinical:* * +/− fever, * vomiting, * self-limited in 24 hrs, • *lab Dx:* food/stool cultures, • *Rx:* none
clinical findings in *Bacillus cereus* food poisoning	• *preformed toxin:* reheated fried rice, • cAMP-mediated, • incubation: 1–6 hours, • *clinical:* * afebrile, * vomiting, * self-limited in 20–24 hours, • *Rx:* none
clinical findings in adult food poisoning due to *Clostridium botulinum*	• *preformed neurotoxin:* home-canned vegetables, fruits, meats, • *neurotoxin:* irreversibly blocks Ach release from cholinergic receptors, • *incubation:* 18–24 hours, • *clinical:* * diplopia first sign (bilateral lateral rectus muscle weakness), * ptosis, * mydriasis, * dysphonia/-arthria/-phagia, * descending

Table continued on following page

Table 9–4. ACUTE AND CHRONIC DIARRHEA *Continued*

Most Common...	Answer and Explanation
Continued	paralysis, * respiratory failure, * $+/-$ diarrhea early and constipation late, • *lab Dx:* * toxin assay of serum/stool (~30% sensitivity), * culture stool (60% sensitivity), * culture suspected food, • *Rx:* * trivalent antitoxin, * respiratory support, • *COD:* * respiratory failure, * mortality <10%, • *prevention:* spores killed by heating in a pressure cooker for 30 minutes at 120°C
clinical findings associated with infectious diarrhea due to enterotoxigenic *E. coli*	• *toxin:* * present in water/salads, * heat labile toxin activates cAMP, * heat stabile toxin activates guanylate cyclase, • *incubation:* 24–72 hours, • *clinical:* * secretory diarrhea, * $+/-$ fever, * self-limited in 24–36 hours, • *lab Dx:* toxin assay of stool, • *Rx:* TMP/SMX or quinolones
clinical findings associated with infectious diarrhea due to *Vibrio cholerae*	• *toxin:* ingested in contaminated water/food/seafood along Gulf Coast, * stimulates cAMP, • *clinical:* * afebrile, * "rice water" stools, * severe volume depletion, * breast-fed infants protected from cholera (antibodies in mother's milk), * may last days to weeks, • *Rx:* * oral hydration with: ♦ glucose or rice (aids in reabsorption of Na^+), ♦ Na^+ ~90 mEq/L, ♦ K^+ ~20 mEq/L, ♦ citrate or bicarbonate ~30 mEq/L, ♦ Cl^- ~80 mEq/L, * tetracycline shortens duration
clinical findings associated with infectious diarrhea due to *Campylobacter jejuni*	• *transmission:* * contaminated water, * unpasteurized milk, * poultry (chickens/turkeys), * seafood, * infected children in day care centers, • *clinical:* * invades jejunum/ileum/colon (crypt abscesses/ulcers resemble UC), * bloody diarrhea/leukocytes, * secretory diarrhea, * abdominal pain, * high fever, * organisms noted in stools, * $+/-$ bacteremia (*C. fetus* more likely), * self-limited in 5–7 days, • *complications:* * HUS, * Reiter's syndrome, * HLA-B27$^+$ ankylosing spondylitis, * toxic megacolon, * pseudomembranous colitis, • *Rx:* * hydration, * erythromycin in severe cases
clinical findings associated with infectious diarrhea due to *Salmonella* non-*typhi* species	• *transmission:* * animal reservoirs (turtles, iguanas), * homosexuals (fecal-oral route), * institutionalized/immunocompromised patients, • *clinical syndromes:* see below • *Rx:* * antibiotics not recommended in enterocolitis

Table 9–4. ACUTE AND CHRONIC DIARRHEA *Continued*

Most Common...	Answer and Explanation
Continued	(prolongs carrier state unless bacteremia is present or patient is immunocompromised), * ciprofloxacin drug of choice
clinical syndromes associated with *Salmonella* non-*typhi* species	• **asymptomatic carrier state:** cholelithiasis often noted, • *enterocolitis:* * S. enteritidis* is MCC of enteritis, * organisms are ingested with poultry, colonize the bowel, and produce toxin (MCC "food poisoning"), * non-bloody diarrhea (leukocytes, fever, vomiting), • *enteric fever:* * simulates typhoid fever, * bacteremia (*S. choleraesuis* most common), * metastatic infection (♦ bones, ♦ meninges)
epidemiologic characteristics of typhoid fever (*Salmonella typhi*)	*transmission:* * fecal-oral route, * usually an asymptomatic human carrier with chronic cholelithiasis
clinical stages/Rx of typhoid fever	• *initial infection:* bacteria penetrate ileal mucosa and enter macrophages in Peyer's patches in first 24 hours, • *first week:* bacteremic phase with: * fever/chills, * abdominal tenderness, * positive blood culture (bone marrow culture most sensitive), • *second week:* * "rose spot" rash on upper anterior trunk (vasculitis), * diarrhea (positive stool culture), * triad of ♦ hepatosplenomegaly, ♦ bradycardia, ♦ absolute neutropenia, • *third week:* complications including * intestinal bleeding, * perforation, • *fourth week:* * resolution, * relapse, * chronic carrier state (see below), • *Rx:* * ciprofloxacin or ceftriaxone, * Rx may encourage a chronic carrier state, • *prevention:* * vaccine, * food precautions
clinical features of chronic carrier state in typhoid fever	• *definition:* persistence of organism 1 year after infection, • *site of infection:* GB, particularly if cholelithiasis is present, • *Rx:* ampicillin and surgery, if stones are present
drugs causing pseudomembranous colitis	• **ampicillin,** • *clindamycin,* • *cephalosporins* [Note: vancomycin cannot cause pseudomembranous colitis.]

Table continued on following page

Table 9–4. ACUTE AND CHRONIC DIARRHEA *Continued*

Most Common...	Answer and Explanation
clinical findings associated with infectious diarrhea due to *Clostridium difficile*	• *clinical:* * fever, * crampy abdominal pain, * watery diarrhea with mucus and blood 1–6 weeks post antibiotics, • *lab Dx:* * gold standard test is CPE of a filtrate of stool and reversal with antitoxin, * rapid ELISA test for toxin A, • *Rx:* * metronidazole (less expensive than oral vancomycin), * oral vancomycin produces resistant strains
clinical findings associated with infectious diarrhea due to *Shigella* species	• *transmission:* * fecal-oral route, * *S. sonnei* most common cause, * no animal reservoirs or carrier state, * extremely high infectivity rate (10 to 100 organisms), • *clinical:* * fever, * bloody diarrhea, * pseudomembranes in rectosigmoid (mistaken for UC), • *complications:* * HUS, * Reiter's syndrome, * bacteremia (*S. dysenteriae* MCC), * rectal prolapse, * HLA-B27+ ankylosing spondylitis, • *lab Dx:* stool culture, • *Rx:* ciprofloxacin in severe cases
strain of *E. coli* associated with HUS	*enterohemorrhagic strain O157:H7 serotype:* often contaminates improperly cooked beef and raw milk
strain of *E. coli* associated with dysentery	*enteroinvasive E. coli:* uncommon in the United States
clinical findings associated with infectious diarrhea due to *Yersinia enterocolitica*	• *transmission:* contaminated food/milk products, • *clinical:* * dysentery with absolute neutrophilic leukocytosis, * chronic enteritis in children (failure to thrive), * RLQ pain simulating acute appendicitis and CD, * mesenteric lymphadenitis (granulomatous microabscesses), * pharyngitis in adults/children, * iron-overloaded patients susceptible to septicemia, • *complications:* * Reiter's syndrome, * HLA-B27 + ankylosing spondylitis, * autoimmune diseases (Graves' disease), * common contaminant in blood transfusions, • *lab Dx:* * stool culture, * culture nodes, • *Rx:* ciprofloxacin
clinical findings associated with infectious diarrhea due to *Vibrio parahaemolyticus*	• *transmission:* toxin ingested in raw or poorly cooked shellfish, • *clinical:* * fever, * watery or bloody diarrhea, * may contaminate open wounds, • *lab Dx:* stool culture, • *Rx:* antibiotics do not shorten the course

Table 9–4. ACUTE AND CHRONIC DIARRHEA *Continued*

Most Common...	Answer and Explanation
clinical findings associated with *Vibrio vulnificus*	• *transmission:* * most invasive *Vibrio* infection in United States, * transmitted by eating raw oysters harvested from water along the Gulf coast or contamination of an open wound by seawater, • *clinical:* * contamination of open wounds with salt water leading to a necrotizing vasculitis/fasciitis/myositis (no underlying disease necessary), * septicemia in alcoholics with liver disease, • *lab Dx:* culture wound/blood, • *Rx:* ceftazidime + doxycycline
parasite-induced cause of dysentery in the United States	*Entamoeba histolytica*
clinical findings associated with infectious diarrhea due to *Entamoeba histolytica*	• *transmission:* * ingestion of cysts (resistant to gastric acid) in water/food, * unprotected anal intercourse, * cysts excyst in alkaline environment of small bowel, * trophozoites burrow into mucosa of cecum, sigmoid colon, and rectum ("flask-shaped" ulcers), • *clinical:* * bloody diarrhea, * absence of fever in 40% (key feature), • *complications:* * hepatic abscess ("anchovy paste" abscess), * direct extension into right pleural cavity, * dissemination, • *lab Dx:* * stool for O/P identify cysts/trophozoites, * indirect hemagglutination titer (80–90% sensitivity), • *Rx:* metronidazole
causes of acute infectious diarrhea associated with bloody stools	• ***Campylobacter jejuni,*** • *Shigella sonnei,* • *Entamoeba histolytica,* • *Vibrio parahaemolyticus,* • *Balantidium coli*
causes of chronic diarrhea	• **osmotic:** e.g., lactase deficiency, • *secretory:* e.g., laxatives, • *inflammatory:* e.g., IBD, • *malabsorption:* e.g., celiac disease, • *motility dysfunction:* e.g., IBS, • *chronic infections:* e.g., diarrhea in AIDS
causes of osmotic diarrhea	• **disaccharidase deficiency:** lactase deficiency (in Native Americans, Asian-Americans, African-Americans), • *ingestion of poorly absorbable solutes:* * magnesium sulfate/hydroxide (laxatives/antacids), * mannitol, * sorbitol (chewing gum/diet candy), * lactulose Rx, • *mucosal malabsorption:* e.g., in celiac disease, undigested CHO acts as osmotic agents

Table continued on following page

Table 9–4. ACUTE AND CHRONIC DIARRHEA *Continued*

Most Common...	Answer and Explanation
mechanism of diarrhea in lactase deficiency	*undigested lactose in the colon is converted by bacteria into fatty acids* (acid stool pH), *methane/hydrogen/CO_2* (bloating, gaseous distention)
tests used to document osmotic diarrhea secondary to lactase deficiency	• **hydrogen breath test:** gold standard, • *fasting:* diarrhea stops with fasting, • *stool osmotic gap:* * normal stool osmolality (use 300 mOsm/kg) and subtract the measured stool electrolytes: 300 mOsm/kg − 2 × (stool Na^+ + stool K^+), * osmotic gap in lactase deficiency is >100 mOsm/kg, • *stool pH <7:* due to fatty acids
Rx of lactase deficiency	• *avoid dairy products,* • *lactase tablets prior to eating dairy products*
causes of secretory diarrheas	• **laxatives:** * phenolphthalein, * senna, * anthraquinones, * castor oil, * bisacodyl, • *medications:* diuretics, • *enterotoxin-induced:* * stimulate cAMP (enterotoxigenic *E. coli, Vibrio cholerae*), * no inflammation of bowel mucosa, • *certain types of invasive diarrhea:* * mucosal injury causes a loss of isotonic fluid, * e.g., *C. jejuni, Y. enterocolitica, S. sonnei,* • *pancreatic cholera:* non-β cell, malignant islet cell tumor secreting vasointestinal peptide, • *carcinoid syndrome:* secretion of serotonin and substance P, • *medullary carcinoma of thyroid:* secretion of calcitonin/serotonin, • *ZE syndrome:* gastrin effect, • *bile acid diarrhea:* see below, • *microscopic collagenous colitis:* * normal gross appearance, * intraepithelial lymphocytes, * subepithelial collagen band
tests used to document secretory diarrheas	• *stool osmotic gap:* * see above formula, * <50 mOsm/kg, • *fasting:* diarrhea continues, • *culture:* R/O invasive types of diarrhea, • *alkalinize stool:* pink color indicates phenolphthalein ingestion (laxative abuse), • *proctoscopy:* R/O melanosis coli from anthracene derivatives (senna, cascara, aloe), • *barium enema:* "cathartic colon" (hypomotile, dilated bowel with absent haustra), • *urine for 5-HIAA:* R/O carcinoid syndrome, • *serum VIP:* R/O VIPoma, • *serum gastrin, BAO/MAO:* R/O ZE

Table 9–4. ACUTE AND CHRONIC DIARRHEA *Continued*

Most Common...	Answer and Explanation
protozoal cause of chronic diarrhea in the United States	*Giardia lamblia:* * ingest cysts in contaminated water, * common in day care centers, * excyst in stomach, * trophozoites attach to small bowel mucosa, * extension into CBD
clinical signs of giardiasis	• **diarrhea,** • *malabsorption,* • *weight loss,* • *association with IgA deficiency,* • *Dx:* * stool for O/P, * Entero-Test (see below)
Rx for giardiasis	*metronidazole*
organisms detected with the Entero-Test (string test)	• *Cryptosporidium parvum,* • *Giardia lamblia,* • *Strongyloides stercoralis* [A string with one end attached to the cheek is swallowed and allowed to remain in the duodenum for a few hours. It is retrieved and the material is examined.]
test to R/O parasitic GI disorders	*stool for O/P:* gold standard test
clinical findings in balantidiasis	• *organism:* * *Balantidium coli,* * ciliate, • *transmission:* ingest cysts, • *clinical:* * colonic ulcers, * bloody diarrhea, • *Dx:* stool O/P, • *Rx:* tetracycline
clinical findings in trichuriasis	• *organism:* * *Trichuris trichiura,* * whipworm, * nematode, • transmission: ingest eggs, • *clinical:* * abdominal pain, * diarrhea, * rectal prolapse, *Dx:* * undeveloped eggs in stool, * eosinophilia, • *Rx:* mebendazole or albendazole
clinical findings in ascariasis	• *organism:* * *Ascaris lumbricoides,* * nematode, • *transmission:* * ingest eggs, * adults live free in small intestine lumen, • *clinical:* * cough/pneumonitis in lung phase, * vague GI complaints, * obstruction, • *Dx:* * undeveloped eggs in stool, * eosinophilia only in lung phase, • *Rx:* mebendazole or pyrantel pamoate
clinical findings in ancylostomiasis	• *organism:* * *Ancyclostoma duodenale,* * *Necator americanus,* * hookworms, * nematodes, • *transmission:* * larvae penetrate skin, * larva transmigrate through the lungs, * adults attach to villi in small intestine and feed on blood, • *clinical:* * dermatitis, *

Table continued on following page

Table 9–4. ACUTE AND CHRONIC DIARRHEA *Continued*

Most Common...	Answer and Explanation
Continued	cough/pneumonitis (lung phase), * diarrhea, * abdominal pain, * iron deficiency, • *Dx:* * undeveloped eggs in stool, * eosinophilia, * low serum ferritin, * positive stool guaiac, • *Rx:* mebendazole or pyrantel pamoate
clinical findings in strongyloidiasis	• *organism:* * *Strongyloides stercoralis,* * nematode, • *transmission:* * larvae penetrate skin, * autoinfection, * larvae transmigrate through the lungs, * female worms burrow into the duodenal mucosa, * rhabditiform larvae birthed in bowel wall and burrow out to the bowel lumen, • *clinical:* * cough/pleuritis (lung phase), * diarrhea, * epigastric pain, * AIDS-defining lesion (often disseminated), • *Dx:* * rhabditiform larvae in stool, * Entero-Test, * eosinophilia, • *Rx:* thiabendazole or ivermectin
clinical findings in anisakiasis	• *organism:* * *Anisakis* species, * nematode, • *transmission:* ingest larvae in marine fish (sushi bar), * larvae penetrate mucosa of stomach/small intestine, • *clinical:* * diarrhea, * epigastric pain, * N/V, • *Dx:* stomach Bx, • *Rx:* endoscopic removal of worms
clinical findings in hymenolepiasis	• *organism:* * *Hymenolepis nana,* * dwarf tapeworm, * cestode, * most common tapeworm infection, • *transmission:* * ingest eggs, * adults attach to small intestine, • *clinical:* * diarrhea, * abdominal pain, * anorexia, • *Dx:* stool for O/P, • *Rx:* praziquantel
clinical findings in diphyllobothriasis	• *organism:* * *Diphyllobothrium latum,* * fish tapeworm, * cestode, • *transmission:* * ingest larvae in lake trout, * adults attach in small intestine, • *clinical:* * diarrhea, * abdominal pain, * B_{12} deficiency, • *Dx:* * stool O/P, * proglottids in stool, • *Rx:* praziquantel
clinical findings in taeniasis	• *organisms:* * *Taenia saginata* (beef tapeworm), * *Taenia solium* (pork tapeworm), * cestodes, • *transmission:* * ingest larvae in beef/pork, * cow/pig intermediate hosts, * adults attach to small intestine, * humans are definitive host, • *clinical:* * digestive disturbances, * anorexia, * weight loss, • *Dx:* * stool for O/P, * proglottids in stool, • *Rx:* praziquantel

Table 9–4. ACUTE AND CHRONIC DIARRHEA *Continued*

Most Common...	Answer and Explanation
clinical findings of schistosomiasis involving the GI tract	• *organism:* * *Schistosoma japonicum,* * trematode, • *transmission:* penetration of skin by larvae in water, * adults present in mesenteric veins of small intestine, • *clinical:* diarrhea, • *Dx:* * stool for O/P, * serologic tests, • *Rx:* praziquantel
clinical findings in fasciolopsiasis	• *organism:* * *Fasciolopsis buski,* * intestinal fluke, * trematode, • *transmission:* * ingest larvae encysted on aquatic plants, * adults attach to small intestine, • *clinical:* * abdominal pain, * diarrhea, * edema, • *Dx:* * stool for O/P, * serologic tests, * eosinophilia, • *Rx:* praziquantel
clinical findings in clonorchiasis in GI tract	• *organism:* * *Clonorchis sinensis,* * Chinese liver fluke, * trematode, • *transmission:* * ingest larvae encysted in freshwater fish, * adults located in bile ducts/GB, • *clinical:* * diarrhea, * jaundice, * cholangiocarcinoma, • *Dx:* * stool O/P, * duodenal aspirate, • *Rx:* praziquantel or albendazole
causes of malabsorption (impaired digestion or absorption of one or more nutrients)	• **small bowel disease:** * mucosal absorptive defect (e.g., celiac disease), * loss of absorptive surface (e.g., resection), * enzyme deficiency (e.g., lactase deficiency), * lymphatic obstruction (e.g., Whipple's disease), • *maldigestion:* * problem with breaking down fat, protein, CHO, e.g., * chronic pancreatitis, • *bile salt deficiency:* bile salts are necessary for lipid absorption, e.g., cirrhosis
S/S suggesting malabsorption	• **diarrhea:** combination of decreased absorption and secretory diarrhea, • *greasy stools:* steatorrhea (increased fat in stool), • *weight loss with good appetite:* calorie loss, • *flatus/bowel distention:* fermentation of unabsorbed CHO, • *intolerance to dairy products:* secondary lactase deficiency, • *water-fat-soluble vitamin deficiencies:* see Table 9–11
screening tests for malabsorption of fat	• **qualitative stool for fat:** Sudan black fat stains, • *quantitative stool for fat:* * gold standard, * use if qualitative test is normal
screening test for small bowel disease	D-*xylose* [Xylose is a five-carbon sugar that does not require pancreatic amylases for absorption. A 25 g oral dose is given and urine is collected for 5 hours (normal is ≥5 g in urine).]

Table continued on following page

Table 9–4. ACUTE AND CHRONIC DIARRHEA *Continued*

Most Common...	Answer and Explanation
causes of decreased D-xylose absorption	• **small bowel disease:** e.g., celiac disease, • *bacterial overgrowth:* breakdown xylose before it is reabsorbed
screening test for bile salt deficiency	*radioactive bile breath test* [The presence of bacterial overgrowth causes the release of radioactive CO_2, which is reabsorbed and measured in the breath. Terminal ileal disease also produces a positive test, since colonic bacteria degrade the radioactive substrate and release radioactive CO_2.]
screening tests for pancreatic insufficiency	• **CT scan of the pancreas:** detect dystrophic calcification, • *bentiromide test:* checks for the ability of chymotrypsin to cleave PABA off bentiromide (liver converts PABA into arylamines, which are excreted and measured in the urine), • *ERCP:* * stimulation tests to measure enzymes, * radiography, • *IV secretin test:* gold standard test for pancreatic insufficiency
screening tests for bacterial overgrowth	• **^{14}C-xylose:** * most sensitive/specific test, * measures $^{14}CO_2$ in the breath, • *^{14}C-glycholate:* measures $^{14}CO_2$ in the breath, • *lactulose-H_2:* measures H_2 in breath
general tests used in evaluating malabsorption	• *serum albumin:* R/O protein loss, • *serum calcium:* R/O vitamin D deficiency, • *CBC:* R/O anemia, • *serum carotenes:* R/O vitamin A deficiency, • *serum electrolytes:* R/O * hypokalemia, * normal AG metabolic acidosis, • *serum folate/B_{12}:* * R/O megaloblastic anemia, * Schilling's test localizes cause of B_{12} deficiency, • *serum iron:* R/O iron deficiency, • *serum magnesium:* common cause of hypocalcemia, • *serum PT:* R/O vitamin K deficiency
small bowel disease causing malabsorption	*celiac disease*
pathogenesis of celiac disease	*autoimmune disease:* * antibodies directed against gliadin (alcohol extract of gluten in wheat), * HLA-B8, Drw3 associations, * women > men, * primarily involves the duodenum/jejunum

Table 9–4. ACUTE AND CHRONIC DIARRHEA *Continued*

Most Common...	Answer and Explanation
screening tests for celiac disease	• **antigliadin antibodies:** * >90% sensitivity, * IgG antibodies are very sensitive, * IgA antibodies are very specific, * combined specificity of >95%, • *antiendomysial antibodies:* * 70–90% sensitivity, * IgG antibodies are more sensitive and IgA antibodies are more specific for celiac disease
confirmatory test for celiac disease	*reappearance of normal villi after a gluten-free diet*
cause of Howell-Jolly bodies in celiac disease	*splenic atrophy:* * occurs in 10–15% of cases, * HJ bodies are remnants of nucleus in RBCs
skin disease associated with celiac disease	*dermatitis herpetiformis:* * autoimmune vesicular skin disease, * see Table 14–1
antibodies associated with DH	*IgA antiendomysial and reticulin antibodies:* ~70% of cases
serious complication of celiac disease	*small bowel T cell malignant lymphoma:* * 8–10%, * may occur after 10–15 years
Rx of celiac disease	*gluten-free diet:* * ~80% response, * refractory cases may respond to glucocorticoids
cause of Whipple's disease	*Trophermyma whippleii:* * defective gram + rod in macrophages, * identified with EM
clinical findings in Whipple's disease	• *male dominant,* • *clinical:* * **recurrent polyarthritis,** * fever, * steatorrhea, * generalized lymphadenopathy, * skin pigmentation
Rx of Whipple's disease	*TMP/SMX:* fatal if left untreated
infectious disease simulating Whipple's disease	*disseminated MAI:* * common cause of diarrhea in AIDS, * occurs when CD_4 T helper count <100 cells/μL
cause of chronic pancreatitis	*alcohol excess*
clinical findings in malabsorption secondary to chronic pancreatitis	• **weight loss:** * anorexia from pain, * maldigestion of nutrients, • *steatorrhea:* 40% after 5–10 yrs, • *B_{12} deficiency:* cannot cleave R factor off of B_{12}

Table continued on following page

Table 9–4. ACUTE AND CHRONIC DIARRHEA *Continued*

Most Common...	Answer and Explanation
mechanism of diarrhea in chronic pancreatitis	• **fat maldigestion:** * >90% of exocrine function destroyed, * diminished lipase/colipase activity, * undigested neutral fats in stool, • *protein maldigestion:* * >90% of exocrine function destroyed, * diminished trypsinogen, chymotrypsinogen, proelastase, procarboxypeptidases A and B, * undigested meat fibers in stool, • *CHO maldigestion:* uncommon owing to predigestion by salivary gland amylase
Rx of pancreatic maldigestion	• *low-fat diet:* use medium chain TG, • *oral enteric-coated pancreatic enzymes,* • *fat-soluble vitamin supplements,* • B_{12} *injections*
causes of bile salt deficiency leading to malabsorption	• **chronic liver disease:** decreased synthesis, • *cholestasis:* decreased delivery, • *bacterial overgrowth:* degraded, • *cholestyramine:* bile salts bound and excreted, • *ileal disease:* decreased reabsorption, e.g., CD, • *ileal resection:* see below
effect of ileal resection on bile salts	• *<100 cm resected:* * mild steatorrhea, * mild decrease in total bile acid pool, * malabsorbed bile salts impair water/electrolyte reabsorption in colon (diarrhea), • *>100 cm resected:* * severe reduction in total bile acid pool, * free long-chain FAs also malabsorbed (secretory diarrhea), * more significant steatorrhea
Rx of bile salt-induced diarrhea	*low-fat diet:* * <50 g/day, * cholestyramine aggravates steatorrhea/decreases bile acid pool
causes of bacterial overgrowth leading to malabsorption	• **intestinal stasis:** e.g., * diverticula, * motility disorders (see Table 9–3), * Billroth II with afferent duodenal loop, • *fistulas:* * gastrocolic, * jejunocolic, • *achlorhydria:* * PA, * H_2-blockers, * gastric resection
clinical findings associated with bacterial overgrowth	• **steatorrhea,** • *bile salt deficiency,* • B_{12} *deficiency*
Rx of bacterial overgrowth	• *surgery:* if anatomic cause, • *antibiotics:* cephalosporin + metronidazole, • *octreotide:* increases bowel motility in motility disorders, • *nutritional Rx:* * medium chained TG (directly reabsorbed), * B_{12}/folate, * Ca^{++}, * Mg^{++}, * iron, * vitamins

Table 9–4. ACUTE AND CHRONIC DIARRHEA *Continued*

Most Common...	Answer and Explanation
GI abnormality in AIDS	*chronic diarrhea with weight loss*
organisms producing diarrhea in AIDS	• ***Cryptosporidium parvum:*** oocysts partially acid-fast, • *CMV,* • *Microsporidia species,* • *MAI,* • *Shigella species,* • *E. histolytica,* • *adenovirus,* • *Histoplasma capsulatum*
sites of CMV infection of the GI tract in AIDS	• **colon:** diarrhea, • *esophagus:* see Table 9–2, • *biliary tract:* MCC cholecystitis, • *pancreas:* MCC pancreatitis
site for disseminated MAI infection in the GI tract in AIDS	*small intestine:* Whipple-like syndrome with * diarrhea, * malabsorption, * weight loss
Rx of MAI in GI tract	• *ethambutol,* • *rifampin,* • *ciprofloxacin,* • *clarithromycin*
site for *Histoplasma capsulatum* in the GI tract in AIDS	*large bowel:* * diarrhea, * weight loss, * fever
Rx of histoplasmosis in GI tract	*amphotericin B or itraconazole*
protozoal infection producing chronic diarrhea in AIDS	*Cryptosporidium parvum:* * 10–20%, * locates in the brush border of intestinal epithelium
clinical signs of cryptosporidiosis	• **watery diarrhea with malabsorption,** • *weight loss,* • *acute cholangitis/cholecystitis:* infects biliary tree, • *lab Dx:* * stool for O/P, * Bx, * Entero-Test, * acid-fast stain
Rx of cryptosporidiosis	*paromomycin*
clinical findings of microsporidiosis in AIDS	• *transmission:* ingest/inhale spores, • *clinical:* * chronic diarrhea, * wasting syndrome, • *Dx:* spores in feces, • *Rx:* albendazole
clinical sign of *Isospora belli* in AIDS	*watery diarrhea with malabsorption:* organisms are partially acid-fast
Rx of *Isospora belli*	*TMP/SMX*
clinical findings of cyclosporiasis	• *organism:* * Cyclospora cayetanensi, * sporozoan, • *transmission:* * ingest oocysts, * invades small intestinal epithelium, • *clini-*

Table continued on following page

Table 9–4. ACUTE AND CHRONIC DIARRHEA *Continued*

Most Common...	Answer and Explanation
Continued	cal: * diarrhea, * abdominal cramps, * weight loss, * cholangitis/cholecystitis, • *Dx:* stool for O/P, • *Rx:* TMP/SMX
intrinsic colonic motility disorder	*irritable bowel syndrome* (IBS)
clinical findings in IBS	• *female dominant disease:* alteration in perception of pain, • *clinical:* * alternating diarrhea/constipation, * constipation alone, * diarrhea alone, * abdominal pain relieved by stooling, * bloating (R/O lactase deficiency), * excessive mucus, * spastic bowel (urgency, tenesmus), • *lab Dx:* * normal flexible sigmoidoscopy, * negative stool cultures/O/P
Rx of IBS	• *stress reduction,* • *high-fiber diet,* • *anticholinergics to relieve spasm*

Question: You would expect steatorrhea in which of the following disorders? **SELECT 4**
    (A) Lactase deficiency
    (B) Celiac disease
    (C) Enterotoxigenic *E. coli* infection
    (D) Crohn's disease
    (E) Cholera
    (F) *Campylobacter jejuni* enteritis
    (G) MAI-induced diarrhea
    (H) Laxative abuse
    (I) Cystic fibrosis

Answers: (B), (D), (G), (I): Steatorrhea refers to the malabsorption of fat, which may be due to mucosal abnormalities in the small bowel (celiac disease, **choice B**), MAI-induced diarrhea (**choice G**), or pancreatic enzyme deficiency in F (**choice I**). Lactase deficiency and certain types of laxatives produce an osmotic diarrhea (**choices A and H are incorrect**). Enterotoxigenic *E. coli* and cholera secondary to *Vibrio cholerae* produce a secretory diarrhea (**choices C and E are incorrect**). *C. jejuni* produces an invasive diarrhea with a secretory component (**choice F is incorrect**).

Ach = acetylcholine, AG = anion gap, AIDS = acquired immunodeficiency syndrome, BAO = basal acid output, Bx = biopsy, cAMP = cyclic adenosine monophosphate, CBC = complete blood count, CBD = common bile duct, CD = Crohn's disease, CHO = carbohydrate, CMV = cytomegalovirus, COD = cause of death, CPE = cytopathic effect, CT = computed tomography, DH = dermatitis herpetiformis, Dx = diagnosis, ELISA = enzyme-linked immunosorbent assay, EM = electron microscopy, ERCP = endoscopic retrograde cholecystopancreatography, FAs = fatty acids, GB = gallbladder, GI = gastrointestinal, 5-HIAA = 5-

hydroxyindoleacetic acid, HJ = Howell-Jolly, HLA = human leukocyte antigen, HUS = hemolytic uremic syndrome, IBD = inflammatory bowel disease, IBS = irritable bowel syndrome, Ig = immunoglobulin, IV = intravenous, MAI = *Mycobacterium avium-intracellulare,* MAO = maximal acid output, MCC = most common cause, N/V = nausea and vomiting, O/P = ova/parasites, PA = pernicious anemia, PABA = paraaminobenzoic acid, PT = prothrombin time, RBC = red blood cell, RLQ = right lower quadrant, R/O = rule out, Rx = treatment, S/S = signs and symptoms, TG = triglyceride, TMP/SMX = trimethoprim-sulfamethoxazole, UC = ulcerative colitis, ZE = Zollinger-Ellison.

Table 9–5. SMALL, LARGE BOWEL, AND PERITONEAL DISORDERS

Most Common...	Answer and Explanation
developmental abnormality in the GI tract	*Meckel's diverticulum:* * persistence of the vitelline duct, * rule of 2's– ♦ 2 inches long, ♦ 2 feet from ileocecal valve, ♦ 2% of population, ♦ 2% symptomatic
clinical findings associated with Meckel's diverticulum	• **bleeding:** bleeding site is at the junction of ectopically located gastric mucosa and ileal mucosa, • *iron deficiency:* MCC in children/ young adults, • *obstruction:* * intussusception, * volvulus, • *perforation,* • *diverticulitis*
test used to identify a Meckel's diverticulum	*99mTc nuclear scan:* technetium concentrates in parietal cells, which are ectopically located in the diverticulum
cause of nontoxic megacolon	*Ogilvie's syndrome:* pseudo-obstruction
clinical findings in Ogilvie's syndrome	• *patient type:* * bedridden, * elderly, • *risk factors:* * spinal cord injuries, * electrolyte imbalance, * drugs reducing bowel motility, • *clinical:* * painless distention of right colon with cutoff at splenic flexure, * normal barium enema
mechanisms of protein-losing enteropathy	• **ulcerative mucosal disease:** e.g., IBD, • *lymphatic obstruction:* e.g., * intestinal lymphangiectasia, * malignant lymphoma, • *malabsorption:* e.g., celiac disease, • *idiopathic:* e.g., * Ménétrier's giant rugal hypertrophy, * villous adenoma
causes of diverticulosis in the colon	• **low-fiber diet with increased constipation,** • *Marfan's syndrome,* • *Ehlers-Danlos syndrome,* • *APKD*

Table continued on following page

Table 9–5. SMALL, LARGE BOWEL, AND PERITONEAL
DISORDERS *Continued*

Most Common...	Answer and Explanation
mechanism of colonic diverticula formation	*herniation of mucosa and submucosa through an area of weakness:* e.g., * constipation leads to high intraluminal pressures, * area of weakness is where the artery penetrates the muscularis propria (danger of hematochezia)
site for acquired diverticular disease in the GI tract	*sigmoid colon* (>90%): * intraluminal pressure highest in this area, * most are asymptomatic, * ~25% symptomatic
diverticular disease causing malabsorption and a macrocytic anemia	*duodenal diverticula:* bacterial overgrowth leading to * bile salt deficiency (malabsorption) and/or * macrocytic anemia (B_{12} deficiency)
collagen vascular disease with wide-mouthed diverticula in the small bowel	*PSS*
complication of diverticular disease	**diverticulitis:** micro/macroperforation of a diverticulum
complication of diverticulitis	*peridiverticular abscess*
clinical presentation for diverticulitis of the colon	• **LLQ pain,** • *fever,* • *constipation/diarrhea,* • *palpable, tender mass,* • *neutrophilic leukocytosis* [Diverticulitis is "left-sided appendicitis."]
method of Dx diverticulitis	• **CT scan:** test of choice for complicated diverticulitis, • *water-soluble barium study:* test of choice for uncomplicated disease, • *plain radiograph:* usually ordered to R/O perforation
Rx of diverticulitis	• *rest bowel,* • *low-fiber diet,* • *antibiotics:* metronidazole + ciprofloxacin, • *surgical consultation*
causes of fistulas in the GI tract	• **diverticular disease,** • *CD*
fistula caused by diverticular disease	*colovesical fistula*
clinical findings of a colovesical fistula	• **pneumaturia,** • *recurrent UTIs*

Table 9–5. SMALL, LARGE BOWEL, AND PERITONEAL
DISORDERS *Continued*

Most Common...	Answer and Explanation
cause of abrupt onset of pain in diverticular disease	*perforation*
clinical findings in diverticular perforation	• **abrupt onset of pain,** • *fever,* • *peritonitis:* * diffuse board-like abdomen, * rebound tenderness, * ileus, • *plain radiograph:* air under diaphragm
causes of hematochezia	• **diverticulosis:** * usually right colon, * bleeding stops spontaneously in 75% of cases, • *angiodysplasia:* see below
method of identifying bleeding site in hematochezia	*inferior mesenteric artery angiography*
GI site for acute ischemia	*small bowel*
vascular supply of small/large bowel	• *celiac artery:* stomach and duodenum, • *SMA:* * remainder of small bowel, * colon up to splenic flexure, * angle of the SMA off the aorta lends itself to embolization, • *IMA:* remaining left colon and rectum
types of acute ischemia involving small bowel	• **acute mesenteric ischemia:** * 50%, * obstruction of SMA by embolus from left heart, * SMA thrombosis over an atheromatous plaque, • *nonocclusive ischemia:* 25%, * hypotension secondary to heart failure, * shock, * ? taking digitalis (? vasospasm), • *SMV thrombosis:* * 25%, * PH, * PRV, * hypercoagulable state
arrhythmia associated with bowel embolism	*atrial fibrillation*
clinical findings in acute mesenteric ischemia due to embolism	• **elderly patient with a sudden onset of severe abdominal pain:** * pain out of proportion to physical findings, * vomiting, * bloody diarrhea, • *history of heart disease with chronic atrial fibrillation,* • *exam:* * hypotension, * ileus, * absence of rebound tenderness, * peritonitis is a late sign

Table continued on following page

Table 9–5. SMALL, LARGE BOWEL, AND PERITONEAL DISORDERS *Continued*

Most Common...	Answer and Explanation
lab/radiographic findings in acute mesenteric ischemia	• *neutrophilic leukocytosis,* • *increased serum amylase:* bowel origin, • *plain abdominal film:* * distention of small bowel, * air/fluid levels, * absence of intestinal gas, * thumbprinting (submucosal edema/hemorrhage), • *mesenteric arteriography:* gold standard
Rx of acute mesenteric ischemia due to embolism	*immediate surgical embolectomy*
clinical findings in chronic ischemic colitis	• **weight loss:** * afraid to eat, * postprandial mesenteric angina (atherosclerosis of mesenteric vessels), • *abdominal pain in splenic flexure area:* watershed area between SMA and IMA, • *bloody diarrhea,* • *abdominal bruit,* • *signs of obstruction:* * late finding, * ischemic stricture from repair of infarcted bowel by fibrosis, • *risk factors:* * HTN, * DM, * artherosclerosis, • *radiography:* * thumbprinting in splenic flexure, * angiography showing vessel stenosis
causes of small bowel obstruction	• **adhesions from previous surgery:** * most commonly produces mid-gut obstruction, * adhesions occur in ~70% of patients postoperatively, * 5% develop obstruction, • *entrapment of small bowel in an indirect hernia sac:* second MCC, • *radiation,* • *KCl:* jejunal strictures, • *gallstone ileus:* see below, • *CD,* • *endometriosis,* • *intussusception*
S/S of small bowel obstruction	• *colicky abdominal pain,* • *vomiting:* * early sign in foregut obstruction, * late sign in hindgut, * vomiting of feculent material with mid to hindgut obstruction, • *obstipation,* • *absence of rebound tenderness:* no peritonitis, unless rupture or strangulation has occurred, • *hypotension:* * third spacing of fluid in bowel lumen/wall, * distention reduces absorption of fluids and increases secretion when pressures >20 mm Hg, • *abdominal distention:* * trapping of swallowed nitrogen gas, * distention is not present in foregut obstruction (gas exits with vomiting), • *hyperperistalsis:* * early sign, * ileus a late sign
initial screening test to R/O obstruction	*plain abdominal radiograph*

Table 9–5. SMALL, LARGE BOWEL, AND PERITONEAL
DISORDERS *Continued*

Most Common...	Answer and Explanation
radiographic findings in small bowel obstruction	• *bowel distention,* • *air/fluid levels:* step-ladder appearance, • *absence of air distal to the obstruction*
S/S of a strangulated bowel	• *fever,* • *rebound tenderness:* peritonitis, • *lactic acidosis:* sign of bowel infarction, • *hypotension:* third spacing, • *vomiting,* • *air under the diaphragm*
causes of colonic obstruction	• **colorectal cancer:** annular constricting mass, • *diverticulitis*
causes of an intussusception in adults	• **polyps,** • *enlarged mesenteric lymph nodes,* • *Meckel's diverticulum*
mechanism of intussusception in adults	• *anatomic lesions are a site for the advancing peristaltic wave to grasp and drag the proximal part of the bowel* (intussusceptum) *into the distal bowel* (intussuscipiens), • *obstruction and compression of vessels leads to infarction and GI bleeding:* "currant jelly" stools
hernia	*indirect inguinal hernia:* * due to protrusion of a new peritoneal process into the inguinal canal, * bowel directly hits the finger
hernia extending through the center of the triangle of Hesselbach	*direct inguinal hernia*
hernia in patients with ascites	*umbilical hernia*
hernia with the highest rate of incarceration	*femoral hernia:* * located below the inguinal ligament, * more common in women
clinical signs of gallstone ileus	• *elderly woman with chronic cholecystitis,* • *intermittent small bowel obstruction,* • *radiograph findings:* * air in biliary tree (fistula between GB/small bowel), * stone lodged at ileocecal valve
cause of intestinal obstruction in pregnancy	*volvulus*

Table continued on following page

Table 9–5. SMALL, LARGE BOWEL, AND PERITONEAL DISORDERS *Continued*

Most Common...	Answer and Explanation
site of a volvulus in elderly and young adults	• *sigmoid colon:* 75% in elderly, • *cecum:* 25% in young adults
causes of volvulus	• **chronic constipation associated with laxative abuse,** • *drugs that reduce motility,* • *adhesions,* • *pregnancy*
clinical findings in volvulus	• *abdominal pain,* • *abdominal distention,* • *vomiting,* • *radiographic findings in a sigmoid volvulus:* * concave portion of dilated bowel points to the LLQ, * BE reveals a "bird's beak" due to tapering of the bowel toward the origin of the volvulus, • *radiographic findings in a cecal volvulus:* distended cecum looks like a coffee bean (concavity points to RLQ)
inflammatory bowel diseases	• **ulcerative colitis** (UC): * chronic relapsing ulceroinflammatory disease, * primarily involves mucosa/submucosa of rectum/left colon, • *Crohn's disease* (CD): * systemic disease, * chronic granulomatous, ulceroconstrictive disease, * transmural inflammation in a discontinuous fashion throughout entire GI tract
epidemiologic features of UC	• *etiology unknown,* • *women > men,* • *whites > blacks,* • *Jews > non-Jews,* • *family members at increased risk*
epidemiologic features of CD	• *etiology unknown,* • *equal sex involvement,* • *risk extends to family members,* • *Jews > non-Jews*
locations of UC and CD	• *rectum:* * 95% in UC, * friable, bloody mucosa, * may involve entire colon in continuity, • *terminal ileum:* * 80% in CD, * 30% terminal ileum alone, * 20% colon alone, * 50% combined, • anal fissures/fistulas: CD
G/M findings in UC	• **mucosal/submucosal inflammation,** • *inflammatory pseudopolyps,* • *neutrophilic crypt abscesses:* active disease, • *lymphocytes/plasma cell inflammation:* chronic disease, • *tendency for dysplasia/adenocarcinoma*
G/M findings in CD	• **transmural inflammation,** • *subserosal lymphoid infiltrates,* • *skip lesions:* discontin-

Table 9–5. SMALL, LARGE BOWEL, AND PERITONEAL DISORDERS *Continued*

Most Common...	Answer and Explanation
Continued	uous spread, • *non-caseating granulomas:* 60%, • *strictures,* • *fistulas,* • *aphthous ulcers:* earliest finding
S/S of UC	• **frequent bloody bowel movements with mucus,** • *LLQ cramping pain,* • *rectal bleeding,* • *tenesmus*
effect of smoking in UC	*improvement:* risks associated with smoking outweigh benefit
S/S of CD	• **intermittent RLQ colicky pain with diarrhea and bleeding** • *anal fistulas/fissures*
extraintestinal findings in IBD	• *arthritis:* * ankylosing spondylitis with/without HLA-B27 relationship, * UC > CD, • *skin lesions:* * erythema nodosum (UC > CD), * pyoderma gangrenosum (UC > CD), * apthous ulcers in mouth (CD > UC), • *primary sclerosing cholangitis:* * UC > CD, * elevated serum ALP, • *uveitis:* UC > CD
findings favoring CD over UC	• *fistula formation,* • *perianal disease,* • *calcium oxalate renal stones,* • *malabsorption:* bile salt deficiency from terminal ileal disease,* • *involvement of other areas of GI tract,* • *obstruction*
findings favoring UC over CD	• *bleeding,* • *greater frequency of diarrhea,* • *toxic megacolon:* * hypotonic, distended bowel >6 cm in diameter, * occurs in 5–10%, • *adenocarcinoma,* • *continuous spread of disease,* • *rectal involvement,* • primary sclerosing cholangitis
factors increasing adenocarcinoma risk in UC	• *early onset of UC,* • *duration >10 years,* • *pancolitis*
causes of toxic megacolon	• *opiates,* • *anticholinergics,* • *hypokalemia,* • *aerophagia,* • *BE*
S/S of toxic megacolon	• *fever,* • *abdominal pain/distention,* • *hemorrhage,* • *volume depletion:* diarrhea, • *gramnegative sepsis/perforation*

Table continued on following page

Table 9–5. SMALL, LARGE BOWEL, AND PERITONEAL DISORDERS *Continued*

Most Common...	Answer and Explanation
Rx of toxic megacolon	• *antibiotics for peritonitis,* • *volume repletion,* • *IV corticosteroids,* • *surgery:* total abdominal colectomy if no response in 48 hours to medical Rx
BE findings in UC	• *"lead pipe" appearance:* due to fibrosis and rigidity of colon • *loss of haustral markings,* • *irregular mucosal lining:* pseudopolyps/ulcers, • *shortening of bowel:* secondary to chronic UC with fibrosis of bowel wall
BE findings in CD	• *"string sign" in terminal ileum:* narrowing of lumen from transmural inflammation, • *fistula formation,* • *cobblestone appearance:* longitudinal/transverse ulcerations, • *skip lesions*
Rx of UC	• **5-aminosalicylic acid (ASA) preparations,** • *glucocorticoids:* * enemas with rectal involvement, * systemic for more extensive disease, • *immunosuppressive agents:* * azathioprine, * 6-MP, * use only for resistant disease or corticosteroid sparing, • *anticholinergic/antidiarrhea drugs:* * reduce pain/diarrhea, * for acute not chronic UC, • *low-fiber diet,* • *surgery:* intractable/life-threatening disease
complications of sulfasalazine	• *fever,* • *rash,* • *aplastic anemia,* • *folate deficiency,* • *hepatitis,* • *male infertility,* • *pancreatitis*
MOA of sulfasalazine	• *metabolized to sulfapyridine* (toxic agent) *and ASA* (active ingredient), • *ASA is an oxygen FR scavenger and inhibits lipoxygenase pathway,* • *mesalamine:* * 5-ASA preparation, * fewer side effects
Rx of CD	• *sulfasalazine:* more effective for colonic than small bowel disease, • *5-ASA:* small bowel disease, • *corticosteroids:* * acute exacerbation, * best for small bowel disease, • *6-MP:* corticosteroid-sparing drug, • *metronidazole:* * perianal disease, * colonic disease, • *surgery:* * 70–90% develop recurrence, * recurrence at anastomosis site, • *nutritional support:* * IM B_{12}, * low fat/low oxalate, * reduce oxalate stone formation with a high-calcium diet

Table 9–5. SMALL, LARGE BOWEL, AND PERITONEAL DISORDERS *Continued*

Most Common...	Answer and Explanation
site of angiodysplasia in young versus older patients	• *young patients:* * stomach, * duodenum, • **elderly patients:** * cecum, * right colon
mechanisms responsible for angiodysplasia	• *vascular ectasias:* increase with age, • *compression of submucosal venules:* vessels dilate where they penetrate the colon owing to intermittent obstruction of submucosal veins by muscle contraction and bowel distention
presentation of angiodysplasia	*lower GI bleeding:* * sometimes massive, * see above
associations with angiodysplasia	• **calcific aortic stenosis,** • *von Willebrand's disease*
methods of diagnosing angiodysplasia	• *colonoscopy:* identifies lesions, * cauterizes lesions, • *angiography:* localizes the disease
malignant tumor of the small bowel	*metastasis:* from the * colon, * rectum, or * ovary
primary malignant tumors of the small bowel	• **carcinoid tumor:** terminal ileum, • *adenocarcinoma:* duodenum, • *malignant lymphoma:* * terminal ileum, * usually B cell origin, * T cell if secondary to celiac disease
site for a carcinoid tumor	*tip of the appendix:* * usually <2 cm, * bright yellow color
G/M features of carcinoid tumors	• *neuroendocrine origin:* * contain neurosecretory granules, * all are malignant, • *risk factors for metastasis:* * <2 cm rarely metastasize, * >2 cm metastasize in 90%, * depth of intramural invasion >50%, • *foregut tumors:* * argentaffin negative, * metastasize to bone, * no risk for carcinoid syndrome, • *midgut tumors:* * argentaffin positive, * metastasize to liver, * MCC of carcinoid syndrome, • *hindgut tumors:* * argentaffin negative, * rarely cause carcinoid syndrome, * metastasize to bone
site for a carcinoid tumor presenting with the carcinoid syndrome	*terminal ileum:* * obstruction due to fibroblast stimulation by serotonin, * metastasize to ♦ regional lymph nodes, ♦ bone (osteoblastic metastasis), ♦ lung, ♦ liver

Table continued on following page

Table 9–5. SMALL, LARGE BOWEL, AND PERITONEAL DISORDERS *Continued*

Most Common...	Answer and Explanation
mechanism of producing carcinoid syndrome	*liver metastasis:* * tumor metastases release serotonin, bradykinin directly into the hepatic vein tributaries (access to systemic circulation) leading to the carcinoid syndrome in 5–10% of cases, * normally, serotonin from terminal ileum is drained by the portal vein to the liver where it is metabolized into 5-HIAA and excreted in the urine
clinical findings in the carcinoid syndrome	• **flushing:** vasodilatation from bradykinin, • *diarrhea:* * increased bowel motility, * serotonin effect, • *right-sided valvular lesions:* fibroblastic effect of serotonin produces tricuspid insufficiency/pulmonic stenosis, • *increased 24-hour urine for 5-HIAA:* diagnostic test
Rx of ileal carcinoid tumors	*en block resection:* * multifocal lesions ~30%, * metastasis in 50%, * 5-year survival ~50%
Rx of carcinoid syndrome	*octreotide:* somatostatin analogue that inhibits release of serotonin and other substances from the tumor
overall site for GI polyps	*sigmoid colon*
polyp in the GI tract	*hyperplastic polyp* [It is a hamartomatous polyp with no malignant potential.]
rectal polyp in children	*juvenile polyp:* solitary hamartomatous polyp that presents with rectal bleeding
syndromes associated with juvenile polyps	• **juvenile polyposis:** * AD or * **nonhereditary,** * small risk for malignancy, • *Cronkhite-Canada syndrome:* * nonhereditary, * polyps + ectodermal abnormalities of the nails, * small cancer risk
polyposis associated with ovarian tumors	*Peutz-Jeghers polyp* (AD): * hamartomatous polyps, * negligible risk for cancer, * associated with sex-cord stromal tumors with annular tubules
location for polyps in PJ syndrome	• **small bowel,** • *stomach,* • *colon* [Mucosal pigmentation of the buccal mucosa, lips, palms/soles is also noted.]

Table 9–5. SMALL, LARGE BOWEL, AND PERITONEAL DISORDERS *Continued*

Most Common...	Answer and Explanation
premalignant dysplastic polyp of the colon	• **tubular adenoma:** * 60%, * stalked polyp, • *tubulovillous adenoma:* 20–30%, • *villous adenoma:* * 10%, * sessile polyp with finger-like projections, * rectosigmoid location
risk factors for malignancy in adenomas	• **size of a tubular adenoma:** >2 cm has 40% risk of malignancy, • *number of polyps:* risk increases with more polyps, • *percent villous component*
clinical/lab findings of a villous adenoma	• **excessive mucus coating stool,** • *hypoalbuminemia,* • *hypokalemia*
polyposis syndrome	*familial polyposis* (AD): * polyps are not present at birth, * begin to develop between 10 and 20 years of age, * >95% will develop colorectal cancer (high penetrance)
pathogenesis of familial polyposis	• **inactivation of APC suppressor gene on chromosome 5:** point mutation, • *activation of ras oncogene:* point mutation, • *inactivation of the p53 suppressor gene:* point mutation
extra-abdominal manifestation of familial polyposis	*congenital hypertrophy of retinal pigment epithelium*
polyposis syndrome with benign bone and soft tissue tumors	*Gardner's syndrome* (AD): associated with * benign osteomas (mandible, skull, long bones), * desmoid tumors (fibromatosis of abdominal sheath), * supernumerary teeth, * thyroid/adrenal tumors, * sebaceous cysts
polyposis syndrome with malignant brain tumors	*Turcot's syndrome* (AR): only AR polyposis syndrome
Rx for patients with familial polyposis syndrome	*prophylactic total colectomy:* usually between 35 and 40 years of age
sites for colorectal cancer	• **rectosigmoid:** 60%, • *cecum/ascending colon:* * 25%, * right-sided cancers are increasing
risk factors for colorectal cancer	• **age >40 years old,** • *low-fiber/high-saturated fat diet,* • *smoking,* • *polyposis syndrome,* • *family Hx in first-degree relative:* * 25% of cases, * 3X greater risk, • *hereditary*

Table continued on following page

Table 9–5. SMALL, LARGE BOWEL, AND PERITONEAL DISORDERS *Continued*

Most Common...	Answer and Explanation
Continued	non-polyposis syndrome: * Lynch syndrome (AD disease, see below), • *past Hx of polyps in the patient or family member,* • *IBD:* see above, • *past Hx of breast/genital cancer in a woman:* 2× increased risk
types of Lynch syndrome	• *type I:* limited to colon (usually right-sided), • *type II:* * family cancer syndrome, * colon plus possible breast, gastric, endometrial, cervical cancers
factors that prevent colorectal cancer	• **FOBT screening annually at ≥50 years of age + flexible sigmoidoscopy at age 50 and every 3–5 years,** • *high-fiber/low saturated-fat diet,* • *aspirin,* • *antioxidants*
screening tests for colon cancer	• *average risk for cancer:* * no family Hx of colon cancer/polyps, * annual rectal exam after age 40, * FOBT annually ≥50 years old, * flexible sigmoidoscopy at age 50 and every 3–5 years, • *high risk for cancer:* * first-degree relative with colon cancer or polyps, * annual FOBT, * colonoscopy age 35–40 and every 2–3 years thereafter, • *UC with pancolitis:* annual colonoscopy with multiple biopsies after 7 years duration, • *Hx of polyposis syndrome:* annual flexible sigmoidoscopy beginning at puberty
procedures for evaluating positive FOBT	• **colonoscopy:** * gold standard, * 75–95% sensitivity for detecting colorectal cancer within its reach, * best test for polyps <1 cm, * evaluates entire colon + distal small bowel, • *flexible sigmoidoscopy:* * evaluates up to 60 cm, * detect ~65–75% of all polyps, * 40–65% of all cancers within its reach, * good for polyps >1 cm, • *barium enema:* * 80–95% sensitivity for detecting cancer within its reach, * 90% sensitivity for polyps >1 cm
S/S of colorectal cancer	• *left-sided cancers obstruct:* * annular, "napkin-ring" appearance, * change in bowel habits (constipation/diarrhea), * decreased stool diameter, • *right-sided cancers bleed:* * polypoid appearance, * melena (slow bleed), * iron deficiency
staging system for colorectal cancer	*Aster-Coller modified Duke's staging system*

Table 9–5. SMALL, LARGE BOWEL, AND PERITONEAL DISORDERS *Continued*

Most Common...	Answer and Explanation
prognostic indicators determining survival in colon cancer	• **depth of invasion and lymph node status:** e.g., * stage A involving mucosa/submucosa has 80–100% 5-year survival, * stage D with metastasis beyond lymph nodes has a 5–10% 5-year survival, * overall 5-year survival is 35%, • *poor prognosis:* * ulceroinfiltrative tumors, * high preoperative levels of serum CEA, * vessel invasion, * high grade, * mucoid tumor (mucus pushes tumor into vessels, poorest prognosis)
site for metastasis of colon cancer	• **liver:** ultrasonogram is best initial screen, • *lungs,* • *bone,* • *brain* [Metastasis or recurrence causes an increase in CEA.]
Rx of colon cancer	*surgery*
postoperative management of colon cancer	• *5-FU and levamisole:* * reduce recurrence risk and mortality for stage C cancer, * ~ 90% of recurrences occur in the first 4 years, • *repeat colonoscopy in 6–12 months:* repeat every 3 years if negative, • *CEA every 3–6 months for 3–4 years,* • *annual FOBT*
cause of a persistently elevated serum CEA after 6 weeks	*incomplete removal of the cancer*
procedure to R/O local recurrence	*CT scan*
disorder of the appendix	*acute appendicitis*
cause of appendicitis	• **lymphoid hyperplasia:** * 60%, * often secondary to a viral infection, * MCC in children, • *fecalith obstructing the proximal lumen:* * 35%, * MCC in adults, * mucus accumulates in the lumen, leading to stasis and bacterial proliferation with invasion of the wall, • *seeds,* • *pinworm infection*
pathogens involved with acute appendicitis	• *Escherichia coli,* • *Bacteroides fragilis,* • *Pseudomonas* species
S/S of acute appendicitis	• **crampy periumbilical pain** → * N/V/low-grade fever; → * shift of pain to RLQ → •

Table continued on following page

Table 9–5. SMALL, LARGE BOWEL, AND PERITONEAL DISORDERS *Continued*

Most Common...	Answer and Explanation
Continued	*rebound tenderness at McBurney's point:* localized peritonitis, • *constipation:* diarrhea is characteristic of a retrocecal appendicitis, • *Rovsing's sign:* pain in RLQ on palpation of LLQ, • *psoas sign:* pain on extension of right thigh, • *obturator sign:* pain on internal rotation of right thigh
disorders simulating appendicitis	• **gastroenteritis,** • *mesenteric lymphadenitis:* * may be associated with *Yersinia enterocolitica,* * submit node for culture, • *PID,* • *ruptured ovarian cyst,* • *torsion of a cystic teratoma,* • *ruptured ectopic pregnancy,* • *mittelschmerz:* peritoneal irritation from blood at ovulation, • *CD,* • *diverticulitis,* • *Meckel's diverticulitis*
test used to exclude gynecologic causes of abdominal pain	*ultrasonography*
complications of appendicitis	• **periappendiceal abscess,** • *perforation:* risk increases with time from onset of symptoms, • *pylephlebitis:* infection of portal vein, • *subphrenic abscess*
clinical findings suggesting perforation in appendicitis	• **high fever,** • *toxic appearance,* • *palpable mass,* • *diffuse abdominal tenderness,* • *neutrophilic leukocytosis* >20,000 cells/μL
clinical findings in retrocecal appendicitis	• *diarrhea,* • *RLQ with sentinel loop:* localized ileus
lab findings of acute appendicitis	• **neutrophilic leukocytosis with left shift:** * 90%, * >11,000 cells/μL, * elderly patients frequently have a normal WBC count but left shift is present, • *hematuria/pyuria:* 25%
Rx of appendicitis	• **appendectomy,** • *prophylactic antibiotics*
FP rate of surgery for appendicitis	*10–20% of appendices are normal:* * acceptable rate, * lower rate of FPs indicates a greater number with peritonitis
tumor of the appendix	*carcinoid tumor:* see above

Table 9–5. SMALL, LARGE BOWEL, AND PERITONEAL DISORDERS *Continued*

Most Common...	Answer and Explanation
cause/S/S/Rx of internal hemorrhoids	• *causes:* * **straining at stool,** * pregnancy, * PH, • *S/S:* painless bleeding, • *Rx:* high-fiber diet [Internal hemorrhoids derive from the superior hemorrhoidal vein. They cannot be palpated during a rectal exam.]
S/S of external hemorrhoids	• **bleeding** • *painful thrombosis*
cause of melanosis coli	*laxative abuse:* laxatives containing phenanthrene pigments are phagocytosed by colonic macrophages in the lamina propria, giving the mucosa a black color
anal cancer	*epidermoid carcinoma:* * increased in homosexual men, * HPV 16, 18 association
cancer located at the squamocolumnar junction	*transitional cell* (basaloid, cloacogenic) *carcinoma*

Question: Which of the following GI disorders are associated with signs and symptoms of obstruction? **SELECT 5**
- (A) CD
- (B) Right-sided colon cancer
- (C) Diverticular disease
- (D) Intussusception
- (E) Hyperplastic polyps
- (F) Ogilvie's syndrome
- (G) UC
- (H) Carcinoid tumor of terminal ileum
- (I) Chronic ischemic colitis
- (J) Angiodysplasia

Answers: (A), (C), (D), (H), (I): CD **(choice A)** involving the distal terminal ileum commonly presents with S/S of obstruction. Right-sided colon cancers are more likely to bleed than obstruct **(choice B is incorrect).** Diverticular disease **(choice C)** associated with diverticulitis may cause obstruction. Intussusception **(choice D)** causes obstruction and strangulation of bowel. Hyperplastic polyps are hamartomas and do not produce any S/S **(choice E is incorrect).** Ogilvie's syndrome is a painless pseudo-obstruction of the colon **(choice F is incorrect).** UC is not associated with obstruction **(choice G is incorrect).** Carcinoid tumors **(choice H)** of the ileum commonly kink the bowel owing to fibrosis in the intestinal wall. Chronic ischemic colitis **(choice I)** commonly leads to stricture formation at the splenic flexure. Angiodysplasia is a vascular ectasia of the cecum and right colon and does not obstruct **(choice J is incorrect).**

AD = autosomal dominant, ALP = alkaline phosphatase, APC = adenomatous polyposis coli, APKD = adult polycystic kidney disease, AR = autosomal recessive, ASA = acetylsalicylic acid, BE = barium enema, CD = Crohn's disease, CEA = carcinoembryonic antigen, CT = computed tomography, DM = diabetes mellitus, Dx = diagnosis, FOBT = fecal occult blood testing, FP = false-positive, FR = free radical, 5-FU = fluorouracil, GB = gallbladder, GI = gastrointestinal, G/M = gross and microscopic, 5-HIAA = 5-hydroxyindoleacetic acid, HLA = human leukocyte antigen, HPV = human papillomavirus, HTN = hypertension, Hx = history, IBD = inflammatory bowel disease, IM = intramuscular, IMA = inferior mesenteric artery, IV = intravenous, LLQ = left lower quadrant, MCC = most common cause, MOA = mechanism of action, MP = mercaptopurine, N/V = nausea and vomiting, PH = portal hypertension, PID = pelvic inflammatory disease, PJ = Peutz-Jeghers polyp, PRV = polycythemia rubra vera, PSS = progressive systemic sclerosis, RLQ = right lower quadrant, R/O = rule out, Rx = treatment, SMA = superior mesenteric artery, SMV = superior mesenteric vein, S/S = signs and symptoms, UC = ulcerative colitis, UTI = urinary tract infection, WBC = white blood cell.

Table 9–6. SIGNS, SYMPTOMS, AND LAB TESTS IN LIVER DISEASE

Most Common...	Answer and Explanation
functions performed by the liver	• *gluconeogenesis:* synthesis of glucose in the fasting state, • *glycogenesis/glycogenolysis:* synthesis and degradation of glycogen, • *synthesis of VLDL:* LDL is derived from VLDL, • *synthesis of ketone bodies:* * acetone, * AcAc, * β-OHB, • *protein synthesis:* * albumin, * transport proteins, * enzymes, * coagulation factors, * APR, • *primary bile acid/salt synthesis,* • *biotransformation of compounds:* cytochrome system, • *clears immunocomplexes,* • *phagocytosis of C3-coated hematopoietic cells*
cause of pruritus in liver disease	*deposition of bile salts in the skin:* complication of cholestatic disease
causes of jaundice	• **cholestatic liver disease,** • *viral hepatitis,* • *EHA*
cause of a dark yellow urine in liver disease	• **increase in CB from cholestatic liver disease,** • *increase in urobilinogen:* EHA
causes of RUQ pain in liver disease	• **rapid enlargement of the liver with swelling of the capsule in viral hepatitis,** • *GB disease*

Table 9–6. SIGNS, SYMPTOMS, AND LAB TESTS IN
LIVER DISEASE *Continued*

Most Common...	Answer and Explanation
causes of light-colored stool in liver disease	• **cholestatic disease,** • *early phase of viral hepatitis*
cause of ascites	*PH secondary to alcoholic cirrhosis*
cause of caput medusae	*PH secondary to alcoholic cirrhosis*
cause of esophageal varices in liver disease	*PH secondary to alcoholic cirrhosis*
cause of hyperestrinism in liver disease	*alcoholic cirrhosis*
mechanisms of hyperestrinism in liver disease	• **decreased metabolism of estrogen in the liver,** • *reduced metabolism of 17-KS with subsequent aromatization into estrogens*
signs of hyperestrinism	• *gynecomastia,* • *palmar erythema,* • *spider angioma:* AV fistulas, • *female secondary sex characteristics,* • *impotence:* increased SHBG decreases free testosterone levels
cause of alterations in sleep patterns and mental status in liver disease	*hepatic encephalopathy secondary to chronic liver disease:* * cirrhosis, * chronic hepatitis, * alcoholic hepatitis
Kayser-Fleisher rings	*Wilson's disease:* AR disease with defect in copper secretion into bile (see below)
cause of xanthelasmas in liver disease	*cholestasis with subsequent increase in serum CH*
cause of Courvoisier's sign	*obstruction of the CBD due to carcinoma of the head of pancreas:* Courvoisier's sign is a palpable GB
cause of asterixis	*hepatic encephalopathy:* asterixis is characterized by a flapping tremor and inability to sustain posture
indices of hepatocellular injury	*transaminases:* * AST, * ALT, * ALT is more specific for liver disease than AST, * in acute hepatitis, transaminase levels range from

Table continued on following page

Table 9–6. SIGNS, SYMPTOMS, AND LAB TESTS IN LIVER DISEASE *Continued*

Most Common...	Answer and Explanation
Continued	500–5000 U/L, * in chronic hepatitis, transaminases are <500 U/L
transaminase used to screen for silent liver disease in blood donors	*ALT:* in chronic HCV, ALT characteristically rises and falls throughout the course of the disease
transaminase pattern in viral hepatitis	*ALT > AST:* * ALT is last to return to normal, * they increase prior to onset of icterus, * they peak at peak of icterus, * they persist after icterus subsides
transaminase pattern in alcohol-related liver disease	*AST > ALT:* * alcohol is a mitochondrial poison, * AST is in the mitochondria, * ALT is in the cytosol
indices of cholestasis or infiltrative liver disease	*ALP, GGT, 5-nucleotidase:* * they are synthesized by bile duct epithelium in the presence of increased local levels of bile acids related to obstruction, * liver infiltration by amyloid raises the ALP, * metastatic tumor or granulomas raise the ALP
types of cholestasis	• **extrahepatic:** CBD, • *intrahepatic*
sources of ALP	• **liver:** * 65%, * heat-stable enzyme, • *bone:* * heat labile enzyme, * only increased during osteoblastic activity, • *intestine,* • *placenta*
liver enzyme increased by drugs enhancing the microsomal system	*GGT:* * e.g., **alcohol,** barbiturates, rifampin, phenytoin, * produce hyperplasia of SER, which houses the cytochrome system and GGT, * GGT is synthesized whenever the system undergoes hyperplasia
method of determining the origin of ALP	*measurement of GGT:* * if ALP/GGT are increased, ALP is most likely of liver origin, * if GGT is normal, ALP is most likely from another source (e.g., bone, placenta)
index of liver excretion	*total bilirubin with fractionation into CB and UCB:* fractionation is expressed as CB% of TB (CB = CB/TB x 100)
metabolic sequence of UCB up to conjugation into CB	• *destruction of senescent RBCs by BM macrophages:* UCB is the lipid soluble end-product of Hb breakdown → • *UCB binds with albumin in blood:* not filtered in urine → • *uptake of UCB by hepatocytes and conjugated into CB:* rendered water soluble

Table 9–6. SIGNS, SYMPTOMS, AND LAB TESTS IN LIVER DISEASE *Continued*

Most Common...	Answer and Explanation
metabolic sequence of CB	• *CB is actively secreted into bile canaliculi →* • *CB enters CBD and is stored/concentrated in GB →* • *CB enters small bowel →* • *CB in terminal ileum/colon is converted by bacteria containing β-glucuronidases back into UCB →* • *small fraction of UCB is reabsorbed back into the blood →* • *remainder of UCB is further reduced to UBG:* colorless pigment → *UBG is oxidized to urobilin:* normal color of stool → • *~20% of UBG is reabsorbed into the circulation → majority of UBG is recycled to the liver (90%) →* • *remainder of UBG enters the urine where urobilin produces the normal color to urine*
initial site of visible jaundice	*sclera:* * elastic tissue has an increased affinity for UCB/CB, * visible scleral icterus when TB is >2.5 mg/dL
cause of jaundice in the United States	*HAV*
bilirubin patterns for jaundice	• **CB** >50%: intra/extrahepatic cholestasis (e.g., stone in CBD) • *CB <20%:* primarily UCB (e.g., * EHA, * decreased uptake/conjugation of UCB), • *CB 20–50%:* mixed UCB/CB (e.g., * hepatitis, * cirrhosis)
urine bilirubin (UB)/urobilinogen (UBG) findings in jaundice	<table><tr><td></td><td>**UB**</td><td>**Urine UBG**</td><td>**Cause**</td></tr><tr><td>*Normal:*</td><td>negative</td><td>slight increase</td><td>—</td></tr><tr><td>*CB<20%:*</td><td>negative</td><td>increased</td><td>EHA</td></tr><tr><td>*CB 20–50%:*</td><td>increased</td><td>increased</td><td>viral hepatitis</td></tr><tr><td>*CB >50%:*</td><td>increased</td><td>absent</td><td>cholestasis</td></tr></table>
genetic cause of jaundice	*Gilberts disease:* * AD disease, * second MCC of jaundice in the United States (~7% of the population)
clinical findings in Gilberts disease	• *defect:* * defect in uptake/conjugation of UCB (CB <20%), * minor element of RBC hemolysis, • *clinical:* * jaundice develops when sick or fasting, * no clinical significance, • *normal liver Bx:* not required to secure Dx
test used to Dx Gilberts disease	*fast the patient:* doubling of the TB over the baseline value

Table continued on following page

Table 9–6. SIGNS, SYMPTOMS, AND LAB TESTS IN LIVER DISEASE *Continued*

Most Common...	Answer and Explanation
genetic cause of a conjugating enzyme deficiency	*Crigler-Najjar syndrome:* * childhood disease, * CB% <20
genetic causes of a defect in the canalicular transport system	• **Dubin-Johnson syndrome** (AR): * black liver (non-melanin pigment), * OCG reveals non-visualization of GB, * CB% >50, * excellent prognosis, • *Rotor's syndrome* (AR): * no pigment, * normal cholecystogram
acquired causes of a CB% <20 in adults	• *extravascular hemolytic anemia:* e.g., * congenital spherocytosis, * AIHA, • *ineffective erythropoiesis:* e.g., BM macrophage RBC destruction (♦ PA, ♦ severe β-thal), • *impaired uptake:* e.g., * rifampin, * portocaval shunt, • *impaired conjugation:* e.g., chronic liver disease
acquired causes of a CB% 20–50	• **viral hepatitis,** • *alcoholic hepatitis*
acquired causes of a CB% >50	• **extrahepatic cholestasis:** e.g., * **CBD stone,** * carcinoma head of pancreas, * PSC, • *intrahepatic cholestasis:* e.g., drugs
cause of a dark urine in viral hepatitis	*increase in urobilin and CB:* * dysfunction in UCB uptake/conjugation, * liver cell necrosis with disruption of bile canaliculi (CB release into blood → urine), * decreased UBG uptake recycled from bowel → urine
cause of a dark urine in extravascular hemolysis	*increased UBG:* * increased production of UBG due to increased production of UCB by macrophage destruction of RBCs, * more UBG recycled into urine
cause of a dark urine in cholestasis	*CB:* * intra/extrahepatic cholestasis leads to a backflow of CB into hepatocytes → leakage into blood, * absent UBG in urine/stool (clay-colored stool)
indices of severity of liver disease	• **PT:** * increased due to decreased coagulation factor synthesis, * best index of severity, • *serum albumin:* * reduced synthesis, * contributes to ascites (decreased oncotic pressure) and peripheral pitting edema
cause of a drop in transaminases and prolongation of PT	*fulminant liver failure*

Table 9–6. SIGNS, SYMPTOMS, AND LAB TESTS IN LIVER DISEASE *Continued*

Most Common...	Answer and Explanation
autoantibodies	• **anti-mitochondrial:** PBC, • *anti-smooth muscle:* AH type I, • *antinuclear antibodies:* AH type I, • *anti-liver/kidney/muscle:* AH type II
tumor markers	• **AFP:** HCC, • *AAT:* HCC, • *CEA:* metastatic disease to liver from colorectal, pancreatic, stomach cancer
cause of an increase in IgM in liver disease	*PBC*
cause of an increase in lipoprotein X	*cholestatic jaundice:* lipoprotein X is high in free (unesterified) CH owing to reduced synthesis of LCAT
cause of a β–γ bridge on an SPE	*alcoholic cirrhosis:* * due to an increase in IgG and IgA in alcoholic cirrhosis, * IgA migrates to the junction of the β/γ-globulin region, * IgG makes up most of the γ-globulin region, * increased IgA obliterates the β/γ junction
lab findings in EHA (arrows indicate magnitude)	• *ALT:* N, • *AST:* * ↑ ↑ * in RBCs, • *ALP:* N, • *GGT:* N, • *TB:* * ↑, * ≤5 mg/dL, • *CB%* <20, • *urine UBG* ↑ ↑, • *urine bilirubin:* neg
lab findings in viral hepatitis (arrows indicate magnitude)	• *ALT:* ↑ ↑ ↑, • *AST:* ↑ ↑, • *ALP:* ↑, • *GGT:* ↑, • *TB:* ↑, • *CB% 20–50,* • *urine UBG:* ↑ ↑, • *urine bilirubin:* ↑ ↑
lab findings in obstructive jaundice (arrows indicate magnitude)	• *ALT:* ↑ ↑, • *AST:* ↑, • *ALP:* ↑ ↑ ↑, • *GGT:* ↑ ↑ ↑, • *TB:* ↑ ↑, • *CB% >50,* • *urine UBG:* neg, • *urine bilirubin:* ↑ ↑
lab findings in alcoholic hepatitis (arrows indicate magnitude)	• *AST:* ↑ ↑, • *ALT:* ↑, • *ALP:* ↑ ↑, • *GGT:* ↑ ↑ ↑, • *TB:* ↑, • *CB% 20–50,* • *urine UBG:* ↑, • *urine bilirubin:* ↑
lab findings in focal metastatic disease to liver (arrows indicate magnitude)	• *ALT:* N, • *AST:* N, • *ALP:* ↑, • *GGT:* ↑, • *LDH:* * ↑ ↑, * nonspecific tumor marker, • *TB:* N [Focal liver disease does not produce enough necrosis to elevate transaminases or bile duct compression to produce cholestasis. In benign disease (e.g., granulomas), LDH is normal.]

Table continued on following page

Table 9–6. SIGNS, SYMPTOMS, AND LAB TESTS IN LIVER DISEASE *Continued*

Question: Which of the following abnormalities would you expect in a patient with carcinoma of the head of pancreas? **SELECT 3**
  (A) Dark stools
  (B) UBG in urine
  (C) Palpable GB
  (D) CB% <20
  (E) Hypercholesterolemia
  (F) ALP proportionately greater than ALT
  (G) AST > ALT

Answers: (C), (E), (F): Carcinoma of the head of pancreas obstructs the CBD, hence CB in bile backs up into the CBD (enlarges the GB, **choice C**), into the hepatocytes, out into the blood (**choice D is incorrect**, CB% >50), and into the urine (**choice B is incorrect**, UBG absent in urine). Absence of CB in the bowel reduces the amount of UBG produced (UBG is oxidized to urobilin, the pigment normally coloring stool), hence the stool color is light (**choice A is incorrect**). Cholestasis causes a marked elevation in ALP (**choice F**) and minor elevation in transaminases, with ALT > AST (**choice G is incorrect**). Serum CH is elevated (**choice E**), since CH is a major component of bile.

AAT = α_1-antitrypsin, AcAc = acetoacetic acid, AD = autosomal dominant, AFP = alpha-fetoprotein, AH = autoimmune hepatitis, AIHA = autoimmune hemolytic anemia, ALT = alanine aminotransferase, ALP = alkaline phosphatase, APRs = acute phase reactants, AR = autosomal recessive, AST = aspartate aminotransferase, AV = arteriovenous, BM = bone marrow, Bx = biopsy, CB = conjugated bilirubin, CBD = common bile duct, CEA = carcinoembryonic antigen, CH = cholesterol, Dx = diagnosis, EHA = extravascular hemolytic anemia, GB = gallbladder, GGT = γ-glutamyl transferase, HAV = hepatitis A virus, Hb = hemoglobin, HCC = hepatocellular carcinoma, HCV = hepatitis C virus, Ig = immunoglobulin, 17-KS = 17-ketosteroids, LCAT = lecithin-cholesterol acyltransferase, LDH = lactate dehydrogenase, LDL = low density lipoprotein, MCC = most common cause, OCG = oral cholecystogram, β-OHB = β-hydroxybutyric acid, PA = pernicious anemia, PBC = primary biliary cirrhosis, PH = portal hypertension, PSC = primary sclerosing cholangitis, PT = prothrombin time, RBC = red blood cell, RUQ = right upper quadrant, SER = smooth endoplasmic reticulum, SHBG = sex hormone binding globulin, TB = total bilirubin, thal = thalassemia, UCB = unconjugated bilirubin, UBG = urobilinogen, VLDL = very low density lipoprotein.

Table 9–7. LIVER INFECTIONS

Most Common...	Answer and Explanation
types of viral hepatitis in descending order of incidence	• **HAV,** • *HBV,* • *HCV,* • *HDV,* • *HEV*

Table 9–7. LIVER INFECTIONS *Continued*

Most Common...	Answer and Explanation
types of viral hepatitis transmitted by fecal-oral route	• **HAV,** • *HEV*
types of hepatitis transmitted by the parenteral route	• **HBV:** * IVDU 25–30%, * heterosexual contact with multiple partners 20–25%, * homosexuals 10%, • *HCV:* IVDU most important risk factor, • *HDV:* IVDU most important risk factor
types of hepatitis that can recur in transplanted livers	• **HBV,** • *HDV*
types of viral hepatitis with the greatest risk for chronic disease	• **HCV:** * 70–90%, * risk increases in alcoholics, * chronicity increased if due to blood transfusion, • *HBV:* * 5–10%, * risk increases with alcohol, • *HDV:* chronic disease in 90% with superinfection
types of hepatitis associated with HCC	• **HBV,** • *HCV:* antibodies found in 40–60% of patients with HCC
types of viral hepatitis without a chronic state	• **HAV,** • *HEV*
cause of traveler's hepatitis	*HAV*
viral causes of fulminant hepatitis	• **HDV:** 5–20%, • *HEV:* 10–30% in pregnant women, • *HAV:* rare, • *HBV:* uncommon, • *HCV:* extremely rare
hepatitis associated with membranous GN and PAN	*HBV:* * membranous GN produces a nephrotic syndrome, * vasculitis in HBV is secondary to PAN
hepatitis associated with autoimmune thyroiditis, cryoglobulinemia, type I MPGN	*HCV:* * type I MPGN produces the nephrotic syndrome, * cryoglobulinemia produces vasculitis and Raynaud's phenomenon
type of icteric viral hepatitis	*HAV*
type of anicteric viral hepatitis	*HCV*

Table continued on following page

Table 9–7. LIVER INFECTIONS *Continued*

Most Common...	Answer and Explanation
types of viral hepatitis with a serum sickness-like (immunocomplex) prodrome	• **HBV,** • *HCV*
clinical findings in serum sickness-like prodrome	• *urticaria,* • *vasculitis/glomerulonephritis:* PAN relationship, • *polyarthritis*
hepatitis requiring HBsAg	*HDV:* incomplete RNA virus
hepatitis transmitted by coinfection and superinfection	*HDV:* * coinfection is HBV/HDV acquired at same time, * superinfection is HDV superimposed on preexisting HBV (more serious infection)
clinical signs of an HDV infection	*sudden appearance of fulminant liver failure in an IVDU with chronic HBV:* unlike HBV, HDV is cytolytic to all hepatocytes infected with HBV
types of chronic hepatitis that progress to cirrhosis	• **HBV:** ~40%, • *HCV:* ~30%
type of chronic hepatitis with fluctuation of ALT levels	*HCV*
hepatitis in day-care centers	*HAV*
cause of post-transfusion hepatitis	*HCV:* 1:3300 risk per unit
hepatitis in homosexuals	*HAV:* * 35%, * occurs via unprotected anal intercourse
beneficial effects of HBV immunization	• **prevents HBV,** • *prevents HDV,* • *prevents HCC secondary to HBV-related postnecrotic cirrhosis:* only tumor vaccine
types of sexually transmitted hepatitis	• **HBV,** • *HCV,* • *HAV:* unprotected anal intercourse
viral infections with no known protective antibodies	• *HCV,* • *HDV* [Presence of antibodies against these viruses indicates infection.]

Table 9–7. LIVER INFECTIONS *Continued*

Most Common...	Answer and Explanation
types of viral hepatitis in which protective antibodies are present	• *HAV:* ∗ anti-HAV IgG, ∗ peaks in 1–2 months, • *HBV:* ∗ anti-HBs appears 2–6 weeks after HBsAg disappears (1–3 months), ∗ 10% do not develop antibodies, • *HEV:* anti-HEV-IgG is protective
clinical phases of viral hepatitis	• *prodromal phase,* • *icteric phase,* • *recovery phase*
S/S of prodromal phase	• **fatigue,** • *"flu-like" symptoms,* • *decreased taste for tobacco/alcohol,* • *serum sickness-like symptoms:* see above, • *RUQ pain/tenderness:* stretching of capsule, • *low-grade fever:* particularly HAV, • *progressive increase in transaminases:* ∗ increase before jaundice appears, ∗ persist after icterus subsides, • *bilirubinuria before jaundice appears:* due to lower renal threshold for bilirubin, • *neutropenia with atypical lymphocytosis*
S/S of icteric phase	• *jaundice:* ∗ most hepatitis is anicteric, ∗ jaundice persists 1–4 weeks, ∗ HAV is most commonly icteric, ∗ HCV is least likely icteric, • *pruritus:* ∗ 50%, ∗ bile salts in skin, • *dark urine:* ∗ bilirubinuria, ∗ absent UBG, • *light stools:* ∗ mild cholestasis, ∗ reduced bile flow decreases production of UBG, • *WBC count begins returning to normal,* • *constitutional symptoms lessen*
S/S of recovery phase	• *return of appetite,* • *decreased jaundice,* • *bilirubinuria disappears,* • *decreased abdominal pain,* • *decreased fatigue*
lab findings in viral hepatitis	• *leukopenia in prodromal phase with atypical lymphocytosis,* • *bilirubinuria precedes jaundice,* • *acholic stools with jaundice,* • *increased ALT/AST:* see above, • *slight increase in ALP/GGT:* particularly in HAV, • *hypoglycemia:* ∗ 50%, ∗ decreased glycogen stores, ∗ decreased gluconeogenesis, • *persistence of increased CB in recovery phase:* due to binding of CB to albumin (δ-bilirubin)
markers of active HAV, HBV, HCV, HDV, and HEV	• *anti-HAV-IgM:* disappears in 1–6 months, • *HBsAg,* • *HBV DNA,* • *HBeAg,* • *anti-HCV,* • *anti-HDV,* • *anti-HEV-IgM*

Table continued on following page

Table 9–7. LIVER INFECTIONS *Continued*

Most Common...	Answer and Explanation
lab findings in HAV	• *anti-HAV-IgM:* * appears 3–4 weeks after exposure, * disappears in 1–6 months, * indicates acute disease, • *anti-HAV-IgG:* * peaks in 3–4 months, * protective
markers of infectivity in HBV	• **HBV-DNA,** • *HBeAg*
sequence of appearance of antigens and antibodies in HBV	• *HBsAg:* * not infective, * may be absent in fulminant hepatitis → • *HBeAg/HBV-DNA:* * infective, * HBeAg may be absent in mutant forms of HBV (Mediterranean countries)→ • *anti-Hbc-IgM:* indicator of viral replication → • *loss of HBeAg/HBV-DNA* → • *loss of HBsAg:* * not infective, * occurs in 90%, * persists in immunocompromised patients → • *persistence of anti-HBc-IgM in window period when anti-HBs is not present:* * serologic gap, * not infective → • *anti-HBs:* protective antibody, • *anti-HBc-IgG:* marker of patient recovery from HBV, • *anti-HBe:* reflects low infectivity
definition for chronic HBV	*persistence of HBsAg >6 months:* * terms CPH, CAH, CLH no longer used to describe chronic hepatitis, * histologic descriptions are based on grading severity of inflammatory response (0–4) and degree of fibrosis (0–4)
serologic marker after receiving recombinant HBV	*anti-HBs*
cause of a positive HBsAg, HBeAg, anti-HBc-IgM	*acute HBV:* indicates high infectivity
cause of a negative HBsAg, HBeAg, anti-HBs and positive anti-HBc-IgM	*patient recovering from HBV who is in the serologic gap*
serologic markers in a patient who has recovered from HBV	• *anti-HBs,* • *anti-HBc-IgG*
cause of a positive HBsAg, negative HBeAg, positive anti-HBc-IgG/IgM, positive anti-HBe	*chronic HBV with low infectivity*

Table 9–7. LIVER INFECTIONS *Continued*

Most Common...	Answer and Explanation
cause of a positive HBsAg, positive HBeAg, positive anti-HBc-IgG/IgM, negative anti-HBe	*chronic HBV with high infectivity*
cause of a positive HBsAg, anti-HBc-IgG, anti-HBs, +/− HbeAg, +/− anti-HBe	*chronic HBV of one subtype and heterotypic anti-HBs:* occurs in ~10%
cause of a negative HBsAg, HBeAg, anti-HBs and positive anti-HBc-IgG, +/− anti-HBe	• *low level HBsAg carrier,* • *remote past infection*
microscopic findings in chronic viral hepatitis indicating a poor prognosis	• *piecemeal necrosis of limiting plate:* necroulceration at the junction of triad with hepatic parenchyma obscured, • *fibrosis between triads, triads and THV, or THV to THV*
lab findings in HBV	• *HBsAg:* acute/chronic HBV, • *HBeAg:* infective, • *HBV-DNA:* infective, • *anti-HBV-IgM:* virus proliferating, • *anti-HBV-IgG:* * recovered from HBV, * nonprotective, • *anti-HBs:* protective, • anti-HBe: • recovered from HBV: * nonprotective
lab findings in HCV	• *screen:* * second generation ELISA, * positive in 2–6 weeks, * present in ~40%, * high FP rate in low prevalence areas, * antibody indicates infection, • *confirm positive ELISA:* * RIBA: more specific but less sensitive than ELISA, * HCV-RNA by PCR: gold standard
lab findings in HDV	• *total anti-HDV:* appears ~50 days after symptoms begin, • *anti-HDV-IgM:* * distinguishes acute from chronic, * appears ~10 days after symptoms begin, • *anti-HDV-IgG:* * does not confer immunity, * chronic infection, • *HDVAg by PCR:* adds little to above testing
lab findings in HEV	• *anti-HEV-IgM:* indicates active disease, • *anti-HEV-IgG:* * indicates recovery, * protective antibody
Rx of acute hepatitis	• *supportive,* • *no need to isolate,* • *handwashing precautions,* • *enteric precautions with HAV,* • *no recapping of needles*

Table continued on following page

Table 9–7. LIVER INFECTIONS *Continued*

Most Common...	Answer and Explanation
prevention modalities for HAV	• *ISG to all household contacts,* • *enteric precautions,* • *HAV vaccine:* * high-risk patients, e.g., ♦ children in day-care centers, ♦ homosexual men, ♦ institutionalized patients, ♦ travelers to high risk areas, * confers immunity in 80–90%
prevention modality for HBV	• *HBV recombinant vaccine:* * all newborns of HbsAG-positive mothers, * all children, * sexually active adolescents not previously immunized, * adults in high-risk groups, • *HBIG:* * newborns of HBsAg-positive mothers, * intimate contacts of patients who are positive for HBsAg or those with needle stick exposure, or mucous membrane exposure of blood from HBsAg-positive patients
prevention modality for HCV exposure	*? ISG*
Rx of chronic HBV and HCV	• **interferon alfa:** * 30–40% of HBV patients lose HBsAg/HBV-DNA, * 40–50% of HCV patients normalize ALT, * 50–75% of HCV patients relapse within 6 mths, * Rx of patients with acute HCV reduces the risk for chronic hepatitis, • *lamivudine:* * oral antiviral agent, * lowers HBV-DNA titers [Note: corticosteroids are not indicated in chronic viral hepatitis.]
cause of "ring granulomas" in the liver	*Q fever due to Coxiella burnetii*
location of a liver abscess	*solitary abscess in right lobe*
S/S of ascending cholangitis	• *fever,* • *jaundice,* • *RUQ pain* [This is called Charcot's triad. It is due to an infection (usually *Escherichia coli*) that ascends from an obstructed CBD (stone or stricture) into the triads.]
cause of a liver abscess in the United States	• **ascending cholangitis,** • *intra-abdominal infection:* e.g., * portal vein, * diverticulitis, * bowel perforation, • *direct extension:* e.g., * subphrenic abscess, • *hematogenous:* e.g., bacterial endocarditis

Table 9–7. LIVER INFECTIONS *Continued*

Most Common...	Answer and Explanation
organisms isolated in liver abscesses	• **gram-negative aerobes:** *E. coli*, • *gram-negative anaerobes: Bacteroides fragilis*, • *gram-positive aerobes: Streptococcus fecalis*
initial test in work-up of a liver abscess	*ultrasonography:* * less expensive than CT, * defines cystic from solid masses in the liver
Rx of pyogenic liver abscess	• *percutaneous drainage*, • *antibiotics:* e.g., * metronidazole (covers anaerobes and amebic abscess), * ampicillin (covers enterococcus), aminoglycoside with anti-pseudomonal coverage (covers gram-negative aerobes)
location for an intra-abdominal abscess	*subdiaphragmatic*
causes of a subdiaphragmatic abscess	• **perforated appendicitis**, • *acute cholecystitis*, • *perforated PUD*, • *acute pancreatitis*
test used to detect an intra-abdominal abscess	• **CT scan:** 95% sensitivity, • *US:* 80% sensitivity, • *plain radiographs:* * ~50% sensitivity, * raised hemidiaphragm, • *radionuclide scan:* 80% sensitivity
infectious cause of granulomatous hepatitis	*TB*
noninfectious cause of granulomatous hepatitis	*sarcoidosis*
cause of hepar lobatum	*Treponema pallidum:* * complication of tertiary syphilis, * granulomatous reaction with diffuse fibrosis and gumma formation
systemic fungus producing miliary spread to the liver	*Histoplasma capsulatum:* commonly produces extensive dystrophic calcifications
cause worldwide of hepatic abscess	*Entamoeba histolytica:* see Table 9–4, * trophozoites from cecum/right colon penetrate portal vein tributaries and infect right lobe of liver (~5% of patients), * trophozoites digest the parenchyma (looks like "anchovy paste"), * ameba may enter the right lung cavity or disseminate
Rx of hepatic amebiasis	*drainage plus IV metronidazole*

Table continued on following page

Table 9–7. **LIVER INFECTIONS** *Continued*

Most Common...	Answer and Explanation
hemoflagellate producing massive hepatosplenomegaly	• *organism:* * *Leishmania donovani* complex, * visceral leishmaniasis, or kala azar, • *transmission:* * bite of sandfly (*Phlebotomus*), * leishmanial forms invade macrophages, • *Dx:* * BM exam of macrophages, * serologic tests, • *Rx:* sodium stibogluconate
cause of "sheep herder's" disease	• *organism:* * *Echinococcus granulosis* or *multilocularis*, * cestode tapeworm, • *transmission:* * sheep dog ingests larva from infected sheep, * larva become adults (dog is definitive host), which lay eggs, * eggs ingested by sheep herder and become larva (sheep herder intermediate host), * larva penetrate bowel and enter liver, * form hydatid cysts (single or multiple) containing scolices (called hydatid sand), * cyst rupture can produce anaphylactic shock, • *Dx:* * calcified cysts on radiograph, * serology, * stool for O/P, • *Rx:* albendazole and surgery
cause of "pipe stem" cirrhosis leading to PH	• *organism:* * *Schistosoma mansoni*, * trematode, • *transmission:* * cercaria penetrate skin and enter mesenteric/portal vein to become adults, * adult eggs produce a hypersensitivity reaction leading to fibrosis and PH, • *Dx:* stool for O/P, • *Rx:* praziquantel [Schistosomiasis is second to malaria as the most common COD due to parasitic disease in the world.]
trematode producing hemobilia and PH	• *organism:* * *Fasciola hepatica*, * sheep liver fluke, • *transmission:* * larvae ingested on aquatic plants, attach to intestinal wall, penetrate bowel, enter the liver and penetrate bile ducts, * adults live in bile ducts/GB, • *clinical:* * blood in bile (hemobilia), * bile duct obstruction leads to PH, cholestasis, jaundice, • *Dx:* * stool for O/P, * serology, * eosinophilia, * adults in bile ducts on ERCP, • *Rx:* bithionol
parasitic cause of cholangiocarcinoma	• *organism:* * *Clonorchis sinensis*, * Chinese liver fluke, • *transmission:* * humans ingest encysted metacercaria larvae in uncooked fish sauce, * larvae enter bile ducts and become adults, • *Dx:* * stool for O/P, * serology, • *Rx:* praziquantel

Table 9–7. LIVER INFECTIONS *Continued*

Question: Which of the following clinical features or laboratory tests are more often associated with HAV hepatitis than hepatitis due to HBV, HCV, and HDV? **SELECT 3**

(A) Fever
(B) Elevated transaminases
(C) Absence of chronic hepatitis
(D) Fecal/oral transmission
(E) Common cause of fulminant hepatitis
(F) Protective antibodies
(G) Vaccination available
(H) Serum sickness-like prodrome
(I) Highest association with IVDU

Answers: (A), (C), (D): Fever (choice A) is a characteristic of HAV hepatitis. Elevated transaminases are present in all types of viral hepatitis (choice B is incorrect). Absence of chronic hepatitis (choice C) occurs only in HAV and HEV. Fecal-oral transmission (choice D) is the primary mode of spread of HAV. Parenteral transmission in HBV, HCV, and HDV. HAV is a very uncommon cause of fulminant hepatitis (choice E is incorrect). Protective antibodies are present in HAV and HBV (anti-HBs, choice F is incorrect) and HEV. Vaccination is available for HBV as well as HAV (choice G is incorrect). A serum sickness-like prodrome is characteristic of HBV and HCV to a lesser extent (choice H is incorrect). IVDU is uncommonly associated with HAV and is more common in HBV, HCV, and HDV (choice I is incorrect).

anti-HBc = anti-hepatitis B core antibody, anti-HBe = anti-hepatitis Be antibody, anti-HBs = anti-hepatitis B surface antibody, ALP = alkaline phosphatase, ALT = alanine aminotransferase, AST = aspartate aminotransferase, BM = bone marrow, CAH = chronic active (aggressive) hepatitis, CB = conjugated bilirubin, CBD = common bile duct, CLH = chronic lobular hepatitis, CPH = chronic persistent hepatitis, CT = computed tomography, Dx = diagnosis, ELISA = enzyme-linked immunosorbent assay, ERCP = endoscopic retrograde cholangiopancreatography, GGT = γ-glutamyl transferase, GN = glomerulonephritis, HAV = hepatitis A virus, HBeAg = hepatitis Be antigen, HBIG = hepatitis immune globulin, HBV = hepatitis B virus, HBsAg = hepatitis B surface antigen, HCC = hepatocellular carcinoma, HCV = hepatitis C virus, HDV = hepatitis D virus, HEV = hepatitis E virus, Ig = immunoglobulin, ISG = immune serum globulin, IVDU = intravenous drug user, MPGN = membranoproliferative glomerulonephritis, O/P = ova/parasite, PAN = polyarteritis nodosa, PCR = polymerase chain reaction, PH = portal hypertension, PUD = peptic ulcer disease, RIBA = radioimmunoblot assay, RUQ = right upper quadrant, Rx = treatment, S/S = signs and symptoms, TB = tuberculosis, THV = terminal hepatic venule, UBG = urobilinogen, US = ultrasonogram, WBC = white blood cell.

Table 9–8. MISCELLANEOUS LIVER DISORDERS

Most Common...	Answer and Explanation
cause of cardiac cirrhosis	*chronic right heart failure:* * chronic back-up of venous blood into the THVs produces the classic "nutmeg" liver, * chronic congestion leads to fibrosis in the areas of congestion
lab abnormalities in hepatic congestion due to RHF	• **marked increase in transaminases:** ALT > AST, • *prolonged PT,* • *jaundice,* • *increased serum ALP:* more likely in chronic congestion
causes of hepatic vein thrombosis (Budd-Chiari syndrome)	• **PRV,** • *oral contraceptives,* • *PNH:* release of TXA$_2$ from platelets, • *hypercoagulable states:* e.g., * ATIII deficiency, * protein C and S deficiency
S/S of Budd-Chiari syndrome	• **rapid onset of ascites:** >90%, • *painful hepatomegaly,* • *splenomegaly,* • *PH*
method of Dx of Budd-Chiari syndrome	• **screen with Doppler US:** * 75% sensitivity in detecting thrombosis, * hypertrophy of caudate lobe (♦ has separate hepatic veins derived from IVC, ♦ they remain patent when hepatic veins draining right and left lobes are thrombosed), • *hepatic vein catheterization/ angiography:* gold standard
Rx of Budd-Chiari syndrome	• **surgical decompression:** shunts, • *fibrino-lytic Rx:* variable results, • *liver transplanta-tion with post-transplant anticoagulation*
causes of veno-occlusive disease	• **GVH reaction post-BM transplantation,** • *ingestion of pyrrolizidine alkaloids*
S/S of veno-occlusive disease	• *hepatomegaly,* • *weight gain,* • *ascites*
causes of portal vein thrombosis in adults	• **pylephlebitis:** e.g., * acute appendicitis, * diverticulitis, • *post-liver transplant,* • *cirrho-sis,* • *HCC:* tumor invasion, • *PRV:* hyper-coagulability, • *pancreatitis:* thrombosis of splenic vein with extension into the portal vein
cause of peliosis hepatis	• **anabolic steroids,** • *oral contraceptives* [Pel-iosis hepatis is RBC accumulation in space of Disse.]
cause of peliosis hepatis in AIDS	*bacillary angiomatosis due to Bartonella henselae:* Rx with erythromycin or doxycy-cline

Table 9–8. MISCELLANEOUS LIVER DISORDERS
Continued

Most Common...	Answer and Explanation
causes of PH	• **cirrhosis,** • *portal vein thrombosis:* prehepatic, • *Budd-Chiari syndrome:* post-hepatic, • *right heart failure:* post-hepatic
causes of PH in cirrhosis	• **obstruction to portal vein blood flow:** intrasinusoidal obstruction by fibrosis and regenerative nodules, • *intrahepatic anastomoses between hepatic arterial and venous systems*
types of alcohol-related disease	• **fatty change:** reversible, • *alcoholic hepatitis:* reversible, • *cirrhosis:* irreversible
risk factors for alcohol-related liver disease	• **amount of alcohol,** • **duration of alcohol intake,** • *female sex:* * cirrhosis occurs faster and with less alcohol, * lower alcohol dehydrogenase in gastric mucosa, • *coexisting HCV,* • *certain genetic tendencies:* * Asians have defective aldehyde dehydrogenase, hence acetaldehyde accumulates faster, * Native Americans metabolize alcohol faster
pathway for alcohol metabolism	alcohol dehydrogenase alcohol → acetaldehyde + $NADH_2$ aldehyde dehydrogenase → acetate + $NADH_2$ → acetyl CoA
S/S of alcoholic fatty liver	*hepatomegaly:* reversible with D/C of alcohol
S/S of alcoholic hepatitis	• **painful hepatomegaly,** • *jaundice,* • *fever,* • *ascites,* • *splenomegaly,* • *hepatic encephalopathy:* in severe cases
lab findings in alcoholic hepatitis	• **AST > ALT,** • *increased serum GGT:* disproportionate increase over ALP, • *mixed hyperbilirubinemia:* CB% 20–50, • *neutrophilic leukocytosis,* • *macrocytic anemia:* * direct effect of alcohol on RBC membrane, * round target cells, • *lactic acidosis* and *β-OHB ketoacidosis:* see Table 1–3, • *hypertriglyceridemia:* see Table 1–3, • *fasting hypoglycemia:* see Table 1–3, • *hyperuricemia:* see Table 1–3, • *prolonged PT:* poor prognostic sign
Rx of alcoholic hepatitis	• **D/C alcohol,** • *corticosteroids:* severe cases

Table continued on following page

Table 9–8. MISCELLANEOUS LIVER DISORDERS
Continued

Most Common...	Answer and Explanation
S/S of autoimmune hepatitis	• *young woman,* • *fever,* • *jaundice,* • *hepatosplenomegaly,* • *diarrhea,* • other *disorders:* e.g., * DM, * AIHA
lab findings in autoimmune hepatitis	• **positive ANA:** 50–80%, • *positive LE prep:* 15%, • *anti-smooth muscle antibody:* * 75%, * type I variant, • *polyclonal gammopathy,* • *elevated transaminases*
Rx of autoimmune hepatitis	*corticosteroids:* * response in 60–80%, * relapse common, * patients may progress into cirrhosis
cause of intrahepatic cholestasis	• **drugs:** e.g., oral contraceptives, • *viral hepatitis:* early cholestatic phase, • *PBC,* • *genetic:* * Dubin-Johnson, * see above, • *alcoholic hepatitis*
cause of extrahepatic cholestasis	• **CBD stone,** • *carcinoma of head of pancreas,* • *PSC*
S/S of cholestasis	• **jaundice,** • *pruritus:* bile salts, • *skin xanthomas:* CH deposition, • *hepatomegaly,* • *secondary biliary cirrhosis,* • *acholic stools:* absent urobilin, • *dark urine:* * CB, * no UBG
lab findings of cholestasis	• **marked elevation of ALP/GGT:** markers of cholestasis, • *mild to moderate increase in ALT/AST,* • *CB% >50,* • *increased CH:* * lipoprotein X, * characteristic of cholestasis
disease associated with PSC	*UC:* * 70% of cases, * multifocal, obliterative fibrosis of extra/intrahepatic bile ducts leading to strictures (beading effect), obstruction, and secondary biliary cirrhosis.
clinical findings of PSC	• *men > women,* • *no relation to severity of UC,* • *clinical:* * fatigue, * pruritus, * jaundice • *lab:* asymptomatic increase in serum ALP
confirmatory test for PSC	*ERCP*
cause of PBC	*autoimmune, granulomatous destruction of the portal triad bile duct radicles, with eventual replacement by fibrosis* (cirrhosis)
clinical findings of PBC	• *disease in middle-aged women,* • *clinical:* * early onset of pruritus (bile salt deposition in

Table 9–8. MISCELLANEOUS LIVER DISORDERS
Continued

Most Common...	Answer and Explanation
Continued	skin), * hepatomegaly, * jaundice late finding, • *associations:* * RA, * Sjögren's, * thyroiditis, * RTA, • *lab:* * markedly elevated ALP/GGT, * CB% >50, * increased IgM, * antimitochondrial antibody (95%)
Rx of PBC	• **ursodeoxycholic acid,** • *cholestyramine,* • *others:* * cyclosporine, * colchicine, * methotrexate
types of drug-induced liver disease	• **idiosyncratic,** • *dose-dependent*
drugs associated with hepatitis (acute/chronic)	• **acetaminophen,** • *isoniazid,* • *halothane:* fever after 1 week, then jaundice, • *methyldopa,* • *salicylates*
drugs associated with intrahepatic cholestasis	• *noninflammatory:* * estrogen derivatives, * anabolic steroids, • *inflammatory:* * erythromycin estolate, * amoxicillin/clavulanate, * chlorpromazine, * thiazides
drugs associated with fatty change	• *amiodarone:* resembles alcoholic hepatitis, • *corticosteroids,* • *tetracycline:* microvesicular, • *valproic acid:* microvesicular
drugs associated with fibrosis	• **methotrexate,** • *hypervitaminosis A*
drugs/chemicals associated with liver tumors	• *liver cell adenoma:* * oral contraceptives, * anabolic steroids, • *nodular hyperplasia:* azathioprine, • *HCC:* * oral contraceptives, * anabolic steroids, • *angiosarcoma:* * vinyl chloride, * arsenic, * Thorotrast
drugs associated with granulomatous hepatitis	• **allopurinol,** • *sulfonamides*
genetic cause of iron overload	*hemochromatosis* (AR): * HLA-A3 relationship, * males > females (menses protective), * abnormal gene on chromosome 6, * unrestricted iron absorption
S/S of hemochromatosis	• **hepatomegaly:** * 95%, * pigment cirrhosis, • *cardiomegaly:* * restrictive cardiomyopathy, * conduction defects, * heart failure, • *diabetes mellitus:* * 70%, * DM (late finding,

Table continued on following page

Table 9–8. MISCELLANEOUS LIVER DISORDERS
Continued

Most Common...	Answer and Explanation
Continued	"bronze diabetes"), * malabsorption, • *hypogonadism:* * pituitary involvement, * testicular atrophy, * weight loss, • *arthritis:* * 50%, * calcium pyrophosphate disease, * chondrocalcinosis, • *metallic gray appearance:* increase in melanocytes plus macrophages with iron in dermis
lab findings in hemochromatosis	• *high serum iron,* • *low TIBC,* • *high percent saturation:* * best screening test, * >55%, • *high serum ferritin:* * screening test, * positive if greater than two times normal, • *liver Bx for quantitation of iron:* confirmatory test, • *screen all family members*
cause of hemosiderosis (acquired iron overload)	• **multiple blood transfusions,** • *drinking well water,* • *alcoholics:* * alcohol increases iron absorption, * red wines contain large amounts of iron
Rx of iron overload	*phlebotomy:* goal is to lower serum ferritin
COD in hemochromatosis	*cirrhosis leading to HCC* (30%)
cause of Wilson's disease	*defect of copper excretion in bile:* * AR disorder, * defective copper-transporting protein leads to an increase of free copper with subsequent deposition in multiple organs
clinical findings in Wilson's disease	• **hepatitis,** • *CNS findngs:* * spasticity, * dementia, * choreoathetosis, • *hemolytic anemia,* • *renal failure,* • *cirrhosis,* • *Fanconi's syndrome:* * normal AG metabolic acidosis, * Fanconi's syndrome (see Table 10–2), • *Kayser-Fleischer ring:* copper in Descemet's membrane of eye
lab findings in Wilson's disease	• **low ceruloplasmin levels,** • *decreased total copper:* * total copper = copper bound to ceruloplasmin + free, * low ceruloplasmin responsible for low total levels, • *increased free copper levels,* • *increased urine copper*
Rx for Wilson's disease	• **penicillamine:** copper chelating agent, • *zinc:* inhibits GI absorption of copper, • *liver transplantation*

Table 9–8. MISCELLANEOUS LIVER DISORDERS
Continued

Most Common...	Answer and Explanation
liver disease in pregnancy	• **viral hepatitis,** • *benign intrahepatic cholestasis:* * estrogen-induced, * benign disease that disappears after delivery, * reappears with birth control pills, • *acute fatty liver:* * abnormality in β-oxidation of fatty acids, * must deliver the baby, • *preeclampsia/eclampsia:* * periportal necrosis, * HELLP syndrome (<u>h</u>emolytic anemia, <u>e</u>levated transaminases, <u>l</u>ow <u>p</u>latelets)
causes of hepatocellular failure	• *fulminant hepatic failure* (FHF): acute liver failure with encephalopathy within 8 wks of hepatic dysfunction, • *cirrhosis:* * see below, * differs from FHF in that it ♦ is associated with PH, ♦ is irreversible, ♦ requires a longer time to develop
causes of FHF	• **viral infections:** 70%, • *drugs:* 25%, • *others:* * Wilson's disease, * acute fatty liver of pregnancy, * Reye's syndrome, * Budd-Chiari syndrome
known viral cause of FHF	• **HBV:** 20% • *undetermined viral hepatitis:* ~40%, • *HDV:* endemic areas
drug causing FHF	*acetaminophen*
risk factors determining poor prognosis in FHF	• *patient* >40 years old, • *drug-induced:* other than acetaminophen, • *grade 3/4 hepatic encephalopathy,* • *PT* >3.5 INR, • *total bilirubin* >18 mg/dL
complications associated with FHF	• **multiorgan failure,** • *infections:* * >90%, * *Staphylococcus aureus,* • *Streptococcus species,* • *intracranial HTN:* >80%
causes of cirrhosis	• **alcohol-related liver disease,** • *postnecrotic cirrhosis:* * **HBV,** * HCV, • *hemochromatosis,* • *PBC,* • *Wilson's disease*
cause of fibrosis related to alcohol	*acetaldehyde binds with lysine residues in proteins to form an acetaldehyde-protein complex:* * complex stimulates myofibroblasts and Ito cells (normally a storage cell for retinoic acid) to produce collagen around the THV (perivenular fibrosis), * collagen replaces necrotic hepatocytes located around islands of regenerating hepatocytes (regenerative nodules of cirrhosis)

Table continued on following page

Table 9–8. MISCELLANEOUS LIVER DISORDERS
Continued

Most Common...	Answer and Explanation
histologic findings in alcoholic cirrhosis	• *regenerative nodules surrounded by fibrosis:* nodules lack normal liver architecture, • *intrasinusoidal HTN:* * due to overall reduction in sinusoids, * compression of existing sinusoids by regenerative nodules, • *anastomoses between venous/arterial system leading to PH*
coagulation defect associated with cirrhosis	*bleeding:* * decreased coagulation factor synthesis (prolonged PT), * platelet dysfunction (decreased clearance of FDPs), * dysfibrinogenemia (abnormal fibrinogen)
CNS abnormality in cirrhosis	*hepatic encephalopathy:* * stage I: ♦ confusion/agitation, ♦ daytime/nighttime reversal, ♦ asterixis, * stage II: ♦ drowsiness, ♦ asterixis, ♦ primitive reflexes; ♦ stage III: ♦ somnolent but rousable, ♦ incomprehensible speech, ♦ hyperreflexia, ♦ hyperventilation, ♦ stage IV: ♦ coma, ♦ no response to stimuli
causes of hepatic encephalopathy	• *toxins:* * ammonia, * mercaptans, • *pathogenesis of toxins:* * portosystemic shunting, * increased ammonia, * decreased degradation of ammonia by liver, • *increased synthesis of false neurotransmitters:* * octopamine, * GABA
risk factors for hepatic encephalopathy	*protein:* * dietary, * blood in GI tract (increases bacterial conversion of urea into ammonia), • *alkalosis:* fewer H^+ ions keep ammonia in NH_3 state (easily reabsorbed into blood), • *diuretics:* produce metabolic alkalosis, • *sedatives,* • *portosystemic shunts:* shunt ammonia away from the liver, • increase in PHY, TRY, TYR: ↑ synthesis of false neurotransmitters PHY, TRY, TYR
Rx of hepatic encephalopathy	• **restrict protein:** reduces ammonia production by colonic bacteria, • *lactulose:* * H^+ ions released by colonic bacteria combine with diffusible NH_3 to produce nondiffusible NH_4, * laxative effect causes loss of nitrogenous compounds, • *neomycin:* reduces colonic bacteria, • *branched chain AAs:* block neurotransmitter synthesis, • *aldosterone blockers for diuresis:* retains H^+ ions, so less NH_3 and more NH_4 is formed, • *avoid sedatives/pain medications:* * oxazepam in the presence of agitation, * flumazenil has also been used

Table 9–8. MISCELLANEOUS LIVER DISORDERS
Continued

Most Common...	Answer and Explanation
causes of ascites in cirrhosis	• **PH:** * see below, * increased hydrostatic pressure, • *hypoalbuminemia:* * decreased albumin synthesis, * decreased oncotic pressure, • *secondary aldosteronism:* * cannot metabolize aldosterone, * stimulation of the RAA system from decreased cardiac output
lab method of distinguishing ascites secondary to cirrhosis from exudates	• **serum albumin–PF albumin gradient:** if gradient is >1.1 g/dL, the fluid is a transudate compatible with cirrhosis, * if <1.1, consider increased vessel permeability (e.g., peritonitis, malignancy), • *PF albumin:* if <2.5 g/dL = transudate, * >2.5 g/dL = exudate
Rx of ascites	• **salt restriction,** • *diuretics:* spironolactone drug of choice, • *paracentesis,* • *peritoneovenous shunt:* * redirects ascitic fluid into blood, * cheaper method of replacing albumin, • *transjugular intrahepatic portosystemic shunt:* stent connects hepatic vein with portal vein
complications of PH	• **ascites:** see above, • *esophageal varices:* * see Table 9–2, * varices are dilated left gastric vein, • *periumbilical varices:* caput medusae, • *hemorrhoids,* • *congestive splenomegaly:* potential for hypersplenism
Rx of PH	*shunting:* * portocaval shunt, * mesocaval shunt (connection of SMV with PV), * splenorenal (♦ most physiologic shunt, ♦ reduces PH/bleeding from varices without bypassing the liver)
cause of hepatorenal syndrome in cirrhosis	*prerenal hypoperfusion secondary to vasoconstriction* (? increased endothelin): * functional renal failure with preservation of tubular function (concentrating ability is intact), * occurs in 40–50% of patients with terminal cirrhosis, * no gross/microscopic changes in kidneys
clinical findings in HRS	• **oliguria,** • *random Una⁺ <10 mEq/L:* indicates intact tubular function, • *UOsm >500 mOsm/kg:* indicates concentration, • *UCr/PCr ratio >30:1,* • *normal urine sediment exam,* • *clinical recovery in 10%,* • *renal transplant reverses renal function to normal*

Table continued on following page

Table 9–8. MISCELLANEOUS LIVER DISORDERS
Continued

Most Common...	Answer and Explanation
mechanism of hyperestrinism in cirrhosis	*see Table 9–6*
signs of hyperestrinism in a male with cirrhosis	• *female secondary sex characteristics:* * female distribution of pubic hair, * soft skin, • *palmar erythema,* • *spider angiomas:* AV fistulas, • *unilateral/bilateral gynecomastia:* breast tissue has different sensitivity to estrogen, • *testicular atrophy/impotence:* increased estrogen, increases synthesis of SHBG, which has an increased affinity for free testosterone
acid-base abnormalities in cirrhosis	• *chronic respiratory alkalosis:* toxic products overstimulate the respiratory center, • *lactic acidosis:* liver cannot metabolize lactic acid, • *hypokalemia:* secondary aldosteronism
lab findings in cirrhosis	• *low BUN/high ammonia:* dysfunctional urea cycle, • *hypoglycemia:* * defective gluconeogenesis, * low glycogen stores, • *low UNa+:* * decreased EABV, * secondary aldosteronism, • *mixed ABG disorders:* chronic respiratory alkalosis + metabolic acidosis (lactic), • *increased PT:* decreased coagulation factor synthesis, • *hypoalbuminemia:* decreased synthesis, • *hypocalcemia:* * hypoalbuminemia, * vitamin D deficiency from decreased first hydroxylation
tumor-like condition in the liver	*focal nodular hyperplasia* (FNH): * 2:1 female/male ratio, * etiology unknown, * no clinical significance
benign tumor of the liver	*cavernous hemangioma:* best diagnosed with enhanced CT
benign tumor of liver associated with birth control pills or anabolic steroids	*liver cell adenoma:* may rupture during pregnancy, * hypovascular on liver scans
malignancy of the liver	*metastasis:* primary sites: * lung, * colorectal, * pancreas, * stomach, * breast
primary malignancy of liver	*HCC*

Table 9–8. MISCELLANEOUS LIVER DISORDERS
Continued

Most Common...	Answer and Explanation
causes of HCC	• **postnecrotic cirrhosis secondary to HBV:** enhanced with aflatoxins, • *postnecrotic cirrhosis secondary to HCV,* • *hemochromatosis,* • *alcoholic cirrhosis,* • *birth control pills,* • *Wilson's disease,* • *AAT deficiency*
clinical findings in HCC	• *invades hepatic/portal vein,* • *early metastasis to lymph nodes, lung, brain, bone,* • *clinical:* * **abdominal pain,** * abdominal mass (hepatomegaly), * fever, * appearance of bloody ascites (tumor invasion of hepatic/portal vein, hemorrhage from tumor), * paraneoplastic syndromes (♦ erythropoietin, ♦ insulin-like factor, ♦ gynecomastia, ♦ hypercalcemia)
lab finding of HCC	• **increased AFP:** * tumor marker, * 75–90%, * >500 ng/mL, • *increased serum AAT:* tumor marker, • *sudden increase in serum ALP/GGT:* very characteristic, • *polycythemia:* ectopic erythropoietin, • *hypoglycemia:* ectopic insulin-like factor
Rx of HCC	• **surgery:** <20% are surgical candidates, • *liver transplantation* [Most patients succumb within 6 months of Dx.]
causes of angiosarcoma	• **vinyl chloride,** • *arsenic,* • *Thorotrast*
bile duct site for primary cancer	*ampulla of Vater:* adenocarcinoma
causes of cholangiocarcinoma	• **PSC,** • *Clonorchis sinensis,* • *Hx of choledochal cyst*
site of a Klatskin's tumor	*cholangiocarcinoma* located at junction of right/left hepatic duct
causes of acute peritonitis	• **ruptured viscus:** e.g., * duodenal ulcer, * diverticula, * appendix, • *ruptured cyst:* e.g., benign follicular cyst, • *ischemic bowel,* • *spontaneous:* ascites in alcoholic cirrhosis (*Escherichia coli* MCC), * ascites in child with nephrotic syndrome (*Streptococcus pneumoniae* MCC)

Table continued on following page

Table 9–8. MISCELLANEOUS LIVER DISORDERS
Continued

Most Common...	Answer and Explanation
S/S of spontaneous bacterial peritonitis in a patient with cirrhosis and ascites	• *fever,* • *abdominal pain,* • *abdominal tenderness* [SBP occurs in 10–20% of cirrhotics with ascites.]
lab findings in SBP	• **PF leukocytes ≥250 cells/μL,** • *positive Gram stain:* * *E. coli* = fat gram-negative rod, * *S. pneumoniae* = gram-positive diplococcus

Question: Which of the following **cause:effect** relationships are correctly matched? **SELECT 4**
    (A) PRV:Budd-Chiari syndrome
    (B) Ruptured viscus:SBP
    (C) PSC:cholangiocarcinoma
    (D) Vinyl chloride:hepatic adenoma
    (E) PH:gynecomastia
    (F) Low ceruloplasmin:Wilson's disease
    (G) PH:esophageal varices
    (H) Anabolic steroids:cholestasis
    (I) Budd-Chiari syndrome:HCC

Answers: (A), (C), (G), (H): PRV is a cause of hepatic vein thrombosis (choice A; Budd-Chiari syndrome). A ruptured viscus is not the cause of SBP. It arises in the setting of cirrhosis complicated by ascites (choice B is incorrect). PSC (choice C) is a cause of cholangiocarcinoma. Vinyl chloride is associated with angiosarcoma not a hepatic adenoma (choice D is incorrect). PH does not cause gynecomastia. Gynecomastia is caused by decreased metabolism of estrogen by the liver and increased aromatization of androstenedione into estrogen (choice E is incorrect). Low ceruloplasmin is an effect, not a cause, of Wilson's disease. The chronic liver disease in Wilson's disease leads to decreased synthesis of ceruloplasmin (choice F is incorrect). PH is a cause of esophageal varices (choice G). Anabolic steroids (choice H) are a cause of intrahepatic cholestasis. Budd-Chiari syndrome is an effect, not a cause, of HCC (choice I is incorrect).

AAs = amino acids, AAT = α₁-antitrypsin, ABG = arterial blood gas, AFP = alpha-fetoprotein, AG = anion gap, AIDS = acquired immunodeficiency syndrome, AIHA = autoimmune hemolytic anemia, ALT = alanine transaminase, ALP = alkaline phosphatase, ANA = antinuclear antibodies, AR = autosomal recessive, AST = aspartate transaminase, ATIII = antithrombin III, AV = arteriovenous, BM = bone marrow, BUN = blood urea nitrogen, Bx = biopsy, CB = conjugated bilirubin, CBD = common bile duct, CH = cholesterol, CNS = central nervous system, CoA = coenzyme A, COD = cause of death, CT = computed tomography, D/C = discontinue, DM = diabetes mellitus, Dx = diagnosis, EABV =

effective arterial blood volume, ERCP = endoscopic retrograde cholangio-pancreatography, FDPs = fibrin degradation products, FHF = fulminant hepatic failure, FNH = focal nodular hyperplasia, GABA = gamma aminobutyric acid, GGT = γ-glutamyl transferase, GI = gastrointestinal, GVH = graft versus host, HBV = hepatitis B, HCC = hepatocellular carcinoma, HCV = hepatitis C, HDV = hepatitis D, HLA = human leukocyte antigen, HTN = hypertension, Hx = history, Ig = immuno-globulin, INR = international normalized ratio, IVC = inferior vena cava, LE = lupus erythematosus, MCC = most common cause, $NADH_2$ = nicotine adenine dinucleotide (reduced form), β-OHB = beta hydroxybu-tyric acid, PBC = primary biliary cirrhosis, PCr = plasma creatinine, PF = peritoneal fluid, PH = portal hypertension, PHY = phenylalanine, PNH = paroxysmal nocturnal hemoglobinuria, PRV = polycythemia rubra vera, PSC = primary sclerosing cholangitis, PT = prothrombin time, PV = portal vein, RA = rheumatoid arthritis, RAA = renin-angiotensin-aldosterone, RBC = red blood cell, RHF = right heart failure, RTA = renal tubular acidosis, Rx = treatment, SBP = spontaneous bacterial peritonitis, SHBG = sex hormone–binding globulin, SMV = superior mesenteric vein, S/S = signs and symptoms, THV = terminal hepatic venule, TIBC = total iron binding capacity, TRY = tryptophan, TYR = tyrosine, TXA_2 = thromboxane A_2, UC = ulcerating colitis, UCr = urine creatinine, UNa^+ = urine sodium, UOsm = urine osmolality, US = ultrasonography.

Table 9–9. GALLBLADDER AND PANCREATIC DISORDERS

Most Common...	Answer and Explanation
cause of stone formation	*supersaturation of bile with CH*
causes of CH supersaturation of bile	• **primary increase in biliary secretion of CH,** • *deficiency of bile salts,* • deficiency of leci-thin (phospholipid)
causes of an increase in biliary secretion of CH	• **obesity,** • *estrogen:* * childbearing, * birth control pills, • *increasing age,* • *Northern European,* • *drugs:* fibric acid derivatives di-rectly stimulate CH secretion into bile
causes of decreased bile salts	• *CD,* • *prolonged fasting,* • *increasing age,* • *drugs:* cholestyramine
causes of both increased biliary secretion of CH and decreased bile salts	• *increasing age,* • *Native Americans,* • *estro-gen Rx in women,* • *leanness*
types of stones	• **CH:** 80%, • *pigment stones:* 20% [Stones occurs in 10–20% of men and 20–40% of women.]

Table continued on following page

Table 9–9. GALLBLADDER AND PANCREATIC DISORDERS *Continued*

Most Common...	Answer and Explanation
causes of black pigment stones	• **EHA:** e.g., * sickle cell disease, * congenital spherocytosis, • *ineffective erythropoiesis with excess UCB:* * severe β-thal, * PA/folate deficiency, • *hypersplenism secondary to cirrhosis:* macrophage destruction of RBCs
causes of brown pigment stones	• **bile stasis in GB,** • *CBD with infection*
complication associated with stones	• **cholecystitis:** acute and chronic, • *CBD obstruction,* • *GB cancer,* • *acute pancreatitis*
cause of acute cholecystitis	• **stone impacted in the cystic duct:** 90%, • *AIDS:* * CMV, * Cryptosporidium [*E. coli* is the most common pathogen in acute cholecystitis.]
S/S of acute cholecystitis	• *fever,* • *RUQ constant, dull pain 15–30 minutes after eating,* • *vomiting:* 75%, • *radiation of pain to right scapula,* • *Murphy's sign:* see Table 9–6, • *jaundice:* 25%, • *palpable GB:* 15%, • *majority resolve in 3–7 days when stone falls out of the duct*
test used to identify stones in cystic duct	*radionuclide scan*
test used to identify stones in the GB	• **ultrasonography:** * gold standard test, * detects stones >1–2 mm in diameter, * detects sludge, * measures GB wall thickness, * not effective in CBD stones, • *plain film:* only 15% are radiopaque, • *CT:* too expensive
lab findings in acute cholecystitis	• *absolute neutrophilic leukocytosis with left shift:* WBC counts >12,000 cells/μL, • *increased serum AST/ALP,* • *increased serum amylase:* suggests pancreatitis
Rx of acute cholecystitis	• *antibiotics:* third-generation cephalosporin + metronidazole, • *laparoscopic cholecystectomy:* usually within 48 hours, • *meperidine for pain:* morphine contracts the sphincter of Oddi and worsens pain
symptomatic disorder of GB	*chronic cholecystitis*

Table 9–9. GALLBLADDER AND PANCREATIC
DISORDERS *Continued*

Most Common...	Answer and Explanation
cause of chronic cholecystitis	*stones in GB with repeated attacks of minor inflammation:* chemical inflammation is more likely than infection
S/S of chronic cholecystitis	• *severe, persistent pain 1–2 hours postprandially in evening,* • *pain radiating into right scapular,* • *epigastric distress, belching, and bloating*
Rx of chronic cholecystitis	*laparoscopic cholecystectomy*
causes of GB cancer	• **gallstones,** • *porcelain GB:* dystrophically calcified GB [It is the most common primary cancer of biliary tract. Porcelain GB is an automatic indication for elective removal.]
defect in cystic fibrosis (CF)	*see Table 6–6 for CF discussion*
cause of acute pancreatitis	• **alcoholism:** * increases permeability of pancreatic duct to enzymes, * thickens pancreatic secretions, • *stone impacted in distal end of the CBD:* ampullary obstruction with bile reflux into pancreatic duct, • *trauma:* MCC in children, • *infection:* e.g., * mumps, * coxsackievirus, * CMV in AIDS, • *drugs:* * azathioprine, * estrogen, * pentamidine, • *hypercalcemia,* • *hypertriglyceridemia,* • *ERCP,* • *obesity:* major risk factor for severe pancreatitis
initiating events responsible for acute pancreatitis	• **zymogen activation:** * intra-acinar autoactivation of trypsinogen to form trypsin, * trypsin activates other enzymes, complement, and kinin system, • *increased duct permeability:* due to obstruction with increased pressure leading to gland fibrosis/atrophy without necrosis
S/S of acute pancreatitis	• **severe, boring mid-epigastric pain with radiation into the back:** * relieved by leaning forward, * worse when supine, • *fever:* low grade, • *dyspnea:* * >50%, * hypoxemia, * intrapulmonary shunting, • *N/V,* • *volume depletion:* third space fluid losses around the

Table continued on following page

Table 9–9. GALLBLADDER AND PANCREATIC
DISORDERS *Continued*

Most Common...	Answer and Explanation
Continued	pancreas, • *Grey-Turner sign:* flank hemorrhage, • *Cullen's sign:* periumbilical hemorrhage, • *tetany:* hypocalcemia from enzymatic fat necrosis
lab finding in acute pancreatitis	• **elevated serum amylase:** * increased in 2–12 h, * returns to normal in 3–4 days (increased renal clearance), * sensitivity 85–90%, * FP increase from bowel infarction, ruptured ectopic pregnancy, mumps, * FN with increased serum TG, • *increased urine amylase:* * elevated 1–10 days, * increased when serum amylase is normal, • *increased serum lipase:* * serum levels increased for 7–10 days, * sensitivity 75–85%, * good test to distinguish origin of increased amylase, • *neutrophilic leukocytosis,* • *hypocalcemia:* * 10–30%, * poor sign, • *hyperglycemia:* ~30%
imaging findings in acute pancreatitis	• *CT scan gold standard for pancreatic imaging:* * not influenced by air in bowel like US, * best test for obese patients, • *plain abdominal film:* sentinel loop, • *left-sided pleural effusion:* * 10%, * contains amylase, which is diagnostic for acute pancreatitis
complications of acute pancreatitis	• **pancreatic necrosis,** • *pseudocyst:* * persistence of hyperamylasemia >1 wk, * CT scan best test, * surgical consult, • *pancreatic abscess:* * fever, * leukocytosis, * persistent hyperamylasemia, * medical emergency, • *ARDS:* destruction of surfactant by increased circulating lecithinase, • *hypovolemic shock:* third space loss of fluids, • *DIC:* activation of prothrombin by trypsin
system used to determine prognosis in acute pancreatitis due to alcohol	*Ransom's criteria* • *admission:* * age >55, * WBC count >16,000 cells/μL, * glucose >200 mg/dL, * LDH >350 IU/L, * AST >250 U/L, • *during first 48 hours:* * Hct drop >10%, * serum BUN rise >5 mg/dL, * Pao$_2$ <60 mm Hg, * base deficit >4 mEq/L, * calcium <8 mg/dL, * fluid sequestration >6 liters, • *prognosis:* <3 signs: 0.9% mortality, 3–4 signs: 16% mortality, 5–6 signs: 40% mortality, >6 signs: 100% mortality

Table 9–9. GALLBLADDER AND PANCREATIC DISORDERS Continued

Most Common...	Answer and Explanation
system used to determine prognosis in acute pancreatitis due to biliary tract disease	*Ransom's criteria* • *admission:* * age >70, * WBC count >18,000 cells/μL, * glucose >220 mg/dL, * LDH >400 IU/L, * AST >250 IU/L, • *during first 48 hours:* * Hct drop >10%, * serum BUN rise >2 mg/dL, * serum calcium <8 mg/dL, * base deficit >5 mEq/L, * fluid sequestration >4 liters, • *prognosis:* same as above
Rx of acute pancreatitis	*supportive therapy:* * crystalloid solutions, * meperidine for pain (less sphincter of Oddi spasm), * NG suction if vomiting severe, * NPO
causes of chronic pancreatitis	• **chronic use of alcohol,** • *CF:* MCC in children, • *hereditary,* • *protein calorie malnutrition:* MCC in third world countries
clinical findings in chronic pancreatitis	• **severe pain:** duct obstruction, • *pancreatic calcifications:* CT best study, • *steatorrhea:* * weight loss, * malnutrition, • *DM:* 70%
lab findings in chronic pancreatitis	• *increased serum amylase:* ~50%, • *increased urine amylase:* more reliable than serum test, • *pancreatic calcifications:* CT best test, • *abnormal bentiromide test:* see Table 9–4, • *abnormal stimulation tests:* IV administration of secretin/cholecystokinin and collection of pancreatic secretions, • *ERCP:* calcified concretions with duct dilatation producing a "chain of lakes" appearance
Rx of chronic pancreatitis	• **abstain from alcohol,** • *pancreatic enzymes,* • *fat-soluble vitamins,* • *meperidine:* addiction is common
type of pancreatic cancer	• **adenocarcinoma,** • *islet cell tumors*
causes of pancreatic carcinoma	• **smoking,** • *chronic pancreatitis,* • *hereditary pancreatitis,* • *DM,* • *high saturated-fat diet* [Point mutations of the p53 suppressor gene and ras oncogene have been strongly implicated.]
pancreatic site for cancer	• **head of the pancreas,** • *body,* • *tail*

Table continued on following page

Table 9–9. GALLBLADDER AND PANCREATIC DISORDERS *Continued*

Most Common...	Answer and Explanation
S/S of carcinoma of the head of pancreas	• **epigastric pain,** • *painless jaundice:* CB% >50, • *acholic stools,* • *weight loss,* • *palpable GB:* Courvoisier's sign, • *Trousseau's superficial thrombophlebitis*
lab findings in pancreatic cancer	*elevated CA19-9:* * gold standard tumor marker, * enzymes not commonly elevated
Rx of pancreatic cancer	*surgery:* 5-year survival is 1%
islet cell tumor	*insulinoma*
clinical findings of an insulinoma	• *benign tumor* (~90%) *arising from* β-*islet cells,* • *MEN I association in 80%,* • *age:* 40–60 year old age bracket, • *clinical:* neuroglycopenia: forgetfulness, mental status abnormalities
lab findings in an insulinoma	• *fasting hypoglycemia:* * insulin normally inhibits gluconeogenesis, * 72-hour fast is the best stimulation test, • *increased serum insulin:* usually >5 μU/mL during fasting, • *increased serum C-peptide:* * excellent marker for endogenous release of insulin, * decreased in patients taking too much insulin, • *radiologic tests:* * CT scan useful in localizing tumor, * selective arteriography most sensitive localizing test
Rx of an insulinoma	• **surgery,** • *drugs:* * diazoxide, * verapamil, * octreotide (somatostatin analogue)
clinical findings of a glucagonoma	• *malignant tumor* (60%) *arising from* α-*islet cells,* • *clinical:* * DM (♦ hyperglycemia, ♦ osmotic diuresis), * weight loss, * classic rash: necrolytic migratory erythema, * diarrhea, * venous thrombosis, • *lab:* * serum glucagon >1000 pg/mL
Rx of a glucagonoma	• **surgery,** • *drugs:* octreotide
clinical findings of a somatostatinoma	• *malignant tumor of* δ-*islet cells,* • *somatostatin normally inhibits insulin, gastrin, secretin, cholecystokinin,* • *clinical:* * DM, * steatorrhea, * gallstones, * achlorhydria
Rx of somatostatinoma	*surgery*

Table 9–9. GALLBLADDER AND PANCREATIC DISORDERS *Continued*

Most Common...	Answer and Explanation
S/S of a VIPoma (pancreatic cholera, Verner-Morrison syndrome)	• *malignant tumor of islets with excessive production of vasointestinal peptide,* • *clinical:* * secretory diarrhea, * achlorhydria, * muscle weakness (hypokalemia), * hypercalcemia (70%), * hyperglycemia (50%)
Rx of a VIPoma	• **surgery,** • *octreotide*

Question: Which of the following disorders have an association with gallbladder disease? **SELECT 4**
(A) Insulinoma
(B) Somatostatinoma
(C) Ascending cholangitis
(D) Gallbladder cancer
(E) AIDS
(F) Ulcerative colitis
(G) Intravascular hemolytic anemia
(H) Dubin-Johnson syndrome
(I) Chronic pancreatitis

Answers: (B), (C), (D), (E): Insulinomas are not associated with gallbladder disease (**chronic A is incorrect**). Somatostatinomas (**choice B**) are associated with gallstones because of the inhibitory effect of somatostatin on the release of cholecystokinin. Ascending cholangitis (**choice C**). Gallstones are the primary risk factor for gallbladder cancer (**choice D**). Both CMV and *Cryptosporidium* produce biliary tract disease in patients with AIDS (**choice E**). Ulcerative colitis is not directly associated with GB disease (**choice F is incorrect**). However, CD is associated with gallstones owing to bile salt deficiency secondary to terminal ileal disease. Intravascular hemolysis is not associated with increased delivery of UCB to the liver. However, extravascular hemolysis is associated with calcium bilirubinate stones (**choice G is incorrect**). Dubin-Johnson syndrome is a genetic hyperbilirubinemia with a defect in secretion of bile. Dye studies show nonvisualization of the GB; however, there is no GB disease (**choice H is incorrect**). Chronic pancreatitis, unlike acute pancreatitis, is not associated with GB disease (**choice I is incorrect**).

AIDS = acquired immunodeficiency syndrome, ALP = alkaline phosphatase, ARDS = adult respiratory distress syndrome, AST = aspartate aminotransferase, BUN = blood urea nitrogen, CBD = common bile duct, CD = Crohn's disease, CF = cystic fibrosis, CH = cholesterol, CMV = cytomegalovirus, CT = computed tomography, DIC = disseminated intravascular coagulation, DM = diabetes mellitus, EHA = extravascular hemolytic anemia, ERCP = endoscopic retrograde cholangiopancreatography, FN = false-negative, FP = false-positive, GB = gallbladder, Hct = hematocrit, IV = intravenous, LDH = lactate dehydrogenase, MCC = most common cause, MEN = multiple endocrine neoplasia, NG =

nasogastric, NPO = Latin term for nothing by mouth, N/V = nausea and vomiting, PaO$_2$ = partial pressure of arterial oxygen, PA = pernicious anemia, RBC = red blood cell, RUQ = right upper quadrant, Rx = treatment, S/S = signs and symptoms, thal = thalassemia, UCB = unconjugated bilirubin, US = ultrasonography, VIP = vasointestinal peptide, WBC = white blood cell.

Table 9–10. NUTRITIONAL ASSESSMENT, EATING DISORDERS, AND PROTEIN ENERGY MALNUTRITION (PEM)

Most Common...	Answer and Explanation
nutritionally related COD	• **heart disease,** • *cancer,* • *stroke* [These three disorders account for two-thirds of all deaths in the United States. Dietary factors (e.g., low fiber/high saturated fat) are the second most common (smoking #1) contributing factor to increased morbidity and mortality in the United States.]
macronutrients	• *protein,* • *fat,* • *CHO*
micronutrients	• *vitamins,* • *minerals,* • *trace elements*
sign of macronutrient deficiency	*progressive weight loss:* * 10% unintended weight loss in 6 months, * 5% unintended weight loss in 1 month
physical findings of macronutrient deficiency	• **wasting of muscle:** * temporal area, * thenar atrophy, * extremity muscles, • *loss of subcutaneous fat*
recommendation for number of kcal to lose, maintain, gain weight	• *lose:* 25 kcal/kg • *maintain:* 30 kcal/kg • *gain:* 35 kcal/kg
formula used to estimate basal energy expenditure (BEE)	*Harris-Benedict equation:* * separate equation for men and women, * based on sex, height, weight, and age
formula to calculate BEE via a Swan-Ganz catheter	*Fick equation:* includes * measured O$_2$ saturation in arterial/venous blood, * cardiac output, * Hb
causes of increased metabolic rate	• **fever,** • *sepsis,* • *severe burn,* • *massive trauma,* • *hyperthyroidism*
formula used to measure ideal body weight (IBW)	• *men:* base of 106 lbs for 5'0", add 6 lbs for each inch over 5'0", • *women:* base of 100 lbs for 5'0", add 5 lbs for each inch over 5'0"

Most Common...	Answer and Explanation
test to evaluate total body fat composition	*caliper skinfold measurements at multiple sites*
tests to evaluate immune competence	• **cutaneous hypersensitivity reactions to common antigens,** • *total lymphocyte count:* * T cells mainly decreased, * no response to common antigens indicates anergy poor CMI
tests to evaluate lean body mass	• *urine creatinine:* metabolic product of creatine in muscle, • *urine 3-methylhistidine:* component of actin and myosin in muscle
tests to evaluate visceral protein mass	• *retinol-binding protein:* 1 day half-life, • *prealbumin:* 2–3 days half-life, • *transferrin:* 8–10 days half-life, • *albumin:* 18–20 days half-life 18–20 days) [The shorter the protein half-life, the greater the correlation with protein mass.]
clinical findings in anorexia nervosa	• **distorted body image,** • *secondary amenorrhea:* * body weight/fat 15% below normal → * decreases GnRH → * decreases FSH/LH → * decreases estrogen → * secondary amenorrhea, • *osteoporosis:* lack of estrogen, • *cardiovascular abnormalities:* * heart failure, * ventricular arrhythmias, • *increased lanugo hair,* • *lab:* stress hormones are increased (ACTH, cortisol, GH)
COD in anorexia nervosa	*ventricular arrhythmias*
clinical findings in bulimia nervosa	• **self-induced vomiting,** • *bruising of knuckles:* Russell's sign, • *acid injury of enamel,* • *enlarged salivary glands,* • *Boerhaave's/Mallory-Weiss syndromes:* distal esophagus/stomach rupture or tear, respectively
acid-base disorder in bulimia nervosa	*hypochloremic, hypokalemic metabolic alkalosis from vomiting*
definition of obesity	*body mass index* (BMI): * >30 kg/m^2 (weight in kilograms divided by height in meters squared), * BMI 27.5–30 kg/m^2 = mild obesity, 31–40 kg/m^2 = moderate obesity, >40 kg/m^2 = morbid obesity
ethnic groups predisposed to obesity	• *Native Americans,* • *blacks,* • *Hispanics,* • *Caucasians*

Table continued on following page

Table 9–10. NUTRITIONAL ASSESSMENT, EATING
DISORDERS, AND PROTEIN ENERGY MALNUTRITION
(PEM) *Continued*

Most Common...	Answer and Explanation
cause of obesity	*genetic factors:* * 50–75%, * energy intake > energy expenditure at rest and exercise, * alterations in hypothalamic feeding/satiety center, * obesity gene in adipose codes for a protein called leptin, which normally controls appetite, * gene inactivation leads to obesity
medical complications in obesity	• **hypertension:** * ? hyperinsulinemia with increased renal sodium reabsorption, * weight loss most effective life modification for lowering blood pressure, • *LVH*, • *thromboembolism*, • *CAD:* waist-to-hip ratio >1 is greatest risk, • *stroke*, • *sleep apnea*, • *gallstones:* increased CH in bile, • *cancer:* * colorectal, * breast, * endometrial, * ovarian, • *osteoarthritis*, • *type II DM:* * increased adipose down-regulates insulin receptor synthesis, * weight loss is most important life modification for controlling glucose, • *lipid abnormalities:* * increased LDL/TG, * decreased HDL
Rx of obesity	• *behavior modification*, • *low-calorie diets*, • *exercise*, • *medication:* * amphetamines, • *surgery:* * vertical banding of stomach, * gastric bypass
COD in calorie-restricted diets	*ventricular arrhythmias*
nutritional problem in developing countries	*protein-energy malnutrition* (PEM): two primary PEM syndromes are kwashiorkor and marasmus
cause of PEM in the United States	*secondary to other diseases:* e.g., * malabsorption, * sepsis, * postoperative state
effect of PEM on nitrogen balance	*negative nitrogen balance:* intake (protein intake 24 hours/6.25) − excretion (urine urea nitrogen 24 hours + 4) ÷ total urine volume in liters, * normal nitrogen balance approaches zero
causes of PEM	• **inadequate protein intake,** • *nutrition losses*, • *increased nutrient requirements*
effect of PEM on hepatic function	*decreased protein synthesis*

Table 9–10. NUTRITIONAL ASSESSMENT, EATING DISORDERS, AND PROTEIN ENERGY MALNUTRITION (PEM) *Continued*

Most Common...	Answer and Explanation
effect of PEM in the heart	*myofiber atrophy with subsequent decrease in cardiac output*
effect of PEM in the lungs	• **atrophy of muscles of respiration:** decreases VC and TV, • *decreased mucociliary clearance:* prone to infections
effect of PEM in GI tract	• *loss of brush border enzymes:* "use it or lose it," • *loss of villi:* malabsorption, • *pancreatic insufficiency:* malabsorption
effect of PEM on the immune system	• *decreases total lymphocyte count:* * <2500 cells/μL, * decreased CD$_4$ T cells, • *decreased C3 and factor B,* • *abnormal phagocytic function:* e.g., * chemotaxis, * phagocytosis, • *decreased secretory IgA*
effect of PEM on wound healing	*all phases adversely affected:* e.g., * neutrophil function, * collagen deposition, * granulation tissue formation, * remodeling of collagen*
clinical findings in marasmus	• **total reduction in caloric intake,** • *muscle wasting,* • *loss of subcutaneous fat,* • *"broomstick extremities"*
clinical findings in kwashiorkor	• **inadequate amount of protein:** normal total caloric intake, • *hypoalbuminemia:* decrease in plasma oncotic pressure → pitting edema/ascites, • *decreased liver synthesis of apolipoproteins:* hepatomegaly with fatty change, • *"flaky paint" dermatitis,* • *diarrhea:* * loss of brush border enzymes, * parasitic diseases, * malabsorption, • *anemia,* • *decreased immune response,* • *reddish hair:* flag sign, • *apathy:* difficult to feed
modes of feeding	• **oral supplementation:** * preferable mode, * less expensive, * fewer complications, • *enteral:* * tube feeding, * maintains mucosal integrity, • *parenteral:* * peripheral IV (short-term Rx <10 days), * TPN via internal jugular/subclavian vein (>10 days anticipated for nutritional support), * danger of infection (♦ *Staphylococcus aureus* most common, ♦ *Candida* sepsis)

Table continued on following page

Table 9–10. NUTRITIONAL ASSESSMENT, EATING DISORDERS, AND PROTEIN ENERGY MALNUTRITION (PEM) *Continued*

Most Common...	Answer and Explanation
complications of enteral feeding	• **diarrhea,** • *electrolyte imbalance:* * hypo/hyperkalemia, * hypo/hypernatremia, * hypomagnesemia, * hypophosphatemia
complications of TPN	• **diarrhea:** * normal AG metabolic acidosis, * hypokalemia, * hypomagnesemia, • *liver dysfunction:* * fatty liver due to excessive CHO and VLDL synthesis, * gallstones, * transaminasemia, • *trace element deficiencies:* zinc, • *increased serum BUN:* protein in TPN mixture, • *hyperglycemia,* • *catheter infection:* * *Staphylococcus aureus* most common, * *Candida* (most common fungus), * culture blood/catheter tip, • *pneumothorax:* * related to placement of catheter (chest radiograph postprocedure)

Question: Which of the following are medical complications directly associated with obesity? **SELECT 5**
   (A) Stomach cancer
   (B) Endometrial cancer
   (C) Anemia of chronic disease
   (D) Type I DM
   (E) Osteoarthritis
   (F) Hypertension
   (G) Hypothyroidism
   (H) Stroke
   (I) Pancreatic carcinoma
   (J) Gallstones

Answers: (B), (E), (F), (H), (J): Stomach cancer and pancreatic cancer are not increased in obesity (choices A and I are incorrect), however, there is an increased incidence of colon cancer. Endometrial cancer (choice B) is increased in obesity owing to increased estrogen synthesis by aromatization of testosterone and androstenedione in the adipose. ACD is not a direct association with obesity, nor is any other type of anemia (choice C is incorrect). Type II DM, not type I DM is directly related to obesity owing to the reduction in insulin receptor synthesis with an increase in adipose (choice D is incorrect). Osteoarthritis (choice E) is common in obesity owing to increased weight on weight-bearing joints. Hypertension (choice F) is the most common complication of obesity. Hypothyroidism may be a cause of obesity, but it is not a complication of obesity (choice G is incorrect). Strokes (choice H) are increased in obesity. Gallstones (choice J) are increased owing to increased CH in bile.

ACD = anemia of chronic disease, ACTH = adrenocorticotropic hormone, AG = anion gap, BEE = basal energy expenditure, BMI = body mass index, BUN = blood urea nitrogen, CAD = coronary artery disease, CH = cholesterol, CHO = carbohydrate, CMI = cell-mediated immunity, COD = cause of death, DM = diabetes mellitus, FSH = follicle-stimulating hormone, GnRH = gonadotropin-releasing hormone, GH = growth hormone, GI = gastrointestinal, Hb = hemoglobin, HDL = high density lipoprotein, IBW = ideal body weight, Ig = immunoglobulin, IV = intravenous, LDL = low density lipoprotein, LH = luteinizing hormone, LVH = left ventricular hypertrophy, PEM = protein-energy malnutrition, Rx = treatment, TG = triglyceride, TPN = total parenteral nutrition, TV = tidal volume, VC = vital capacity, VLDL = very low density lipoprotein.

Table 9–11. VITAMIN DISORDERS

Most Common...	Answer and Explanation
types of vitamins associated with toxicity	*fat-soluble vitamins A, D, E, K:* * fat-soluble vitamins are stored in fat, * water-soluble vitamins, when in excess, are excreted in urine
vitamins involved in biochemical reactions	*water-soluble vitamins*
functions of vitamin A	• *prevents squamous metaplasia,* • *maintains visual purple:* rods/cones in retina, • *wound healing,* • *spermatogenesis,* • *normal growth*
causes of vitamin A deficiency	• **malnutrition:** alcoholics, • *malabsorption syndromes,* • *laxative abuse with mineral oils,* • *drugs:* * aluminum hydroxide antacids, * neomycin, * cholestyramine, * clofibrate, • *nephrotic syndrome:* lose RBP in urine
clinical findings in vitamin A deficiency	• **nyctalopia:** night blindness, • *blindness:* * keratomalacia of cornea, * very common cause of global blindness, • *follicular hyperkeratosis,* • *poor wound healing*
clinical findings in vitamin A toxicity	• **intracranial HTN:** * papilledema, * pseudotumor cerebri (headache, diplopia, papilledema, sixth nerve palsy), • **liver necrosis:** elevated transaminases, • *hypercalcemia:* enhances PTH activity [Vitamin A is in very high concentration in polar bear livers and has produced toxicity in hunters and Alaskan natives.]
lab test used to diagnose vitamin A deficiency/toxicity	• *serum retinol,* • *serum retinol esters, respectively*

Table continued on following page

Table 9–11. VITAMIN DISORDERS *Continued*

Most Common...	Answer and Explanation
functions of vitamin D	• **reabsorb calcium/phosphorus from small intestine:** * vitamin D activation of receptors on osteoblasts causes the release of ALP, * ALP establishes a high solubility product $(Ca^{++} \times PO_4^{--})$ by increasing local PO_4^{--} concentration, * mineralizes bone/cartilage, • *stimulates conversion of marrow macrophages into osteoclasts*
sites involved in vitamin D synthesis	• **skin:** synthesis of 7-dehydrocholesterol, • *small intestine:* reabsorption, • *liver:* first hydroxylation to 25-(OH)-D_3 cholecalciferol calcidiol, • *kidneys:* second hydroxylation to 1,25 (OH)$_2$-D_3 cholecalciferol (calcitriol), • *vitamin D receptors on target organs:* * duodenum, * osteoblasts
causes of vitamin D deficiency	• **chronic renal failure:** decreased second hydroxylation, • *lack of sun exposure:* decreased synthesis of skin-derived 7-dehydrocholesterol, • *malnutrition:* * decreased intake, * unfortified milk, * breast milk, • *malabsorption:* decreased absorption, • *liver disease:* decreased first hydroxylation, • *hyperphosphatemia:* decreased synthesis of 1-α-hydroxylase, • *hypoparathyroidism:* decreased synthesis of 1-α-hydroxylase, • *drugs enhancing liver cytochrome system causing increased metabolism of 25-(OH)-D_3:* e.g., * phenytoin, * phenobarbital, • *mineral oil cathartics:* * malabsorption, * common in the elderly, • *cholestyramine:* malabsorption
stimuli for synthesis of 1-α-hydroxylase	• **PTH,** • *hypophosphatemia* [The enzyme is synthesized in the proximal tubules. 1,25 (OH)$_2$-D_3 and hyperphosphatemia inhibit enzyme synthesis.]
clinical finding in vitamin D deficiency in adults	• *osteomalacia:* * soft bone, * reduced bone mineralization leads to an excess of osteoid, • *clinical:* * bowing of legs, * bone pain, * pathologic fractures
radiologic findings in vitamin D deficiency	• **osteopenia:** rarefied bone, • *pseudofractures:* * Looser's lines, * milkman's fractures, * linear lines in the metaphysis where blood vessels push aside the soft osteoid
lab test to assess vitamin D status	25-(OH)-D_2 (calcidiol): longer circulating half-life (3 weeks) than calcitriol (4–6 hours)

Table 9–11. VITAMIN DISORDERS *Continued*

Most Common...	Answer and Explanation
lab findings in vitamin D deficiency due to chronic renal disease	• **hypocalcemia,** • *normal to high serum phosphorus:* * kidneys are the main excretory route of phosphorus, * "normalizes" owing to phosphaturic effect of increased PTH from stimulus for PTH release, • *high ALP:* response to reduced bone mineralization, • *increased PTH:* * stimulus of hypocalcemia, * called secondary hyperparathyroidism, • *normal 25-(OH)-D₃,* • *low 1,25 (OH)₂-D₃*
lab findings in vitamin D deficiency due to malabsorption	• **hypocalcemia,** • *hypophosphatemia,* • *high ALP,* • *increased PTH,* • *low 25-(OH)-D₃,* • *low 1,25 (OH)₂-D₃*
cause of type I vitamin D–dependent rickets	*low 1-α-hydroxylase*
lab findings in type I vitamin D–dependent rickets	• *hypocalcemia,* • *hypophosphatemia,* • *high ALP:* osteomalacia, • *high PTH,* • *normal/ high 25-(OH)-D₃,* • *low 1,25 (OH)₂-D₃*
cause of type II vitamin D–dependent rickets	*absent receptors for vitamin D*
lab findings in type II vitamin D–dependent rickets	• *hypocalcemia,* • *hypophosphatemia,* • *high ALP:* osteomalacia, • *high PTH,* • *normal 25- (OH)-D₃,* • *high 1,25 (OH)₂-D₃:* key distinction from type I
cause of hypervitaminosis D	• **Rx with vitamin D in renal disease,** • overuse in vitamin faddists
clinical findings in vitamin D toxicity	• *hypercalcemia,* • *soft tissue metastatic calcification,* • *nephrocalcinosis:* renal dysfunction, • *altered mental status*
Rx of vitamin D toxicity	*glucocorticoids*
functions of vitamin E	*antioxidant:* * inhibits lipid peroxidation of cell membranes, * acts in conjunction with selenium
causes of vitamin E deficiency	• **chronic fat malabsorption:** e.g., CF, • *abetalipoproteinemia:* absent apo B decreases formation of chylomicrons carrying fat-soluble vitamins

Table continued on following page

Table 9–11. VITAMIN DISORDERS *Continued*

Most Common...	Answer and Explanation
clinical finding in vitamin E deficiency	• **spinocerebellar ataxia**, • *hemolytic anemia*, • *posterior column disease:* * proprioception abnormalities, * areflexia, • *retinopathy*
lab test to confirm vitamin E deficiency	*RBC fragility test:* * vitamin E maintenance of lipids in RBC cell membrane, * increased hemolysis indicates deficiency
clinical findings in vitamin E toxicity	*low levels of vitamin K–dependent coagulation factors II, VII, IX, X, protein C and protein S*
functions of vitamin K	γ-*carboxylates vitamin K–dependent factors synthesized by the liver:* * vitamin K–dependent factors are II, VII, IX, X, protein C, protein S, * γ-carboxylation sites are where calcium binds to the factor in a clot
causes of vitamin K deficiency	• **broad-spectrum antibiotics:** kill colon bacteria synthesizing vitamin K_2, • *malabsorption*, • *newborns:* no bacterial colonization, • *drugs:* warfarin inhibits epoxide reductase, which normally keeps vitamin K active, • *rat poison:* contains warfarin, • *excess vitamin E:* * decreases levels of vitamin K–dependent coagulation factors, * potentiates warfarin
clinical findings in vitamin K deficiency	*hemorrhagic diathesis:* * ecchymoses, * petechiae, * GI bleeding [In newborns, it is called hemorrhagic disease of the newborn.]
lab test to confirm vitamin K deficiency	*prothrombin time:* functional assessment of vitamin K
clinical findings of vitamin K toxicity	• *dyspnea,* • *cardiovascular collapse:* this primarily occurs with IV administration
functions of thiamine (B_1)	• *cofactor in pyruvate dehydrogenase:* * conversion of pyruvate to acetyl CoA, * generates ATP, • *cofactor in* α-*ketoglutarate dehydrogenase:* * converts α-ketoglutarate to succinyl CoA, * generates ATP
causes of thiamine deficiency	• **alcohol excess,** • *populations eating polished rice,* • *renal dialysis,* • *high CHO diet:* uses up thiamine in the pyruvate dehydrogenase reaction, • *diuretics*
clinical findings of thiamine deficiency	• *wet beriberi:* * high output cardiac failure, * congestive cardiomyopathy, • *dry beriberi:* * Wernicke's encephalopathy (confusion,

Table 9–11. VITAMIN DISORDERS Continued

Most Common...	Answer and Explanation
Continued	ataxia, nystagmus, ophthalmoplegia), * Korsakoff's psychosis (antegrade/retrograde memory deficits, confabulation), * peripheral neuropathy, • *muscle weakness*
lab test to confirm thiamine deficiency	*RBC transketolase activity:* an increase in transketolase activity after adding thiamine indicates deficiency
functions of riboflavin (B_2)	• *component of flavin mononucleotide* (FMN): oxidative phosphorylation, • *component of flavin adenine dinucleotide* (FAD): oxidative phosphorylation, • *component of glutathione reductase:* production of glutathione
causes of riboflavin deficiency	*conjunction with other vitamin deficiencies*
clinical findings of riboflavin deficiency	• **neovascularization of cornea,** • *facial dermatitis:* resembles seborrheic dermatitis, • *scrotal dermatitis,* • *magenta tongue:* glossitis, • *cheilosis:* dryness of vermilion border of lips, • *angular stomatitis:* cracking in angles of the mouth
lab test to confirm riboflavin deficiency	*RBC glutathione reductase activity:* increased activity after FAD stimulation indicates deficiency
functions of niacin (B_3)	*formation of nicotinamide adenine dinucleotide* (NAD^+) *and nicotinamide adenine dinucleotide phosphate* ($NADP^+$): * key cofactors for oxidation reduction reactions, * nicotinic acid also lowers lipids
essential amino acid used to synthesize niacin	*tryptophan:* also used to synthesize serotonin (neurotransmitter, vasodilator)
causes of niacin deficiency	• **diets high in corn:** lack tryptophan, • *tryptophan deficiency:* * carcinoid syndrome, * Hartnup's disease (decreased intestinal/renal reabsorption of neutral amino acids)
clinical findings in niacin deficiency (pellagra)	• **triad of diarrhea, dementia, dermatitis** (Casal's necklace: hyperpigmented area resembling a necklace), • *glossitis,* • *cheilosis,* • *burning dysesthesias*

Table continued on following page

Table 9–11. VITAMIN DISORDERS *Continued*

Most Common...	Answer and Explanation
lab test to confirm niacin deficiency	*urine metabolites of niacin:* N-methylnicotin-amide
clinical findings of nicotinic acid toxicity	• **cutaneous flushing:** * vasodilatation, * prevented by pretreatment with aspirin, • *liver necrosis,* • *hyperglycemia,* • *gout*
functions of pyridoxine (B$_6$)	• *heme synthesis:* glycine + succinyl CoA → δ-ALA, • *synthesis of neurotransmitters:* * GABA, * serotonin, * NOR, • *transamination reactions:* amino acids ↔ α-ketoacid conversions, • *niacin synthesis from tryptophan*
causes of pyridoxine deficiency	• **drugs:** * INH, * hydralazine, * penicillamine, * diuretics, * birth control pills, * theophylline, • *alcohol excess*
clinical findings of pyridoxine toxicity	• *glossitis,* • *angular stomatitis,* • *sideroblastic anemia:* * defect in heme synthesis, * ringed sideroblasts in marrow, • *CNS signs:* * irritability, * depression, * abnormal EEG, * convulsions (particularly infants), • *peripheral neuropathy*
lab method to confirm pyridoxine deficiency	• *serum pyridoxal phosphate,* • *RBC enzyme activity testing using transaminases*
clinical findings of pyridoxine toxicity	• **convulsions,** • *peripheral neuropathy,* • *photosensitivity reactions:* excess porphyrin synthesis, • *nasolabial seborrhea*
functions of vitamin C (ascorbic acid)	• *hydroxylation of proline/lysine in collagen synthesis:* hydroxylation site is binding site for cross-bridging to produce strong collagen, • *reduction of ferric to ferrous ions:* * important in GI absorption of iron, * metHb → reduced Hb, • *reduction of dihydrofolate →THF,* • *synthesis of NOR,* • *blocks formation of nitrosamines:* these are carcinogenic agents implicated in esophageal/stomach cancer, • *traps reactive oxygen FRs*
causes of vitamin C deficiency	• **poor diet:** common in elderly, • *smoking*

Table 9–11. VITAMIN DISORDERS *Continued*

Most Common...	Answer and Explanation
clinical findings of vitamin C deficiency (scurvy)	• **hemorrhagic diathesis:** * ecchymoses, * petechiae, * bleeding gums after brushing teeth, * hemarthroses, • *bone pain:* hemorrhage into periosteum, • *perifollicular hemorrhage,* • *corkscrew hairs,* • *loss of teeth,* • *poor wound healing,* • *fatigue/depression,* • *stomach cancer:* increase in nitrosamines, • *iron/folate deficiency,* • *glossitis*
lab method to confirm vitamin C deficiency	*estimating amount of ascorbic acid in leukocytes:* * women have 20% higher levels than men, * smoking lowers ascorbic acid
clinical findings of vitamin C excess	• **diarrhea,** • *increased oxalate synthesis:* ? increased calcium oxalate renal stones, • *false-positive Clinitest reactions in urine:* ascorbic acid is a reducing agent, • *false-negative reactions in urine dipstick reactions:* * blood, * glucose, * bilirubin, * nitrites, * leukocyte esterase
functions/causes of folate and vitamin B_{12}	*see Table 8–5*
functions of biotin	*carboxylase reactions:* pyruvate → oxaloacetate
cause of biotin deficiency	*eating large quantities of raw eggs:* * avidin in raw eggs binds biotin, * requires ~20 eggs on a continual basis to produce deficiency
vitamin toxicities producing hypercalcemia	• *vitamin A:* enhances the action of vitamin D, • *vitamin D*
vitamin deficiencies with eye abnormalities	• **vitamin A:** * squamous metaplasia of conjunctiva (Bitot's spot), * keratomalacia, * nyctalopia, • *riboflavin:* corneal neovascularization
vitamin deficiencies with skin/hair abnormalities	• **vitamin A:** follicular hyperkeratosis, • *vitamin C:* * perifollicular hemorrhages, * corkscrew hairs, • *biotin:* alopecia, • *niacin:* * pellagra, * hyperpigmentation in sun-exposed areas, • *riboflavin:* flaky dermatitis

Table continued on following page

Table 9–11. VITAMIN DISORDERS *Continued*

Most Common...	Answer and Explanation
vitamin deficiencies producing anemia	• **folate:** * macrocytic, * most commonly noted in alcoholics, • *B_{12}:* * macrocytic, * most commonly due to PA, • *vitamin E:* hemolytic anemia, • *vitamin C:* iron/folate deficiency, • *pyridoxine:* sideroblastic anemia
vitamin deficiency manifested after infusion of glucose	*thiamine:* * infusion of glucose uses up the already low stores of thiamine when pyruvate dehydrogenase converts pyruvate to acetyl CoA, * precipitates acute Wernicke's encephalopathy (see above), * IV thiamine should be administered before infusing glucose to prevent this complication
vitamin deficiencies producing diarrhea	• *niacin:* pellagra, • *B_{12}/folate:* reduction in DNA synthesis causes malfunction of intestinal cells leading to malabsorption
vitamin deficiencies produced by drinking goat's milk	• **folate,** • *pyridoxine* [Goat's milk is commonly used as a substitute in milk-allergic children and as substitute for breast milk in Third World countries.]
vitamin deficiency causing atrophic gastritis and achlorhydria	*B_{12}:* * specifically PA, * in PA, autoantibodies destroy parietal cells, which synthesize acid and intrinsic factor
antioxidant vitamins	• *vitamin E:* inhibits lipid peroxidation in cell membrane, • *vitamin C:* FR scavenger
endocrine disorder producing β-carotenemia	*primary hypothyroidism:* * thyroxine enhances small intestine conversion of β-carotenes into retinoic acid, * hypothyroidism causes a buildup β-carotenes and production of yellow-colored skin (not conjunctiva), * β-carotenes are not toxic in high doses
supplements required in pregnancy	• *folate:* folate stores last ~3–4 months, • *iron:* * women have ~400 mg of iron stores, * normally lose 500 mg per pregnancy
mechanism of folate deficiency with phenytoin	*blocks intestinal conjugase:* enzyme converts polyglutamates (form of folate in food) into monoglutamates for reabsorption
mechanism of folate deficiency with birth control pills	*blocks uptake of monoglutamates in the jejunum*

Table 9–11. VITAMIN DISORDERS *Continued*

Most Common...	Answer and Explanation
mechanism of alcohol in producing folate deficiency	• **decreased intake,** • *blocks reabsorption of monoglutamates in jejunum*
mechanism of folate deficiency with methotrexate	*block in dihydrofolate reductase:* enzyme that converts DHF into THF

Question: Which of the following signs of vitamin deficiency would you expect in a patient with cystic fibrosis who has steatorrhea?
SELECT 5
- (A) Nyctalopia
- (B) Congestive cardiomyopathy
- (C) Osteomalacia
- (D) Skin hyperpigmentation
- (E) Corneal neovascularization
- (F) Tetany
- (G) Spinocerebellar ataxia
- (H) Ecchymoses

Answers: (A), (C), (F), (G), (H): All fat-soluble vitamins (A, D, E, K) are deficient in CF owing to exocrine pancreas insufficiency and maldigestion of fats. Nyctalopia **(choice A)** is the first sign of vitamin A deficiency. Congestive cardiomyopathy is found in thiamine deficiency, which is not present in CF **(choice B is incorrect)**. Osteomalacia **(choice C)** and tetany **(choice F)** are signs of vitamin D deficiency, the former due to lack of bone mineralization and the latter to hypocalcemia. Hyperpigmentation of skin is a sign of niacin deficiency and is not seen in CF **(choice D is incorrect)**. Corneal neovascularization is a sign of riboflavin deficiency, which is not present in CF **(choice E is incorrect)**. Spinocerebellar ataxia **(choice G)** is noted in vitamin E deficiency. Ecchymoses **(choice H)** are a sign of vitamin K deficiency.

δ-ALA = delta aminolevulinic acid, ALP = alkaline phosphatase, apo = apolipoprotein, ATP = adenosine triphosphate, CF = cystic fibrosis, CHO = carbohydrate, CNS = central nervous system, CoA = coenzyme A, DHF = dihydrofolate, EEG = electroencephalogram, FAD = flavin adenine dinucleotide, FMN = flavin mononucleotide, FR = free radical, GABA = γ-aminobutyric, GI = gastrointestinal, Hb = hemoglobin, HTN = hypertension, INH = isoniazid, IV = intravenous, metHb = methemoglobin, NAD = nicotinamide adenine dinucleotide, NADP = nicotinamide adenine dinucleotide phosphate, NOR = norepinephrine, PA = pernicious anemia, PTH = parathormone, RBC = red blood cell, RBP = retinol-binding protein, Rx = treatment, THF = tetrahydrofolate.

Table 9–12. TRACE ELEMENT DISORDERS, DIETARY
FIBER, NUTRITION AND CANCER, NUTRITIONAL
CHANGES WITH AGING, SPECIAL DIETS

Most Common...	Answer and Explanation
cause of trace element deficiencies	• **TPN,** • *decreased absorption:* malabsorption, • *increased excretion:* * chelation Rx, * nephrotic syndrome, * diuretics, * diarrhea, • *increased requirement:* * elderly, * DM
functions of zinc	• *cofactor in enzymes:* * SOD (neutralizes superoxide FR), * ALP (bone mineralization), * collagenases (remodeling collagen in wounds), • *immune functions:* macrophage function, • *nucleic acid/protein synthesis,* • *spermatogenesis,* • *embryonic development,* • *normal growth*
causes of zinc deficiency	• **TPN,** • *DM,* • *chronic malabsorption,* • *acrodermatitis enteropathica,* • *diet rich in phytic acid,* • *miscellaneous:* * AMI, * infection, • *drugs:* BCPs
S/S of zinc deficiency	• **poor wound healing,** • *dysgeusia:* lack of taste, • *growth retardation,* • *hypogonadism,* • *alopecia,* • *nyctalopia,* • *dry, scaly skin around eyes/mouth,* • *acrodermatitis enteropathica:* * AR disease, * decreased intestinal absorption of zinc, * growth retardation
functions of copper	• *cofactor in enzymes:* e.g., lysyl oxidase (forms collagen cross-links), • *Hb synthesis,* • *connective tissue metabolism*
causes of copper deficiency	• **TPN,** • *nephrotic syndrome,* • *kwashiorkor,* • *malabsorption*
S/S of copper deficiency	• *iron deficiency,* • *growth retardation,* • *defective hair pigmentation:* flag sign in kwashiorkor, • *dissecting aortic aneurysm,* • *osteoporosis*
S/S of Wilson's disease	*see Table 9–8*
functions of chromium	*glucose tolerance factor that enhances insulin activity*
S/S of chromium deficiency	• **glucose intolerance,** • *peripheral neuropathy*

**Table 9–12. TRACE ELEMENT DISORDERS, DIETARY
FIBER, NUTRITION AND CANCER, NUTRITIONAL
CHANGES WITH AGING, SPECIAL DIETS** *Continued*

Most Common...	Answer and Explanation
functions of selenium	• **antioxidant:** neutralizes peroxide, • *enhances immune system,* • *enhances conversion of T_4 to T_3*
functions of fluoride	*incorporates itself into bone/enamel*
abnormality in fluoride deficiency	*dental caries*
S/S of fluoride excess	• **mottling of teeth,** • *calcification ligaments/tendons,* • *increases brittleness of bones*
insoluble fibers	• *wheat bran,* • *wheat germ:* * insoluble fiber is nonfermentable, * composed of lignin, hemicellulose, cellulose
soluble fibers	• *oat bran,* • *fruits,* • *psyllium seeds:* * soluble fiber is fermentable, * composed of pectins, gums, mucilages, hemicellulose
fiber type that has a hypoglycemic/ hypocholesterolemic effect	*soluble fiber:* hypoglycemic effect enhances insulin activity
effects of fiber on stool	• **stool eliminated faster,** • *increases stool bulk,* • *decreases stool pH:* increase excretion of carcinogenic secondary bile acids (lithocholic acid), • *deconjugation of estrogen delivered in bile:* decrease amount of estrogen reabsorbed
cancers that are decreased owing to a high-fiber diet	• **colorectal,** • *endometrial,* • *ovarian,* • *breast* [Increased excretion of estrogen protects against endometrial, ovarian, breast cancers.]
cancers associated with high-fat diets	• *breast,* • *endometrial,* • *ovarian,* • *prostate,* • *colon:* * saturated fats plus ω-6 polyunsaturated fats increase the amount of free estrogen and estrogen metabolites, * saturated fats are converted into secondary bile acids, which are carcinogenic
functions of linoleic/ linolenic essential FAs	• synthesis of ω-3 polyunsaturated fats: * linolenic, * cardioprotective, • *linoleic acid is utilized in the synthesis of arachidonic acid and ω-6 fats*

Table continued on following page

Table 9–12. TRACE ELEMENT DISORDERS, DIETARY FIBER, NUTRITION AND CANCER, NUTRITIONAL CHANGES WITH AGING, SPECIAL DIETS *Continued*

Most Common...	Answer and Explanation
S/S of essential FA deficiency	• *dry skin,* • *thrombocytopenia,* • *hair loss,* • *impaired wound healing*
group of vegetables linked to a reduction in cancer	*cruciferous vegetables:* * e.g., broccoli, cauliflower, * contain increased amounts of β-carotenoids, vitamin C, vitamin E
food contaminant associated with HCC	*aflatoxins:* this mold is a cocarcinogen with hepatitis B in producing HCC
effects of FRs in promoting cancer	• *inititiate:* produce mutations in DNA, • *promote:* clonal expansion of initiated cell, • *enhance progression:* neoplastic cells develop heterogeneous populations with different functions
effects of a high saturated-fat diet	• *enhance atherosclerosis,* • *carcinogenic* [A saturated-fat diet contains saturated fat + ω-6 polyunsaturated lipids.]
role of monounsaturated fats in nutrition	*protective effect on hormone metabolism:* monounsaturated fats include canola oil and olive oil
vitamins that reduce cancer risk	• **vitamin C:** * prevents nitrosamination, * decreases incidence of oral, esophageal, stomach cancer, • *vitamin E,* • β-*carotenoids*
dietary recommendations to prevent cancer	• *avoid obesity,* • *decrease total fat intake to <25% of total calories,* • *decrease saturated fat to <7% of total calories,* • *increase intake of whole-grain foods,* • *increase intake of vegetables rich in* β-*carotenes:* dark green, yellow, deep orange vegetables, • *increase intake of cruciferous vegetables,* • *reduce amount of smoked meats, salt-cured meats, nitrite-cured foods,* • *avoid/reduce alcohol intake*
nutritional changes associated with aging	• *decrease in body weight,* • *decrease in lean body mass:* relative increase in fat, • *decrease in energy requirements*

Table 9–12. TRACE ELEMENT DISORDERS, DIETARY FIBER, NUTRITION AND CANCER, NUTRITIONAL CHANGES WITH AGING, SPECIAL DIETS *Continued*

Most Common...	Answer and Explanation
dietary inadequacies associated with aging	• *pyridoxine,* • *vitamin D,* • *folate,* • *calcium,* • *zinc*
supplements not recommended for the elderly	• *iron:* generates FRs and formation of oxidized LDL, • *vitamin A:* liver cannot clear retinoic acid out of the blood very well
recommendations for prevention of osteoporosis in postmenopausal women	• **estrogen,** • *calcium:* 1000–1500 mg, • *vitamin D:* 400–800 IU, • *exercise*
indications for a low-sodium diet	• *essential HTN,* • *CHF,* • *chronic renal disease:* if the patient has pitting edema, • *cirrhosis*
indications for a low-protein diet	• *chronic renal disease:* low-protein diet decreases urea load on the kidneys, • *cirrhosis:* low-protein diet decreases formation of ammonia by urease-producing bacteria in bowel [Diet should contain ~0.6 g/kg/d of protein.]
use of a high-fiber diet	• *lower CH,* • *decrease incidence of cancer,* • *decrease diverticular disease,* • *reduce blood glucose,* • *reduce IBS*
use of a fat-restricted diet	*fat malabsorption*
use of a low-CH, low saturated-fat diet	• **Rx of hyperlipidemia,** • *DM,* • *cancer prevention,* • *Rx of essential HTN*
use of a high-potassium diet	• **compensate for potassium loss due to diuretics,** • *lower blood pressure*
use of a high-calcium diet	• *prevent postmenopausal osteoporosis,* • *lower blood pressure,* • *prevent colon cancer* (binds with secondary bile acids)
problem associated with a pure vegan diet	B_{12} *deficiency:* B_{12} is only in animal products

Table continued on following page

Table 9–12. TRACE ELEMENT DISORDERS, DIETARY FIBER, NUTRITION AND CANCER, NUTRITIONAL CHANGES WITH AGING, SPECIAL DIETS *Continued*

Question: Which of the following reduce the risk for cancer? **SELECT 3**

- (A) Vitamin C
- (B) Thiamine
- (C) Unopposed estrogen
- (D) ω-6 polyunsaturated fats
- (E) ω-3 polyunsaturated fats
- (F) Wheat bran
- (G) Nitrite-cured foods
- (H) Aflatoxin

Answers: (A), (E), (F): Vitamin C **(choice A)** prevents nitrosamination, hence preventing the formation of nitrosamines, which increase the risk for esophageal and stomach cancers. Thiamine is not associated with cancer **(choice B is incorrect)**. Unopposed estrogen increases the risk for endometrial cancer **(choice C is incorrect)**. ω-6 polyunsaturated fats are cancer promoters and alter estrogen metabolism **(choice D is incorrect)**. ω-3 polyunsaturated fats (fish oils, canola oil) have a protective effect on hormone metabolism **(choice E)**. Wheat bran **(choice F)** is an insoluble fiber, which decreases the risk for cancer. Nitrite-cured foods increase the risk for cancer **(choice G is incorrect)**. Aflatoxin is a cocarcinogen with hepatitis B and increases the risk for hepatocellular carcinoma **(choice H is incorrect)**.

ALP = alkaline phosphatase, AMI = acute myocardial infarction, AR = autosomal recessive, BCP = birth control pill, CH = cholesterol, CHF = congestive heart failure, DM = diabetes mellitus, FA = fatty acid, FR = free radical, Hb = hemoglobin, HCC = hepatocellular carcinoma, HTN = hypertension, IBS = irritable bowel syndrome, LDL = low density lipoprotein, Rx = treatment, SOD = superoxide dismutase, S/S = signs and symptoms, TPN = total parenteral nutrition.

CHAPTER

10

NEPHROLOGY

CONTENTS

Table 10–1. SIGNS AND SYMPTOMS OF RENAL DISEASE, RENAL FUNCTION STUDIES

Most Common...	Answer and Explanation
cause of costovertebral angle pain	*renal disease:* e.g., * APN, * adenocarcinoma [Renal pain may radiate to the umbilicus, testicle, labium. Pain is related to swelling of the capsule and is usually constant. Pain related to obstruction (e.g., stone) is colicky (rises/falls). N/V commonly occur.]
systemic diseases associated with renal disease	• **essential HTN:** * BNS, * malignant HTN, • *DM:* * CRF, * APN, * renal papillary necrosis, • *shock:* ATN, • *peripheral vascular disease:* renal artery stenosis, • *collagen vascular disease:* * SLE, * PSS, * PAN
UUT (kidneys, ureter) causes of hematuria	• **renal stone:** ~40%, • *GN/medullary sponge kidney/renal papillary necrosis:* ~20%, • *renal adenocarcinoma:* * 10%, * most common initial finding, • *renal pelvis transitional cell carcinoma* (TCC): 7%
LUT (bladder, urethra, prostate) causes of hematuria	• **infection,** • *TCC:* MCC gross hematuria in absence of infection, • *BPH*

Table continued on following page

Table 10–1. SIGNS AND SYMPTOMS OF RENAL DISEASE, RENAL FUNCTION STUDIES *Continued*

Most Common...	Answer and Explanation
cause of microscopic hematuria in adult males	*BPH*
drugs associated with hematuria	• **anticoagulants:** e.g., * warfarin, * heparin, • *cyclophosphamide:* hemorrhagic cystitis, • *drugs causing interstitial nephritis:* e.g., * methicillin, * analgesic nephropathy
initial steps in evaluating hematuria	• **complete UA,** • *urine culture,* • *others pending results of UA/culture:* * IVP (upper urinary tract), * cystoscopy (gross hematuria), * urine cytology (R/O bladder cancer)
lab abnormalities indicating renal disease	• **proteinuria,** • *hematuria,* • *pyuria,* • *elevated serum creatinine*
uses of US in renal disease	• **solid versus cystic renal mass,** • *R/O hydronephrosis/APKD,* • *assess kidney size,* • *stone work-up*
uses of an IVP in renal disease	• **evaluate anatomic features of urinary excretory system:** e.g., * stones, * cysts, * calyceal deformities, * ureteral obstruction, • *work-up of hematuria*
causes of radiocontrast-induced nephropathy	• **DM,** • *CRF,* • *multiple myeloma*
use of retrograde pyelography	*evaluate urinary collecting system if IVP not helpful*
uses of renal arteriography	• **evaluate cause of renovascular hypertension:** e.g., * atherosclerosis, * fibromuscular hyperplasia, • *identify:* * embolization, * thrombosis, • *evaluate vascularity of tumors*
use of CT scan in renal disease	*evaluate renal masses*
use of MRI in renal disease	• **evaluate renal masses,** • *staging of renal adenocarcinoma*
use of radionuclide scan	• **measure function of one kidney versus the other:** useful in work-up of renovascular HTN, • *follow renal function in transplant kidneys*

Table 10–1. SIGNS AND SYMPTOMS OF RENAL DISEASE, RENAL FUNCTION STUDIES *Continued*

Most Common...	Answer and Explanation
uses of renal biopsy	• **workup of GN,** • *evaluate post-transplant kidney for rejection*
tests used to evaluate renal function	• **urinalysis** (UA), • *serum BUN,* • *serum creatinine,* • *BUN/creatinine ratio,* • *CCr,* • *UOsm,* • *FENa$^+$*
source of urea	*end-product of amino acid/pyrimidine metabolism*
causes of an increased serum BUN	• **decreased GFR:** e.g., * CHF, * shock, * hypovolemia, • *renal failure,* • *postrenal obstruction,* • *increased intake of protein:* * bacterial ureases convert urea into ammonia, which is reabsorbed and converted into urea in liver urea cycle, e.g., * TPN, * GI bleed (blood is protein), • *glucocorticoids:* breakdown muscle protein, • *tetracyclines:* * inhibit protein synthesis, * more amino acids are shunted into the urea cycle, * serum creatinine is normal
causes of a low serum BUN	• **chronic liver disease:** dysfunctional urea cycle, • *pregnancy:* * dilutional effect, * increased renal clearance, • *SIADH:* * dilutional effect, * increased renal clearance, • *malnutrition:* decreased protein intake
source of creatinine	*metabolism of creatine in muscle:* * underscores why creatinine is used as a measure of muscle mass, * creatinine is excreted in the kidneys at a constant rate and is neither reabsorbed nor secreted
pathologic causes of an elevated creatinine	• **prerenal azotemia:** decreased GFR, • *renal failure,* • *postrenal obstruction* [Creatinine is a poor screen for renal disease, since >50–70% of renal mass must be destroyed before it increases. Serum creatinine increases when GFR is <40% of normal. Creatinine increases 0.5–1.0 mg/dL/d in patients with acute renal failure.]
causes of a falsely high serum creatinine	• **ketoacids,** • *increased meat intake:* organic acid interference with the test, • *vitamin C,* • *drugs:* * cefoxitin, * TMP, * aspirin, * cimetidine, • *rhabdomyolysis*

Table continued on following page

Table 10–1. SIGNS AND SYMPTOMS OF RENAL DISEASE, RENAL FUNCTION STUDIES *Continued*

Most Common...	Answer and Explanation
causes of a low serum creatinine	• **advancing age:** loss in muscle mass, • *cachexia:* loss in muscle mass, • *chronic liver disease:* decreased synthesis of creatine
clearance substance used in clinical medicine	*creatinine:* * creatinine clearance formula is: CCr = UOsm × V/POsm, where V = volume of a 24 h urine collection in mL/min, * creatinine is not a perfect clearance substance, (some is secreted, some is excreted in the GI tract)
causes of a decreased CCr	• **increasing age:** * age-dependent finding, * CCr declines by 1 mL/minute/year over the age of 40, • *inadequate 24 h urine collection:* decreases urine volume in numerator, • *renal failure*
causes of an increased CCr	• **pregnancy:** increase in plasma volume increases GFR and CCr, • *early diabetic nephropathy:* * hyperfiltration is early feature of DM, * efferent arteriole is hyalinized, which decreases blood flow out of the glomerular capillaries and increases GFR
effect of a decreased GFR on BUN/ creatinine ratio	*increases normal 10/1 ratio to >15/1* [A decrease in GFR increases proximal reabsorption of urea. Urea reabsorption is flow dependent (up to 80% reabsorbed when GFR is decreased). Creatinine is not reabsorbed, however, a drop in the GFR reduces its clearance by the kidneys, so it is mildly increased. There is a disproportionate increase in urea over creatinine, leading to an increased ratio.]
effect of renal failure on serum BUN/ creatinine ratio	*maintenance of 10/1 ratio* [Serum BUN and creatinine are equally affected by intrinsic renal disease. Both increase at same rate and maintain the normal 10/1 ratio (e.g., serum BUN 80 mg/dL, creatinine 8 mg/dL). This is called *renal azotemia* (uremia).]
effect of post-renal obstruction on serum BUN/ creatinine ratio	*>15–20/1 ratio* [In post-renal obstruction (e.g., ureters, bladder, urethra), there is a back diffusion of urea from urine into the blood and a decrease in the GFR (see below). This is called postrenal azotemia.]
indicator of tubular dysfunction	*inability to concentrate urine*

Table 10–1. SIGNS AND SYMPTOMS OF RENAL DISEASE, RENAL FUNCTION STUDIES *Continued*

Most Common...	Answer and Explanation
use of UOsm	• *evaluate renal concentration:* usually >800 mOsm/kg, • *evaluate diluting capacity of the kidneys:* <100 mOsm/kg, • *clinical use in oliguria* (urine flow <400 mL/d, <20 mL/h): * UOsm <350 mOsm/kg indicates tubular dysfunction, * UOsm >500 mOsm/kg indicates intact tubular function
use of FENa$^+$ (fractional excretion of sodium)	*work-up of oliguria:* * FENa$^+$ = (UNa$^+$ × PCr)/(PNa$^+$ × UCr) × 100, * values <1 indicate intact tubular function, * values >1 (usually >2) indicate tubular dysfunction
use of urine Na$^+$	• **evaluation of hypo/hypernatremia:** * UNa$^+$ <10 mEq/L indicates a nonrenal cause of hypo/hypernatremia, * UNa$^+$ >20 mEq/L indicates a renal cause of hypo/hypernatremia, • *work-up of oliguria:* * UNa$^+$ <20 mEq/L indicates good tubular function, * UNa$^+$ >40 mEq/L indicates poor tubular function
changes in UNa$^+$ in metabolic alkalosis	• *early phase:* UNa$^+$ >20 mEq/L, since excess HCO$_3^-$ anions filtered by kidney are excreted as NaHCO$_3$, • *late phase:* when volume depletion occurs, proximal tubule HCO$_3^-$ reclamation and reabsorption of Na$^+$ increases (UNa$^+$ <10 mEq/L)
use of urine Cl$^-$	• *identify Cl$^-$ responsive metabolic alkalosis*: * UCl$^-$ <10 mEq/L, * e.g., vomiting, * Cl$^-$ responsive means the metabolic alkalosis is corrected by infusing isotonic saline, • *identify Cl$^-$ resistant metabolic alkalosis*: * UCl$^-$ >20 mEq/L, * e.g., primary aldosteronism, * Cl$^-$ resistant means that isotonic saline will not correct the metabolic alkalosis
use of urine K$^+$	*identify causes of hypokalemia:* * UK$^+$ <20 mEq/L indicates a nonrenal cause (e.g., diarrhea), * UK$^+$ >20 mEq/L indicates a renal cause (e.g., diuretics)
causes of a dark yellow urine	• **concentrated urine,** • *coloring from vitamins,* • *CB:* e.g., obstructive jaundice, • *increased UBG:* e.g., EHA

Table continued on following page

**Table 10–1. SIGNS AND SYMPTOMS OF RENAL
DISEASE, RENAL FUNCTION STUDIES** *Continued*

Most Common...	Answer and Explanation
causes of a red urine	• **hematuria:** e.g., urinary stone, • *myoglobin:* e.g., rhabdomyolysis, • *drugs:* e.g., phenazopyridine, • *porphyrias:* e.g., AIP, • *beets*
causes of a black urine	• *alkaptonuria:* * AR, * homogentisic acid must be oxidized on exposure to air before urine turns black, • *blackwater fever:* * P. falciparum infection, * Hb changed into hematin, which is a black color
urine dipstick components	• *specific gravity,* • *pH,* • *protein,* • *glucose,* • *ketones,* • *bilirubin,* • *UBG,* • *leukocyte esterase,* • *nitrites*
use of urine specific gravity	*crude indicator of UOsm:* * hypotonic urine has specific gravity <1.015 (~ UOsm 220 mOsm/kg), * concentrated urine has specific gravity >1.023 (~ UOsm 900 mOsm/kg), * UOsm is best indicator of urine concentration/dilution
causes of a falsely high urine specific gravity	• **glucosuria,** • *proteinuria*
causes of isosthenuria (fixed specific gravity)	• **chronic renal failure:** * complete loss of concentration/dilution, * plasma is isosmotic with the urine at all times, • *sickle cell trait/ disease:* microinfarcts in renal medulla destroy tubular function, • *chronic interstitial nephritis:* e.g., analgesic abuse
dipstick urine pH findings in meat eaters and vegans	• *meat eater:* acid pH due to inorganic/organic acids from meat, • *vegan:* alkaline pH due to citrate conversion into bicarbonate
uses of urine pH	• *alter pH to prevent renal stones:* e.g., alkalinize urine in uric acid stones, • *alter pH to excrete drugs:* e.g., alkalinize urine to excrete salicylates, • *diagnose RTA:* urine pH >5.5 in type I distal RTA
cause of an alkaline urine that smells like ammonia	*urease producing bacterial infection:* * e.g., *Proteus/Pseudomonas* species, * urease breaks urea down into ammonia, which alkalinizes urine

Table 10–1. SIGNS AND SYMPTOMS OF RENAL DISEASE, RENAL FUNCTION STUDIES *Continued*

Most Common...	Answer and Explanation
dipstick finding indicating primary renal disease	*proteinuria:* * dipstick protein detects albumin (not globulins), * unreliable in detecting albumin <10–30 mg/dL, * a +1 reading is equivalent to 30 mg/dL, which ~ equals 150 mg/d, the cut-off point for normal protein excretion per day
confirmatory test for a positive dipstick for protein	*SSA:* * detects albumin and globulins, * detects Bence-Jones protein (light chains)
pathologic cause of a negative dipstick protein and strongly positive SSA	*Bence-Jones proteinuria in multiple myeloma:* * dipstick and SSA reading for protein should be the same if only albumin is present, * a disproportionate increase in SSA over dipstick protein indicates globulin in the urine (possibility of BJ protein)
tests to detect microalbuminuria (30–300 mg albumin/day)	• **quantitative immunoassays,** • *microalbumin dipsticks* [Dipsticks are used as screens and are sensitive to 1.5–8 mg/dL, unlike the standard urine dipsticks, which only detect as low as 30 mg/dL. Microalbuminuria is the first sign of diabetic nephropathy.]
causes of a positive dipstick for glucose	• **DM,** • *normal pregnancy:* * low renal threshold for glucose, * normal serum glucose, • *benign glucosuria:* * low threshold, * serum glucose is normal, • *proximal RTA* [Normal threshold for glucose is 165–200 mg/dL. The test is specific for glucose, since it uses glucose oxidase.]
causes of a false-negative dipstick glucose	• **elevated urinary ascorbic acid:** excessive dose of vitamin C, • *increased ketones,* • *increased specific gravity*
use of Clinitest	*detect urine-reducing substances:* * e.g., glucose, galactose, lactose, ascorbic acid, fructose, * sucrose is not a reducing sugar [Test is too nonspecific for detection of glucose. Commonly used in pediatrics as a screen for some inborn errors of metabolism.]

Table continued on following page

**Table 10–1. SIGNS AND SYMPTOMS OF RENAL
DISEASE, RENAL FUNCTION STUDIES** Continued

Most Common...	Answer and Explanation
causes of a positive dipstick for ketones	• **volume depletion,** • *DKA,* • *normal pregnancy,* • *ketogenic diets,* • *isopropyl alcohol poisoning,* • *von Gierke's disease* [Nitroprusside in the test system only reacts with AcAc and acetone, not β-OHB.]
causes of a positive dipstick for bilirubin	• **viral hepatitis,** • *obstructive jaundice* [Only CB is detected. UCB is lipid soluble.]
cause of a false-negative test for CB in the urine	*high urine ascorbate levels*
causes of an increased dipstick reaction for UBG	• **viral hepatitis:** see Table 9–6. • *EHA:* see Table 9–6
cause of an increase in urine UBG and bilirubin	*viral hepatitis:* see Table 9–6
cause of an increase in urine bilirubin, no change in UBG	*viral hepatitis:* * this pattern occurs in the early cholestatic phase of hepatitis, * see Table 9–6
causes of a positive dipstick for blood	• **hematuria:** e.g., * **cystitis,** * renal stone, * renal adenocarcinoma, * bladder cancer, • *hemoglobinuria,* • *myoglobinuria:* * dipstick reagents are positive for myoglobin or Hb, * elevated serum CK is expected in myoglobinuria but not hemoglobinuria
cause of a positive dipstick for leukocyte esterase	**cystitis:** neutrophils contain esterase
cause of a positive dipstick for leukocyte esterase and a negative standard urine culture	*sterile pyuria* [Pyuria refers to ≥10 WBCs/HPF in a centrifuged specimen or ≥5 WBCs/HPF in an uncentrifuged specimen. If a standard urine culture for uropathogens is negative, the term *sterile pyuria* is applied. Infectious causes include *Chlamydia trachomatis, Mycoplasma hominis, Ureaplasma urealyticum,* or *renal TB.* Acute or chronic interstitial nephritis due to drugs or other noninfectious causes may also cause sterile pyuria.]

Table 10–1. SIGNS AND SYMPTOMS OF RENAL DISEASE, RENAL FUNCTION STUDIES *Continued*

Most Common...	Answer and Explanation
cause of a false-negative leukocyte esterase	*high urinary tetracycline levels*
cause of a positive dipstick for nitrites	*cystitis:* * most urinary pathogens reduce nitrates to nitrites, * the test has greater specificity than sensitivity, * *Escherichia coli* is the most common nitrate reducer and uropathogen
cause of a false-negative dipstick for nitrites	• **collection of urine <4 h after last void:** * it requires at least 4 h for a nitrate reducer to convert nitrates into nitrites, * most patients have increased frequency of urination, • *high urine ascorbate levels*
cause of dysmorphic (abnormal shapes) RBCs in the urine	*GN:* * dysmorphic RBCs are best seen with a phase contrast microscope, * indicate a glomerular origin for the RBCs, * hematuria is >2–3 RBCs per HPF
causes of WBCs in the urine	• **infection:** * **cystitis,** * pyelonephritis, * urethritis, • *drug-induced interstitial nephritis* [>10 WBCs/HPF in a spun sediment is abnormal in women and >1–3 WBCs/HPF is abnormal in men.]
cause of eosinophiluria	*drug-induced interstitial nephritis*
cause of oval fat bodies and free lipid in the urine	*nephrotic syndrome* (proteinuria > 3.5 g/24 h) [Epithelial cells or macrophages with lipid are designated oval fat bodies. If urine polarization reveals Maltese crosses in oval fat bodies, casts, or free, CH rather than TG is present. TG is identified with Sudan stains.]
cause of hemosiderinuria	*chronic intravascular hemolytic anemia:* * e.g., microangiopathic hemolytic anemia in a patient with aortic stenosis, * iron deficiency may occur
location of urine cast formation	*diseases originating in the kidneys:* e.g., * GN, * pyelonephritis [Casts are formed in tubular lumens. They are composed of a protein matrix (Tamm-Horsfall protein) within which is entrapped cells, debris, or protein leaking through the glomeruli. Their presence proves a renal origin of the disease.]

Table continued on following page

Table 10–1. SIGNS AND SYMPTOMS OF RENAL DISEASE, RENAL FUNCTION STUDIES *Continued*

Most Common...	Answer and Explanation
cast in the urine	*hyaline casts:* * acellular, * clear casts, * composed of Tamm-Horsfall protein [They usually have no clinical significance, unless present in great numbers.]
casts associated with the nephritic syndrome	• **RBC casts,** • *WBC casts*
cast associated with the nephrotic syndrome	*fatty casts with or without Maltese crosses*
cast associated with acute pyelonephritis	*WBC cast*
cast associated with ATN	*pigmented (Hb) renal tubular cast*
casts in chronic renal disease	• *broad casts:* also called renal failure casts, • *waxy casts*
progression of degeneration of a cellular cast in a renal tubule	• *cellular cast:* e.g., WBC cast → • *coarsely granular cast* → • *finely granular cast* → • *waxy cast:* usually after 3 months, which is why it is an indicator of chronic renal disease
clinically important crystals in an acid urine	• *uric acid:* e.g., gout, • *calcium oxalate:* * look like the back of an envelope, e.g., * Crohn's disease, * ethylene glycol poisoning (see Table 7–4)
clinically important crystal in an alkaline urine	*triple phosphate:* * looks like a coffin lid, * present in urine containing urease-producing organisms (e.g., *Proteus* species)
inborn error of metabolism with a pathognomonic urine crystal	*cystinuria:* hexagonal crystal
types of proteinuria	• **hemodynamic:** * exercise, * fever, * CHF, • *glomerular:* * selective (only albumin), * nonselective (albumin + globulins), • *overflow:* * normal glomerular and tubular function, * excess amount of LMW proteins (e.g., amino acids) in plasma, • *tubular:* * normal glomerular function, * tubules are damaged and cannot reabsorb normally filtered proteins

Table 10–1. SIGNS AND SYMPTOMS OF RENAL DISEASE, RENAL FUNCTION STUDIES *Continued*

Most Common...	Answer and Explanation
causes of proteinuria	• **loss of negative charge of GBM:** * e.g., nephrotic syndrome, * negative charge due to heparan sulfate, * repels albumin, • **alteration in size barrier of GBM:** * nonselective loss of albumin + globulins, * e.g., glomerular disease, • *proximal tubule abnormality:* * tubular proteinuria, * loss of ♦ amino acids, ♦ transferrin, ♦ β_2-microglobulins, * e.g., proximal RTA, * heavy metal poisoning, • *protein overload:* * overflow type, * e.g., loss of BJ proteins in multiple myeloma, * aminoacidurias, * liver disease (tyrosine, leucine)
benign cause of proteinuria	*postural* (orthostatic) *proteinuria:* * proteinuria with standing, * disappears after lying down, * first AM void is free of protein

Question: In post-streptococcal glomerulonephritis, you would expect which of the following laboratory abnormalities? **SELECT 4**

(A) FENa$^+$ >1
(B) UOsm >500
(C) Positive urine dipstick for blood
(D) 24 h urine protein >3.5 g
(E) Primarily WBC casts
(F) Decrease CCr
(G) UNa$^+$ <10 mEq/L

Answers: (B), (C), (F), (G): A FENa$^+$ <1 implies a loss in tubular function (kidneys cannot concentrate urine). Acute post-streptococcal GN is a glomerular disease, which does not alter tubular function, hence the FENa$^+$ is <1 **(choice A is incorrect).** A UOsm >500 mOsm/kg **(choice B)** indicates normal tubular function. A positive dipstick for blood **(choice C)** is expected in inflammation of the glomerulus. A sediment exam in post-streptococcal GN usually uncovers RBC casts **(choice E is incorrect).** Proteinuria is present in post-streptococcal GN, however it is not in the nephrotic range **(choice D is incorrect).** The CCr is decreased **(choice F)** in post-streptococcal GN, since the GFR is decreased from inflamed glomerular capillaries. Since tubular function is intact, the UNa$^+$ is <10 mEq/L.

AcAc = acetoacetic acid, AIP = acute intermittent porphyria, APKD = adult polycystic kidney disease, APN = acute pyelonephritis, AR = autosomal recessive, ATN = acute tubular necrosis, BJ = Bence-Jones, BNS = benign nephrosclerosis, β-OHB = beta-hydroxybutyric acid, BPH = benign prostatic hyperplasia, BUN = blood urea nitrogen, CB = conjugated bilirubin, CCr = creatinine clearance, CH = cholesterol, CHF = congestive heart failure, CK = creatine kinase, CRF = chronic renal failure, CT = computed tomography, DKA = diabetic ketoacidosis, DM = diabetes mellitus, EHA = extravascular hemolytic anemia, FENa$^+$ =

fractional excretion of sodium, GBM = blomerular basement membrane, GFR = glomerular filtration rate, GI = gastrointestinal, GN = glomerulo-nephritis, Hb = hemoglobin, HPF = high-power field, HTN = hyperten-sion, IVP = intravenous pyelogram, LMW = low molecular weight, LUT = lower urinary tract, MCC = most common cause, MRI = magnetic resonance imaging, N/V = nausea and vomiting, PAN = polyarteritis nodosa, PCr = plasma creatinine, PNa^+ = plasma sodium, POsm = plasma osmolality, PSS = progressive systemic sclerosis, RBC = red blood cell, R/O = rule out, RTA = renal tubular acidosis, SIADH = syndrome of inappropriate antidiuretic hormone, SLE = systemic lupus erythematosus, SSA = sulfosalicylic acid, TB = tuberculosis, TCC = transitional cell carcinoma, TG = triglyceride, TMP = trimethoprim, TPN = total parenteral nutrition, UA = urinalysis, UBG = urobilinogen, UCB = unconjugated bilirubin, UCl^- = urine chloride, UCr = urine creatinine, UK^+ = urine potassium, UNa^+ = urine sodium, UOsm = urine osmolality, UUT = upper urinary tract, WBC = white blood cell.

Table 10–2. VOLUME AND POTASSIUM DISORDERS

Most Common...	Answer and Explanation
sites housing total body water (TBW) and total body sodium ($TBNa^+$)	• *TBW:* distributed in both ECF/ICF, • *$TBNa^+$*: limited to ECF compartment (plasma/intersti-tial fluid) [The ICF contains two-thirds of TBW, and ECF the remaining one-third. Inter-stitial fluid is two-thirds and vascular com-partment one-third of ECF.]
clinical index of a patient's TBW status	*serum Na^+ concentration* [Serum Na^+ does not directly correlate with $TBNa^+$. It is only one component of total body osmolality. Total body osmolality is the sum of $TBNa^+$ + TBK^+ ÷ TBW. Simplifying the formula, se-rum Na^+ = $TBNa^+$/TBW. Since sodium is limited to the ECF, it controls water move-ment between the ECF and ICF by osmosis (water moves from low to high concentra-tion). In hyponatremia, water moves from ECF to ICF. In hypernatremia, water moves from ICF to ECF. A normal serum Na^+ has no gradient for water movement.]
clinical index of $TBNa^+$	*physical examination*
clinical index of a decrease in $TBNa^+$	*signs of volume depletion* [Since $TBNa^+$ is limited to the ECF and the ISF fluid accounts for two-thirds of the ECF, a decrease in $TBNa^+$ in ISF is reflected as a decrease in skin turgor: tenting of skin, dry mucous mem-branes, dry axilla. In the vascular compart-ment, volume depletion is associated with

Table 10–2. VOLUME AND POTASSIUM DISORDERS
Continued

Most Common...	Answer and Explanation
Continued	increased thirst (function of increased ATII), orthostatic hypotension, oliguria (decreased GFR), flat neck veins, and sinus tachycardia.]
clinical indices of an increase in TBNa$^+$	• **dependent pitting edema:** increased TBNa$^+$ in ISF, • *transudates in body cavities:* e.g., * ascites, * pleural effusion
clinical index of a normal TBNa$^+$	*absence of above clinical signs*
lab test evaluating plasma solute concentration	*plasma osmolality:* POsm in mOsm/kg
formula for calculating POsm	*POsm = (2) Na$^+$ + serum glucose/18 + serum blood urea nitrogen (BUN)/2.8 = 275–295 mOsm/kg:* normally, the calculated POsm and measured POsm are within 10 mOsm/kg of each other
cause of a decreased POsm	*hyponatremia*
cause of an increased POsm	• **hyperglycemia,** • *hypernatremia,* • *azotemia:* increased serum BUN
pathologic causes of water movement between ECF and ICF	• **hyponatremia,** • *hypernatremia,* • *hyperglycemia* [Sodium and glucose establish osmotic gradients between the ECF and ICF, since both are limited to the ECF. Urea equalizes itself between the two compartments (osmolality is the same in both compartments) without establishing a gradient.]
formula used to evaluate the tonicity of ECF causing water movements between the ECF and ICF	*effective osmolality (EOsm) = 2 (serum Na$^+$) + glucose/18* [A *normal EOsm* represents an isotonic state, where there is no gradient for water movements. A *low EOsm* indicates a hypotonic state, in which water moves from ECF to ICF (ICF expansion). A *high EOsm* represents a hypertonic state (hypernatremia/hyperglycemia), in which water moves from ICF to ECF (ICF contraction).]
effect of hyperglycemia on serum Na$^+$	*dilutional hyponatremia:* * osmotic gradient established by hyperglycemia favors water movement from ICF to ECF, * excess water dilutes serum Na$^+$ in ECF

Table continued on following page

Table 10–2. VOLUME AND POTASSIUM DISORDERS
Continued

Most Common...	Answer and Explanation
formula used to correct serum Na$^+$ for dilutional effect of hyperglycemia	*corrected serum sodium = measured serum sodium + (glucose mg/dL/100 × 1.6):* * e.g., serum Na$^+$ = 132 mEq/L (136–145 mEq/L), serum glucose = 1000 mg/dL (70–110 mg/dL), the corrected serum sodium = 132 + (1000/100 × 1.6) = 148 mEq/L, which is elevated, * the correction indicates what the serum Na$^+$ would be if serum glucose were normal, * serum Na$^+$ would be 148 mEq/L due to osmotic diuresis and loss of more water than Na$^+$ in the urine
factors controlling plasma volume	• **kidney reabsorption of salt/water,** • *thirst:* * low POsm inhibits thirst, * high POsm stimulates thirst, * high ATII stimulates thirst, • *low/high pressure baroreceptors,* • *RAA system,* • *ADH*
factors activating the RAA system	• **increase in catecholamines:** activation of baroreceptors from decreased cardiac output, • *decrease in renal blood flow:* decrease in cardiac output [They both stimulate the JG apparatus to release renin (an enzyme) → renin cleaves angiotensinogen into ATI → ACE converts ATI into ATII (* stimulates thirst, * increases TPR) → ATII stimulates release of ATIII and aldosterone (increases Na$^+$ reabsorption).]
clinical term reflecting volume status	*effective arterial blood volume* (EABV): total circulating volume of blood necessary to stimulate volume receptors
cause of a proportional decrease in EABV and ECF	*isotonic loss of fluid:* * loss of isotonic fluid (equal loss of Na$^+$/water), * e.g., blood loss, * ECF contraction and drop in EABV, * ICF compartment is normal (no osmotic gradient)
cause of a decrease in EABV and increase in ECF	*Starling's force abnormality* [Normally, EABV and ECF parallel each other (decreased EABV ↔ decreased ECF). If plasma hydrostatic pressure is increased or oncotic pressure (serum albumin) is decreased, a transudate moves out of the vascular compartment into the ISF. The increase in ECF volume is manifested as dependent pitting edema and body cavity

Table 10–2. VOLUME AND POTASSIUM DISORDERS
Continued

Most Common...	Answer and Explanation
Continued	effusions (e.g., ascites). Fluid trapped in the ISF compartment decreases venous return to the right heart, which decreases EABV.]
sites of the low and high pressure baroreceptors	• *low-pressure types:* * left atrium, * major intrathoracic veins, • *high-pressure types:* * aortic arch, * carotid sinus [Baroreceptors are innervated by cranial nerves IX and X.]
physiologic events associated with a decreased EABV	• *stimulation of baroreceptor reflex → increased sympathetic activity with catecholamine release → catecholamines:* * venoconstrict (increase venous return to the heart), * increase cardiac output and heart rate (increases systolic BP), * increase TPR (increases diastolic BP), * stimulate RAA system along with decreased RBF → *activated RAA system increases ATII* (* stimulates thirst, * increases TPR, * stimulates aldosterone release) → *aldosterone increases renal Na^+ reabsorption,* • *neural reflexes in left atrium stimulate ADH release:* reabsorbs free water in collecting tubules, • *decrease in RBF decreases peritubular capillary hydrostatic pressure* (P_H) *and increases peritubular capillary oncotic pressure* (P_O) → *increase in P_O increases proximal tubule reabsorption of salt/water as well as other solutes* (* urea, * called prerenal azotemia), • *tonicity of fluid reabsorbed by the kidneys into the ECF to restore volume is slightly hypotonic* (more water than salt)
physiologic events associated with an increased EABV	• *no activation of baroreceptor reflex,* • *no release of ADH,* • *no activation of RAA system,* • $P_H > P_O$: *no proximal reabsorption of salt/water,* • *renal loss of a hypotonic solution*
stimulus for release of ANP	*distention of the left/right atrium:* e.g., * CHF, * volume overload
functions of ANP	• *suppresses baroreceptor events listed above,* • *vasodilates peripheral vessels,* • *directly inhibits renal Na^+ reabsorption* [ANP counters an increase in ECF volume and offsets the actions of ATII/aldosterone.]

Table continued on following page

Table 10–2. VOLUME AND POTASSIUM DISORDERS
Continued

Most Common...	Answer and Explanation
functions of prostaglandin E_2 (synthesized in the kidneys)	• *inhibits ADH,* • *blocks renal Na^+ reabsorption,* • *vasodilates afferent arterioles*
nephron site for Na^+ reabsorption	*proximal tubule:* * reabsorb 60–80% of filtered Na^+, * P_O must be greater than P_H to reabsorb Na^+ into peritubular capillaries
MOA of acetazolamide	*carbonic anhydrase inhibitor in proximal tubule:* acts as a diuretic by inhibiting reclamation of sodium bicarbonate
acid-base/electrolyte abnormalities associated with acetazolamide	• *hyperchloremic, normal anion gap metabolic acidosis:* see Table 6–2, • *kaluresis:* hypokalemia, • *natriuresis:* hyponatremia
nephron site for generation of free water	*thick ascending limb* (TAL) *in the medullary segment* [TALs segment contains Na^+-K^+-$2Cl^-$ co-transport pump, which produces free water (solute-free water). Water that must accompany solute for excretion (20 mL water per mOsm of solute) is called *obligated water*. Up to the TAL segment, all water is obligated. Free water is generated by actively separating Na^+, K^+, and Cl^- from their obligated water, which leaves their free water behind. For normal dilution to occur, free water must be excreted in the absence of ADH. For normal concentration to occur, free water must be reabsorbed in the presence of ADH.]
MOA of loop diuretics	*blocks Na^+-K^+-$2Cl^-$ co-transport pump:* also blocks calcium reabsorption
effect of loop diuretics on calcium reabsorption	*decreases calcium reabsorption:* useful in Rx of hypercalcemia
MOA of thiazide diuretics	*blocks Na^+/Cl^- pump in cortical segment of TAL*
effect of thiazides on calcium reabsorption	*increases calcium reabsorption:* * calcium uses the same channel as Na^+ for PTH-enhanced absorption, * blocking Na^+ enhances calcium reabsorption, * useful in Rx of hypercalciuria in calcium stone formers

Table 10–2. VOLUME AND POTASSIUM DISORDERS
Continued

Most Common...	Answer and Explanation
nephron site where aldosterone-enhanced ATPase pumps for Na$^+$/K$^+$ are located	*DCT/collecting tubules:* * aldosterone increases Na$^+$ reabsorption in exchange for either K$^+$ or H$^+$ ions, * primary site for K$^+$ secretion, * exchange of Na$^+$ for H$^+$ results in reclamation of HCO$_3^-$
nephron site where aldosterone-enhanced H$^+$/K$^+$ pump is located	*collecting tubule:* * H$^+$/K$^+$ pump is primary mechanism for secreting excess H$^+$ ions, * pump also regenerates (de novo synthesis) HCO$_3^-$
cause of hypokalemia with loop or thiazide diuretic	*increased distal delivery of unreabsorbed Na$^+$ to aldosterone-enhanced Na$^+$/K$^+$ pumps:* * greater exchange of Na$^+$ for K$^+$ than usual, * hypokalemia will occur unless K$^+$ supplements are taken
acid-base/electrolyte abnormalities with loop or thiazide diuretics	• *metabolic alkalosis,* • *hyponatremia,* • *hypokalemia* [Once tubular K$^+$ is depleted in exchange for Na$^+$ (leads to hypokalemia), Na$^+$ exchanges with H$^+$ ions. H$^+$ ions increase HCO$_3^-$ reclamation resulting in metabolic alkalosis. Urine Na$^+$ loss is hypertonic (more Na$^+$ lost than water), causing hyponatremia.]
MOA of spironolactone	*aldosterone blocker:* * collecting duct diuretic, * loss of Na$^+$ (hyponatremia), * retention of K$^+$ (hyperkalemia), * retention of H$^+$ ions (metabolic acidosis)
MOA of triamterene and amiloride	• *act independent of aldosterone,* • *directly block Na$^+$ reabsorption by DCT/collecting ducts:* * urine Na$^+$ loss (hyponatremia), * retention of K$^+$ (hyperkalemia) and H$^+$ ions (metabolic acidosis)
variables affecting K$^+$ loss in DCT and collecting tubule	• *increased distal delivery of Na$^+$ from more proximally acting diuretics:* e.g., * carbonic anhydrase inhibitor, * loop/thiazide diuretics, • *presence of aldolsterone:* * increased exchange of Na$^+$ for K$^+$, * e.g., primary aldosteronism, • *respiratory/metabolic alkalosis:* * H$^+$ ions from tubules enter the blood (mechanism to combat alkalosis) in exchange for K$^+$, * Na$^+$ in urine primarily exchanges with K$^+$ ions in tubules, leading to hypokalemia

Table continued on following page

Table 10–2. VOLUME AND POTASSIUM DISORDERS
Continued

Most Common...	Answer and Explanation
nephron site for dilution/ concentration	*collecting ducts:* depends on the absence (dilution) or presence (concentration) of ADH
nephron site for secretion of H^+ ions	*collecting ducts:* * contain aldosterone-enhanced H^+/K^+ ATPase pumps, * H^+ ions combine with HPO_4^- to form $Na_2H_2PO_4$ (titratable acid) and NH_3 to form NH_4Cl
factors that disrupt generation/ excretion of free water in order to dilute urine	• *decreased delivery of Na^+ to TALs segment:* e.g., decreased EABV with increased proximal tubule reabsorption of Na^+, • *inhibition of $Na^+/K^+/2\ Cl^-$ co-transport pump:* loop diuretic, • *presence of ADH:* * presence of ADH reabsorbs free water, * e.g., SIADH
patient parameter that best reflects volume depletion or gain	*daily weight:* indirectly reflects $TBNa^+$
organs most sensitive to volume depletion	• **kidneys:** particularly renal medulla, • brain: neurons
extrarenal losses resulting in volume depletion	• **hemorrhage,** • *cutaneous losses:* * sweat, * burn fluid, • *GI losses:* * vomiting, * diarrhea, • *third spacing:* e.g., isotonic fluid around the pancreas in pancreatitis
renal causes of volume depletion	• **diuretics,** • *aldosterone deficiency:* e.g., * Addison's disease, * spironolactone, * 21-OHase deficiency, • *osmotic diuresis:* * glucosuria, * mannitol, • *RTA,* • *salt-losing renal disease:* e.g., cystic disease
type of fluid loss with the greatest hemodynamic effect	• **whole blood:** contains albumin for oncotic pressure and sodium, • *loss of isotonic fluid,* • *loss of solute-free water:* * loss of pure water has very little effect on volume status (loss mainly in ICF), * loss of any Na^+ has marked effects on volume status (loss restricted to ECF)
fluid used to restore volume	*isotonic saline/Ringer's lactate:* 1 out of 3 liters remains in vascular compartment (other 2 liters in ISF)

Table 10–2. VOLUME AND POTASSIUM DISORDERS
Continued

Most Common...	Answer and Explanation
methods of uncovering volume deficits that are not clinically detectable	• **volume challenge with 500 mL of isotonic saline infused over 1–3 h:** improvement in BP/heart rate indicates volume depletion, • *tilt test:* * evaluates BP/pulse lying down/ sitting up, * further drop in BP/increase in pulse when sitting up indicates volume deficit, • *SGC measurement of PCWP* (measure of LVEDP) *and cardiac output:* most precise method
group of drugs that should be avoided in a volume depletion state	*NSAIDs:* block renal vasodilation effect of prostaglandin E_2 (important in maintaining renal blood flow), which counters vasoconstrictive effects of ATII
Rx of volume depletion	• *massive hemorrhagic shock:* * infuse whole blood, * crystalloid solutions used to maintain BP while blood is being crossmatched, • *less massive blood loss:* combination of * packed RBCs and infusion of * crystalloid solutions, • *loss of solute free water* (pure water): 5% dextrose and water, • *loss of hypotonic fluid* (more water than salt): infuse isotonic saline first if the patient is hypotensive and then switch to 0.45 saline, • *loss of isotonic fluid* (equal amounts of salt and water): infuse crystalloid solutions
conditions with signs of volume depletion unrelated to obvious fluid losses	• **decreased cardiac output:** e.g., * AMI, * pericardial tamponade, • *increased venous capacitance:* e.g., * septic shock, * cirrhosis, • *fluid shifts into ISF:* "third space" shifts, e.g., ♦ acute pancreatitis, ♦ bowel infarction, ♦ tissue trauma
causes of volume excess	• **Starling's force alterations:** * increased hydrostatic pressure and/or decrease in oncotic pressure, * EABV decreased, * ECF increased, * e.g., CHF, cirrhosis, • *primary mineralocorticoid excess:* EABV increased, • *primary excess in solute-free water:* * EABV increased, * e.g., SIADH, • *primary renal retention of salt:* * EABV increased, * e.g., CRF
causes of volume excess secondary to an increase in hydrostatic pressure	• **LHF:** increase in pulmonary vein hydrostatic pressure, • **RHF:** increase in systemic venous pressure, • *constrictive pericarditis:* increase in systemic venous pressure

Table continued on following page

Table 10–2. VOLUME AND POTASSIUM DISORDERS
Continued

Most Common...	Answer and Explanation
causes of volume excess secondary to a decrease in oncotic pressure	• **malnutrition:** * decreased protein intake, e.g., * kwashiorkor, • *nephrotic syndrome:* loss of albumin, • *malabsorption:* protein loss in stool, • *cirrhosis:* decreased albumin synthesis
cause of volume excess due to increased hydrostatic pressure/decreased oncotic pressure	*cirrhosis:* * decreased oncotic pressure from decreased albumin synthesis, * increased portal vein hydrostatic pressure
causes of volume excess due to a primary increase in mineralocorticoids	• **primary aldosteronism,** • *Cushing's syndrome,* • *11-hydroxylase deficiency*
causes of volume excess due to an increase in solute-free water	• **SIADH,** • *psychogenic polydipsia*
causes of volume excess due to primary retention of salt	• **renal failure,** • *salt overload:* e.g., * $NaHCO_3$ infusions, * antibiotics containing sodium (e.g., carbenicillin)
Rx of volume excess states	• *excess solute-free water:* e.g., SIADH, * **restrict water,** * demeclocycline (produces nephrogenic DI), * infusion of 3% hypertonic saline + loop diuretic (loop diuretic causes salt/water loss, replace salt with 3% saline), * see calculation below, • *excess in TBNa+:* * e.g., salt overload, renal failure, * restrict salt, * diuretics, • *excess TBNa+ and water:* * e.g., RHF, cirrhosis, * restrict salt and water, * diuretics, • *primary mineralocorticoid excess:* * e.g., primary aldosteronism, * Rx underlying condition, * aldosterone blockers
cause of normonatremia and volume depletion: ↓ TBNa+, ↓ TBW, ↓ EABV, isosmotic hypovolemic normonatremia	*isotonic fluid loss:* * ↔ serum Na+ = ↓ TBNa+/↓ TBW, e.g., * secretory diarrhea, * third degree burns, * third spacing of fluid, * TBNa+ loss produces volume depletion, * random UNa+ <10 mEq/L (increased renal reabsorption of Na+)

Table 10–2. VOLUME AND POTASSIUM DISORDERS
Continued

Most Common...	Answer and Explanation
effect of access to water on serum Na^+ concentration in isotonic fluid loss	*hyponatremia:* * TBW increases without any change in $TBNa^+$, * $\downarrow$ serum Na^+ = $\downarrow TBNa^+/\uparrow\uparrow$ **TBW**
cause of normonatremia and volume excess with pitting edema: $\uparrow TBNa^+$, $\uparrow$ TBW, $\uparrow$ EABV, isosmotic hypervolemic normonatremia	*isotonic fluid gain:* * $\leftrightarrow$ serum Na^+ = $\uparrow TBNa^+/\uparrow$ TBW, * e.g., excess infusion of isotonic saline, * ECF expanded, * normal ICF (no osmotic gradient), * random UNa^+ >20 mEq/L ($P_H > P_O$, Na^+ not reabsorbed), * patient is edematous
electrolyte disturbance in hospitalized population	*hyponatremia:* * serum Na^+ <136 mEq/L, * a rapid onset of hyponatremia is more likely to be symptomatic than a slow onset
pathophysiologic mechanisms responsible for hyponatremia in volume-depleted state	• **volume depletion stimulates ADH release:** * volume depletion overrides osmolality as stimulus for ADH, * ADH increases free water reabsorption, • *increased proximal tubule reabsorption of sodium* ($P_O > P_H$): reduces distal delivery of Na^+ necessary for generating free water (necessary for dilution), • *excessive water intake:* patient retains water due to impaired free water generation
S/S of hyponatremia	• *seizures,* • *lethargy,* • *cramps,* • *decreased DTRs*
renal cause of hyponatremia with volume depletion: $\downarrow\downarrow TBNa^+$, $\downarrow$ TBW, $\downarrow$ EABV, hyposmotic hypovolemic hyponatremia	*hypertonic loss of fluid:* * $\downarrow$ serum Na^+ = $\downarrow\downarrow TBNa^+/\downarrow$ TBW, e.g., * **diuretics,** * Addison's disease, * 21-OHase deficiency, * salt-losing renal diseases
extrarenal cause of hyponatremia with volume depletion: $\downarrow TBNa^+$, $\uparrow\uparrow$ TBW, $\downarrow$ EABV, hyposmotic hypovolemic hyponatremia	*hypotonic/isotonic loss of fluid with patient access to water:* * sweating (hypotonic loss)—initially: $\uparrow$ serum Na^+ = $\downarrow TBNa^+/\downarrow\downarrow$ TBW, after access to water: $\downarrow$ serum Na^+ = $\downarrow TBNa^+/\uparrow$ **TBW,** * isotonic loss—initially: $\leftrightarrow$ serum Na^+ = $\downarrow TBNa^+/\downarrow$ TBW, after access to water: $\downarrow$ serum Na^+ = $\downarrow TBNa^+/\uparrow\uparrow$ **TBW**

Table continued on following page

Table 10–2. VOLUME AND POTASSIUM DISORDERS
Continued

Most Common...	Answer and Explanation
formula used to calculate the Na^+ deficit in volume depletion causing hyponatremia	Na^+ *deficit = 0.6 × weight in kg × (140 − measured serum Na^+):* * e.g., 70 kg man with serum Na^+ 120 mEq/L: Na^+ deficit = 0.6 (70) × (140 − 120) = 840 mEq/L, * 0.9% normal saline contains 154 mEq/L: infuse 840/154 or ~5.5 liters
cause of hyponatremia and volume excess with pitting edema, and ↓EABV: ↑TBNa⁺, ↑↑TBW, hyposmotic hypervolemic hyponatremia	alteration in Starling's forces with a *hypotonic gain of more water than salt:* * ↓ serum Na^+ = ↑TBNa⁺/↑↑TBW, * e.g., ♦ CHF, ♦ cirrhosis, * TBNa⁺ limited to ECF (pitting edema), * TBW distributed in both ICF and ECF, * random UNa⁺ <10 mEq/L (P_O > P_H), * Rx is water/salt restriction and diuretics
cause of hyponatremia and volume excess with pitting edema, and ↑EABV: ↑TBNa⁺, ↑↑TBW, hyposmotic hypervolemic hyponatremia	*hypotonic gain of more water than salt:* * ↓ serum Na^+ = ↑TBNa⁺/↑↑TBW, * e.g., renal failure with salt excess (problem with salt excretion), * no alteration in Starling's forces, * since EABV is increased, random UNa⁺ >20 mEq/L (P_H > P_O), * Rx is a loop diuretic or dialysis
cause of hyponatremia and normal physical exam: normal TBNa⁺, ↑↑TBW, ↔/↑EABV, hyposmotic euvolemic hyponatremia	*hypotonic gain of pure water:* * ↓ serum Na^+ = TBNa⁺/↑↑TBW, e.g., * increased TBW distributes in both ECF/ICF, * since EABV is increased, random UNa⁺ >20 mEq/L (P_H > P_O), * gain in TBW alone never produces pitting edema (must be a gain in TBNa⁺), * continual presence of ADH leads to concentration of urine and reabsorption of free water
causes of SIADH	• **small cell carcinoma of lung,** • *other neoplastic diseases:* * leukemia/lymphoma, * pancreatic cancer, • *drugs enhancing ADH production:* e.g., * cyclophosphamide, * phenothiazines, * carbamazepine, * vincristine, * amitriptyline, • *drugs enhancing ADH activity:* e.g., * oxytocin drip, * NSAIDs, * chlorpropamide, * carbamazepine, • *CNS disease:* * trauma, * infection, • *pulmonary disease:* * TB, * pneumonia, * PEEP therapy

Table 10–2. VOLUME AND POTASSIUM DISORDERS
Continued

Most Common...	Answer and Explanation
lab findings in SIADH	• **severe hyponatremia:** usually <120 mEq/L, • *low serum BUN:* * increased plasma volume has dilutional effect, * urea lost in urine due to $P_H > P_O$, • *hypouricemia:* lost in urine due to $P_H > P_O$, • *UNa$^+$ >40 mEq/L:* no proximal tubule reabsorption of Na$^+$ • *UOsm > POsm*
Rx of SIADH	• **water restriction,** • *demeclocycline:* * blocks ADH effect in kidneys (acquired nephrogenic DI), * use in severe hyponatremia or small cell carcinoma, • *loop diuretic:* replace salt lost in urine with 3% hypertonic saline
CNS disorder due to overzealous infusions of saline in patients with hyponatremia	*central pontine myelinolysis* [In hyponatremia, the brain is edematous as water moves into brain cells by osmosis. Brain cells synthesize idiogenic osmoles which when secreted into the ISF draw fluid out of brain cells and normalize brain hydration. Rapid administration of isotonic fluid is "hypertonic" in relation to osmolality in the brain cells, causing an irreversible demyelinating disease called central pontine myelinolysis.]
pathophysiologic events causing hypernatremia (serum Na$^+$ >145 mEq/L)	• **pure water loss:** TBNa$^+$/↓ ↓ TBW, • *hypotonic fluid loss:* * lose more water than salt, * ↓ TBNa$^+$/↓ ↓ TBW, • *hypertonic gain in salt:* ↑ ↑ TBNa$^+$/↑ TBW [Hypernatremia is most often the result of inability of the patient to have access to water (e.g., too young, too old, too sick). Access to water increases TBW, which could change a hypernatremia into a normonatremia or hyponatremia.]
S/S of hypernatremia	• *irritability,* • *seizures,* • *hyperreflexia,* • *ataxia,* • *mental status abnormalities*
cause of hypernatremia with volume depletion: ↓ TBNa$^+$, ↓ ↓ TBW, ↓ EABV, hyperosmotic hypovolemic hypernatremia	*hypotonic loss of more water than salt:* * ↑ serum Na$^+$ = ↓ TBNa$^+$/↓ ↓ TBW, * e.g., ◆ osmotic diuresis (DKA, mannitol, urea), ◆ sweating, * random UNa$^+$ <10 mEq/L in extrarenal fluid loss and >20 mEq/L in osmotic diuresis

Table continued on following page

Table 10–2. VOLUME AND POTASSIUM DISORDERS
Continued

Most Common...	Answer and Explanation
Rx of hypernatremia due to hypotonic fluid loss	• **isotonic saline to raise BP into normal range,** • *once BP is stabilized, use 0.45% saline* (see calculation below)
cause of hypernatremia with volume excess and pitting edema: $\uparrow\uparrow$TBNa$^+$, $\uparrow$TBW, $\uparrow$EABV, hyperosmotic hypervolemic hypernatremia	*hypertonic gain of more salt than water:* * $\uparrow$ serum Na$^+$ = $\uparrow\uparrow$TBNa$^+$/$\uparrow$TBW, * e.g., ♦ excessive NaHCO$_3$ infusions, ♦ infusion of Na$^+$ salt antibiotics, * random UNa$^+$ >20 mEq/L
Rx of hypernatremia from a hypertonic gain of salt	• *salt restriction,* • *diuretics*
cause of hypernatremia with a normal physical exam: normal TBNa$^+$, $\downarrow\downarrow$TBW, $\leftrightarrow$/$\downarrow$EABV, hyperosmotic euvolemic hypernatremia	*pure water loss:* * $\uparrow$ serum Na$^+$ = $\leftrightarrow$TBNa$^+$/$\downarrow\downarrow$TBW, * e.g., ♦ insensible water loss (evaporation of water without salt, e.g., fever, respirators), ♦ central/nephrogenic DI, * water loss alone does not decrease skin turgor or drop BP, * random UNa$^+$ <10 mEq/L in insensible water loss and >20 mEq/L in DI
Rx of hypernatremia from pure water loss	• **oral administration of water,** • *if oral hydration is not feasible:* infuse 5% dextrose and water
formula used to calculate the fluid deficit in hypernatremia associated with volume depletion/pure water loss	*fluid deficit = 0.6 × weight in kg × (measured serum Na$^+$/140 − 1):* * e.g., 70 kg man with serum Na$^+$ 160 mEq/L: fluid deficit = 0.6 (70) × (160/140 − 1) = ~6 liters, * if hypernatremia due to pure water loss, give IV 5% dextrose/water or water by mouth, * if hypernatremia due to a hypotonic loss of more water than salt, give IV 0.45% saline
CNS abnormality produced with overzealous infusions of saline in patients with hypernatremia	*cerebral edema leading to herniation* [In hypernatremia, brain cells are initially contracted from water loss. Idiogenic osmoles (see above) are manufactured, which draw fluid back into brain cells over time and rehydrate the brain. Rapid IV infusion may cause cerebral edema and herniation. IV fluids must be administered slowly over 24–48 h. Serum Na$^+$ should not drop ≥0.5 mEq/L/h.]

Table 10–2. VOLUME AND POTASSIUM DISORDERS
Continued

Most Common...	Answer and Explanation
cause of isosmotic euvolemic hyponatremia	*pseudohyponatremia* [Pseudohyponatremia is due to hypertriglyceridemia (>1500 mg/dL) or excess γ-globulins (e.g., multiple myeloma). Since 93% of plasma is water and 7% contains nonaqueous components (lipids, proteins), an increased nonaqueous phase reduces the amount of water (<93%). On some lab instruments, this results in a falsely low serum Na^+. POsm is normal, since the Na^+ distributed in plasma water is still normal.]
cause of hyperosmotic hypovolemic hyponatremia	• **hyperglycemia:** * DKA, * HNKC, • *mannitol:* * used to reduce intracranial/intraocular pressure, * Rx of HTR, • *glycine:* prostate surgery [All the above are limited to ECF and produce a dilutional hyponatremia.]
electrolyte disorder in AIDS	*hyponatremia:* 50%
causes of hyponatremia in AIDS	• **SIADH,** • *GI losses:* diarrhea, • *adrenal insufficiency:* CMV, • *Na^+ transport defect*
compartment site for potassium	*ICF*
causes of hypokalemia (serum K^+ <3.5 mEq/L)	• **renal loss:** * UK^+ >20 mEq/L, e.g., * **diuretics,** * mineralocorticoid excess (Conn's, chronic licorice ingestion), * osmotic diuresis, * type I/II RTA, * increased urine anions (HCO_3^-, ketoacids), • *GI loss:* UK^+ <20 mEq/L, e.g., * vomiting/diarrhea, • *transcellular shift:* see below
factors promoting K^+ shift into cells (transcellular shift into ICF) leading to hypokalemia	• **insulin:** * enhances Na^+/K^+ ATPase pump, * reduces Na^+ permeability favoring K^+ gradient shift into cells, • *epinephrine,* • *alkalosis:* H^+ moves out of cells/K^+ moves in, • $β_2$-*agonists:* e.g., * albuterol, * enhances Na^+/K^+ ATPase pump, • *aldosterone:* enhances Na^+/K^+ pump, • *hypokalemic periodic paralysis:* intermittent K^+ shifts into cells after high CHO meals
S/S of hypokalemia	• **muscle weakness:** changes intracellular/extracellular K^+ membrane potential, • *constipation,* • *paralytic ileus:* absent bowel

Table continued on following page

Table 10–2. VOLUME AND POTASSIUM DISORDERS
Continued

Most Common...	Answer and Explanation
Continued	sounds, • *polyuria:* * vacuolar nephropathy, * tubules resistant to ADH, * acquired nephrogenic DI, • *rhabdomyolysis:* hypokalemia inhibits insulin, which decreases muscle glycogenesis, • *ventricular arrhythmias:* common in patients taking digitalis, • *precipitate hepatic encephalopathy in chronic liver disease:* hypokalemia increases renal ammoniagenesis
ECG findings in hypokalemia	• **U waves:** positive wave after T wave, • *sagging ST segment,* • *T wave depression*
Rx of hypokalemia	• **oral replacement safest:** enteric coated preparations produce jejunal strictures, • *IV:* add KCl to IV solutions to a final concentration of 40 mEq/L not to exceed an infusion rate of 10–20 mEq/h, • *use of aldosterone blockers in patients on diuretics:* conserves K^+, • *dietary Na^+ restriction:* less Na^+ delivery to distal tubule/collecting duct, hence less K^+ exchanged with Na^+
nonpathologic cause of hyperkalemia	*pseudohyperkalemia secondary to iatrogenic hemolysis of RBCs:* occurs with an increase in WBCs or platelets
pathophysiologic causes of hyperkalemia	• **decreased renal excretion:** e.g., * renal failure, * aldosterone deficiency (e.g., Addison's, hyporeninemic hypoaldosteronism, aldosterone blockers), • *increased tissue release:* e.g., rhabdomyolysis, • *transcellular shift:* see below
factors promoting K^+ shift out of cells leading to hyperkalemia	• **inorganic metabolic acidoses:** e.g., * renal failure (not ketoacidosis/lactic acidosis), * intracellular buffering of H^+ ions causes K^+ to move out of cells to maintain electroneutrality, • *insulin deficiency,* • *hypertonicity:* e.g., hyperglycemia, • β-*antagonists:* e.g., propranolol, • *digitalis toxicity:* inhibits Na^+/K^+ ATPase pump, • *succinylcholine:* muscle relaxant, • *hyperkalemic periodic paralysis:* * AD disease with periodic K^+ shift out of cells, * often precipitated by cold or exercise
S/S of hyperkalemia	• **cardiac arrhythmias:** e.g., * ventricular arrhythmias, * heart stops in diastole, • *muscle weakness:* hyperkalemia partially depolarizes

Table 10–2. VOLUME AND POTASSIUM DISORDERS
Continued

Most Common...	Answer and Explanation
Continued	cell membrane, which interferes with membrane excitability, • *impairs renal acid excretion leading to metabolic acidosis:* * K^+ moves into the distal/collecting duct tubules in exchange for H^+ ions moving into ECF
early ECG findings in hyperkalemia	*peaked narrow T waves:* accelerated repolarization of cardiac muscle [Serum K^+ between 7 and 8 mEq/L decrease cardiac excitability owing to inactivation of Na^+ permeability during the initial spike in the action potential. This results in widening of PR interval and QRS. Serum K^+ levels >8 mEq/L results in cardiac standstill in diastole.]
Rx of hyperkalemia	• **IV calcium gluconate:** * decreases membrane excitability, * protects heart, • *IV $NaHCO_3$:* create metabolic alkalosis to shift K^+ into ICF, • *insulin + glucose:* shifts K^+ into ICF, • *β_2-agonists:* shifts K^+ into ICF, • *cation exchange resins:* * Na^+ polystyrene promotes Na^+ exchange for K^+ in GI tract, * increases excretion K^+, • *loop diuretics:* increase K^+ excretion

Table continued on following page

Table 10–2. VOLUME AND POTASSIUM DISORDERS
Continued

Question: In which of the following clinical situations would you expect hyposmotic hypervolemic hyponatremia with a UNa^+ <10 mEq/L? **SELECT 2**
- (A) Loop diuretic
- (B) Untreated RHF
- (C) SIADH
- (D) Chronic renal failure
- (E) Sweating
- (F) Diabetic ketoacidosis
- (G) Cirrhosis

Answers: (B), (G): Loop diuretics produce a hyposmotic hypovolemic hyponatremia with a UNa^+ >20 mEq/L (choice A is incorrect). Untreated RHF (choice B) produces a hyposmotic hypervolemic hyponatremia with a UNa^+ <10 mEq/L (increased renal reabsorption). If the patient were on diuretics, the UNa^+ would be >20 mEq/L. SIADH produces a hyposmotic euvolemic hyponatremia with a UNa^+ >20 mEq/L ($P_H > P_O$, choice C is incorrect). CRF usually produces a hyposmotic hypervolemic hyponatremia with a UNa^+ >20 mEq/L, the latter owing to tubular dysfunction (choice D is incorrect). Sweating normally produces a hyperosmotic hypovolemic hypernatremia, UNa^+ is < 10 mEq/L due to increased renal reabsorption ($P_O > P_H$, choice E is incorrect). Diabetic ketoacidosis is most commonly associated with a hyperosmotic hypovolemic hyponatremia and a UNa^+ >20 mEq/L (choice F is incorrect). Hyponatremia is due to water moving out of the ICF into the ECF, causing a dilutional hyponatremia with a UNa^+ >20 mEq/L. Cirrhosis (choice G) produces a hyposmotic hypervolemic hyponatremia with a UNa^+ <10 mEq/L, since EABV is decreased and Na^+ is reabsorbed in proximal tubule.

AD = autosomal dominant, ADH = antidiuretic hormone, AIDS = acquired immunodeficiency syndrome, AMI = acute myocardial infarction, ANP = atrial natriuretic peptide, ATI = angiotensin I, ATII = angiotensin II, BP = blood pressure, BUN = blood urea nitrogen, CHF = congestive heart failure, CHO = carbohydrate, CMV = cytomegalovirus, CNS = central nervous system, CRF = chronic renal failure, DCT = distal convoluted tubule, DI = diabetes insipidus, DKA = diabetic ketoacidosis, DTRs = deep tendon reflexes, EABV = effective arterial blood volume, ECF = extracellular fluid, ECG = electrocardiogram, EOsm = effective osmolality, GFR = glomerular filtration rate, GI = gastrointestinal, HNKC = hyperosmolar nonketotic coma, HTR = hemolytic transfusion reaction, ICF = intracellular fluid, ISF = interstitial fluid, IV = intravenous, JG = juxtaglomerular, LHF = left heart failure, LVEDP = left ventricular end-diastolic pressure, MOA = mechanism of action, NSAIDs = nonsteroidal anti-inflammatory drugs, OHase = hydroxylase, PCWP = pulmonary capillary wedge pressure, PEEP = positive end-expiratory pressure, P_H = peritubular capillary hydrostatic pressure, P_O = peritubular capillary oncotic pressure, POsm = plasma osmolality, PTH = parathormone, RAA = renin-angiotensin-aldosterone, RBC = red blood cell, RBF = renal blood flow, RHF = right heart failure, RTA =

renal tubular acidosis, Rx = treatment, SGC = Swan Ganz catheter, SIADH = syndrome of inappropriate antidiuretic hormone, S/S = signs and symptoms, TAL = thick ascending limb, TB = tuberculosis, TBK$^+$ = total body potassium, TBNa$^+$ = total body sodium, TBW = total body water, TPR = total periphreal resistance, UK$^+$ = urine potassium, UNa$^+$ = urine sodium, WBC = white blood cell.

Table 10–3. CYSTIC DISORDERS, GLOMERULAR DISORDERS, DIALYSIS, RENAL TRANSPLANTATION

Most Common...	Answer and Explanation
congenital kidney disorder associated with Turner's syndrome	*horseshoe kidney:* * fused at lower pole, * danger of infection owing to VUR
nonhereditary cystic disease in adults that shows up as an IVP abnormality	*medullary sponge kidney:* striations in the papillary portion of the medulla are noted in an IVP
S/S of medullary sponge kidney	• **recurrent UTIs,** • *microscopic hematuria,* • *recurrent renal stones,* • *abnormal urinary concentrating ability,* • *nephrocalcinosis*
cause of acquired polycystic kidney disease	*renal dialysis:* * occurs in ~50% of patients on hemodialysis/peritoneal dialysis >3 y, * small risk for renal carcinoma
type of cyst in adults	*simple retention cysts:* * derived from tubular obstruction, * located in cortex/medulla, * confused with cystic renal adenocarcinoma
clinical findings in medullary cystic disease in adults	• *AD disease:* first manifests in adults, • *gross:* * small kidneys, * cysts at corticomedullary junction, • *clinical:* * **polyuria,** * HTN uncommon, * salt wasting, * renal failure
hereditary adult kidney disease	*adult polycystic kidney disease* (APKD): * AD disease, * high penetrance, * abnormal gene on chromosome 16, * cysts noted by 20–25 years of age
S/S of APKD	• **HTN:** >80%, • *abdominal/flank pain:* * 60%, * pain from bleeding into cysts, • *bilaterally palpable kidneys:* cysts in cortex/medulla, • *hematuria:* 50%, • *renal defects in concentration,* • *hepatic cysts:* * 40–60%, * cysts in spleen/pancreas, • *intracranial berry aneurysms:* * 10–30%, * subarachnoid hem-

Table continued on following page

**Table 10–3. CYSTIC DISORDERS, GLOMERULAR
DISORDERS, DIALYSIS, RENAL TRANSPLANTATION**
Continued

Most Common...	Answer and Explanation
Continued	orrhage, • *diverticulosis:* 80%, • *risk for renal adenocarcinoma,* • *MVP:* 30%, • *recurrent UTIs,* • *renal stones:* uric acid and calcium oxalate stones, • *secondary polycythemia:* increased EPO, • *CRF by 70 y:* account for 10% of all dialysis patients
imaging study to diagnose APKD	• **US,** • *CT*
Rx of APKD	• **dialysis,** • *renal transplantation*
COD in APKD	• **renal failure:** 50%, • *HTN complications:* * ~30%, * AMI, * stroke (intracerebral bleed, ruptured berry aneurysm)
mechanisms producing GN	• **immune-complex deposition:** * ICs activate complement system, * C5a chemotactic to neutrophils, * neutrophils damage glomeruli, • *CMI,* • *NEG:* DM, • *hyperfiltration:* DM
mechanisms of antibody-mediated GN	• **circulating ICs:** * type III hypersensitivity, * antigens include ♦ DNA (SLE), ♦ bacterial products (group A strep), ♦ viral products (HBsAg, HCV), ♦ malarial antigens, ♦ tumor antigens (CEA), • *antibodies:* * directed against antigens normally present in glomerulus (GBM), * directed against "planted" antigens (trapped in glomerulus, e.g., DNA, drugs, bacterial products)
studies performed on renal biopsy specimens	• *H&E stains:* classify type of GN, • *IF:* * linear and granular patterns, * identify type of deposits (e.g., IgA, C3), • *EM:* * location of immune deposits, * structural abnormalities: e.g., podocyte fusion
cause of a linear IF glomerular pattern	*Goodpasture's syndrome:* * anti-GBM antibodies against α_3 type IV collagen, * deposit on endothelial side of GBM producing smooth IF pattern
cause of a granular ("lumpy-bumpy") IF glomerular pattern	*IC deposition:* location of deposit is dependent on charge, size, solubility

Table 10–3. CYSTIC DISORDERS, GLOMERULAR DISORDERS, DIALYSIS, RENAL TRANSPLANTATION
Continued

Most Common...	Answer and Explanation
GN where IF confirms Dx	*IgA GN* (Berger's disease)
type of glomerular disease with podocyte fusion	*nephrotic syndrome:* e.g., minimal change disease
EM appearance of IC deposits	*densities:* * subendothelial, * subepithelial, intramembranous, * mesangial
general subtypes of GN	• **nephritic,** • *nephrotic*
S/S and lab findings of nephritic syndrome	• *oliguria,* • *HTN,* • *periorbital edema,* • *hematuria,* • *proteinuria:* not in nephrotic range, • *RBC casts,* • *WBCs in sediment*
S/S and lab findings of the nephrotic syndrome	• **generalized pitting edema:** albumin loss, • *spontaneous peritonitis:* Streptococcus pneumoniae, • *hypogammaglobulinemia:* increased infection risk, • *renal vein thrombosis:* * ATIII loss in urine, * increased factor V, VIII, fibrinogen, platelets, • *HTN:* exception: minimal change disease, • *osteomalacia:* loss of vitamin D binding protein, • **proteinuria:** >3.5 g/24 h, • *fatty casts,* • *oval fat bodies,* • *high CH,* • *iron deficiency:* transferrin loss
primary GN	*IgA GN* (Berger's disease): * primarily nephritic (nephrotic in some cases), * pathogenesis due to an exaggerated increase in mucosal IgA, * polymeric IgA deposits in mesangium
secondary causes of IgA GN	• *chronic liver disease,* • *celiac sprue,* • *ankylosing spondylitis*
S/S and lab findings of IgA GN	• **gross** (children) **or asymptomatic microscopic hematuria** (adults): often follows a URI, • *increased serum IgA:* 50%, • *normal complement levels,* • *IgA in mesangium,* • *clinical:* * HTN uncommon, * same renal lesion as HSP
Rx of IgA GN	*fish oil capsules with ω-3 fatty acid:* * slows disease progression, * 20% reach end-stage renal disease in 20 y, * recurs in renal transplant

Table continued on following page

Table 10–3. CYSTIC DISORDERS, GLOMERULAR
DISORDERS, DIALYSIS, RENAL TRANSPLANTATION
Continued

Most Common...	Answer and Explanation
S/S and lab findings of post-streptococcal GN	• *primarily nephritic,* • *hematuria 2–4 wks following streptococcal type 49 skin infection or 1–3 wks following type 12 pharyngeal infection,* • *periorbital edema,* • *oliguria,* • *HTN,* • *granular IF,* • *subepithelial deposits,* • *low C3:* alternative pathway activation, • *anti-ASO titers:* increased in pharyngeal infections, • *anti-DNAase titers:* increased in skin infections
Rx of post-streptococcal GN	• *supportive,* • *penicillin for patient and contacts* [Children fare better than adults. CRF is uncommon.]
type of renal diseases in SLE	• **diffuse proliferative GN,** • *acute/chronic interstitial nephritis,* • *vasculitis* [50% have renal disease at presentation. 90% develop renal disease in the course of their disease.]
S/S and lab findings of SLE diffuse proliferative GN	• *nephritic >70% with or without progression to nephrotic syndrome,* • *disease activity correlates with anti-dsDNA antibody titers,* • *exacerbations occur with pregnancy:* delay pregnancy until renal disease under control for 6 mths, • *granular IF,* • *subendothelial deposits,* • *low C3:* classical pathway activation
Rx of SLE diffuse proliferative GN	*steroids + cyclophosphamide:* * SLE GN usually evolves into end-stage disease, * no recurrence in transplanted kidney, * membranous SLE (type V) is nephrotic and resistant to steroids
genetic GN with nerve deafness and ocular abnormalities	*Alport's syndrome:* * SXD, * defect in α_5 type IV collagen in GBM, * anti-GBM antibodies present but glomeruli lack Goodpasture's antigen so no IF pattern is present
clinical findings in Alport's syndrome	• *primarily nephritic,* • *ocular abnormalities:* * anterior lenticonus, * cataracts, • *worse prognosis in males,* • *end-stage disease occurs by 15–30 yrs*
type of GN in renal transplants in patient's with Alport's syndrome	*anti-GBM disease:* * transplant kidneys have Goodpasture's antigen, * anti-GBM antibodies react against the antigen

Table 10–3. CYSTIC DISORDERS, GLOMERULAR DISORDERS, DIALYSIS, RENAL TRANSPLANTATION
Continued

Most Common...	Answer and Explanation
GBM abnormality in Goodpasture's syndrome	*anti-basement membrane antibodies:* antibodies directed against non-collagen domain of α_3 type IV collagen in GBM/pulmonary capillaries
S/S and lab findings in Goodpasture's syndrome	• *primarily nephritic,* • *male dominant:* * 90%, * usually young smoking adults, • *begins with hemoptysis:* * 70%, * precedes or coincides with renal disease, • *progresses to glomerular disease:* * usually progresses into RPGN, * linear IF, • *Dx:* * based on finding anti-GBM antibodies in plasma or linear IF, * normal complement levels
Rx of Goodpasture's syndrome	• **plasmapheresis:** removes antibodies, • *steroids,* • *cyclophosphamide,* • *poor prognosis if oliguria is present or serum creatinine >6 mg/dL,* • *35% develop end-stage renal disease with a 25% mortality*
causes of primary RPGN	• **type I:** anti-GBM antibody disease with pulmonary disease (Goodpasture's syndrome), • *type II:* IC-mediated: * IgA GN, * MPGN, • *type III:* * no immune deposits or anti-GBM antibodies, * pauci-immune GN, * usually ANCA positive: ♦ Wegener's granulomatosis (c-ANCA), ♦ PAN (p-ANCA)
causes of secondary RPGN	• *SLE,* • *HSP,* • *post-infectious GN,* • *mixed cryoglobulinemic GN*
S/S and lab findings in RPGN	• *primarily nephritic,* • *acute deterioration in renal function:* * days to weeks to months, * oliguria present, • *abnormal urinary sediment:* * hematuria, * RBC casts, • *crescents in >50% of glomeruli:* parietal cell proliferation
Rx of RPGN	*depends on disease causing RPGN*
cause of nephrotic syndrome in children	*minimal change disease:* * nil disease/lipoid nephrosis, * occurs in 20% of adults
mechanism of minimal change disease	*cellular immune reaction against visceral epithelial cells:* * lymphokines destroy negative charge in GBM (called polyanion loss), * lymphokines cause podocyte fusion

Table continued on following page

Table 10–3. CYSTIC DISORDERS, GLOMERULAR DISORDERS, DIALYSIS, RENAL TRANSPLANTATION
Continued

Most Common...	Answer and Explanation
secondary causes of minimal change disease	• *nodular sclerosing HD,* • *NSAIDs,* • *atopic individuals,* • *CLL*
S/S and lab findings in minimal change disease	• *often follows URI,* • *normotensive,* • *generalized pitting edema,* • *normal glomeruli on H&E staining:* most children do not require renal biopsies to confirm Dx, • *podocyte fusion,* • *negative IF,* • *normal complement levels,* • *relapsing course*
Rx of minimal change disease	• *children:* respond well to steroids, • *adults:* * 80% respond to steroids, * 60% have relapsing course, * cyclophosphamide prolongs remissions/lowers steroid dose to control disease, * poor response to Rx requires a renal Bx to R/O FSG
nephrotic syndrome in adults	*diffuse membranous GN:* * 25–30%, * IC disease with in-situ deposition of cationic antigens causing subepithelial deposits ("spike and dome" appearance visible with stains)
causes of membranous GN	• **idiopathic,** • *drugs:* * captopril, * gold therapy, * penicillamine, * probenecid, * some NSAIDs, • *infections:* * **HBV,** * *Plasmodium malariae,* * schistosomiasis, * leprosy, * secondary syphilis, • *malignancy:* * **colorectal** (CEA-anti-CEA ICs), * non-Hodgkin's lymphoma, * melanoma, • *sickle cell disease*
S/S of membranous GN	• *25% not in nephrotic range of proteinuria,* • *HTN:* 40%, • *highest association with malignancies of all GN types,* • *highest association with renal vein thrombosis,* • *normal complement levels*
Rx of membranous GN	• *steroids,* • *cyclophosphamide,* • *ACE inhibitors:* control degree of proteinuria, * prognosis worse with massive proteinuria and HTN, * without Rx, ♦ ~25% spontaneously remit, ♦ ~50% partially remit, ♦ ~20% progress to end-stage disease
GN in AIDS	• **FSG,** • *post-infectious GN,* • *HIV-associated IgA GN,* • *MPGN,* • *membranous GN,* • *HUS*

Table 10–3. CYSTIC DISORDERS, GLOMERULAR
DISORDERS, DIALYSIS, RENAL TRANSPLANTATION
Continued

Most Common...	Answer and Explanation
secondary causes of FSG other than AIDS	• **IV heroin abuse,** • *reflux nephropathy,* • *massive obesity* [FSG accounts for ~15–20% of adult nephrotic syndrome.]
S/S of FSG	• **nephrotic syndrome:** 90%, • *HTN,* • *IgM/C3 in mesangium,* • *normal complement*
Rx of FSG	• *steroids,* • *cyclosporine,* • *ACE inhibitors:* reduce proteinuria, • *50–80% progress to CRF,* • *recurs in renal transplant*
types of MPGN	• **type I:** commonly follows URI, • *type II:* also known as dense deposit disease, • primarily nephrotic syndrome: * 50%, * 5–10% of cases of adult nephrotic syndrome
secondary causes of type I MPGN	• **HCV,** • *HBV,* • *cryoglobulinemia,* • *sickle cell disease*
S/S and lab findings of type I MPGN	• *IC disease with subendothelial deposits,* • *tram tracks noted on EM:* mesangium splits GBM, • *high association with HCV,* • *HTN,* • *low C3 levels*
S/S and lab findings in type II MPGN	• *"dense deposit disease":* intramembranous deposit of C3, • *autoantibody against alternative pathway C3 convertase:* * called C3 nephritic factor, * persistent breakdown of C3 causes very low C3 levels, • *HTN*
Rx of MPGN	• *? use of steroids,* • *dipyramidole/aspirin slow progression of disease,* • *recurs in renal transplants:* type II > type I, • *poor prognosis*
systemic disease secondarily affecting the glomerulus	*DM:* type I DM (30–40%) > type II DM (20–30%)
initial lab finding in DM nephropathy	*microalbuminuria:* proteinuria may be in nephrotic range later in the disease
mechanisms of microalbuminuria	*see Table 10–1*
extrarenal abnormalities in DM nephropathy	• **HTN:** type I and II, • *retinopathy:* * universal in type I, * 60–70% of type II

Table continued on following page

**Table 10–3. CYSTIC DISORDERS, GLOMERULAR
DISORDERS, DIALYSIS, RENAL TRANSPLANTATION**
Continued

Most Common...	Answer and Explanation
stages of diabetic nephropathy	• **hyperfiltration:** increased GFR → *microalbuminuria* → • *normalization of GFR, mesangial/capillary BM damage evident* → • *HTN* → • *overt proteinuria, HTN, decline in GFR:* lasts 10–15 y → • *ESRD with heavy proteinuria:* 5–7 y
Rx for early DM nephropathy	• *ACE inhibitors:* e.g., * captopril, * independent of BP-lowering effect, • *tight glycemic control,* • *control HTN,* • *decrease protein intake,* • *aldose reductase inhibitors:* decrease production of sorbitol, which may play a minor role in producing glomerular disease
beneficial effects of ACE inhibitors in DM nephropathy	• *reduce ATII effect of increasing intraglomerular pressure,* • *slows progression of microalbuminuria to overt proteinuria,* • *lowers BP in HTN,* • *decrease LVH*
type of renal disease in amyloidosis	*nephrotic syndrome:* * most common with primary amyloidosis due to light chains, * light chain myeloma associated with renal disease, * enlarged kidneys
causes of chronic GN in descending order of incidence	• **RPGN,** • *FSG,* • *type I MPGN*
types of dialysis	• **hemodialysis,** • *peritoneal dialysis*
complications associated with both types of dialysis	• *hepatitis:* **HCV most common,** • *infection,* • *osteodystrophy:* * decreased 1,25 $(OH)_2D$, * increased PTH, * aluminum toxicity, • *heart disease:* * **AMI,** * HTN, * LVH
complication associated with peritoneal dialysis	*peritonitis*
complications associated with hemodialysis	• **N/V and headache,** • *hypotension,* • *air embolism,* • *aluminum intoxication*
complications associated with long-term dialysis	• **AMI/CVA:** * 50% of deaths, * risk factors: ♦ HTN, ♦ accelerated atherosclerosis, ♦ LVH, • *dialysis dementia:* relation to aluminum, • *acquired cystic disease:* see above, • *hemodi-*

Table 10–3. CYSTIC DISORDERS, GLOMERULAR DISORDERS, DIALYSIS, RENAL TRANSPLANTATION
Continued

Most Common...	Answer and Explanation
Continued	*alysis-related amyloidosis:* * β_2-microglobulin deposition, * spondylitis, * carpal tunnel syndrome
source for a living donor	*siblings:* * 25% chance for 2-haplotype match, * 50% chance for 1-haplotype match, * 25% chance for 0-haplotype match, * parents are 1-haplotype matches
type of renal transplant	• **cadaver:** 1 y graft survival rate is 80%, • *living donor:* 1 y graft survival rate is 90%, • *transplantation is Rx of choice for ESRD*
types of compatibility necessary for renal transplantation	• *ABO compatible,* • *class I, class II compatible:* should be at least 6 antigen matches in both class I and II HLA antigens for cadaveric kidney transplantation
tests employed for renal transplantation	• *cross-match test:* patient serum against donor leukocytes to R/O anti-HLA antibodies against donor leukocytes, • *HLA typing*
types of renal disease requiring transplantation in descending order	• **DM with renal failure,** • *hypertensive renal disease,* • *GN*
type of GN with highest rate of recurrence in graft	• **FSG:** 20–30%, • *MPGN,* • *membranous GN,* • *DM,* • *HUS,* • *IgA GN:* mild and not usually significant
absolute contraindications for renal transplantation	• *malignancy,* • *severe atherosclerosis,* • *pulmonary disease,* • *active hepatitis*
immunosuppressants used in renal transplant patients	• *cyclosporine:* inhibits IL-2 release from CD_4 T helper cells, • *azathioprine:* inhibits proliferation of activated T cells, • *prednisone:* blocks IL-1 and cytokine production from T cells, • *OKT3:* monoclonal antibody against T cell antigen receptor
side effects of cyclosporine	• **dose-related nephrotoxicity:** interstitial fibrosis, • *gum hyperplasia,* • *hypertrichosis,* • *HUS,* • *TTP,* • *hepatotoxicity,* • *HTN,* • *lymphoproliferative malignancy,* • *hyperkalemia*

Table continued on following page

Table 10–3. CYSTIC DISORDERS, GLOMERULAR DISORDERS, DIALYSIS, RENAL TRANSPLANTATION
Continued

Most Common...	Answer and Explanation
causes of hyperacute rejection	• **anti-HLA antibodies**, • *ABO incompatibility* [It is a type II hypersensitivity reaction with vessel thrombosis developing within hours of transplant surgery.]
cause of acute rejection	• *primarily CMI:* lymphocyte infiltrate in parenchyma, • *humoral component:* vessel thrombosis/fibrosis [Acute rejections occur after the first week or after a few years.]
Rx of acute rejection	• *IV methylprednisolone*, • *antithymocyte globulin or OKT3*
cause of allograft rejection	*chronic rejection:* * leads to total renal failure in months to years, * interstitial fibrosis and vessel fibrosis (ischemia), * no specific Rx
tests to evaluate renal transplant rejection	• **renal biopsy**, • *renal scans*
COD in renal transplant patients	• **opportunistic infections:** * CMV, *Aspergillus*, • *AMI*

Question: Which of the following more likely occur in the nephrotic rather than nephritic syndrome? **SELECT 4**
(A) Generalized pitting edema
(B) RBC casts
(C) Fatty casts
(D) Hypertension
(E) Podocyte fusion
(F) Renal vein thrombosis
(G) Low complement levels

Answers: (A), (C), (E), (F): Generalized pitting edema **(choice A)** is a key feature of nephrotic syndrome owing to hypoalbuminemia secondary to massive proteinuria (>3.5 g/24 h). RBC casts are more commonly noted in the nephritic syndrome owing to a greater degree of neutrophilic damage to the glomeruli **(choice B is incorrect).** Fatty casts **(choice C)** are a classic feature of the nephrotic syndrome. Hyperlipidemia with increased CH is commonly present as well as lipiduria. Hypertension is present in both the nephritic and nephrotic syndrome **(choice D is incorrect).** Fusion of the podocytes **(choice E)** is a classic EM finding in the nephrotic syndrome. Renal vein thrombosis **(choice F)** is more likely to accompany the nephrotic syndrome (particularly membranous GN) owing to an increase in fibrinogen and factors V and VIII, and a decrease in ATIII. Low complement levels are present in both the nephritic and nephrotic syndrome **(choice G is incorrect).**

ACE = angiotensin converting enzyme, AD = autosomal dominant, AIDS = acquired immunodeficiency syndrome, AMI = acute myocardial infarction, ANCA = antineutrophil cytoplasmic antibody, APKD = adult polycystic kidney disease, ATII = angiotensin II, ATIII = antithrombin III, BM = basement membrane, BP = blood pressure, Bx = biopsy, CEA = carcinoembryonic antigen, CH = cholesterol, CLL = chronic lymphocytic leukemia, CMI = cell-mediated immunity, CMV = cytomegalovirus, COD = cause of death, CRF = chronic renal failure, CT = computed tomography, CVA = cerebrovascular accident, DM = diabetes mellitus, Dx = diagnosis, EM = electron microscope, EPO = erythropoietin, ESRD = end-stage renal disease, FSG = focal segmental glomerulosclerosis, GBM = glomerular basement membrane, GFR = glomerular filtration rate, GN = glomerulonephritis, HBsAg = hepatitis B surface antigen, HBV = hepatitis B virus, HCV = hepatitis C virus, HD = Hodgkin's disease, H&E = hematoxylin and eosin, HLA = human leukocyte antigen, HSP = Henoch-Schönlein purpura, HTN = hypertension, HUS = hemolytic uremic syndrome, IC = immunocomplex, IF = immunofluorescent, IV = intravenous, IVP = intravenous pyelogram, LVH = left ventricular hypertrophy, MPGN = membranoproliferative glomerulonephritis, MVP = mitral valve prolapse, NEG = nonenzymatic glycosylation, NSAIDs = nonsteroidal anti-inflammatory drugs, N/V = nausea and vomiting, PAN = polyarteritis nodosa, PTH = parathormone, RBC = red blood cell, R/O = rule out, RPGN = rapidly progressive crescentic glomerulonephritis, Rx = treatment, SLE = systemic lupus erythematosus, S/S = signs and symptoms, SXD = sex-linked dominant, TTP = thrombotic thrombocytopenic purpura, URI = upper respiratory infection, US = ultrasonography, UTI = urinary tract infection, VUR = vesicoureteral reflux, WBC = white blood cell.

Table 10–4. TUBULAR, TUBULOINTERSTITIAL, VASCULAR, OBSTRUCTIVE, AND NEOPLASTIC DISEASES OF THE KIDNEYS

Most Common...	Answer and Explanation
causes of ARF	• **hypovolemia:** leads to ischemic ATN, • *AMI/CHF,* • *ureteral obstruction:* * least common cause of ARF, * most treatable, • *vascular disease:* e.g., * HTN, * vasculitis, • *rhabdomyolysis with myoglobinuria,* • *GN,* *tubular injury:* e.g., drugs, • *tubulointerstitial disease:* e.g., drugs
patterns of ATN	• **ischemic ATN:** * oliguric (<400 mL/d or <20 mL/h), * polyuric most common type (>800 mL/d), • *nephrotoxic ATN* [Most cases of ATN are multifactorial.]
cause of ischemic ATN	*prerenal azotemia:* * reversible disease associated with a reduced GFR, * greatest potential for ischemic tubular damage

Table continued on following page

**Table 10–4. TUBULAR, TUBULOINTERSTITIAL,
VASCULAR, OBSTRUCTIVE, AND NEOPLASTIC DISEASES
OF THE KIDNEYS** *Continued*

Most Common...	Answer and Explanation
causes of nephrotoxic ATN	• **drugs:** e.g., * **aminoglycosides**, * cisplatin, * cyclosporine, • *radiocontrast agents:* patients at risk include: * **DM**, * multiple myeloma, * old age, * volume depleted
mechanisms of oliguria in ATN	• **vasoconstriction of afferent arterioles**, • *tubular cells blocking lumen*, • *increased interstitial pressure from fluid leaking out through damaged BMs*, • *decreased permeability of glomerulus*
tests used in work-up of oliguria	• **FENa⁺**, • *UOsm*, • *random UNa⁺*, • *serum BUN/serum Cr ratio*, • *UA* [See Table 10–1.]
profile for good tubular function (ability to concentrate urine)	• **FENa⁺ <1**, • *UOsm >500 mOsm/kg*, • *random UNa⁺ <20 mEq/L*, • *BUN/serum Cr ratio >20/1*, • *normal UA*
profile for poor tubular function (inability to concentrate urine)	• **FENa⁺ >1:** usually *>2*, • *UOsm <350 mOsm/kg*, • *random UNa⁺ >40 mEq/L*, • *BUN/serum Cr ratio <15/1*, • *UA with renal tubular casts*
causes of oliguria	• **prerenal azotemia**, • *ATN*, • *postrenal azotemia*, • *acute GN* (see Table 10–3)
causes of prerenal azotemia	• **decreased EABV:** e.g., * CHF, * hypovolemia, * hypotension, • *drugs:* e.g., * NSAIDs (block intrarenal prostaglandin production), * ACE inhibitors (block ATII and aldosterone production)
cause of postrenal azotemia in kidneys	*intratubular obstruction by crystals:* e.g., * **uric acid**, * oxalate, * drug crystals
causes of postrenal azotemia in ureters	• **kidney stone,** • *blood clot,* • *retroperitoneal fibrosis*, • *TCC*, • *cervical cancer*
causes of postrenal azotemia in bladder	• **trauma,** • *stones*, • *TCC*
causes of postrenal azotemia in the urethra	• **benign prostatic hyperplasia,** • *cervical cancer*
causes of oliguria with preserved tubular function	• **prerenal azotemia:** normal UA, • *acute GN:* * RBC casts, * hematuria

Table 10–4. TUBULAR, TUBULOINTERSTITIAL, VASCULAR, OBSTRUCTIVE, AND NEOPLASTIC DISEASES OF THE KIDNEYS *Continued*

Most Common...	Answer and Explanation
causes of oliguria with tubular dysfunction	• **ATN:** * pigmented renal tubular casts, * "dirty urine," • *postrenal azotemia:* * normal UA, * only prolonged postrenal obstruction leads to tubular damage
clinical problems associated with ARF	• **excess sodium/water retention:** cause weight gain/hyponatremia, respectively, • *hyponatremia:* excess water intake, • *increased AG metabolic acidosis:* decreased excretion of H^+ ions (~1 mEq/kg/d), • *hyperkalemia:* * transcellular shift secondary to metabolic acidosis, * decreased renal excretion, • *GI bleeding:* hemorrhagic gastritis, • *hyperphosphatemia:* decreased excretion, • *hypocalcemia:* * decreased synthesis of 1,25 (OH)$_2$D, * metastatic calcification, • *hyperuricemia:* decreased excretion, • *anemia:* decreased EPO, • *uremic pericarditis:* * usually hemorrhagic, * may produce cardiac tamponade, • *uremic syndrome:* accumulation of toxic products with multiorgan dysfunction
phases of ARF	• *oliguric phase:* * 1–2 weeks, * azotemia, * hyperkalemia, * metabolic acidosis, • *diuretic phase:* * usually 3rd week, * hypokalemia may occur, * severe hypercalcemia may occur in rhabdomyolysis, • *recovery phase:* GFR improves over subsequent 3–12 mths
Rx of ARF	• *fluid challenge:* useful in nonvolume overloaded oliguric patients, • *loop diuretic:* * attempts to convert an oliguric into polyuric ARF, * flushes tubular cells out of lumen, • *keep hemodynamically stable:* * Rx volume depletion with 0.45 saline, * Rx volume excess with loop diuretics, • *low-dose dopamine:* renal vasodilator, • *daily weight:* restrict sodium if weight increases, • *limit dietary protein:* 0.5 g/kg/d, • *Rx hyperphosphatemia:* * calcium carbonate with meals, * low phosphate diet, • *Rx hyperkalemia:* * see Table 10–2, * Rx when serum K^+ >6.5 mEq/L or * abnormal ECG, • *Rx metabolic acidosis:* if HCO_3^- <15–16 mEq/L, • *avoid nephrotoxic drugs,* • *dialyze when necessary:* * keep serum BUN <100 mg/dL, * Rx for hemor-

Table continued on following page

Table 10–4. TUBULAR, TUBULOINTERSTITIAL, VASCULAR, OBSTRUCTIVE, AND NEOPLASTIC DISEASES OF THE KIDNEYS *Continued*

Most Common...	Answer and Explanation
Continued	rhagic pericarditis, * Rx for peripheral neuropathy, * Rx for volume overload resistant to diuretics, * Rx for hyperkalemia/hyperphosphatemia when medical management is inadequate
COD in ARF	• **infection:** sepsis, • *cardiopulmonary disease*
time-frame for aminoglycoside-induced ATN	*5–10 d:* * some degree of ARF occurs in 10–15%, * gentamicin/amikacin most toxic, * streptomycin least toxic, * polyuric ATN, * K^+ and magnesium wasting commonly occur
types of nephrotoxic ATN in which alkalinization of urine is helpful	• *amphotericin B:* * distal tubule dysfunction, * volume depletion major risk factor, • *methotrexate:* precipitates in renal tubules (similar to acyclovir and some sulfa drugs), • *rhabdomyolysis:* * heme pigments produce intrarenal vasoconstriction/tubular obstruction
clinical findings in myoglobin-induced ATN	• *clinical settings:* * **crush injuries,** * alcoholism, * prolonged unconsciousness (particularly CO poisoning, post-seizures), * heat stroke, * brown recluse spider bite, * cocaine, • *usually polyuric,* • *lab findings:* * hypocalcemia, * hyperuricemia, * hyperphosphatemia, * hyperkalemia in acute phase, * hypercalcemia in diuretic phase
Rx of myoglobin-induced ATN	• **forced diuresis (mannitol) to remove heme pigments,** • *alkalinize urine*
mechanisms of ARF due to radiocontrast dyes	• *intrarenal vasoconstriction,* • *tubular obstruction,* • *direct tubular toxicity* [Patients become oliguric 1–2 d after dye injection. $FENa^+ <1$. Usually reversible within a week.]
preventive methods to avoid radiocontrast dye-induced ARF	• *decreased dose of dye,* • *forced diuresis with normal saline,* • *adequate hydration*
clinical findings of atheroembolic-induced ARF	• *most common in elderly population,* • *spontaneous or post-invasive procedure:* e.g., angiogram, • *cardiac source of emboli is common:* particularly with chronic AF, • *livedo reticularis,* • *CH emboli on retinal exam,* • *lab findings:* * increased ESR, * low complement

Table 10–4. TUBULAR, TUBULOINTERSTITIAL, VASCULAR, OBSTRUCTIVE, AND NEOPLASTIC DISEASES OF THE KIDNEYS *Continued*

Most Common...	Answer and Explanation
Continued	levels, * eosinophilia/eosinophiluria, * thrombocytopenia, • *renal Bx demonstrates CH emboli in vessels*, • *minimal reversibility*
causes of ARF in pregnancy	• **severe pre-eclampsia**, • *abruptio placenta:* hypotension, • *sepsis*, • *DIC*, • *retained placenta*
renal manifestation of ARF in pregnancy	*diffuse cortical necrosis:* * infarction of renal cortex, * anuria, * poor prognosis
causes of anuria (<50 mL/d)	• **complete obstruction**, • *RPGN*, • *renal cortical necrosis*, • *bilateral renal artery occlusion*
known causes of CRF in descending order	• **DM nephropathy**, • *HTN*, • *GN:* e.g., * **RPGN**, * FSG, * MPGN, • *cystic renal disease*, • *interstitial nephritis*
presentation of CRF	*reduction in GFR >3–6 months:* * symptomatic when GFR <10–15 mL/min, * constellation of findings is called the uremic syndrome, * kidneys are shrunken
hematologic findings in CRF	• **anemia:** * **decreased EPO**, * iron deficiency (inadequate intake, loss in dialysis, GI bleeds), • *qualitative platelet defects:* * ecchymoses/epistaxis/bleeding after trauma, * guanidinosuccinic acid inhibits platelet aggregation, * reversible with dialysis
manifestations of renal osteodystrophy in CRF	• **osteitis fibrosa cystica:** * secondary HPTH from hypocalcemia, * increased PTH resorption of bone, • *osteomalacia:* * hypocalcemia from hypovitaminosis D, * hyperphosphatemia (drives calcium into tissue), • *osteoporosis:* bone buffers excess H^+ ions in metabolic acidosis
clinical findings in renal osteodystrophy in CRF	• *spontaneous fractures/bone pain:* present in above disorders, • *skeletal deformities:* * primarily in osteomalacia, * bowed legs, • *pseudofractures:* * primarily in osteomalacia, * see Table 9–11, • *radiograph:* * subperiosteal resorption, * cysts, * patchy osteosclerosis (primarily in osteitis fibrosa cystica)

Table continued on following page

Table 10–4. TUBULAR, TUBULOINTERSTITIAL, VASCULAR, OBSTRUCTIVE, AND NEOPLASTIC DISEASES OF THE KIDNEYS *Continued*

Most Common...	Answer and Explanation
cardiac findings in CRF	• **HTN:** * **sodium retention with volume expansion**, * RAA activation, • *uremic pericarditis:* * chest pain, * friction rub, * Rx with dialysis, • *CHF:* * **volume expansion**, * HTN heart disease, * metabolic acidosis (decreases cardiac contractility), * butterfly fluid distribution around hilum, • *accelerated atherosclerosis:* high TG levels
GI findings in CRF	• **anorexia,** • *N/V,* • *chronic hiccups,* • *hemorrhagic gastritis,* • *PUD*
neurologic findings in CRF	• *irritability,* • *inability to concentrate,* • *decreased libido,* • *asterixis,* • *peripheral neuropathy:* * less common with advent of dialysis, * restless leg syndrome, * sensory type of neuropathy, • *myoclonus*
muscle findings in CRF	*proximal myopathy:* * weakness/atrophy, * Rx with dialysis, • *cramps/twitching*
dermatologic findings in CRF	• **pruritus:** * metastatic calcification in dermal adnexal structures, * high calcium/phosphate solubility product, • *uremic frost:* urea crystals, • *sallow, yellow skin:* increased urobilin deposition, • *soft tissue metastatic calcification*
endocrine findings in CRF	• **insulin resistance:** hyperglycemia, • *hypothermia:* * often 35.5°C, * problem in recognizing infection, since a "normal" temperature may be abnormal, • *impotence*
causes of normal to large kidneys in CRF	• **APKD,** • *DM,* • *amyloidosis*
causes of acute deterioration in CRF	• **volume depletion,** • *infection,* • *HTN,* • *urinary tract obstruction,* • *nephrotoxic drugs,* • *CH embolization:* see above
lab findings in CRF	• *hyponatremia:* * excess water intake, * salt wasting in some CRF cases, • *hyperkalemia:* ECG is best monitor, • *increased AG metabolic acidosis:* AG 20–24 mEq/L, • *hypocalcemia:* * **hypovitaminosis D**, * hyperphosphatemia, • *hyperphosphatemia:* * major cause of secondary HPTH, * increases calcium × phosphorous solubility product (met-

Table 10–4. TUBULAR, TUBULOINTERSTITIAL, VASCULAR, OBSTRUCTIVE, AND NEOPLASTIC DISEASES OF THE KIDNEYS Continued

Most Common...	Answer and Explanation
Continued	astatic calcification), • increased intact PTH: PTH cannot be excreted by diseased kidneys, • prolonged BT: decreased platelet aggregation, • normocytic anemia: decreased EPO, • isosthenuria: see Table 10–1, • broad/waxy casts: see Table 10–1, • increased TG • hyperuricemia: * decreased excretion, * may precipitate gout, • hypermagnesemia: * decreased excretion, * avoid magnesium containing antacids
salt losing types of CRF	• chronic PN, • medullary cystic disease, • hydronephrosis, • chronic interstitial nephritis, • milk-alkali syndrome: absorbable calcium antacid + increased ingestion of milk
Rx of CRF	• R/O postrenal obstruction: e.g., * prostate hyperplasia, * order renal US, • correct volume depletion: due to: * diuretics, * decreased intake, * N/V, • limit protein intake: * 0.6–0.7 g/kg/d, * supplement with water soluble B vitamins (not fat soluble), vitamin C, calcitriol (dihydrotachysterol: analogue of calcitriol), folate, iron, calcium, • restrict sodium: only if pitting edema present, • restrict potassium, phosphorous, magnesium, • control HTN: * ACE inhibitors best unless hyperkalemia is present, * loop diuretics (best diuretic for CRF), • Rx anemia with EPO: keep Hct between 30–33%, • Rx metabolic acidosis if bicarbonate <18 mEq/L, • dialysis
causes of acute interstitial nephritis	• APN, • drug-induced, • systemic infections: e.g., * Legionnaire's disease, * CMV, * leptospirosis, • immune disease: e.g., * Sjögren's syndrome, * SLE, * acute transplant rejection, • heavy metals: e.g., * Pb, * arsenic, * cadmium, * mercury
clinical findings of acute interstitial nephritis	• sterile pyuria: * 100%, * WBCs/WBC casts, • hematuria: * 95%, * RBC casts rare, • fever: 90%, • tubular proteinuria: * 75%, * <2 g/d, * LMW proteins, • renal insufficiency: * 60%, * oliguria, * azotemia, * FENa$^+$ >1, • eosinophilia: * 50%, * eosinophiluria, • skin rash: * 25%, * mainly drug-induced type, • renal

Table continued on following page

Table 10–4. TUBULAR, TUBULOINTERSTITIAL, VASCULAR, OBSTRUCTIVE, AND NEOPLASTIC DISEASES OF THE KIDNEYS *Continued*

Most Common...	Answer and Explanation
Continued	*osteodystrophy:* see above, • *proximal tubule dysfunction:* type II proximal RTA, • *distal tubule dysfunction:* * type I RTA, * type IV RTA, * nephrogenic DI, • *hematologic abnormalities:* anemia (decreased EPO)
causes of APN	• **ascending infection:** * urethra initial entry site, * *Escherichia coli* derived from enteric organisms, * low O_2 tension in renal medulla, • *hematogenous:* * *Staphylococcus aureus*, * cortical location
predisposing causes of APN	• **VUR:** * incompetent ureterovesical junction, * microabscesses in tubules and interstitium, • *urinary tract obstruction,* • *DM,* • *cystic kidney disease,* • *pregnancy,* • *previous LUT instrumentation*
test used to identify VUR	*cystourethrogram*
clinical and lab findings in APN	• **young woman with sudden onset of spiking fever,** • *flank pain,* • *LUT signs of infection:* * increased frequency, * dysuria, * urgency, • *UA findings:* * pyuria, * bacteria, * WBC casts, * hematuria, * positive dipstick for esterase/nitrite, • *absolute neutrophilic leukocytosis/left shift*
complications of APN	• **septicemia:** * blood cultures positive in 20%, * potential for endotoxic shock, • *chronic PN,* • *renal papillary necrosis,* • *perinephric abscess,* • *pyonephrosis:* pus in renal pelvis, • *stone formation:* urease-producing organisms produce struvite stones
Rx of APN	• *uncomplicated APN:* * FQ (orally) or * TMP/SMX for 2 wks, • *complicated APN:* * AMP/GENT IV or * FQ IV for 2 wks
causes of CPN	• **reflux:** * due to VUR, * initially targets children, * more common in boys in first yr. of life (usually a congenital abnormality), • *obstruction:* * e.g., tumors, prostatic hyperplasia, stones, * leads to hydronephrosis, calyceal blunting, cortical scars
clinical and lab findings in CPN	• **HTN,** • *renal insufficiency,* • *tubular dysfunction:* see above

**Table 10–4. TUBULAR, TUBULOINTERSTITIAL,
VASCULAR, OBSTRUCTIVE, AND NEOPLASTIC DISEASES
OF THE KIDNEYS** *Continued*

Most Common...	Answer and Explanation
pathogenesis of acute drug-induced interstitial nephritis	• **type IV cellular immune reaction:** * delayed type, * cytotoxic T cells, • *antibodies directed against basement membranes:* e.g., methicillin
causes of acute drug-induced IN	• **methicillin,** • *rifampin,* • *sulfonamides,* • *NSAIDs:* interstitial nephritis is accompanied by nephrotic syndrome, • *allopurinol,* • *diuretics:* * thiazides, * loop diuretics, • *cimetidine,* • *cyclosporine:* see above
Rx of acute drug-induced IN	• **withdraw the drug:** never use drug again, • *corticosteroids may be useful*
cause of chronic drug-induced interstitial nephritis	*analgesic nephropathy*
mechanisms of analgesic nephropathy	• *acetaminophen:* FR injury of tubules and interstitium, • *aspirin:* decreases synthesis of intrarenal prostaglandin leading to ischemia in renal medulla, • *cumulative ingestion* ≥ 3 *kg or* ≥ 1 *g/d for 3 y produces renal damage*
clinical findings of analgesic nephropathy	• **woman (85%) with a long history of pain:** * chronic headaches (80%), * arthritis, * myalgia, • *anemia:* 85%, • *HTN:* 40%, • *renal papillary necrosis:* 30%, • *PUD:* 40%, • *UTI with dysuria:* 25%, • *history of urinary tract obstruction:* 10%, • *lab findings:* * sterile pyuria, * proteinuria (<2 g/d), * normal AG metabolic acidosis (distal tubule RTA), * small kidneys (50%)
complications of analgesic nephropathy	• **renal papillary necrosis,** • *HTN,* • *accelerated atherosclerosis:* increased TG, • *renal pelvic, ureter, bladder transitional cell carcinoma:* bladder cancer is less common than in other sites
causes of renal papillary necrosis	• **analgesic nephropathy,** • *DM,* • *APN,* • *sickle cell trait/disease,* • *chronic alcoholism with cirrhosis,* • *urinary tract obstruction,* • *TB*
clinical and lab findings of renal papillary necrosis	• *sudden onset of colicky flank pain,* • *gross hematuria,* • *IVP:* * calyceal clubbing, * ring sign (filling defect left behind from sloughed papilla)

Table continued on following page

Table 10–4. TUBULAR, TUBULOINTERSTITIAL, VASCULAR, OBSTRUCTIVE, AND NEOPLASTIC DISEASES OF THE KIDNEYS *Continued*

Most Common...	Answer and Explanation
tubular abnormalities associated with aminoglycosides	*potassium/magnesium wasting*
tubular abnormalities associated with tetracyclines	• **nephrogenic DI:** particularly demeclocycline, • *Fanconi syndrome:* * type II proximal tubule RTA (see below), * outdated tetracycline
tubular abnormalities associated with amphotericin B	• **distal tubule dysfunction:** * type I distal tubule RTA (see below), * nephrogenic DI, * renal potassium wasting, • *nephrotoxic ATN*
tubular abnormalities associated with cisplatin	• **magnesium wasting,** • *nephrotoxic ATN,* • *potassium wasting,* • *mild proteinuria*
causes of urate nephropathy	**tumor lysis syndrome after Rx of disseminated cancers:** * increased production of purines, * e.g., Rx of ALL and malignant lymphomas, • *Pb poisoning:* Pb decreases uric acid secretion, • *MPD:* e.g., PRV
pathogenesis of urate nephropathy	*tubular obstruction by crystals:* * serum uric acid usually >15 mg/dL, * urine uric acid >1000 mg/d, * urine uric acid/plasma creatinine ratio >1 on random urine
Rx of urate nephropathy	• **allopurinol:** inhibits xanthine oxidase involved in uric acid synthesis, • *establish urinary output >3 liters/d,* • *alkalinize urine:* uric acid soluble in alkaline pH
causes of Pb nephropathy	*see Table 7–4*
clinical signs of Pb nephropathy	• *gout:* * Pb decreases uric acid secretion, * Pb produces a chronic interstitial nephritis, • *HTN,* • *chronic renal insufficiency*
method of evaluating Pb stores	*IV ethylenediaminetetraacetic acid* (EDTA): * chelates Pb, * collect urine and measure Pb
heavy metals other than Pb producing interstitial nephritis	• *arsenic,* • *mercury:* organic salt of mercury, • *cadmium:* alkaline battery workers, • *gold*

**Table 10–4. TUBULAR, TUBULOINTERSTITIAL,
VASCULAR, OBSTRUCTIVE, AND NEOPLASTIC DISEASES
OF THE KIDNEYS** *Continued*

Most Common...	Answer and Explanation
clinical signs of lithium nephropathy	• **polyuria:** * nephrogenic DI, * usually clinically insignificant, • *incomplete distal RTA:* see below, • *renal sodium wasting,* • *chronic interstitial nephritis:* microcystic changes in renal tubules
causes of oxalate nephropathy	• **ethylene glycol poisoning,** • *high doses of ascorbic acid,* • *methoxyflurane:* * metabolized to fluoride and oxalate, * produces nephrogenic DI, • *pyridoxine deficiency,* • *increased GI absorption:* CD
causes of nephrocalcinosis	• **primary HPTH,** • *multiple myeloma:* hypercalcemia, • *distal tubule RTA:* see below, • *hyperphosphatemia:* renal failure [Calcium deposits in mitochondria within the tubules and within the tubular lumens.]
renal effects of hypercalcemia	• **nephrocalcinosis,** • *nephrogenic DI,* • *produces intrarenal vasoconstriction*
clinical findings of nephrocalcinosis	• **polyuria:** * loss of urine concentration, * nephrogenic DI, • *HTN,* • *renal failure*
renal findings in multiple myeloma	• **hypersensitivity reaction to BJ protein,** • *nephrocalcinosis:* hypercalcemia-induced, • *amyloid nephropathy:* light chains are nephrotoxic, • *metastasis*
types of renal tubular acidosis	• **distal RTA:** type I, • *proximal RTA:* type II, • *hyporeninemic hypoaldosteronism:* type IV
causes of distal RTA (type I)	• **multiple myeloma,** • *cystinosis,* • *amphotericin B,* • *Pb poisoning,* • *outdated tetracycline,* • *lithium,* • *Sjögren's syndrome,* • *sickle cell disease*
pathogenesis of distal RTA (type I)	• **defect in aldosterone-enhanced H^+/K^+ ATPase pump in the collecting tubule:** major site for excreting excess H^+ ions and regeneration of bicarbonate, • *inability to maintain a steep urine-to-blood H^+ gradient:* * H^+ ions recycle back into blood, * mechanism of amphotericin B

Table continued on following page

Table 10–4. TUBULAR, TUBULOINTERSTITIAL, VASCULAR, OBSTRUCTIVE, AND NEOPLASTIC DISEASES OF THE KIDNEYS *Continued*

Most Common...	Answer and Explanation
clinical findings in distal RTA	• **muscle weakness:** hypokalemia from kaluresis, • *polyuria:* * nephrogenic DI from hypokalemic nephropathy, * nephrocalcinosis, • *nephrolithiasis:* * due to calcium loss in urine, * usually occurs with incomplete type of distal RTA (calcium phosphate stones)
lab findings in distal RTA	• **hyperchloremic normal AG metabolic acidosis:** H^+ ions are retained and combine with Cl^- anions to form HCl, • *severe hypokalemia:* * H^+/K^+ pump blocked, * K^+ lost in urine, • *urine pH >5.5:* H^+ ions are not excreted into urine to combine with ammonia or HPO_4^-, • *no urine acidification after infusion of NH_4Cl:* H^+ pump is defective, • *kidneys can reclaim infused bicarbonate:* predominantly a proximal not a distal tubule function, • *urine anion gap O or positive:* * urine AG = (random urine Na^+ + random urine K^+) − random urine Cl^-, * urine Cl^- is an indirect measure of NH_4Cl excretion, * inability to excrete H^+ in urine leads to less NH_4Cl in the urine and a O to positive value for urine AG, * urine AG is negative value in normal AG metabolic acidosis due to diarrhea since urine acidification is normal
Rx of distal RTA	• **sodium bicarbonate tablets,** • *bicarbonate alternative:* Shoal's solution, which contains citrate (converted into bicarbonate)
causes of proximal RTA (type II)	• **carbonic anhydrase inhibitors,** • *acute/chronic interstitial nephritis,* • *primary HPTH:* excess PTH inhibits reclamation of bicarbonate, • *toluene sniffing,* • *heavy metal poisoning*
pathogenesis of proximal RTA	*lower proximal tubule renal threshold for reclaiming bicarbonate:* * renal threshold drops to 15–18 mEq/L, * excess filtered HCO_3^- lost in urine with Na^+/K^+ (urine pH is initially >5.5 from bicarbonaturia), * plasma HCO_3^- eventually drops to same level as renal threshold, * HCO_3^- reclaimed up to new threshold (not lost in urine, urine pH <5.5)

Table 10–4. TUBULAR, TUBULOINTERSTITIAL, VASCULAR, OBSTRUCTIVE, AND NEOPLASTIC DISEASES OF THE KIDNEYS *Continued*

Most Common...	Answer and Explanation
clinical findings of proximal RTA	• **related to normal AG metabolic acidosis:** * growth failure, * renal osteodystrophy, • *hypokalemia:* * muscle weakness, * polyuria, * nocturia, * nephrogenic DI, • *osteomalacia:* * skeletal deformities, * fractures
lab findings of proximal RTA	• **hyperchloremic normal AG metabolic acidosis,** • *hypokalemia,* • *fractional excretion of infused bicarbonate >15%:* lost in urine owing to lower renal threshold for HCO_3^-, • *urine pH >5.5 in early stages and <5.5 when serum and renal threshold values equilibrate,* • *urine AG O to positive:* see above, • *generalized Fanconi syndrome:* * proximal RTA, * uricosuria (hypouricemia), * phosphaturia (hypophosphatemia), * aminoaciduria, * glucosuria
Rx of proximal RTA	• **volume contraction with thiazides:** raises renal threshold for reclaiming HCO_3^-, • *oral administration of potassium* HCO_3^-, • most cases are not severe enough to warrant HCO_3^- Rx
causes of type IV RTA	• **DM,** • *chronic interstitial nephritis,* • *obstructive uropathy,* • *drugs:* spironolactone, • *AIDS*
pathogenesis of type IV RTA	*destruction of JG apparatus:* * low PRA and aldosterone, * hypoaldosteronemia: ♦ Na^+ loss, ♦ retention H^+ ions (metabolic acidosis), ♦ retention K^+ (hyperkalemia)
clinical finding of type IV RTA	*increased susceptibility to hyperkalemia:* hyperkalemia develops quickly when patients take K^+ supplements, NSAIDs, ACE inhibitors
lab findings in type IV RTA	• **hyperkalemia,** • *hyperchloremic normal AG metabolic acidosis,* • *urine AG O to positive* [Only normal AG metabolic acidosis with hyperkalemia.]
Rx of type IV RTA	• **fludrocortisone:** mineralocorticoid replacement, • *loop diuretic,* • *restriction of K^+ or drugs predisposing to K^+ sparing,* • *oral administration of $NaHCO_3$*

Table continued on following page

**Table 10–4. TUBULAR, TUBULOINTERSTITIAL,
VASCULAR, OBSTRUCTIVE, AND NEOPLASTIC DISEASES
OF THE KIDNEYS** *Continued*

Most Common...	Answer and Explanation
causes of visible renal calcifications on radiographs	• **stones,** • *nephrocalcinosis,* • *calcified tumors/cysts,* • *infections:* e.g., * *histoplasmosis,* • *medullary sponge kidney*
renal disease in essential HTN	*benign nephrosclerosis:* due to ischemic changes associated with hyaline arteriolosclerosis: ♦ tubular atrophy, ♦ glomerular sclerosis, ♦ small kidneys
lab findings in BNS	• **proteinuria,** • *hematuria,* • *renal azotemia,* • *hyaline casts*
causes of malignant HTN	• **preexisting BNS,** • *PSS,* • *HUS,* • *TTP:* see Table 5–4
cause of diffuse cortical necrosis	*pregnancy complicated by DIC*
causes of obstructive uropathy in UUT (above UV junction)	• **nephrolithiasis,** • *pregnancy,* • *TCC,* • *renal papillary necrosis,* • *intratubular obstruction:* e.g., uric acid, • *retroperitoneal fibrosis*
causes of LUT obstruction	• **prostate hyperplasia,** • *cervical cancer:* * ureterovesical junction obstruction, • *TCC,* • *phimosis:* cannot retract prepuce over glans, • *urethral strictures*
kidney finding in UUT obstruction	*hydronephrosis:* * renal pelvis dilatation, * compression atrophy of cortex/medulla
sequence of events in renal function in postrenal obstruction	**increased tubular hydrostatic pressure** → *increased intraglomerular hydrostatic pressure* → *drop in GFR* → *ischemia secondary to vasoconstriction of mesangial cells and efferent arterioles by ATII/TXA$_2$* → *tubular necrosis/atrophy*
clinical finding in complete obstruction	*anuria leading to ARF*
causes of complete urinary tract obstruction	• **urethral obstruction:** prostate hyperplasia, • *bilateral UUT obstruction:* see above

Table 10–4. TUBULAR, TUBULOINTERSTITIAL, VASCULAR, OBSTRUCTIVE, AND NEOPLASTIC DISEASES OF THE KIDNEYS Continued

Most Common...	Answer and Explanation
clinical/lab findings in partial obstruction	• **polyuria**, • *flank pain*, • *tubular dysfunction:* see above, • *UTI*, • *HTN*, • *palpable mass:* hydronephrosis, • *lab findings:* * BUN/creatinine ratio >15:1, * FENa$^+$ <1, * UOsm >500 mOsm/kg, * hypernatremia (♦ hypotonic fluid loss, ♦ urea osmotically active), * type IV RTA: see above
tests to confirm urinary tract obstruction	• **renal ultrasonography:** * sensitivity ~98%, * specificity ~75%, • *abdominal CT with contrast + renal US:* * 100% sensitivity, * specificity confirming cause of obstruction ~85%, • *KUB:* initial step for stone evaluation, • *IVP:* good test if KUB is normal
Rx of urinary tract obstruction	*depends on the cause*
clinical findings in postobstructive diuresis	*osmotic diuresis leading to volume depletion and loss of electrolytes:* e.g., * Na$^+$, * K$^+$, * Mg^{++}
metabolic cause of renal calculi	*hypercalciuria*
causes of hypercalciuria	• **increased GI absorption**, • *increased renal absorption*, • *increased bone resorption*
risk factors for renal calculi	• **low urine volume**, • *hypercalciuria*, • *male sex*, • *reduced urine citrate:* normally chelates calcium, • *primary HPTH:* * increased bone resorption, * increased vitamin D synthesis, • *diet high in dairy products:* calcium phosphate stones, • *diet high in oxalates:* calcium oxalate stones, • *diet high in sodium:* * increases urine calcium excretion, * lowers urine citrate, • *diet high in protein:* * increases calcium, oxalate, uric acid excretion, * lowers urine citrate, • *CD:* increased oxalate reabsorption, • *tumor lysis syndrome:* urate stones, • *distal RTA:* calcium phosphate stones, • *UTIs secondary to urease producers:* struvite stones, • *cystic disease*, • *genetic diseases:* * **cystinuria**, * gout (25% have stones), * xanthinuria, * primary hyperoxaluria

Table continued on following page

Table 10–4. TUBULAR, TUBULOINTERSTITIAL, VASCULAR, OBSTRUCTIVE, AND NEOPLASTIC DISEASES OF THE KIDNEYS *Continued*

Most Common...	Answer and Explanation
renal stones	• **calcium oxalate,** • *calcium phosphate*, • *magnesium ammonium phosphate:* * struvite stone, * "staghorn calculus," • *uric acid*, • *cystine*, • *xanthine*
S/S of renal calculus	• **sudden onset of colicky pain in the flank with radiation into groin,** • *patient constantly moving owing to pain,* • *N/V,* • *gross/microscopic hematuria*
initial tests to identify stones	• **UA:** * confirms hematuria, * identify crystals, * urine pH, • *KUB:* 85% of stones contain calcium, • *renal ultrasonogram:* if KUB is normal
confirmatory test for a stone	*stone analysis by x-ray diffraction:* patients must strain their urine
stones that are radiolucent	• **uric acid,** • *xanthine*, • *cystine:* occasionally radiodense
lab tests for recurrent stone formers	• *24 h urine collections:* * Ca^{++}, * phosphate, * uric acid, * Na^+, * Mg^{++}, * citrate, • *calcium load test:* see below, • *serum PTH:* R/O primary HPTH, • *serum calcium/phosphorus:* R/O primary HPTH, • *serum electrolytes:* R/O distal RTA, • *serum BUN/creatinine:* R/O renal disease
method of distinguishing cause of hypercalciuria	*calcium load test:* distinguishes three main causes: * absorptive hypercalciuria (**most common overall type**), * resorptive hypercalciuria, * primary renal disease causing hypercalciuria
mechanism/Rx of type I absorptive hypercalciuria	• *mechanism:* * increased jejunal reabsorption of calcium, * <u>independent</u> of calcium intake, * normal: serum calcium, phosphorous, PTH, vitamin D, • *Rx:* * cellulose phosphate: binds GI calcium, * hydrochlorothiazide: increases renal calcium reabsorption, * potassium citrate
mechanism/Rx of type II absorptive hypercalciuria	• *mechanism:* * increased jejunal reabsorption of calcium, * <u>dependent</u> on calcium intake, * normal: serum <u>calcium</u>, phosphorous, PTH, vitamin D, • *Rx:* * dietary restriction of calcium, * potassium citrate

Table 10–4. TUBULAR, TUBULOINTERSTITIAL, VASCULAR, OBSTRUCTIVE, AND NEOPLASTIC DISEASES OF THE KIDNEYS *Continued*

Most Common...	Answer and Explanation
mechanism/Rx of type III absorptive hypercalciuria	• *mechanism:* * increased renal loss of phosphate, * hypophosphatemia stimulates synthesis of 1-α hydroxylase enzyme and vitamin D, * vitamin D increases GI calcium reabsorption, * serum calcium/PTH normal, * serum phosphorous low, * serum vitamin D high, • *Rx:* * oral orthophosphate: increases serum phosphate which inhibits vitamin D synthesis, * potassium citrate
mechanism/Rx of resorptive hypercalciuria due to primary HPTH	• *mechanism:* * increased PTH increases bone resorption causing hypercalcemia, * calcium excreted in urine > amount reabsorbed in urine, * serum calcium/PTH/vitamin D high, * serum phosphorous low, • *Rx:* remove parathyroid adenoma
mechanism/Rx of hypercalciuria due to primary renal disease	• *mechanism:* * kidney cannot reabsorb calcium, * serum calcium/phosphorus normal, * serum PTH/vitamin D high, • *Rx:* * hydrochlorothiazide, * potassium citrate
general Rx of stones	• **increased fluid intake:** urine output >2.5 liters/d, • *analgesia,* • *stones <5 mm usually pass,* • *50% of stones 5–7 mm pass,* • *stones >7 mm usually do not pass and require surgical intervention:* * percutaneous extraction for struvite stones, * extracorporeal shock wave lithotripsy for large stones or stones in upper one-third of ureter, * extraction of stones located in lower pole of ureter
Rx of uric acid stones	*overproduction of uric acid* (24 h urine uric acid >1000 mg/d): * **allopurinol** (blocks xanthine oxidase), * alkalinize urine
Rx of hyperoxaluria	• **avoid foods high in oxalates,** • *potassium citrate,* • *magnesium gluconate*
Rx of hypocitruria	*potassium citrate*
Rx of struvite stones	• *eradicate infection,* • *extracorporeal shockwave lithotripsy,* • *surgical removal*
Rx of cystine stones	• *low methionine diet,* • *potassium citrate*

Table continued on following page

Table 10–4. TUBULAR, TUBULOINTERSTITIAL, VASCULAR, OBSTRUCTIVE, AND NEOPLASTIC DISEASES OF THE KIDNEYS *Continued*

Most Common...	Answer and Explanation
renal finding in tuberous sclerosis	*angiomyolipoma:* * 50% of cases (see Table 15–8), * they are hamartomas
malignant kidney tumor in adults	*renal adenocarcinoma:* * alias Grawitz tumor, hypernephroma, * arise from proximal tubules, * >3 cm in 75–80%, * men > women, * sixth–seventh decade
causes of renal adenocarcinoma	• **smoking,** • *von Hippel-Lindau disease:* * bilateral renal cancer develops in 50–60%, • *APKD,* • *obesity,* • *acquired renal cystic disease,* • *phenacetin abuse*
S/S of a renal adenocarcinoma	• **hematuria:** 90%, • *pain:* 45%, • *flank mass:* 30%, • *fever,* • *leukemoid reaction:* benign neutrophil elevation >50,000 cells/μL, • *amyloidosis,* • *Staufer's syndrome:* * hepatic cell necrosis unrelated to metastasis, * hepatic lesions after nephrectomy, • *HTN:* increased renin secretion
ectopic hormone relationships in renal adenocarcinoma	• **erythropoietin:** polycythemia, • *PTH-like peptide:* hypercalcemia, • *renin:* HTN, • *gonadotropins:* feminization/masculinization, • *cortisol:* ectopic Cushing's syndrome
metastatic sites	• **lungs:** * classic "cannon ball" metastases, * hemoptysis common, • *bone:* always lytic, • *skin:* one of a few cancers that metastasize to skin, • *liver,* • *brain,* • *general comments:* * metastasis present in one-third when initially discovered, * renal vein invasion in 50%, * regional lymph node involvement 20%, * metastases commonly occur after 10–20 y
primary organ sites that metastasize to the kidney	• **lung,** • *breast,* • *stomach,* • *malignant lymphoma* [Kidney metastasis is uncommon.]
method for diagnosing renal adenocarcinoma	• **CT scan,** • *US* [Most solid masses in the kidneys are renal adenocarcinoma. US is most useful in distinguishing cystic from solid masses. Percutaneous FNA is commonly performed to obtain tissue for diagnosis.]

Nephrology **523**

Table 10–4. TUBULAR, TUBULOINTERSTITIAL, VASCULAR, OBSTRUCTIVE, AND NEOPLASTIC DISEASES OF THE KIDNEYS *Continued*

Most Common...	Answer and Explanation
Rx of renal adenocarcinoma	• **radical nephrectomy,** • *metastatic disease:* * progestational agents, * α-interferon, * IL-2, * vinblastine, • *renal vein invasion does not adversely affect prognosis,* • *average 5 y survival 45%*
cancers of renal pelvis	• **TCC:** ~50% have TCC in other areas of GU tract, • *SCC*
risk factors for TCC of renal pelvis	• **smoking,** • *phenacetin abuse:* high risk, • *aromatic amines:* * benzidine, * naphthyl-amine, • *cyclophosphamide*
risk factors for SCC of renal pelvis	• **stones,** • *chronic infection*

Question: Which of the following conditions are associated with a FENa$^+$ <1, UOsm >500 mOsm/kg, and a serum BUN/creatinine ratio >15:1? **SELECT 3**
  (A) Acute interstitial nephritis
  (B) CHF
  (C) Nephrotoxic ATN
  (D) Acute proliferative glomerulonephritis
  (E) Acute pyelonephritis
  (F) Volume depletion secondary to GI bleed

Answers: (B), (D), (F): Acute interstitial nephritis produces ARF with tubular dysfunction (FENa$^+$ >1, UOsm <350 mOsm/kg, BUN/creatinine ratio <15:1, **choice A is incorrect**). CHF **(choice B)** is associated with a decreased EABV and a low GFR with preservation of tubular function (prerenal azotemia). Nephrotoxic ATN is associated with tubular dysfunction. It is most commonly caused by drugs **(choice C is incorrect).** Acute proliferative GN **(choice D)** has preservation of tubular function but oliguria. Acute PN has preservation of renal function, but the serum BUN/creatinine ratio is normal (<15:1, **choice E is incorrect**). Volume depletion **(choice F)** in general is associated with prerenal azotemia with preservation of tubular function. If left untreated, it will progress into ischemic ATN.

ACE = angiotensin converting enzyme, AF = atrial fibrillation, AG = anion gap, ALL = acute lymphoblastic leukemia, AMI = acute myocardial infarction, AMP = ampicillin, APKD = adult polycystic kidney disease, APN = acute pyelonephritis, ARF = acute renal failure, ATII = angiotensin II, ATN = acute tubular necrosis, BJ = Bence-Jones, BM = basement membrane, BNS = benign nephrosclerosis, BT = bleeding time, BUN = blood urea nitrogen, CD = Crohn's disease, CH = cholesterol, CHF = congestive heart failure, CMV = cytomegalovirus, COD = cause of death, CPN = chronic pyelonephritis, Cr = creatinine, CRF =

chronic renal failure, CT = computed tomography, DI = diabetes insipidus, DIC = disseminated intravascular coagulation, DM = diabetes mellitus, EABV = effective arterial blood volume, ECG = electrocardiogram, EPO = erythropoietin, ESR = erythrocyte sedimentation rate, $FENa^+$ = fractional excretion of sodium, FNA = fine needle aspiration, FQ = fluoroquinolones, FR = free radical, FSG = focal segmental glomerulosclerosis, GENT = gentamicin, GFR = glomerular filtration rate, GI = gastrointestinal, GN = glomerulonephritis, GU = genitourinary, Hct = hematocrit, HPTH = hyperparathyroidism, HTN = hypertension, HUS = hemolytic uremic syndrome, IL-2 = interleukin 2, IN = interstitial nephritis, IV = intravenous, IVP = intravenous pyelogram, JG = juxtaglomerular, KUB = kidney/ureter/bladder radiographs, LMW = low molecular weight, LUT = lower urinary tract, MPD = myeloproliferative disease, MPGN = membranoproliferative glomerulonephritis, NSAIDs = nonsteroidal anti-inflammatory drugs, N/V = nausea and vomiting, PN = pyelonephritis, PRA = plasma renin activity, PRV = polycythemia rubra vera, PSS = progressive systemic sclerosis, PTH = parathyroid hormone, PUD = peptic ulcer disease, RAA = renin angiotensin aldosterone, RBC = red blood cell, R/O = rule out, RPGN = rapidly progressive glomerulonephritis, RTA = renal tubular acidosis, Rx = treatment, SCC = squamous cell carcinoma, SLE = systemic lupus erythematosus, S/S = signs and symptoms, TB = tuberculosis, TCC = transitional cell carcinoma, TG = triglyceride, TMP/SMX = trimethoprim-sulfamethoxazole, TTP = thrombotic thrombocytopenic purpura, UA = urinalysis, UNa^+ = urine sodium, UOsm = urine osmolality, US = ultrasonography, UTI = urinary tract infection, UUT = upper urinary tract, UV = ureterovesical, VUR = vesico-ureteral reflux, WBC = white blood cell.

Table 10–5. MISCELLANEOUS BLADDER, PROSTATE, TESTICLE DISORDERS, MALE HYPOGONADISM, AND IMPOTENCE

Most Common...	Answer and Explanation
cause of acute cystitis	*ascending infection secondary to Escherichia coli* (80–90%): acute cystitis is more common in women (short urethra) than men
viral cause of hemorrhagic cystitis	*adenovirus*
cause of acute cystitis in sexually active women	*Staphylococcus saprophyticus:* * coagulase negative, * accounts for ~10–20% of UTIs
causes of acute urethral syndrome in women (pyuria, <10^5 CFU/mL)	• ***Chlamydia trachomatis:*** PCR of voided urine is currently recommended to detect the organism, • *Mycoplasma hominis*, • *Ureaplasma urealyticum*, • *Neisseria gonorrhoeae*

Table 10–5. MISCELLANEOUS BLADDER, PROSTATE, TESTICLE DISORDERS, MALE HYPOGONADISM, AND IMPOTENCE *Continued*

Most Common...	Answer and Explanation
bacterial infection in the elderly	*lower UTIs*
general risk factors for a LUT infection	• **female sex,** • *indwelling urinary catheter,* • *sexual intercourse:* "honeymoon cystitis," • *DM,* • *pregnancy,* • *neurogenic bladder,* • *cystic renal disease,* • *instrumentation*
risks of indwelling urinary catheters	• **sepsis:** * indwelling catheters are MCC of sepsis in hospitalized patients, * account for 50% of all nosocomial UTIs, * >90% have infection by 3–4 d, * prophylactic antimicrobial Rx is ineffective, * Rx if symptomatic infection
risk factors for LUT infections in men	• **lack of circumcision,** • *anal intercourse,* • *intercourse with a woman whose vagina is colonized with uropathogens*
S/S of LUT infection	• **dysuria:** painful urination, • *increased frequency,* • *urgency,* • *nocturia,* • *suprapubic discomfort,* • *gross hematuria* [Fever is not a feature of LUT infection.]
lab findings of a LUT infection	• **pyuria:** * WBCs in urine, * definition: ≥10 WBCs/HPF in a centrifuged specimen or ≥5 WBCs in uncentrifuged specimen, • *bacteriuria,* • *hematuria,* • *positive dipstick leukocyte esterase,* • *positive dipstick nitrite,* • $≥10^5$ *colony forming units/mL:* * gold standard criterion of infection, * mid-stream clean catch urine, * low colony counts with symptoms are significant, * $≥10^5$ CFU/mL correlates with 1 or more organisms/OPF on a Gram stain of unspun urine
urine contaminants	• *Lactobacillus,* • α-*hemolytic streptococci*
causes of asymptomatic bacteriuria in women	• **pregnancy,** • *elderly women in nursing homes,* • *DM,* • *sickle cell trait,* • *cystic renal disease* [Asymptomatic bacteriuria is defined as two successive cultures with $≥10^5$ CFU/mL in an asymptomatic patient.]
cause of recurrent UTIs within 1–2 weeks of Rx in women	*usually exogenous reinfection in >90%*

Table continued on following page

Table 10–5. MISCELLANEOUS BLADDER, PROSTATE, TESTICLE DISORDERS, MALE HYPOGONADISM, AND IMPOTENCE *Continued*

Most Common...	Answer and Explanation
preventive measures recommended in recurrent UTIs	• **void immediately after coitus,** • *one dose of TMP/SMX* (40 mg/400 mg) *after coitus,* • *avoid intercourse while on Rx*
Rx of uncomplicated, symptomatic UTI in women and men	• *women:* * empiric Rx with TMP/SMX for 3 d, * symptoms plus microscopic examination of urine compatible with a UTI are all that is necessary to Rx the patient, • *men:* * pretreatment urine culture is necessary (UTIs uncommon in men), * Rx with TMP/SMX for 14 d
Rx of asymptomatic bacteriuria	• *Rx in pregnant women:* * ampicillin or cephalosporin, * avoid sulfa drugs or tetracycline, * Rx for 10–14 days, * APN may occur in 1–2%, • *Rx in patients undergoing urologic surgery,* • *Rx in DM* [Rx is not necessary in elderly, otherwise healthy women.]
Rx of acute urethral syndrome	• **azithromycin:** * single dose, * patient more likely to take drug with single dose regimen, • *doxycycline:* 100 mg, PO, bid, for 7 d
types of bladder cancer	• **TCC:** * men > women, * majority are papillary (low-grade), * multifocality is the rule (common malignant stem cell abnormality or reimplantation of the tumor from another site), • *SCC: Schistosoma hematobium* relationship, • *adenocarcinoma*
causes of TCC involving bladder	• **smoking,** • *aniline dyes,* • *aromatic amines,* • *cyclophosphamide:* also causes hemorrhagic cystitis, • *phenacetin abuse:* less common cause in bladder than in renal pelvis TCC
S/S of bladder cancer	• **painless gross/microscopic hematuria:** 70–90%, • *irritative bladder complaints:* * dysuria, * increased frequency of urination
metastatic sites	• **regional lymph nodes,** • *liver,* • *lung,* • *bones*
methods to diagnose bladder cancer	• **cystoscopy with Bx,** • *urine cytology*

**Table 10–5. MISCELLANEOUS BLADDER, PROSTATE,
TESTICLE DISORDERS, MALE HYPOGONADISM,
AND IMPOTENCE** *Continued*

Most Common...	Answer and Explanation
Rx of bladder cancer	• *unifocal disease:* cystoscopy with fulguration, • *multifocal disease:* intravesical therapy with * bacille-Calmette-Guerin, * mitomycin C, or * thiotepa, • *invasive disease:* * total cystectomy, * adjuvant chemotherapy if nodal involvement is present, • *prognosis:* 5 y survival with superficial disease 85–90%
causes of acute/ chronic prostatitis	• *acute prostatitis:* * ***E. coli***, * *Pseudomonas aeruginosa,* * *Klebsiella pneumoniae,* • *chronic prostatitis:* most cases abacterial, • *prostate infections linked to infections of urethra and/or bladder*
S/S of prostatitis	• **pain:** * low back, * perineal, * suprapubic, • *painful/swollen gland on rectal exam,* • *dysuria,* • *hematuria*
lab Dx of prostatitis	• *collect four specimens for culture:* * first 10 mL of urine is urethral component, * second specimen is midstream (bladder component), * third specimen is at the end of voiding (prostatic secretions), * fourth specimen represents prostatic secretions milked out of the penis after prostate massage, • *>20 WBCs/HPF in third specimen suggests acute prostatitis,* • *confirmatory test is bacterial count:* bacterial count 1 or more logarithms higher in 3rd and 4th specimens than in specimens 1 and 2 indicates prostatitis
Rx of acute prostatitis	*TMP/SMX* (double strength), *bid, for 14 d*
Rx for chronic prostatitis	*as above for 3 mths or FQ for 1 mth*
benign disorder of the prostate	*BPH*
cause of BPH	*slight excess of DHT enhanced by estrogen:* * DHT causes gland/stromal/smooth muscle hyperplasia, * estrogen sensitizes prostatic tissue to androgens, * age-dependent

Table continued on following page

Table 10–5. MISCELLANEOUS BLADDER, PROSTATE, TESTICLE DISORDERS, MALE HYPOGONADISM, AND IMPOTENCE *Continued*

Most Common...	Answer and Explanation
location for BPH	*transitional zone:* zone closest to prostatic urethra
clinical/lab findings in BPH	• **signs of obstruction:** * trouble initiating stream, * dribbling, * incomplete emptying, * nocturia, • *hematuria,* • *PSA:* * increased in 25% of men, * rarely >10 ng/mL (0–4 ng/mL)
complications of BPH	• **obstructive uropathy:** * postrenal azotemia, * bilateral hydronephrosis, • *bladder infections,* • *prostatic infarcts:* * pain, * indurated gland, * high PSA values, • *bladder wall hypertrophy,* • *bladder diverticula,* • *no risk for progression into carcinoma*
Rx of symptomatic BPH	• **α_1-adrenergic blockers:** * e.g., terazosin, * reduce smooth muscle tone in bladder neck, • *5 α-reductase inhibitors:* * e.g., finasteride, * blocks conversion of testosterone to DHT, * libido maintained, • *gonadotropin agonists:* * e.g., leuprolide, * sustained release of LH decreases androgen synthesis, * impotence, • *block androgen receptor:* * e.g., flutamide, * libido maintained, * gynecomastia, • *saw palmetto,* • *TUR:* retrograde ejaculation common
cancer in males	*prostate adenocarcinoma:* * age-dependent, African-Americans > whites, * uncommon <40 y old, * asymptomatic until advanced
risk factors for prostate cancer	• **age,** • *family history:* first degree relatives, • *African-American,* • *smoking,* • *high saturated fat diet,* • *occupational exposures:* * pesticides, * rubber, * cadmium
location for prostate cancer	*peripheral zone:* * palpable by DRE, * obstructive uropathy not an early finding
S/S of symptomatic prostate cancer	• **obstructive uropathy,** • *low back/pelvic pain:* metastases, • *compression of spinal cord:* vertebral metastasis
screening program for prostate cancer	*DRE/PSA annually beginning at 50 years of age:* * DRE does not falsely increase PSA but does increase PAP (no longer used), * rate of PSA change/y is important (e.g., >0.75 ng/mL change/y highly predictive of cancer), * ~70% with PSA >10 ng/mL have cancer

Table 10–5. MISCELLANEOUS BLADDER, PROSTATE, TESTICLE DISORDERS, MALE HYPOGONADISM, AND IMPOTENCE *Continued*

Most Common...	Answer and Explanation
confirmatory test for prostate cancer	*transrectal US with needle biopsies of suspicious sites if screening tests are abnormal*
spread of prostate cancer	• **perineural invasion:** method of extension of tumor to capsule, seminal vesicles, bladder neck, • *lymphatic spread to regional lymph nodes:* obturator and iliac nodes first, • *hematogenous:* * **bone** (♦ increases serum ALP, ♦ radiodense, ♦ radionuclide scans more sensitive than plain films), * lungs, * liver
extranodal metastatic site of prostate cancer	*vertebral column:* * 40% to lumbar spine, * osteoblastic in most cases
grading system for prostate cancer	*Gleason system:* higher the score, the more undifferentiated the cancer
staging system for prostate cancer	• *stage A:* * cannot palpate, * organ-confined, * A1 ≤5% of specimen involved, * A2 ≥5% specimen involved, • *stage B:* * organ-confined, * palpable, • *stage C:* local extension (periprostatic tissue, seminal vesicles), • *stage D:* * pelvic nodal involvement (D1), * distant metastasis (D2)
Rx for stage A1	*observed without Rx*
Rx of organ-confined prostate cancer (stage A2 or B)	*radical prostatectomy:* some clinicians prefer watchful waiting if patient has <10 y of life expectancy, • *prognosis:* 15-y tumor-free survival rate for organ-confined cancer ~85–90%
Rx of locally advanced disease (stage C)	*irradiation*
Rx of stage D1 prostate cancer (positive pelvic nodes)	*irradiation plus androgen deprivation:* * some clinicians only use androgen deprivation, e.g. * bilateral orchiectomy, * anti-androgen drugs * DES
Rx of stage D2 prostate cancer (distant metastasis)	• *androgen deprivation:* * radiation Rx for bone metastasis, * ketoconazole Rx for spinal cord compression, • *prognosis:* 10–40% 10-y survival rate

Table continued on following page

Table 10–5. MISCELLANEOUS BLADDER, PROSTATE, TESTICLE DISORDERS, MALE HYPOGONADISM, AND IMPOTENCE *Continued*

Most Common...	Answer and Explanation
methods for follow-up of prostate cancer	• **PSA**, • *radionuclide bone scan*
cause of left scrotal enlargement in an adult·	*varicocele:* * left sided (testicular vein drains into left renal vein not the inferior vena cava), * common cause of male infertility
cause of scrotal enlargement	*hydrocele:* * persistence of tunica vaginalis, * transillumination distinguishes scrotal from testicular mass, * US more accurate
cause of abrupt testicular pain	*testicular torsion:* * loss of cremasteric reflex, * testicle higher on involved side
causes of acute epididymitis	• *<35 y old:* * Neisseria gonorrhoeae, * Chlamydia trachomatis, • *>35 y old:* * E. coli, * Pseudomonas aeruginosa
S/S of acute epididymitis	• **variable onset of scrotal pain with radiation into spermatic cord or flank,** • *scrotal swelling,* • *epididymal tenderness,* • *urethral discharge:* if STD, • *Prehn's sign:* elevation of scrotum decreases pain
Rx for acute epididymitis	• *STD:* ceftriaxone + doxycycline, • *STD ruled out:* FQ
location for cryptorchid testis	*inguinal canal*
complication of cryptorchid testis	*potential for infertility and dysgerminoma:* risk for dysgerminoma applies to both the affected testicle and normal testicle
cause of orchitis	• **extension of acute epididymitis,** • *syphilis,* • *mumps,* • *HIV*
functions of the detrusor muscle	• *relaxed:* storage of urine in bladder, • *contracted:* emptying of bladder
functions of sympathetic nervous system in bladder control	• *relaxes detrusor muscle,* • *contracts internal sphincter:* increases urine storage
function of parasympathetic nervous system in bladder control	• *contracts detrusor muscle:* internal sphincter muscle relaxes owing to sympathetic inhibition, hence allowing emptying of the bladder

Table 10–5. MISCELLANEOUS BLADDER, PROSTATE, TESTICLE DISORDERS, MALE HYPOGONADISM, AND IMPOTENCE *Continued*

Most Common...	Answer and Explanation
bladder changes that occur with aging	• *smaller bladder,* • *early contractions of detrusor muscle:* increased voiding, • *increased nocturnal urination,* • *decreased ability to suppress detrusor muscle contraction* [Urinary incontinence is not a normal age-related finding.]
factors that affect urination and urinary continence	• *diuretics:* bladder fills quickly, • *anticholinergics/narcotics impair detrusor contraction:* retain urine, • α-*adrenergics increase internal sphincter tone:* retain urine, • α-*adrenergic antagonists impair internal sphincter tone:* leak urine
types of urinary incontinence	• **urge incontinence:** 40–70%, • *overflow incontinence,* • *stress incontinence,* • *functional incontinence*
mechanism of urge incontinence	*overactivity of detrusor muscle:* early detrusor contractions with low volumes of urine
S/S of urge incontinence	• *increased urinary frequency/urgency,* • *small volume voids,* • *nocturia*
causes of urge incontinence	• **bladder irritation:** * BPH, * atrophic urethritis, * infection, • *CNS disease:* * Parkinson's disease, * mass lesions, * stroke
Rx of urge incontinence	• **anticholinergics:** inhibit parasympathetic stimulation of detrusor contraction, • *behavioral training,* • *topical estrogen in urethral atrophy in women*
mechanism of overflow incontinence	• **outflow obstruction:** e.g., * BPH, * pelvic tumor, • *detrusor underactivity/hypotonic bladder:* e.g., autonomic neuropathy
S/S of overflow incontinence	• *dribbling,* • *low urine flow*
Rx of overflow incontinence	• *cholinergic drugs to enhance muscle tone:* increase detrusor contraction, • *Rx obstruction:* e.g., * α-adrenergic antagonist (decrease internal sphincter tone), * TUR of prostate tissue, • *indwelling urinary catheter:* try to avoid this

Table continued on following page

Table 10–5. MISCELLANEOUS BLADDER, PROSTATE, TESTICLE DISORDERS, MALE HYPOGONADISM, AND IMPOTENCE *Continued*

Most Common...	Answer and Explanation
mechanism of stress incontinence	• *laxity of pelvic floor muscles with lack of bladder support:* posterior urethrovesical angle of 90–100 degrees is not maintained, • *lack of estrogen* [Primarily a disease of women.]
S/S of stress incontinence	*loss of urine with increases in intra-abdominal pressure:* e.g., laughing, coughing, sneezing
Rx of stress incontinence	• *increase internal sphincter tone with α-adrenergic agonists,* • *topical estrogen therapy,* • *Kegel pelvic floor muscle exercises,* • *surgery*
mechanism of functional incontinence	*inability to reach toilet facilities in time:* * patients are normally continent, * commonly occurs when patients are on diuretics or drink too many caffeinated beverages
cause of a painless mass in the testicle	*malignancy:* * most common malignancy between 15–35 y old, * majority are of germ cell origin, * seminomas most common
risk factors for testicular cancer	• **cryptorchid testicle:** highest risk is an intra-abdominal cryptorchid testis, • *DES exposure of male infant*
clinical sign of testicular cancer	*painless enlargement of testicle*
tumor markers to work up testicular cancer	• *AFP:* yolk sac tumor origin, • *β-hCG:* choriocarcinoma (syncytiotrophoblast origin of β-hCG), • *LDH:* elevated in cancer
classification of testicular cancer	• **seminomas:** * 60%, * 30–50 y old, * 10% have positive β-hCG (does not alter prognosis), * spread by lymphatics, • *non-seminomas:* * 40% (mixed type most common) * spread by lymphatics/hematogenous routes, * embryonal (♦ 20–30 y olds, ♦ AFP elevated), * teratoma, * teratocarcinoma (see below), * choriocarcinoma (see below)
bilateral testicular cancer	*metastatic malignant lymphoma:* most commonly occurs in men >50 y old
testicular cancer producing gynecomastia	*choriocarcinoma secreting β-hCG:* * most aggressive cancer, * usually mixed with other non-seminoma types, * pure choriocarcinomas do not enlarge the testicle

**Table 10–5. MISCELLANEOUS BLADDER, PROSTATE,
TESTICLE DISORDERS, MALE HYPOGONADISM,
AND IMPOTENCE** Continued

Most Common...	Answer and Explanation
testicular cancer in adults containing derivatives from more than one germ layer	*teratocarcinoma:* * mixture of embryonal carcinoma and teratoma, * both AFP/β-hGG elevated in 90% of cases, * teratomas more common in children and tend to be benign
means of Dx of testicular cancer	• **US:** * screen for testicular cancer, * distinguish the mass as solid or cystic, • *orchiectomy:* establishes Dx
Rx of seminomas	• *low-stage disease:* * orchiectomy + irradiation of the para-aortic lymph nodes (first site of metastasis), * most radiosensitive of testicular cancers, * >95% cure rate, • *high-stage disease:* platinum-based chemotherapy
Rx of non-seminomas	• *low-stage disease and negative marker studies:* orchiectomy + ? observation, • *high-stage disease and positive markers:* platinum-based chemotherapy + bilateral retroperitoneal lymph node dissection, • *prognosis:* 50–90% have long-term remissions
cancer of penis	*SCC:* HPV 16, 18 link in two-thirds of cases
risk factors for squamous cancer of the penis	• **lack of circumcision,** • *Bowen's disease:* shaft of the penis, • *erythroplasia of Queyrat:* red lesion(s) on glans
definition of male hypogonadism	• *decreased testosterone production,* • *resistance to testosterone:* e.g., * androgen receptor deficiency (testicular feminization), * 5 α-reductase deficiency (Reifenstein's syndrome)
clinical presentations of male hypogonadism	• **impotence:** failure to sustain an erection during attempted vaginal intercourse, • *loss of male secondary sex characteristics,* • *decreased energy/stamina,* • *osteoporosis:* testosterone inhibits excessive release of interleukin-1 (osteoclast activating factor) from osteoblasts, • *gynecomastia:* estrogen is unopposed, • *hypogonadal facies:* * facial pallor, * fine wrinkling around mouth and eyes, • *infertility:* * not always synonymous with testosterone deficiency, * seminiferous tubule dysfunction (spermatogenesis) may be abnormal in presence of normal Leydig cell function (testosterone synthesis)

Table continued on following page

Table 10–5. MISCELLANEOUS BLADDER, PROSTATE,
TESTICLE DISORDERS, MALE HYPOGONADISM,
AND IMPOTENCE *Continued*

Most Common...	Answer and Explanation
classification of male hypogonadism	• *primary hypogonadism:* * problem with Leydig cell function, * hypergonadotropic (increased gonadotropins) hypogonadism, • *secondary hypogonadism:* * hypothalamic/pituitary dysfunction, * hypogonadotropic hypogonadism
tests to evaluate male hypogonadism/infertility	• **semen analysis:** * gold standard test for infertility, * best collected by masturbation, * components: ♦ volume, ♦ sperm count (20–150 million sperm/mL), ♦ morphology, ♦ motility, • *hormone evaluation:* * FSH (spermatogenesis in seminiferous tubules), * LH (testosterone synthesis in Leydig cells), * prolactin (enhances testosterone synthesis), * total testosterone with fractionation (bound and free testosterone), * estradiol (useful in Klinefelter's syndrome), • *chromosome analysis:* useful in Klinefelter's syndrome, • *gonadotropin stimulation test:* * GnRH used to stimulate FSH/LH, * distinguishes pituitary from hypothalamic problem, • *testicular biopsy:* primarily for infertility
test to distinguish types of hypogonadism	*gonadotropins:* * increase in serum FSH/LH indicates a primary testicular disorder, * decrease in FSH/LH is hypothalamic/pituitary disorder
components of semen	• *spermatozoa:* derive from seminiferous tubules, • *coagulant:* seminal vesicles, • *enzymes to liquefy semen:* prostate gland
primary causes of seminiferous tubule dysfunction	• **varicocele:** increased heat reduces spermatogenesis, • *Klinefelter syndrome*, • *orchitis*
lab findings in pure seminiferous tubule failure	• *high FSH:* * loss of inhibin from Sertoli cells, * inhibin normally has negative feedback on FSH, • *normal LH:* Leydig cells are synthesizing testosterone, • *normal serum testosterone*, • *decreased sperm count* [90% of all cases of male infertility are due to seminiferous tubule dysfunction. Spermatogenesis is affected before Leydig cell dysfunction in testicular disorders.]

Table 10–5. MISCELLANEOUS BLADDER, PROSTATE, TESTICLE DISORDERS, MALE HYPOGONADISM, AND IMPOTENCE *Continued*

Most Common...	Answer and Explanation
causes of Leydig cell failure	• *chronic liver disease,* • *chronic renal failure,* • *irradiation,* • *orchitis:* postpubertal males
lab findings in pure Leydig cell failure	• *normal FSH:* inhibin present, • *high LH:* * low testosterone, * testosterone has negative feedback on LH, • *low serum testosterone,* • *low sperm count*
causes of seminiferous and Leydig cell failure	• *chronic liver disease,* • *chronic renal failure,* • *irradiation,* • *orchitis*
lab findings in mixed seminiferous/ Leydig cell failure	• *high FSH:* inhibin absent, • *high LH:* low testosterone, • *low serum testosterone,* • *low sperm count*
lab findings in Klinefelter's syndrome	• *high FSH:* loss of inhibin, • *high LH:* low testosterone, • *low serum testosterone,* • *high serum estradiol,* • *azoospermia:* no active seminiferous tubules [See Table 3–1.]
causes of hypothalamic/ pituitary male hypogonadism	• *constitutional delay in puberty:* testicular volume usually >4 mL indicates puberty has begun, • *Kallmann's syndrome:* see below, • *hypopituitarism:* * pituitary adenoma (adult), * craniopharyngioma (child), * see Table 11–1, • *anorexia nervosa:* see Table 9–10
cause of Kallmann's syndrome	*AD disorder with maldevelopment of olfactory bulbs and GnRH-producing cells*
clinical findings in Kallmann's syndrome	• **delayed puberty,** • *anosmia:* 80%, • *color blindness,* • *cryptorchidism,* • *lab findings:* * decreased serum FSH, LH, testosterone, * due to GnRH deficiency
Rx of Kallmann's syndrome	• *pulsatile GnRH,* • *androgen replacement*
tests to evaluate hypogonadotropic hypogonadism	• *serum gonadotropins:* FSH/LH evaluate degree of impairment, • *serum testosterone,* • *serum prolactin,* • *MRI of the head:* exclude mass lesions, • *pituitary stimulation tests:* see Table 11–1

Table continued on following page

Table 10–5. MISCELLANEOUS BLADDER, PROSTATE, TESTICLE DISORDERS, MALE HYPOGONADISM, AND IMPOTENCE *Continued*

Most Common...	Answer and Explanation
types of androgen Rx used in male hypogonadism	• *GnRH:* induces spermatogenesis/restores fertility, • *17-hydroxyl esters of testosterone:* * long-acting, * danger of prematurely closing epiphyses in pubertal males, * R/O prostate cancer in older males
mechanisms of male infertility	• **decreased or abnormal sperm count:** * **idiopathic**, * primary testicular dysfunction (see above), * secondary hypogonadism (see above), • *ductal obstruction:* e.g., * previous vasectomy, * CF (atretic or absent vas deferens), • *disorders associated with accessory sex organs, ejaculation, or technique* [Regarding infertility in couples, one-third is related to female dysfunction, one-third male dysfunction, and one-third is a combination of the two.]
tests performed in work-up of male infertility	• **sperm count/morphology:** * gold standard, * see above, • *gonadotropins:* increased serum FSH/normal LH defect in spermatogenesis, • *serum testosterone:* see above, • *serum prolactin:* R/O prolactinoma, • *vasographic studies:* R/O obstruction, • *testicular Bx:* evaluate seminiferous tubules/Leydig cells
causes of male impotence	• **psychogenic,** • *low testosterone:* see above, • *vascular disease*, • *neurologic disease:* * parasympathetic system for erection (S2–S4), * sympathetic system for ejaculation (T12–L1), • *drug effects*, • *endocrine disease*, • *alcohol* • *penis disorders*
cause of impotence in young men	*psychogenic:* * stress at work, * marital conflicts, * performance anxiety
sign compatible with psychogenic-induced impotence	*presence of nocturnal penile tumescence:* * organic/drug-induced causes lose nocturnal erections, * other causes lose erections
cause of impotence in men >50-y-old	*vascular insufficiency*
causes of vascular insufficiency	• *Leriche syndrome:* * aortoiliac atherosclerosis involving hypogastric arteries, * calf claudication, * calf atrophy, * diminished femoral pulse, • *penile vascular insufficiency*, • *venous leaks in corpus cavernosum*

Table 10–5. MISCELLANEOUS BLADDER, PROSTATE, TESTICLE DISORDERS, MALE HYPOGONADISM, AND IMPOTENCE Continued

Most Common...	Answer and Explanation
neurogenic causes of male impotence	• *multiple sclerosis*, • *peripheral neuropathy:* * DM, * alcoholic, • *stroke*, • *spinal cord injury*, • *radical prostatectomy*
drugs causing male impotence	• *leuprolide*, • *methyldopa*, • *psychotropics*, • *cimetidine*, • *spironolactone*
endocrine disorders causing male impotence	• **DM**, • *hypothyroidism*, • *prolactinoma*
mechanism of alcohol-induced male impotence	• *directly inhibits release of LH/FSH from anterior pituitary*, • *inhibits binding of LH to Leydig cells:* decreases testosterone synthesis, • *increased liver synthesis of SHBG:* * related to hyperestrinism, * SHBG has greater affinity for testosterone than estrogen, hence lowering free testosterone levels
penile disorders	• *Peyronie's disease:* * type of fibromatosis, * painful contractures of penis, • *trauma*, • *priapism:* e.g., sickle cell disease

Question: A physically active 75-year-old man with a past history of a radical prostatectomy presents with lower lumbar back pain. A radionuclide bone scan reveals increased uptake in the lower lumbar vertebrae, femoral heads, and focal areas throughout the pelvic girdle. The PSA is undetectable and serum alkaline phosphatase is mildly elevated. What is your next step in the management of this patient? SELECT 1
(A) Bone marrow biopsy
(B) Bone irradiation
(C) DES
(D) Anti-androgen therapy
(E) Bilateral orchiectomy
(F) Patient reassurance

Answer: (F): The patient has osteoarthritis involving the lower lumbar vertebrae, pelvic girdle, and femoral heads. Metastatic prostate cancer is ruled out by absence of PSA elevation. Osteoarthritis produces sclerotic changes in bone that can easily be confused with prostate cancer and osteoblastic metastasis. Alkaline phosphatase is mildly elevated in osteoarthritis owing to reactive bone formation (osteophytes). No further testing or therapy is necessary in this patient (choice F).

AD = autosomal dominant, AFP = alpha-fetoprotein, APN = acute pyelonephritis, BPH = benign prostate hyperplasia, Bx = biopsy, CF =

cystic fibrosis, CFU = colony forming units, CNS = central nervous system, DES = diethylstilbestrol, DHT = dihydroxytestosterone, DM = diabetes mellitus, DRE = digital rectal examination, Dx = diagnosis, FSH = follicle-stimulating hormone, FQ = fluoroquinolones, GnRH = gonadotropin-releasing hormone, β-hCG = human chorionic gonadotropin, HIV = human immunodeficiency virus, HPF = high-power field, HPV = human papillomavirus, LH = luteinizing hormone, LUT = lower urinary tract, MCC = most common cause, MRI = magnetic resonance imaging, OPF = oil-power field, PAP = prostatic acid phosphatase, PCR = polymerase chain reaction, PSA = prostate-specific antigen, R/O = rule out, Rx = treatment, SCC = squamous cell carcinoma, SHBG = sex-hormone binding globulin, S/S = signs and symptoms, STD = sexually transmitted disease, TCC = transitional cell carcinoma, TMP/SMX = trimethoprim/sulfamethoxazole, TUR = transurethral resection, US = ultrasonography, UTI = urinary tract infection, WBC = white blood cell.

Table 10–6. SEXUALLY TRANSMITTED DISEASES

Most Common...	Answer and Explanation
STD	*Chlamydia trachomatis:* frequently coexists with GC
STD associated with *C. trachomatis*	• **urethritis:** not detected with a Gram stain, • *PID,* • *cervicitis:* * ~5–25% of pregnant women are infected, * fetus develops infection (conjunctivitis, pneumonia) from passing through infected cervix, • *proctitis,* • *prostatitis,* • *epididymitis*
Rx for STDs due to *C. trachomatis*	*doxycycline:* recently, a single dose of azithromycin has been recommended, since doxycycline requires three doses over 7–10 d
STD producing urethritis/PID in first week after exposure	*GC:* * gram-negative, coffee-bean shaped diplococcus, * *C. trachomatis* is symptomatic 7–10 d after sexual exposure
STDs associated with GC	• **urethritis/cervicitis,** • *PID:* late menses or shortly after, • *vulvovaginitis:* prepubescent females who lack estrogen, • *proctitis:* untreated GC in homosexual partner can be a source for recurrent penile GC, • *pharyngitis,* • *disseminated GC,* • *Bartholin's gland abscess,* • *epididymitis,* * *prostatitis* [Women are more likely to be asymptomatic carriers (75–80%) than men (10–15%). ~20% chance of infection with each sexual exposure. ~20% are reinfections. No immunity against future attacks of GC. BCPs protect against GC but not *Chlamydia* infections.]

Table 10–6. SEXUALLY TRANSMITTED DISEASES
Continued

Most Common...	Answer and Explanation
methods used to diagnose GC	• *urethral swabs:* male/female, • *cervical swab* [After collection, the material should be directly inoculated onto a Thayer-Martin plate (chocolate agar). Positive Gram stain of a penis discharge in a male is confirmatory (presumptive Dx in a female).]
cause of Rx failure in GC	*chromosomal mutations and* β-*lactamase production* (plasmid mediated)
Rx of GC	*ceftriaxone* (for GC) + *doxycycline* (for *Chlamydia trachomatis*): ~30–60% of patients with GC have *Chlamydia* as a coinfection.
drug used for GC Rx failures	*spectinomycin*
cause of FitzHugh-Curtis syndrome	• **C. trachomatis**, • *GC*
clinical findings of FitzHugh-Curtis syndrome	• *complication of PID*, • perihepatitis (adhesions between liver capsule and peritoneum) that develop from pus collecting under diaphragm, * recurrent RUQ pain
S/S of disseminated GC	• **tenosynovitis:** * wrist, * foot, • *septic arthritis:* * knee, * wrist, * foot, • *dermatitis:* pustules on wrist, foot
complications of GC and *C. trachomatis* infections	• **sterility:** male/female, • *ectopic pregnancy*
cause of genital *Herpes*	*HSV type 2*
S/S of primary/ recurrent *Herpes* genitalis	• *primary disease:* * fever, * regional lymphadenopathy, * painful ulcerating vesicles, • *recurrent herpes:* * not systemic, * vesicles located on penis, labia, vulva, cervix (mucopurulent cervicitis), • *culture is recommended*
Rx to reduce recurrences of *Herpes* genitalis	*acyclovir*

Table continued on following page

Table 10–6. SEXUALLY TRANSMITTED DISEASES
Continued

Most Common...	Answer and Explanation
cause of venereal warts (condyloma acuminatum)	*HPV types 6 and 11:* * fern-like lesions that develop in moist anogenital areas, * usually flat condyloma on the cervix
histologic finding in HPV	*koilocytosis:* nucleus of squamous cells is pyknotic and surrounded by a clear halo
HPV type associated with cervical, anal, vaginal squamous cancers	**HPV 16,** *18, 31*
Rx for venereal warts	• **topical podophyllin,** • *liquid nitrogen,* • *5-fluorouracil*
cause of LGV	*Chlamydia trachomatis subspecies*
S/S of LGV	• *genital papules:* no ulceration, • *painful lymphadenopathy with draining sinuses:* granulomatous microabscesses, • *lymphedema of scrotum/vulva,* • *rectal strictures in women*
Rx of LGV	*doxycycline*
cause of chancroid	*Haemophilus ducreyi:* * gram-negative rod, * "school of fish" orientation on Gram stain
S/S of chancroid	*painful genital ulcer with suppurative inguinal lymph nodes*
Rx of chancroid	• **IM ceftriaxone:** single dose, • *azithromycin:* single dose
cause of granuloma inguinale	*Calymmatobacterium granulomatis* (Donovan's bacillus): gram-negative coccobacillus found in macrophages
S/S of granuloma inguinale	*creeping ulcers:* heal by scarring
Rx of granuloma inguinale	*doxycycline*
cause of syphilis	*Treponema pallidum:* spirochete
S/S in primary syphilis	• **solitary painless chancre on shaft of penis or labia of female,** • *anus,* • *mouth* [Chancre occurs 3–4 wks post exposure. Persists 1–5 weeks before resolving.]

Table 10–6. SEXUALLY TRANSMITTED DISEASES
Continued

Most Common...	Answer and Explanation
S/S of secondary syphilis	• **diffuse maculopapular rash:** also includes palms/soles, • *generalized lymphadenopathy*, • *condyloma latum:* raised pink lesions in moist anogenital areas, • *pericholangitis*, • *alopecia:* "moth-eaten" appearance, • *meningitis*, • *nephrotic syndrome:* membranous GN [Usually occurs 6 wks to 6 mths after primary syphilis. Most contagious stage of the disease.]
S/S of latent syphilis	*asymptomatic:* * develops 4–12 wks after secondary syphilis, * *early latent syphilis* has a positive serology for <1 y, * *late latent syphilis* has a positive serology for >1 y
Rx of latent syphilis	*penicillin:* after 4 y, latent syphilis is noninfective except in pregnancy (can be transmitted to fetus)
S/S of tertiary syphilis	• **neurosyphilis:** see Table 15–7, • *aortitis involving aortic arch*, • *gummas*
tests for syphilis	• **darkfield microscopy:** gold standard for primary/secondary syphilis with mucocutaneous lesions, • *direct IF*, • *RPR*, • *VDRL*, • *FTA-ABS:* confirmatory test
cause of a false-positive syphilis serology	*anti-cardiolipin antibodies:* * ACA antibodies react against cardiolipin antigen in RPR/VDRL test system, * always exclude SLE, since some patients have ACA antibodies
cause of a false negative syphilis serology	*antibody excess:* * prozone effect, * most often occurs in secondary syphilis, * serum dilution optimizes antibody/antigen concentration in test system leading to agglutination
effect of Rx on RPR, VDRL, FTA-ABS	• *non-treponemal tests:* either become nonreactive or low-titered, • *FTA-ABS:* * usually remains positive, * positive test does not distinguish active from inactive disease
Rx of syphilis	*penicillin*
S/S of a Jarisch-Herxheimer reaction	*generalized rash, fever, headache after Rx of syphilis with penicillin:* * reaction occurs 6–8 h after Rx with penicillin, * reaction due to proteins released from dead treponemes, * not an allergic penicillin reaction

Table continued on following page

Table 10–6. SEXUALLY TRANSMITTED DISEASES
Continued

Most Common...	Answer and Explanation
cause of bacterial vaginosis	*Gardnerella vaginalis:* gram-negative rod
pathogenesis of bacterial vaginosis	*alteration of vaginal pH:* * pH >4.5 due to reduction in lactobacilli (acid producers of vagina), * not an inflammatory vaginitis
S/S and lab findings in bacterial vaginosis	• **malodorous discharge:** amine smell with KOH, • *no inflammation,* • *presence of clue cells:* squamous cells with adherent bacteria
Rx of bacterial vaginosis	*metronidazole:* Rx of partner is not recommended
S/S/lab findings in vaginal candidiasis	• **pruritic vaginitis,** • *red inflamed vaginal mucosa,* • *cottage cheese-like discharge,* • *external dysuria,* • *yeasts/pseudohyphae*
conditions predisposing to vaginal candidiasis	• **oral contraceptives,** • **post-antibiotics,** • *DM,* • *pregnancy,* • *summer months*
Rx of vaginal candidiasis	*fluconazole:* PO or intravaginal, single dose
protozoal cause of vaginitis	*Trichomonas vaginalis*
S/S/lab findings in trichomonas vaginitis	• **pruritic vaginitis,** • *inflamed vaginal mucosa:* strawberry-colored, • *greenish-frothy discharge,* • *vaginal pH >4.5,* • *dysuria:* urethritis, • *motile organisms in hanging drop preparation*
Rx of trichomonas vaginitis	*metronidazole:* treat both partners

Table 10–6. SEXUALLY TRANSMITTED DISEASES
Continued

Question: Which of the following primarily occur in *Neisseria gonorrhoeae* infections rather than *Chlamydia trachomatis* infections? **SELECT 3**

    (A) PID
    (B) Urethritis 1–2 weeks after exposure
    (C) Perihepatitis
    (D) Positive Gram stain
    (E) Protection with birth control pills
    (F) Vulvovaginitis

Answers: (D), (E), (F): PID and perihepatitis may be secondary to both GC and *Chlamydia* (**choices A and C are incorrect**). Urethritis 1–2 weeks after exposure is more likely due to *Chlamydia* urethritis (**choice B is incorrect**). A positive Gram stain (**choice D**) is present only with GC. Chlamydia must be cultured or detected by PCR. BCPs only protect against GC not *Chlamydia* (**choice E**). Vulvovaginitis (**choice F**) is only seen in prepubertal girls with GC.

ACA = anti-cardiolipin antibody, BCP = birth control pill, DM = diabetes mellitus, Dx = diagnosis, FTA-ABS = fluorescent treponema antibody absorption test, GC = gonorrhea, GN = glomerulonephritis, HPV = human papilloma virus, HSV = *Herpes simplex* virus, IF = immunofluorescence, IM = intramuscular, KOH = potassium hydroxide, LGV = lymphogranuloma venereum, PCR = polymerase chain reaction, PID = pelvic inflammatory disease, RPR = rapid plasma reagin, RUQ = right upper quadrant, Rx = treatment, SLE = systemic lupus erythematosus, S/S = signs and symptoms, STD = sexually transmitted disease, VDRL = Veneral Disease Research Laboratory.

CHAPTER

ENDOCRINOLOGY

CONTENTS

Table 11–1. GENERAL CONCEPTS, HYPOTHALAMIC/ PITUITARY DISORDERS

Most Common...	Answer and Explanation
functional type of endocrine disorder	*hypofunctioning gland*
causes of a hypofunctioning gland	• **autoimmune destruction:** e.g., Hashimoto's thyroiditis, • *decreased stimulation:* e.g., secondary hypocortisolism, • *enzyme defects:* e.g., adrenogenital syndrome, • *neoplasms:* e.g., pituitary adenoma, • *infections:* e.g., Waterhouse-Friderichsen syndrome, • *infarction:* e.g., Sheehan's postpartum necrosis
causes of a hyperfunctioning endocrine gland	• **benign adenoma:** e.g., prolactinoma, • *primary hyperplasia:* e.g., adrenal Cushing's syndrome, • *cancer:* e.g., parathyroid cancer
endocrine gland with a primary cancer	*thyroid*
type of lab tests used to evaluate hypofunctioning endocrine glands	*stimulation tests:* e.g., ACTH stimulation test in hypocortisolism

Table continued on following page

545

Table 11–1. GENERAL CONCEPTS, HYPOTHALAMIC/
PITUITARY DISORDERS *Continued*

Most Common...	Answer and Explanation
type of lab tests used to evaluate hyperfunctioning endocrine glands	*suppression tests:* e.g., * dexamethasone suppression test for hypercortisolism, * most hyperfunctioning glands are nonsuppressible (autonomous), * exceptions: prolactinoma and pituitary Cushing's syndrome
tumors affecting the hypothalamus	• **pituitary adenoma,** • *craniopharyngioma:* * second most common tumor, * suprasellar location, • *suprasellar dysgerminoma,* • *midline hamartoma:* not a true neoplasm
inflammatory disorders affecting the hypothalamus	• **sarcoidosis,** • *hystiocytosis X:* childhood disease, • *meningitis:* * neonates, * 2–10 y olds
nutritional disorder affecting the hypothalamus	*Wernicke's encephalopathy:* * thiamine deficiency, * see Table 9–11
effects of head trauma on pituitary hypothalamus	• **hypothalamic hemorrhages/infarct,** • *posterior pituitary hemorrhages,* • *anterior pituitary hemorrhage/infarction*
clinical findings in hypothalamic disease	• **hypopituitarism:** * no releasing hormones to stimulate anterior pituitary, * target organ dysfunction, • *central DI:* * polyuria, * hypernatremia, • *hyperprolactinemia:* * loss of dopamine inhibition, * galactorrhea, • *precocious puberty:* due to midline hamartomas, • *visual field disturbances:* e.g., bitemporal hemianopia, • *mass effects:* e.g., * seizures, * obstructive hydrocephalus, • *growth disorders:* dwarfism in children
anterior pituitary hormone affected by hypothalamic lesions	*GH*
congenital lesion causing prepubertal GnRH deficiency	*Kallmann's syndrome:* see Table 10–5
causes of true precocious puberty in boys	• **midline hypothalamic hamartoma:** 38%, • *CNS lesions:* 31%, • *familial:* 23%, • *idiopathic:* 8% [True precocious puberty in boys is the onset of puberty <9 years old. "True" implies a central origin of the disorder, while pseudo-precocious implies a peripheral cause (e.g., testicular, adrenal).]

Table 11–1. GENERAL CONCEPTS, HYPOTHALAMIC/ PITUITARY DISORDERS *Continued*

Most Common...	Answer and Explanation
causes of true precocious puberty in girls	• **idiopathic:** 65%, • *midline hamartomas:* 15%, • *CNS lesions:* 14%, • *McCune-Albright syndrome:* * 6%, * polyostotic fibrous dysplasia, * precocious puberty, * cafe-au-lait spots
clinical effect of destruction of supraoptic/ paraventricular nuclei	• **central DI:** destructive lesions include * sarcoidosis, * histiocytosis X, * craniopharyngioma, • *SIADH:* due to irritative lesions in this area
clinical effect of destruction of mediobasal portion of hypothalamus	*hypothalamic obesity:* lesions inhibit satiety and lead to hyperphagia
site for melatonin production	*pineal gland:* * midline location above quadrigeminal plate behind posterior commissure, * postganglionic neurons from superior cervical ganglia stimulate β_1-adrenergic receptors on pinealocytes causing synthesis/release of melatonin into CSF and venous circulation
purported function of melatonin	*chemical messenger of darkness:* * nighttime release (light suppresses release), * important in sleep/moods and circadian rhythms
use of melatonin	*Rx of chronobiologic sleep/mood disorders*
abnormality affecting pineal gland	*calcification:* * begins in childhood, * useful in showing shifts due to mass lesions
types of pineal tumors	• **germ cell tumors:** * 75%, * most resemble seminomas (see Table 10–5), * teratomas account for remainder of tumors, • *pinealoma:* well-differentiated pinealocytoma in adults
clinical findings in pineal tumors	• **headache,** • *visual disturbances:* paralysis of upward conjugate gaze (Parinaud's syndrome), • *obstructive hydrocephalus:* compression of aqueduct of Sylvius in third ventricle, • *precocious puberty in boys:* * teratoma (50%), * pinealoblastoma (40%)
radiologic imaging study used to evaluate pituitary gland	• **MRI,** • *CT*

Table continued on following page

Table 11–1. GENERAL CONCEPTS, HYPOTHALAMIC/ PITUITARY DISORDERS *Continued*

Most Common...	Answer and Explanation
cause of hypopituitarism in children	*craniopharyngioma:* * benign tumor, * cystic, calcifications, * derived from Rathke's pouch remnants
causes of hypopituitarism in adults	• **nonfunctioning pituitary adenomas:** hypopituitarism due to * direct destruction, * compression atrophy, * hemorrhage/infarction (pituitary apoplexy), • *removal (surgery)/ablation* (radiation) *for Rx of pituitary tumors,* • *Sheehan's postpartum necrosis:* * cessation of lactation, * pituitary infarction, • *lymphocytic hypophysitis:* see below, • *empty sella syndrome:* see below, • *suprasellar craniopharyngioma,* • *pituitary stalk disease:* trauma, • *hypothalamic disease:* see above
clinical findings in lymphocytic hypophysitis	• *probable autoimmune disease,* • *female dominant,* • *occurs during pregnancy/postpartum,* • *presents as hypopituitarism or sellar mass with hyperprolactinemia*
defect in empty sella syndrome	• *defect in diaphragmatic sella with arachnoid herniation into fossa,* • *compression of pituitary,* • *enlargement of sella*
clinical findings of primary empty sella syndrome	• *usually an obese woman with headaches:* may be related to increased intracranial pressure, • *no visual disturbances,* • *hypopituitarism uncommon*
clinical findings in secondary empty sella syndrome	• *causes:* * previous pituitary tumor surgery/radiation, * hypophysitis, * Sheehan's syndrome, • *signs of hypopituitarism,* • *visual defects*
extrasellar cause of hypopituitarism in adults	*craniopharyngioma*
sequence of trophic hormone loss due to an expanding mass	$FSH/LH \rightarrow GH \rightarrow TSH \rightarrow ACTH \rightarrow prolactin$
functions of FSH and LH	• *FSH (woman):* * prepare follicle, * stimulate aromatase synthesis in granulosa cells (converts testosterone into estradiol), * stimulates LH receptor synthesis, • *FSH (man):* induces spermatogenesis in conjunction with testos-

Most Common...	Answer and Explanation
Continued	terone, • *LH (woman):* * stimulates 17-KS/ testosterone synthesis in theca interna of developing follicle, * testosterone is aromatized into estradiol in granulosa cells, * maintains corpus luteum and progesterone synthesis, • *LH (man):* stimulates testosterone synthesis in Leydig cells
functions of estradiol	• *maintains secondary sex characteristics,* • *main hormone of proliferative phase of menstrual cycle,* • *stimulates maturation of vaginal superficial squamous cells,* • *rise in estrogen at midcycle leads to LH surge and ovulation,* • *negative and positive feedback on FSH/LH, respectively,* • *stimulates prolactin secretion,* • *blocks prolactin action on the breast during pregnancy,* • *increases tubal motility,* • *increases synthesis of SHBG, TBG, angiotensinogen, transcortin*
functions of progesterone	• *main hormone of secretory phase of menstrual cycle,* • *breast development,* • *negative feedback on FSH/LH,* • *increases basal body temperature 0.6°F,* • *decreases estrogen receptor formation:* inhibits gland proliferation, • *increases Na⁺ reabsorption,* • *stimulates respiratory center:* respiratory alkalosis of pregnancy
functions of GH/IGF-1 (somatomedin)	• *GH:* * increases AA uptake in muscle, * decreases uptake of glucose in muscle/adipose, * stimulates gluconeogenesis: glucose synthesis in fasting state, * decreases FA synthesis/increases lipolysis, * promotes erythropoiesis, * stimulates liver synthesis/release of IGF-1, * stimulated by stress/hypoglycemia, * inhibited by hyperglycemia (basis of suppression test), * somatostatin inhibits GH release, • *IGF-1:* * stimulates ♦ linear bone growth, ♦ chondrogenesis, ♦ soft tissue growth, * negative feedback on GH, * malnutrition lowers SMM without affecting GH
function of TSH	• *stimulates synthesis/release of thyroid hormones:* increases trapping of iodide, • T_4/ T_3: * negative feedback on TSH/TRH, * T_3 metabolically active form, * T_3 primarily derived from peripheral conversion of T_4 into T_3 by an outer ring deiodinase

Table continued on following page

Table 11–1. GENERAL CONCEPTS, HYPOTHALAMIC/ PITUITARY DISORDERS *Continued*

Most Common...	Answer and Explanation
function of thyroid hormone in the cardiovascular system	*increases synthesis of β-adrenergic receptors:* * enhances catecholamine effects of increased heart rate/contractility, * regulates protein metabolism in muscle
function of thyroid hormone in vitamin A metabolism	*promotes intestinal conversion of β-carotene to retinoic acid:* in hypothyroidism, the skin turns yellow due to build-up of β-carotenes
function of thyroid hormone in CHO metabolism	• *increases glucose reabsorption in GI tract,* • *promotes glycogenolysis/glycolysis,* • *increases degradation of insulin* [The above lead to hyperglycemia in hyperthyroidism.]
function of thyroid hormone in lipid metabolism	*increases LDL receptor synthesis:* * in hyperthyroidism, serum CH is decreased, * in hypothyroidism, CH is increased
functions of ACTH	*stimulates steroidogenesis in adrenal cortex:* * stimulates fasciculata/reticularis (cortisol, 17-KS), * no primary effect on glomeruli, which synthesize aldosterone, * negative feedback of cortisol on ACTH
function of cortisol in protein metabolism	• *increases protein catabolism,* • *decreases AA uptake:* AAs are used for gluconeogenesis [In hypercortisolism, increased protein catabolism is responsible for loss of muscle mass in extremities and supplies AA as fuel for gluconeogenesis causing hyperglycemia.]
function of cortisol in CHO metabolism	• *decreases muscle/adipose uptake of glucose,* • *increases gluconeogenesis,* • *enhances glycogenolysis* [In hypocortisolism, fasting hypoglycemia occurs. In hypercortisolism, hyperglycemia occurs.]
function of cortisol in lipid metabolism	• *enhances lipolysis:* releases FAs, • *inhibits phospholipase:* * anti-inflammatory action, * decreases prostaglandin/leukotriene synthesis, • *increases surfactant synthesis*
function of excess cortisol in collagen synthesis	*decreases collagen synthesis:* decreased collagen synthesis leads to poor wound healing/ vascular instability (ecchymoses)
function of cortisol in immune system	• *stabilizes mast cell membrane:* prevents histamine release, • *hypercortisolism:* * neutrophilic leukocytosis (decreases adhesion molecule synthesis), * reduces eosinophil count

Table 11–1. GENERAL CONCEPTS, HYPOTHALAMIC/
PITUITARY DISORDERS *Continued*

Most Common...	Answer and Explanation
Continued	(eosinopenia), * reduces lymphocyte count (lymphopenia), * decreases size of thymus/ lymph nodes, * decreases antibody production
function of excess cortisol in bone metabolism	• **increases bone resorption:** leads to osteoporosis, • *decreases calcium/phosphorus reabsorption in kidneys*
function of cortisol in volume control	*inhibits ADH activity:* in hypocortisolism, loss of inhibitory effect on ADH leads to SI-ADH
functions of prolactin	• *promotes breast development:* in concert with estrogen/progesterone, at puberty it * stimulates proliferation/branching of mammary ducts, in pregnancy it * stimulates growth/development of mammary alveoli, • *promotes lactogenesis:* * stimulates milk production/secretion, * *inhibits ovulation:* inhibits synthesis/release of GnRH, • *assists LH stimulation of testosterone synthesis in Leydig cells*
S/S of gonadotropin deficiency in adults	• *women:* * secondary amenorrhea, * infertility, * loss of secondary sex characteristics, * diminished libido, • *men:* * impotence, * diminished libido, * loss of secondary sex characteristics, * atrophy of testes/prostate
S/S of GH deficiency in adults	• **decreased vigor,** • *weakness,* • *increased body fat,* • *fasting hypoglycemia*
S/S of TSH deficiency in adults (secondary hypothyroidism)	• **muscle weakness,** • *cold intolerance,* • *dry/ brittle hair,* • *facial puffiness,* • *impaired memory,* • *constipation,* • *predisposes to mild SIADH:* * mild hyponatremia, * thyroid hormone inhibits ADH activity [In secondary hypothyroidism there is a low serum T_4/low serum TSH.]
S/S of ACTH deficiency in adults (secondary hypocortisolism)	• **fatigue/weakness,** • *inability to tan:* loss of ACTH's intrinsic MSH properties, • *adrenal crises with stress,* • *mild SIADH:* * mild hyponatremia, * cortisol inhibits ADH activity, • *orthostatic hypotension,* • *fasting hypoglycemia:* cortisol normally enhances gluconeogenesis [ACTH does not stimulate adrenal re-

Table continued on following page

Table 11–1. GENERAL CONCEPTS, HYPOTHALAMIC/ PITUITARY DISORDERS *Continued*

Most Common...	Answer and Explanation
Continued	lease of aldosterone. Electrolyte disturbances are not as profound as they are with primary adrenal insufficiency. Secondary hypocortisolism has low serum cortisol/ACTH (primary disease has a high ACTH).]
lab findings in hypogonadism (hypogonadotropic hypogonadism)	• *hypogonadism* (women): * low FSH/LH, * low estradiol, * GnRH stimulation test: ♦ no significant increase in FSH/LH in hypopituitarism, ♦ eventual increase in FSH/LH in hypothalamic disease, • *hypogonadism* (man): * low FSH/LH, * low testosterone, * low sperm count, * similar GnRH stimulation results
lab findings in GH deficiency	• *low IGF-1:* * most sensitive screening test, • *low GH,* • *fasting hypoglycemia:* 50%, • *insulin tolerance test:* * induce hypoglycemia (stimulus for GH release and ACTH release), * no increase in GH/IGF-1 or ACTH/cortisol, • L-*dopa and* L-*arginine test:* no increase in GH/IGF-1, • *sleep:* * normally stimulates GH in early morning, * no GH/IGF-1 response in hypopituitarism
lab findings in Laron dwarfism	• *high GH,* • *low IGF-1:* mutant receptor cannot transduce signal from GH
lab findings in TSH deficiency (secondary hypothyroidism)	• *low serum TSH,* • *low serum T_4/T_3,* • *hypercholesterolemia:* decreased LDL receptor synthesis, • *hyponatremia:* loss of inhibitory effect of thyroid hormone on ADH, • *TRH stimulation test:* * decreased TSH response in hypopituitarism, * eventual TSH response in hypothalamic dysfunction
test for ACTH reserve in anterior pituitary	*metyrapone* [Metyrapone blocks 11-OHase in the adrenal cortex, • this blocks conversion of 11-deoxycortisol → cortisol. The low cortisol increases ACTH (loss of negative feedback) and increases 11-deoxycortisol, which is proximal to the block. No increase in ACTH or 11-deoxycortisol indicates hypopituitarism. [An increase in ACTH and decrease in 11-deoxycortisol indicates a primary adrenal hypocortisolism.]

Table 11–1. GENERAL CONCEPTS, HYPOTHALAMIC/ PITUITARY DISORDERS *Continued*

Most Common...	Answer and Explanation
lab findings in ACTH deficiency (secondary hypocortisolism)	• *decreased ACTH,* • *abnormal metyrapone test:* see above, • *fasting hypoglycemia:* decreased gluconeogenesis/glycogenolysis, • *hyponatremia:* loss of ADH inhibition, • *insulin tolerance test* (induce hypoglycemia): * diminished ACTH/cortisol response, • *short ACTH (cosyntropin) test:* * no significant increase (does not distinguish secondary from primary hypocortisolism [see below], * in primary disease, ACTH is increased
test to distinguish secondary from primary hypocortisolism (Addison's disease)	*3-day IV ACTH stimulation test:* * in secondary hypocortisolism (hypopituitarism), urine for 17-hydroxycorticoids eventually increases (adrenal glands are atrophic and not destroyed), * in Addison's disease, 17-hydroxycorticoids do not increase (gland is destroyed)
general Rx of hypopituitarism	*treat cause and replace deficient hormones:* e.g., surgical removal of pituitary adenoma
Rx of gonadotropin deficiency	• *ovulation/spermatogenesis:* * pulsatile GnRH (for GnRH deficient patients), * FSH, * hCG (LH analogue), • *conjugated estrogens with supplemental progestational agent:* if uterus present, • *long-acting parenteral testosterone for men*
Rx of GH deficiency	• *GH replacement primarily recommended for children to improve impaired linear growth,* • *experimental in adults:* does increase muscle mass and decrease adipose
Rx of TSH deficiency	T_4: * initiate glucocorticoid replacement before thyroid hormone replacement to prevent acute adrenocortical crisis, * use free T_4 hormone levels to monitor effectiveness of Rx, since TSH is already low
Rx of ACTH deficiency	*prednisone:* begin prednisone Rx before replacing thyroid hormone in order to prevent acute adrenocortical crisis

Table continued on following page

Table 11–1. GENERAL CONCEPTS, HYPOTHALAMIC/ PITUITARY DISORDERS *Continued*

Most Common...	Answer and Explanation
Rx of prolactin deficiency	*not necessary*
types of diabetes insipidus (DI)	• **central:** ADH deficiency, • *nephrogenic:* end-organ defect [See Table 10–2 for discussion of ADH excess.]
mechanisms of central DI	*disorders of* • **anterior hypothalamus,** • *median eminence,* • *upper pituitary stalk*
mechanism of nephrogenic DI	*end-organ unresponsiveness to ADH*
causes of central DI	• **idiopathic hypothalamic DI:** probably autoimmune disease, • *trauma:* * closed head injury (basilar skull fracture), * neurosurgery, • *inflammation:* * histiocytosis X, * TB, * sarcoidosis, • *tumors:* * craniopharyngioma, * metastatic breast/lung cancer
causes of nephrogenic DI	• **chronic renal disease,** • *electrolyte disorders:* * severe hypokalemia, * metastatic calcification in hypercalcemia, • *drugs inhibiting ADH action:* * demeclocycline, * lithium, * amphotericin B, • *SXR familial nephrogenic DI*
symptoms/lab findings of DI	• *polyuria,* • *increased thirst:* preference for ice-cold water, • *nocturia,* • *dilute urine:* UOsm <100 mOsm/kg, • *normal serum Na+:* * access to water usually compensates for renal loss of water, * hypernatremia occurs when there is no access to water
causes of polyuria other than DI	• **diuretics:** e.g., thiazides, • *osmotic diuresis:* e.g., glucosuria, • *primary polydipsia:* * compulsive water drinker, * low serum osmolality and suppression of ADH
lab findings in DI pre/post-ADH injection after water deprivation	POsm/UOsm UOsm post-ADH CDI: increased/ decreased UOsm increases >50% over UOsm post-water deprivation NDI: increased/ decreased UOsm increases <45% over UOsm post-water deprivation

Table 11-1. GENERAL CONCEPTS, HYPOTHALAMIC/ PITUITARY DISORDERS *Continued*

Most Common...	Answer and Explanation
Continued	[Note: In CDI, the urine becomes concentrated after giving ADH, while in NDI, the degree of concentration is less depending on the severity of the disease.]
lab findings in primary polydipsia post-water deprivation and ADH injection	POsm/UOsm UOsm post-ADH <hr> normal/increased UOsm not significantly increased [Note: Restricting water produces normal urine concentration and a POsm that is at the upper limit of normal.]
Rx of central DI	• *Rx underlying disease,* • *severe central DI:* * desmopressin (nasal insufflation, spray, parenteral), • *partial central DI:* * chlorpropamide, * carbamazepine
Rx of nephrogenic DI	*thiazides:* produce volume contraction and increased proximal tubule reabsorption of water (decreases polyuria)
cause of GH excess	*GH secreting pituitary adenoma:* prolactin is also increased in ~25% of cases
manifestations of GH excess in children/adults	• *children:* gigantism due to increased linear bone growth (epiphyses not fused), • *adults:* acromegaly with increased lateral bone growth
musculoskeletal signs of excess GH/IGF-1	• **acral enlargement hands/feet,** • **frontal bossing:** increased hat size due to enlarged sinuses, • *arthritis,* • *prognathism:* prominent jaw ("lantern jaw"), • *muscle weakness*
cutaneous signs of excess GH/IGF-1	• **increased thickness of soft tissue,** • *increased heel pad thickness,* • *oily skin,* • *hyperhidrosis,* • *acanthosis nigricans*
oral cavity signs of excess GH/IGF-1	• *wide-spacing of teeth:* due to jaw growth, • *macroglossia,* • *enlarged lips,* • *obstructive sleep apnea:* increased pharyngeal soft tissue
cardiovascular signs of excess GH/IGF-1	• **cardiomegaly:** * heart failure, * angina, * hypertrophy, • *HTN:* 25–35%

Table continued on following page

Table 11–1. GENERAL CONCEPTS, HYPOTHALAMIC/ PITUITARY DISORDERS *Continued*

Most Common...	Answer and Explanation
CNS signs of excess GH/IGF-1	• **headache,** • *visual field defects*
metabolic signs of excess GH/IGF-1	• **DM:** 20%, • *hyperphosphatemia*
disease associations in acromegaly	• *goiter:* * Graves' disease, * multinodular, • *MEN I syndrome,* • *increased risk for colorectal cancer/premalignant polyps*
lab findings in acromegaly	• **increased IGF-1:** confirms Dx if adolescence/pregnancy excluded, • *increased GH,* • *oral glucose tolerance test* (suppression test): * no significant decrease in GH, * most reliable confirmatory test, • *paradoxical increase in GH with TRH stimulation:* 60%, • *suppression of GH with* L-*dopa,* • *increased size of sella:* most are macroadenomas, • *hyperglycemia,* • *hyperphosphatemia*
Rx of acromegaly	• **surgery:** 60% successful, • *recurrent tumor:* * radiation, * drugs (bromocriptine, octreotide [somatostatin analogue])
COD in acromegaly	*heart failure*
pituitary tumors	• **prolactinoma:** 40–50%, • *non-functioning pituitary adenoma:* 30–40%, • *ACTH-secreting tumors:* * 10–15%, * Cushing's disease, • *GH tumors:* 10–15%
S/S of a prolactinoma	• *female:* * secondary amenorrhea (prolactin inhibits GnRH), * galactorrhea, • *male:* impotence, • *adolescent:* delayed puberty [Microadenomas are more common in women of reproductive age, while macroadenomas occur in men and postmenopausal women.]
causes of galactorrhea other than prolactinoma	• **primary hypothyroidism:** * 15–30%, * low T_4 increases TSH/TRH, the latter a potent prolactin stimulator, • *drugs:* * estrogen, * phenothiazines, * tricyclics, * reserpine, * calcium channel blockers, * cimetidine, • *pregnancy,* • *pituitary stalk transection:* loss of inhibitory effect of dopamine on prolactin, • *metabolic conditions:* * **primary hypothyroidism,** * pregnancy, * cirrhosis, * renal failure

Table 11–1. GENERAL CONCEPTS, HYPOTHALAMIC/
PITUITARY DISORDERS *Continued*

Most Common...	Answer and Explanation
lab findings in prolactinoma	• **high serum prolactin:** * serum levels >200 ng/mL diagnostic, * height of prolactin correlates with tumor mass, • *low FSH/LH,* • *low estradiol,* • *low testosterone*
Rx of prolactinomas	• **bromocriptine:** * dopamine analogue, * restores gonadal function 70–80%, * shrinks tumor mass in <50%, • *cabergoline:* dopamine analogue, • *surgery for macroadenomas*
side-effects of bromocriptine	• *postural hypotension,* • *dizziness,* • *nasal stuffiness*

Question: In an adult patient with panhypopituitarism, you would expect which of the following laboratory abnormalities? **SELECT 2**
(A) Severe hyponatremia
(B) Hypoglycemia
(C) Hyperkalemia
(D) Increased GH with insulin tolerance test
(E) Cortisol response to single dose of ACTH
(F) No increase in gonadotropins after GnRH stimulation

Answer: (B), (F): Severe hyponatremia is not a feature of hypopituitarism because ACTH does not stimulate aldosterone, hence mineralocorticoid deficiency is not present (**choice A is incorrect**). Mild hyponatremia does occur and relates to the loss of inhibition cortisol and T_4 normally have on ADH. Hypoglycemia (**choice B**) is related to loss of GH and cortisol, both of which enhance gluconeogenesis. Hyperkalemia is present in Addison's disease, since there is no mineralocorticoid deficiency (hyperkalemia is present in Addison's disease, **choice C is incorrect**). GH does not increase with the insulin tolerance test, since the anterior pituitary is destroyed (**choice D is incorrect**). Cortisol does not increase with a single dose of ACTH, because the adrenal gland is atrophic (**choice E is incorrect**). A 3-day ACTH stimulation test will, in most cases, bring the adrenal cortex back into a functional condition. FSH and LH will not increase with GnRH stimulation, since the anterior pituitary is destroyed (**choice F**). In a hypothalamic cause of deficiency, the gonadotropins would increase.

AA = amino acid, ACTH = adrenocorticotropic hormone, ADH = antidiuretic hormone, CDI = central diabetes insipidus, CHO = carbohydrate, CNS = central nervous system, COD = cause of death, CSF = cerebrospinal fluid, CT = computed tomography, DI = diabetes insipidus, DM = diabetes mellitus, dopa = dopamine, FA = fatty acid, FSH = follicle-stimulating hormone, GH = growth hormone, GI = gastrointestinal, GnRH = gonadotropin-releasing hormone, hCG = human chorionic gonadotropin, HTN = hypertension, IGF-1 = insulin growth factor, IV = intravenous, 17-KS = 17-ketosteroids, LDL = low density lipoprotein, LH = luteinizing hormone, MEN = multiple endocrine neoplasia,

MRI = magnetic resonance imaging, MSH = melanocyte-stimulating hormone, NDI = nephrogenic diabetes insipidus, 11-OHase = 11-hydroxylase, POsm = plasma osmolality, Rx = treatment, SIADH = syndrome of inappropriate antidiuretic hormone, SHBG = sex hormone binding globulin, SMM = somatomedin, S/S = signs and symptoms, SXR = sex-linked recessive, T_3 = triiodothyronine, T_4 = thyroxine, TB = tuberculosis, TBG = thyroid binding globulin, TRH = thyrotropin releasing hormone, TSH = thyroid-stimulating hormone, UOsm = urine osmolality.

Table 11–2. THYROID DISORDERS

Most Common...	Answer and Explanation
tests included in a thyroid profile	• *serum T_4,* • *resin T_3 uptake* (RTU), • T_4 *binding ratio:* T_4BR = RTU/30%, • *free-T_4 index* (FT$_4$-I), • *TSH:* best overall test
factors controlling serum T_4 concentration	• *hypothalamic/pituitary function,* • *thyroid gland function,* • *TBG concentration* [The total serum T_4 = sum of T_4 bound to TBG and free T_4, which is the metabolically active fraction once converted to T_3.]
causes of an elevated/decreased serum T_4	• **increased/decreased free T_4 hormone level:** e.g., hyperthyroidism/hypothyroidism, respectively, • *increased/decreased TBG level:* former increases serum T_4, latter decreases serum T_4, * free T_4/TSH are normal with TBG alterations [In *normal conditions,* one-third of the binding sites of TBG are occupied by T_4. If additional TBG is synthesized by the liver, one-third of their binding sites must be bound by T_4. This increases total T_4 without altering free T_4 levels, since the thyroid gland replaces the T_4 used to bind to the extra TBGs. Similarly, a decrease in TBG leads to a decrease in total T_4 without affecting the free T_4 level.]
causes of an increase in TBG	• **estrogen:** increases liver synthesis of TBG, • *acute hepatitis:* increases TBG release
causes of a decrease in TBG	• *androgens:* breaks them down, • *chronic liver disease:* decreased synthesis, • *high doses of salicylate,* • *corticosteroids*
effect of TBG alterations on serum TSH	*no effect:* free T_4 levels are normal

Table 11–2. THYROID DISORDERS *Continued*

Most Common...	Answer and Explanation
effect of alterations of free T_4 levels due to thyroid disease on TSH	• *low free T_4:* increase serum TSH, • *increased free T_4:* decrease serum TSH
indication for ordering RTU	*indirect measurement of TBG* [The RTU reflects the number of binding sites available on TBG. Radioactive T_3 ($*T_3$) is added to a tube of patient plasma and binds to all available TBG sites. A resin is added to the tube to bind any residual $*T_3$. The amount of $*T_3$ bound to the resin (not the TBG) is measured and reported as a percent (normally 30%).]
effect of an increase in TBG on RTU	*lowers RTU:* * more TBG sites available to bind $*T_3$, * less binds with resin
effect of a decrease in TBG on RTU	*increases RTU:* * less TBG leaves fewer sites available for $*T_3$ and more is left over to bind with resin, * an increase in TBG lowers RTU, * a decrease in TBG increases RTU
effect of an increase in free T_4 on RTU	*increases RTU:* * excess in T_4 saturates most of TBG binding sites, * fewer sites available for $*T_3$ and more binds with the resin
effect of a decrease in free T_4 on RTU	*decreases RTU:* * decrease in T_4 leaves more sites available on TBG for $*T_3$, * less $*T_3$ binds to resin
method of calculating T_4BR	*T_4BR = measured RTU ÷ 30%:* e.g., patient RTU = 15%, T_4BR = 0.5 (15/30)
use of T_4BR	*calculate FT_4-I* (free T_4 level): * FT_4-I = T_4BR × total serum T_4, * e.g., RTU = 15%, serum T_4 = 10, T_4BR = 15%/30% = 0.5, FT_4-I = 0.5 × 10 = 5
effect of an excess of free T_4 on RTU, T_4BR, FT_4-I	• *RTU increased,* • *T_4BR increased,* • *FT_4-I increased*
effect of a decrease in free T_4 on RTU, T_4BR, FT_4-I	• *RTU decreased,* • *T_4BR decreased,* • *FT_4-I decreased*

Table continued on following page

Table 11–2. THYROID DISORDERS *Continued*

Most Common...	Answer and Explanation
effect of an increase in TBG on serum T_4, RTU, T_4BR, FT_4-I, TSH	• *serum T_4 increased,* • *RTU decreased,* • *T_4BR decreased,* • *FT_4-I normal:* change in RTU "normalizes" FT_4-I, • *TSH normal:* no alteration in free T_4 level
effect of a decrease in TBG on serum T_4, RTU, T_4BR, FT_4-I, TSH	• *serum T_4 decreased,* • *RTU increased,* • *T_4BR increased,* • *FT_4-I normal:* change in RTU "normalizes" FT_4-I, • *TSH normal:* no alteration in free T_4 level
indication for measuring serum T_3	*R/O T_3 toxicosis*
indications for ordering serum TSH	• **Dx of primary hypothyroidism:** TSH usually >20 μU/mL (normal 0.3–6.0 μU/mL), • *Dx of subclinical hypothyroidism:* * gland about to fail, * TSH 6–20 μU/mL, • *Dx of hyperthyroidism:* TSH <0.3 μU/mL, • *follow T_4 Rx in primary hypothyroidism:* * goal is to bring TSH into normal range, * use free T_4 levels to monitor secondary hypothyroidism, • *distinguish alterations in TBG on serum T_4 concentration versus true free hormone abnormalities:* TSH is normal when TBG is altered
indications for ordering ^{131}I uptake	• **Dx of primary hyperthyroidism:** excess production of T_4 (e.g., Graves' disease), • *distinguish thyrotoxicosis due to inflammation/factitious intake of hormone from hyperthyroidism:* * thyrotoxicosis refers to end-organ effects of excess thyroid hormone regardless of cause, • *radionuclide scanning:* distinguish "cold" from "hot" nodules, • *identify metastatic thyroid cancer:* follicular thyroid cancers concentrate ^{131}I, • *identify lingual thyroid:* nodular mass at base of tongue, • *calculate dose for thyroid ablation:* Rx of hyperthyroidism
^{131}I findings in primary hyperthyroidism	*increased ^{131}I uptake:* gland is synthesizing excess hormone and requires iodine for T_4 synthesis
^{131}I findings in thyroiditis/excess intake of T_4	*decreased ^{131}I uptake:* * in thyroiditis, excess T_4 is released from damaged tissue (not synthesized), * with excessive hormone intake, suppression of TSH causes gland atrophy and decreased ^{131}I uptake

Table 11–2. THYROID DISORDERS *Continued*

Most Common...	Answer and Explanation
¹³¹I findings with "cold"/"hot" nodules	• **"cold" nodules:** * nonfunctioning nodules, * no uptake of ¹³¹I, * there is ¹³¹I uptake by functioning tissue, • *"hot" nodules:* * increased ¹³¹I uptake by nodule, * remainder of gland is not visualized
uses of serum thyroglobulin	• **tumor marker for thyroid cancer recurrence:** increased, • *differentiate silent postpartum thyroiditis from factitious thyrotoxicosis:* * increased in former, * low in latter [Thyroglobulin does not accurately differentiate benign from malignant thyroid disease.]
indications for ordering serum reverse T_3	*Dx of nonthyroidal illness syndrome:* * normally, a peripheral tissue outer ring deiodinase converts T_4 into metabolically active T_3, * in nonthyroidal illness, outer ring deiodinase is blocked and inner ring deiodinase converts T_4 into inactive reverse T_3
lab findings of variants of nonthyroidal illness syndrome	• **most common variant:** * normal serum T_4, * low serum T_3, * normal TSH, * high reverse T_3, • *less common variant:* * low serum T_4/T_3, * normal/low TSH, * high reverse T_3
indications for ordering thyroid stimulating immunoglobulins (TSI)	• **immune marker for Graves' disease:** * IgG immunoglobulin attaches to TSH receptors and stimulates hormone synthesis, * only increased in Graves' disease, • *differentiate proptosis secondary to euthyroid Graves' disease from other causes of proptosis:* in Graves' disease, low serum TSH, normal serum T_4, high TSI, • *predict remission/relapse in patients treated with thiourea drugs for Graves' disease:* * low TSI in remission, * high TSI in relapse, • *identify neonatal thyrotoxicosis due to Graves' disease:* IgG antibody crosses placenta and causes transient neonatal thyrotoxicosis
indications for ordering antithyroid antibodies	*Dx autoimmune thyroiditis:* two antibodies are * antimicrosomal (best overall test) and * antithyroglobulin antibodies, * antimicrosomal (peroxidase) antibodies have highest titers in Hashimoto's thyroiditis (moderately elevated in Graves' disease)

Table continued on following page

Table 11–2. THYROID DISORDERS *Continued*

Most Common...	Answer and Explanation
causes of thyroiditis	• **Hashimoto's thyroiditis:** see below, • *acute thyroiditis,* • *subacute painful thyroiditis,* • *subacute painless lymphocytic thyroiditis,* • *Reidel's thyroiditis*
causes of acute thyroiditis	*bacterial infection:* e.g., * *Streptococcus pneumoniae,* • *Staphylococcus aureus,* * *Pneumocystis carinii*
S/S of acute thyroiditis	• **enlarged, tender gland,** • *cervical adenopathy,* • *fever,* • *thyrotoxicosis:* gland destruction
cause of subacute painful thyroiditis (de Quervain's thyroiditis)	*coxsackievirus:* granulomatous inflammation
clinical findings in subacute painful thyroiditis	• *women 40–50 y old,* • *often preceded by URI,* • *enlarged, tender gland,* • *cervical adenopathy not prominent,* • *thyrotoxicosis:* * 50%, * due to gland destruction, • *self-limited,* • *permanent hypothyroidism uncommon,* • *Rx:* NSAIDs or corticosteroids
lab findings in subacute painful thyroiditis	• **high ESR,** • *antithyroid antibodies:* 10–20%, • *high serum T_4,* • *low serum TSH,* • *low ^{131}I uptake*
cause of subacute painless lymphocytic thyroiditis	*autoimmune disease:* commonly occurs 3–6 mths postpartum
clinical findings in subacute painless thyroiditis	• *abrupt onset of thyrotoxicosis:* gland destruction, • *gland minimally enlarged and painless,* • *no previous URI,* • *mild lymphocytic infiltrate without germinal follicles:* unlike Hashimoto's thyroiditis, • *40–50% progress into Hashimoto's thyroiditis with goiter or hypothyroidism,* • *Rx:* beta blockers if thyrotoxicosis is present
lab findings in subacute painless thyroiditis	• **normal TSI:** high in Graves' disease, • *low titer of antimicrosomal antibodies,* • *high serum thyroglobulin,* • *lab findings of thyrotoxicosis:* see above, • *low ^{131}I uptake*

Table 11–2. THYROID DISORDERS *Continued*

Most Common...	Answer and Explanation
clinical findings in Reidel's thyroiditis	• *thyroid replaced by fibrous tissue,* • *rock-hard thyroid mimics thyroid cancer,* • *fibrous tissue extends into periglandular tissue:* may obstruct trachea, • *associations:* * sclerosing mediastinitis, * retroperitoneal fibrosis, • *hypothyroidism may occur*
cause of hypothyroidism	*Hashimoto's thyroiditis:* * autoimmune chronic thyroiditis, * HLA-Dr5 relationship
mechanism of hypothyroidism in Hashimoto's thyroiditis	• **cytotoxic T cells:** type IV hypersensitivity, • *antimicrosomal/thyroglobulin antibodies:* type II hypersensitivity, • *blocking autoantibodies against TSH receptor:* type II hypersensitivity, • *possible outcome of subacute painless lymphocytic thyroiditis*
clinical associations of Hashimoto's thyroiditis	• *Sjögren's syndrome,* • *PA*
G/M findings in Hashimoto's thyroiditis	• *gross:* symmetrically enlarged, nodular, painless gland, • *microscopic:* heavy lymphocytic infiltrate with germinal follicles
general clinical findings in Hashimoto's thyroiditis	• **weight gain:** * hypometabolic, * retain water and salt, • *daytime somnolence,* • *fatigue,* • *cold intolerance*
musculoskeletal findings in Hashimoto's thyroiditis	• **weakness:** proximal muscle myopathy with elevated serum CK, • *delayed recovery of Achilles reflex,* • *carpal tunnel syndrome*
cutaneous/soft tissue findings in Hashimoto's thyroiditis	• **periorbital puffiness:** GAG deposition, • *coarse yellow skin:* β-carotenemia due to less conversion of β-carotenes into retinoic acid in intestinal cells (function of thyroid hormone), • *dry/brittle hair,* • *brittle nails,* • *loss of lateral eyebrows,* • *pretibial myxedema:* * GAG deposition, * non-pitting
cardiorespiratory findings in Hashimoto's thyroiditis	• *diastolic HTN:* * 10%, * due to salt/water retention, * resolves with thyroid hormone replacement, • *sinus bradycardia,* • *congestive cardiomegaly/heart failure,* • *hoarse voice:* GAG deposition in vocal cords, • *CAD:* increased LDL (decreased LDL receptor synthesis), • *obstructive sleep apnea*

Table continued on following page

Table 11–2. THYROID DISORDERS *Continued*

Most Common...	Answer and Explanation
CNS findings in Hashimoto's thyroiditis	• **mental/emotional slowing,** • *uncommon findings:* * dementia, * deafness, * depression
hematologic findings in Hashimoto's thyroiditis	• **macrocytic anemia:** * PA, * membrane abnormalities, • *iron deficiency:* menorrhagia, • *increased incidence of malignant lymphoma of thyroid*
GI findings in Hashimoto's thyroiditis	• **constipation:** bowel hypomotility, • *macroglossia*
reproductive system findings in Hashimoto's thyroiditis	• *women:* * **menorrhagia** (amenorrhea less common), * *infertility,* • *men:* impotence
metabolic findings in Hashimoto's thyroiditis	• **hypercholesterolemia:** decreased LDL receptor synthesis, • *SIADH:* see Table 11–1, • *early S/S of thyrotoxicosis:* * early phase when gland is inflamed, * called hashitoxicosis
lab findings in primary hypothyroidism	• **high serum TSH:** best marker, • *low serum T_4,* • *low RTU/T_4BR,* • *low FT_4-I,* • *^{131}I:* not performed, • *high serum CH,* • *high serum CK:* myopathy
Rx of primary hypothyroidism	*levothyroxine:* goal is to bring serum TSH into normal range
Rx of primary hypothyroidism in pregnancy	*increase levothyroxine dose:* clearance of thyroxine increases in pregnancy (increase in TSH is noted)
Rx of primary hypothyroidism in patients with angina	*slow incremental increase in levothyroxine from low doses to higher doses depending on patient's tolerance*
causes of myxedema coma	• **idiopathic,** • *cold exposure,* • *use of sedatives/opiates,* • *acute illness*
S/S of myxedema coma	• **progressive stupor,** • *hypothermia,* • *bradycardia,* • *hypoventilation,* • *hypoglycemia,* • *hypocortisolism,* • *hyponatremia:* SIADH
Rx of myxedema coma	• **ventilatory support,** • *Rx hypothermia,* • *maintain hydration:* watch for SIADH, • *IV levothyroxine,* • *high doses of corticosteroid,* • *mortality:* 20–50%

Table 11–2. **THYROID DISORDERS** *Continued*

Most Common...	Answer and Explanation
causes of hyperthyroidism	• **Graves' disease,** • *toxic multinodular goiter:* Plummer's disease, • *toxic adenoma,* • *T₃ toxicosis* [Hyperthyroidism is defined as excess synthesis and release of thyroid hormone. Thyrotoxicosis refers to the end-organ effects of excess hormone regardless of cause (includes Graves' disease and others listed above).]
cause of Graves' disease	• **autoimmune disease with TSI antibodies directed against TSH receptor:** type II hypersensitivity, * HLA Dr3 relationship, • *inciting events:* * viral/bacterial infection, * *Yersinia enterocolitica* infection, * withdrawal of corticosteroids, * iodide excess, * lithium Rx, * postpartum
causes of thyrotoxicosis other than Graves' disease	• **acute/subacute thyroiditis,** • *factitious hyperthyroidism:* * excessive intake of hormone, * weight loss clinics, * eating ground meat with thyroid tissue, • *struma ovarii:* ovarian teratoma with functional thyroid tissue, • *choriocarcinoma:* hCG has TSH-like activity, • *metastatic follicular carcinoma,* • *Jodbasedow effect:* * common in iodide-deficient areas, * excess iodine induces hyperthyroidism (particularly in patients with toxic nodular goiter or on certain drugs; see below)
drug associated with Jodbasedow effect	*amiodarone* (antiarrhythmic drug): contains iodine
S/S unique to Graves' disease	• **exophthalmos,** • *pretibial myxedema,* • *thyroid acropachy:* nail separation, • *bruit heard over the gland:* very vascular
general findings in thyrotoxicosis	• **weight loss with increased appetite,** • *heat intolerance,* • *fatigue,* • *fine tremor of hands,* • *diffuse gland enlargement*
CNS findings in thyrotoxicosis	• **nervousness,** • *emotional lability*
GI findings in thyrotoxicosis	• **hyperdefecation,** • *diarrhea*

Table continued on following page

Table 11–2. THYROID DISORDERS *Continued*

Most Common...	Answer and Explanation
cardiovascular findings in thyrotoxicosis	• **sinus tachycardia,** • *palpitations,* • *atrial fibrillation:* common in the elderly, • *systolic HTN,* • *increased pulse pressure,* • *high output cardiac failure,* • *dyspnea*
cutaneous findings in thyrotoxicosis	• **warm, moist skin,** • *fine hair,* • *increased sweating,* • *hair loss*
musculoskeletal findings in thyrotoxicosis	• **proximal muscle weakness,** • *increased DTRs,* • *muscle atrophy,* • *osteoporosis:* increased bone turnover
eye findings in thyrotoxicosis	• **lid stare:** * present in any cause of thyrotoxicosis, * retraction of upper lid from excess sympathetic stimulation, • *exophthalmos:* * unique to Graves', * 20–40%, * infiltrative ophthalmopathy (GAGs infiltrate muscle, fat, soft tissue), * proptosis of eye, * impaired upward gaze, * periorbital edema, * ophthalmoplegia, * conjunctival irritation
clinical findings in apathetic hyperthyroidism	• *Graves' disease of elderly,* • *cardiac abnormalities:* * atrial fibrillation, * CHF, • *weakness,* • *apathy,* • *weight loss due to loss of appetite,* • *goiter:* no goiter in 20%
lab findings in hyperthyroidism/ thyrotoxicosis	• **low serum TSH:** <0.3 μU/mL, • *high serum T_4,* • *high RTU/T_4BR,* • *high FT_4-I,* • *increased ^{131}I uptake:* * Graves', * toxic multinodular goiter, * other hyperthyroid disorders, • *decreased ^{131}I uptake:* * thyroiditis, * patient taking excess hormone, • *low CH:* increased LDL receptor synthesis, • *hyperglycemia:* increased glycogenolysis/gluconeogenesis, • *absolute lymphocytosis,* • *hypercalcemia:* increased bone turnover
Rx of Graves' disease	• **ablation with ^{131}I:** * most common Rx for adults, * 80–90% reduced euthyroid/hypothyroid, * all eventually develop hypothyroidism, • *beta-blockers:* * decrease catecholamine effects, * Rx for all patients, • *thionamides:* see below, • *surgery:* * subtotal thyroidectomy, * primarily for Graves' disease in young patients or in pregnancy
side-effect of ablation Rx with ^{131}I	*hypothyroidism*

Table 11–2. THYROID DISORDERS *Continued*

Most Common...	Answer and Explanation
antithyroid drugs	• **PTU**, • *methimazole*
MOA of antithyroid drugs	• *block hormone synthesis:* * PTU also blocks peripheral conversion of T_4 to T_3, * PTU preferred in pregnancy (low doses due to teratogenic effects), • *side effects:* * agranulocytosis, * hepatitis, * vasculitis, • *Rx:* * 6–12 mths and stop drug, * some spontaneously revert to normal, *>50% have recurrence and are candidates for ^{131}I ablation
drugs used to prepare for thyroid surgery	• *antithyroid drugs:* render euthyroid, • *Rx with iodide:* * decreases vascularity, * decreases hormone release from colloid
causes of thyroid storm (thyrotoxic crisis)	• **inadequately treated patients with Graves' disease undergoing surgery,** • *infection,* • *trauma,* • *iodine,* • *pregnancy*
S/S of thyroid storm	• *hyperpyrexia,* • *tachyarrhythmias,* • *shock,* • *acute metabolic encephalopathy*
Rx of thyroid storm	• *inhibit hormone synthesis:* * PTU, * iodide, • *sympathetic blockade:* beta-blockers (not if CHF or asthma present), • *hydrocortisone,* • *IV fluids,* • *temperature cooling*
thyroid disorder in the United States	*nontoxic goiter*
types of nontoxic goiter	• **endemic,** • *sporadic* [A goiter refers to thyroid enlargement from excess colloid.]
cause of an endemic goiter	*iodide deficiency*
causes of sporadic goiter	• **goitrogens:** e.g., * turnips, * Brussels sprouts, * lithium, * thionamides, • *enzyme deficiencies,* • *puberty,* • *pregnancy,* • *elderly:* increasing incidence with age
mechanism of goiter formation	*absolute or relative deficiency of thyroid hormone:* * relative/absolute deficiency of hormone causes alternating hyperplasia/involution of gland, * initially diffusely enlarged and then becomes multinodular

Table continued on following page

Table 11–2. THYROID DISORDERS *Continued*

Most Common...	Answer and Explanation
complications associated with multinodular goiters	• **hemorrhage into a cyst:** sudden, painful, enlargement of gland, • *hoarseness:* laryngeal nerve compression, • *dyspnea:* tracheal compression, • *jugular vein compression:* neck congestion (Pemberton's sign), • *hypothyroidism,* • *toxic multinodular goiter:* Plummer's disease (not a Graves' variant)
lab test ordered in a patient with a goiter	*serum TSH:* evaluates functional status of thyroid (e.g., overactive, underactive, normal)
Rx of a goiter	• **thyroxine:** * reduces gland size, * achieves euthyroid state, • *surgery:* if compressive symptoms persist
causes of a "cold" solitary thyroid nodule in a woman	• **non-neoplastic cyst:** 60%, • *follicular adenoma:* 25%, • *cancer:* 15% [85–90% of solitary nodules are nonfunctional.]
cause of a "hot" nodule	*toxic nodular goiter*
risk factors for a nodule representing cancer	• **previous history of radiation to head/neck area:** papillary cancer most common, • *child,* • *adult male,* • *nodule with palpable cervical lymph nodes*
initial steps in evaluation of a solitary nodule	*FNA:* * sensitivity 95–98%, * benign FNA report → periodic follow-up, * suspicious aspirate → thyroid scanning: excise cold nodules, observe/ablate hot nodules, * malignant aspirate → surgery
benign thyroid tumor	*follicular adenoma:* "cold" nodules
endocrine gland cancer	*papillary adenocarcinoma:* ~70–80%
histologic findings in papillary adenocarcinoma	• **papillary fronds,** • *psammoma bodies,* • *multicentricity:* 25–50%, • *often contains follicular cancer:* still considered papillary cancer, • *lymphatic invasion with spread to cervical lymph nodes*
extranodal sites of papillary cancer metastasis	• **lungs,** • *bone*

Table 11–2. THYROID DISORDERS *Continued*

Most Common...	Answer and Explanation
Rx of papillary cancer	• **near total/total thyroidectomy with removal of suspicious lymph nodes:** surgery followed by suppressive T_4 therapy which reduces tumor recurrence, • *ablative ^{131}I therapy depending on extent of tumor,* • *prognosis:* 20-y mortality rate 5–15%, * thyroglobulin levels detect cancer recurrence
thyroid cancer associated with vessel invasion	*follicular carcinoma:* * ~10%, * invasive or encapsulated variants, * vessel invasion (~60%), * lymphatic invasion with lymph node metastasis uncommon (<10%), * lung/bone common metastatic sites
Rx of follicular carcinoma	• **near total/total thyroidectomy:** surgery followed by suppressive T_4 therapy (reduces tumor recurrence), • *ablative ^{131}I therapy depending on extent of tumor:* * follicular cancers concentrate ^{131}I, * ^{131}I used in metastasis, • *prognosis:* * 10-y survival ~60%, * serum thyroglobulin detects cancer recurrence
cell of origin of medullary carcinoma	*parafollicular C cells:* * parafollicular cells synthesize calcitonin (tumor marker), * most cases sporadic (80%), * 20% MEN IIa/IIb AD syndromes
clinical differences distinguishing hereditary from sporadic medullary carcinoma	• *younger age bracket,* • *C cell hyperplasia:* precursor for medullary cancer, • *multicentric,* • *better 5-y survival than sporadic cancer*
products secreted by medullary carcinoma	• **calcitonin,** • *ACTH,* • serotonin, • histaminase
stimulation test to detect C cell hyperplasia	*IV infusion of pentagastrin and calcium gluconate:* in patients with C cell hyperplasia calcitonin levels increase
genetic testing to R/O familial medullary carcinoma	*PCR detection of DNA mutation of RET-proto-oncogene*
Rx of medullary carcinoma	• **near total to total thyroidectomy with a modified lymph node dissection,** • *calcitonin used to detect tumor recurrence,* • *prognosis:* * 5-y survival for sporadic cancer ~50%, * MEN IIa 80%, * MEN IIb 50%

Table continued on following page

Table 11–2. THYROID DISORDERS *Continued*

Most Common...	Answer and Explanation
cause of primary malignant lymphoma of the thyroid	*pre-existing Hashimoto's thyroiditis:* majority are diffuse, B cell, large cell type
Rx of malignant lymphoma of thyroid	*radiotherapy:* 5-y survival ~50%

Question: Which of the following clinical or laboratory findings occur more often in Graves' disease rather than in thyrotoxicosis secondary to excessive intake of thyroxine? **SELECT 4**
- (A) Increased ^{131}I uptake
- (B) Suppressed serum TSH
- (C) Lid stare
- (D) Pretibial myxedema
- (E) Systolic hypertension
- (F) Thyroid-stimulating antibodies
- (G) High RTU
- (H) Enlarged thyroid

Answers: (A), (D), (F), (H): The ^{131}I uptake (choice A) is increased in Graves' disease and decreased in patients taking excess hormone. Both conditions have suppressed TSH (choice B is incorrect), lid stare (choice C is incorrect), systolic hypertension (choice E is incorrect), and a high RTU (choice G is incorrect). Graves' disease is more likely to have pretibial myxedema (choice D), thyroid-stimulating antibody (choice F), and thyromegaly (choice H). The thyroid gland is nonpalpable in patients taking excess hormone.

ACTH = adrenocorticotropic hormone, AD = autosomal dominant, CAD = coronary artery disease, CH = cholesterol, CHF = congestive heart failure, CK = creatine kinase, CNS = central nervous system, DTRs = deep tendon reflexes, Dx = diagnosis, ESR = erythrocyte sedimentation rate, FNA = fine needle aspiration, FT₄-I = free T₄-index, GAG = glycosaminoglycans, GI = gastrointestinal, G/M = gross and microscopic, hCG = human chorionic gonadotropin, HLA = human leukocyte antigen, HTN = hypertension, [131]I = radioactive iodine uptake, IV = intravenous, LDL = low density lipoprotein, MEN = multiple endocrine neoplasia, MOA = mechanism of action, NSAIDs = nonsteroidal anti-inflammatory drugs, PA = pernicious anemia, PCR = polymerase chain reaction, PTU = propylthiouracil, R/O = rule out, RTU = resin T₃ uptake, Rx = treatment, SIADH = syndrome of inappropriate antidiuretic hormone, S/S = signs and symptoms, T₃ = triiodothyronine, T₄ = thyroxine, *T₃ = radioactive T₃, TBG = thyroid binding globulin, T₄BR = thyroxine binding ratio, TSH = thyroid stimulating hormone, TSI = thyroid stimulating immunoglobulin, URI = upper respiratory infection.

Table 11–3. CALCIUM/PHOSPHORUS DISORDERS AND METABOLIC BONE DISEASE

Most Common...	Answer and Explanation
functions of PTH	• *increases proximal renal tubule reabsorption of calcium,* • *decreases proximal reabsorption of phosphate and reclamation of* HCO_3^-, • *increases 1 α-hydroxylase synthesis:* second hydroxylation of vitamin D, • *increases bone resorption to maintain serum ionized calcium* [PTH receptors are on osteoblasts. When activated, osteoblasts release IL-1 (osteoclast activating factor). IL-1 stimulates osteoclasts to remove calcium from bone. Estrogen and testosterone have an inhibitory effect on IL-1.]
functions of vitamin D	*increases jejunal reabsorption of calcium/phosphorus*
parathyroid disorder	*primary hyperparathyroidism* (HPTH)
cause of ambulatory hypercalcemia	*primary HPTH:* >50% are asymptomatic and are discovered as an incidental finding
cause of primary HPTH	• **parathyroid adenoma:** * 85%, * female dominant, * right inferior gland most often involved, • *primary parathyroid hyperplasia,* • *parathyroid cancer*
cardiovascular findings in primary HPTH	• **diastolic HTN,** • *arrhythmias,* • *potentiates digitalis toxicity,* • *short QT interval*
GI findings in primary HPTH	• **constipation,** • *PUD:* calcium stimulates gastrin release, • *pancreatitis:* calcium activates pancreatic enzymes
renal findings in primary HPTH	• **renal stones:** * most common symptomatic presentation, * 5% of patients with a first renal stone have HPTH, * 15% chance of HPTH if recurrent calcium stones, • *polyuria:* nephrocalcinosis leads to tubular dysfunction and nephrogenic DI, • *CRF:* nephrocalcinosis
skeletal findings in primary HPTH	• **subperiosteal bone resorption of radial side of phalanges,** • *bone resorption of tooth socket,* • *osteitis fibrosa cystica:* * late bone finding, * hemorrhage into cyst, * jaw common site, * pathologic fractures, • *"salt and pepper" appearance of skull on radiograph,* • *increased incidence of chondrocalcinosis/ pseudogout of knee*

Table continued on following page

Table 11–3. CALCIUM/PHOSPHORUS DISORDERS AND METABOLIC BONE DISEASE *Continued*

Most Common...	Answer and Explanation
CNS findings in primary HPTH	• **personality changes**, • *depression*, • *psychosis*
sites for metastatic calcification in primary HPTH	• **kidneys:** nephrocalcinosis, • *skin;* pruritus, • *cornea:* band keratopathy
lab findings in primary HPTH	• **hypercalcemia**, • *hypophosphatemia*, • *high PTH:* * >90%, * 10% have "normal" PTH ("normal" PTH is abnormal in hypercalcemia), • *normal AG metabolic acidosis:* HCO_3^- loss in urine counterbalanced by gain in Cl^- ions, • *hypercalciuria:* amount filtered > amount reabsorbed, • *phosphaturia*, • Cl^-/ *phosphate ratio >33/1:* ratio <29/1 excludes HPTH
localizing studies used to confirm primary HPTH	• *noninvasive:* * CT scan, * US, * thallium-technetium subtraction scintigraphy, • *invasive:* selective venous sampling
Rx of primary HPTH	*surgery* [Total excision of parathyroid adenoma. In primary hyperplasia (all four glands involved), a small amount of tissue is left behind or some tissue is autotransplanted in the forearm or cryopreserved if the patient develops hypoparathyroidism.]
cause of hypercalcemia in hospitalized patients	*malignancy*
mechanisms of malignancy-induced hypercalcemia	• **metastasis to bone:** tumor releases osteoclast-activating factors (IL-1, prostaglandins), which resorb bone, • *secretion of PTH-like peptide:* increase calcium/decrease phosphorus reabsorption
cancer associated with hypercalcemia	*metastatic breast cancer to bone*
cancers secreting PTH-like peptide	• **squamous carcinoma of lung**, • *renal adenocarcinoma*, • *breast cancer*

Table 11–3. CALCIUM/PHOSPHORUS DISORDERS AND METABOLIC BONE DISEASE *Continued*

Most Common...	Answer and Explanation
lab findings in malignancy-induced hypercalcemia	• *hypercalcemia*, • *low PTH:* hypercalcemia suppresses endogenous PTH release [Assays are available for measuring PTH-like peptide.]
mechanism of hypercalcemia in sarcoidosis	*macrophages in granulomas synthesize 1 α-hydroxylase:* increases 1,25 [OH]$_2$D synthesis
mechanism of hypercalcemia in HTLV-1 malignant lymphoma	*similar to sarcoidosis:* see above
mechanism of hypercalcemia with thiazides	• **increased calcium reabsorption from urine**, • *volume depletion increases proximal tubule reabsorption of calcium*, • *subclinical HPTH is often present, which enhances calcium reabsorption*
mechanism of hypercalcemia in multiple myeloma	*intra-marrow release of IL-1* (osteoclast activating factor) *from malignant plasma cells*
mechanism of hypercalcemia in hypervitaminosis D	• **increased calcium reabsorption from the jejunum**, • *conversion of macrophages in the bone marrow into osteoclasts leading to increased bone resorption*
clinical findings in familial hypercalciuric hypercalcemia (FHH)	• *AD disease*, • *mechanism:* exaggerated renal calcium/magnesium from urine, * hypercalcemia does not suppress PTH (PTH slightly elevated), * hypermagnesemia enhances PTH activity, • *clinical:* hypercalcemia/renal stones develop <10 y of age
lab findings in FHH	• **hypercalcemia/low urine calcium**, • *calcium/creatinine clearance ratio <0.01/1*, • *slight PTH elevation*, • *hypermagnesemia*
mechanism of hypercalcemia in milk-alkali syndrome	*combination of absorbable calcium antacid* (baking soda) + *excess milk ingestion:* sequence of events: hypercalcemia (increased calcium reabsorption) → metabolic alkalosis (bicarbonate in antacid) → nephrocalcinosis → renal failure → hyperphosphatemia from renal failure drives calcium into soft tissue

Table continued on following page

Table 11–3. CALCIUM/PHOSPHORUS DISORDERS AND METABOLIC BONE DISEASE *Continued*

Most Common...	Answer and Explanation
mechanism of hypercalcemia in thyrotoxicosis	*increased bone resorption*
mechanism of hypercalcemia in Addison's disease	*volume contraction:* leads to increased proximal tubule reabsorption of calcium
Rx of hypercalcemia	• **induce diuresis with isotonic saline and follow-up with a loop diuretic,** • *bisphosphonates:* * drug of choice in severe hypercalcemia, * pamidronate most often used, • *calcitonin:* * receptors on osteoclasts, * inhibits osteoclastic activity, * blocks renal calcium reabsorption, • *plicamycin:* inhibits osteoclast resorption, • *gallium nitrate:* inhibits osteoclast resorption, • *glucocorticoids:* mainly for hypercalcemia due to: * hypervitaminosis D (e.g., sarcoidosis), * IL-1 (e.g., HTLV-1 lymphoma)
cause of hypocalcemia	*hypoalbuminemia* [Total calcium is calcium bound to albumin (40%), phosphates/sulfates (13%), and free (47%, ionized, metabolically active calcium). Hypoalbuminemia reduces total calcium without altering ionized calcium (no tetany). Formula to correct total calcium for hypoalbuminemia: corrected calcium = (measured calcium − serum albumin) + 4.]
pathologic cause of hypocalcemia in a hospitalized patient	*hypomagnesemia* [Magnesium enhances PTH activity, increases PTH release from the parathyroids, and is a cofactor for adenylate cyclase (necessary for PTH function). Hypomagnesemia causes an acquired hypoparathyroidism with decreased renal reabsorption of calcium.]
causes of hypomagnesemia	• **diuretics,** • *diarrhea,* • *alcoholism,* • *drugs:* e.g., * aminoglycosides, * cisplatin
cause of primary hypoparathyroidism	• **previous thyroid surgery,** • *autoimmune destruction:* second MCC
sign of hypoparathyroidism	*tetany:* * due to a low ionized calcium, * see clinical findings below

Table 11–3. CALCIUM/PHOSPHORUS DISORDERS AND METABOLIC BONE DISEASE *Continued*

Most Common...	Answer and Explanation
neuromuscular findings in hypoparathyroidism	• **tingling of the circumoral area, hands/feet**, • *Trousseau's sign:* carpopedal spasm while measuring blood pressure, • *Chvostek's sign:* facial muscle twitching with tapping of facial nerve, • *laryngeal stridor*, • *muscle cramping*
cardiovascular finding in hypoparathyroidism	*prolonged QT interval*
CNS findings in hypoparathyroidism	• **basal ganglia calcification:** high serum phosphate drives calcium into brain tissue, • *apathy*, • *benign intracranial HTN*, • *extrapyramidal signs*
skin findings in hypoparathyroidism	• *alopecia*, • *candidal infections*
eye findings in hypoparathyroidism	*cataracts*
lab findings in primary hypoparathyroidism	• **hypocalcemia:** low ionized calcium, • *hyperphosphatemia*, • *low PTH*
cause of pseudohypo- parathyroidism	*AD disease with a defective receptor for PTH* (type I) or *post-receptor problem* (type II)
S/S of pseudohypo- parathyroidism	• *tetany*, • *mental retardation*, • *short 4th/5th metacarpal bones:* "knuckle-knuckle-dimple-dimple" sign, • *basal ganglia calcification*
lab findings in pseudohypo- parathyroidism	• **hypocalcemia**, • *hyperphosphatemia*, • *normal to high PTH*, • *increased urine cAMP after PTH infusion in type II*, • *no increase in cAMP in type 1*
cause of tetany when total calcium is normal	*alkalosis* [Alkalosis (respiratory primarily, metabolic less commonly) increases negative charges on albumin. This further increases calcium binding to albumin at the expense of the ionized calcium pool. Total calcium level is unaltered.]
mechanism of hypocalcemia in hypovitaminosis D	*decreased calcium reabsorption from the jejunum*

Table continued on following page

Table 11–3. CALCIUM/PHOSPHORUS DISORDERS AND METABOLIC BONE DISEASE *Continued*

Most Common...	Answer and Explanation
mechanism of hypocalcemia in acute pancreatitis	*enzymatic fat necrosis:* calcium is consumed by binding to fatty acids
mechanism of hypocalcemia in CRF	• **hypovitaminosis D**, • *hyperphosphatemia:* * drives calcium into soft tissue/bone, * called metastatic calcification
mechanism of hypocalcemia in malabsorption	*malabsorption of vitamin D*
Rx of hypocalcemia	• *oral calcium*, • *IV calcium:* emergency conditions, • *vitamin D:* in hypovitaminosis D
causes of secondary HPTH	• **CRF**, • *malabsorption:* hypovitaminosis D, • *hyperphosphatemia:* drives calcium into soft tissue/bone [In CRF, the second hydroxylation of vitamin D does not occur, leading to hypovitaminosis D → hypocalcemia → stimulus for PTH synthesis (all four glands are hyperplastic).]
cause of tertiary HPTH	*CRF* [Secondary HPTH from CRF may raise serum calcium levels into normal and then into an elevated range, the latter referred to as tertiary HPTH. Parathyroid glands eventually become resistant to normal physiologic stimuli (glands become autonomous).]
causes of hyperphosphatemia	• **CRF**, • *increased phosphate load:* transfusion of old blood, • *primary hypoparathyroidism*, • *normal childhood*
clinical finding associated with hyperphosphatemia	• **metastatic calcification:** drives calcium into kidneys (renal failure), skin/soft tissue, • *hypovitaminosis D:* * high $PO_4^=$ inhibits 1-α hydroxylase synthesis, * leads to hypocalcemia, • *secondary HPTH:* due to hypocalcemia, • *renal osteodystrophy:* due to * secondary HPTH, * renal failure (metabolic acidosis), * see Table 10–4
Rx of hyperphosphatemia	• **oral calcium bicarbonate with meals**, • *dialysis*

Table 11–3. CALCIUM/PHOSPHORUS DISORDERS AND METABOLIC BONE DISEASE *Continued*

Most Common...	Answer and Explanation
acquired causes of hypophosphatemia	• **respiratory/metabolic alkalosis:** alkalosis activates PFK with enhanced glycosis and phosphorylation of glucose, • *insulin Rx in DKA:* glucose requires phosphorus to remain in adipose/muscle, • *excess fructose intake:* phosphorus moves into cells to phosphorylate fructose, • *ingestion of phosphate binders:* aluminum, calcium, magnesium antacids, • *phosphaturic drugs:* * diuretics, * corticosteroids, • *hypovitaminosis D:* * malabsorption, * inadequate intake, * decreased sunlight, • *primary HPTH:* phosphaturia
genetic causes of hypophosphatemia	• **Fanconi syndrome:** see Table 10–4, • *vitamin D resistant rickets:* * SXD, * primary defect in reabsorption of $PO_4^=$ in kidneys/GI tract
clinical findings in hypophosphatemia	• **muscle weakness:** * respiratory paralysis (levels <1.0 mg/dL), * low ATP, • *RBC hemolysis:* spectrin must be phosphorylated, • *rhabdomyolysis:* muscles need ATP
Rx of hypophosphatemia	**oral replacement:** preferred route, • *parenteral:* for severe depletion
metabolic bone disease	*osteoporosis:* * reduction in bone mass, * bone remaining behind is normally mineralized
causes of osteopenia	• **osteoporosis**, • *osteomalacia* [Osteopenia ("poverty of bone") is a bone mass value 1–2.5 SD below the young adult mean. Osteomalacia is decreased bone mineralization with normal to excess amounts of structurally normal osteoid. Osteoporosis/osteomalacia have "washed out" bone on radiography.]
mechanisms of osteoporosis	• **increased resorption of bone matrix:** osteoporosis develops in areas of *high turnover* of trabecular matrix/cortical bone (e.g., vertebral column), • *decreased formation of bone matrix:* low turnover

Table continued on following page

Table 11–3. CALCIUM/PHOSPHORUS DISORDERS AND METABOLIC BONE DISEASE *Continued*

Most Common...	Answer and Explanation
primary types of osteoporosis	• **type I, or postmenopausal osteoporosis:** high turnover, • *type II, or senile osteoporosis*
mechanism involved in postmenopausal (type I) osteoporosis	*increased resorption of trabecular bone:* * estrogen normally dampens release of osteoclast activating factor (OAF) from PTH-stimulated osteoblasts, * estrogen lack leads to greater osteoclastic breakdown of trabecular bone than formation of bone by osteoblasts
fracture sites for postmenopausal osteoporosis	• **vertebral column:** compression fractures, • *Colles' fracture of distal radius*
mechanism involved in senile (type II) osteoporosis	• **low bone turnover,** • *decreased bone formation* [There is a reduction in trabecular/cortical bone. Axial appendicular skeletal fractures are more prevalent.]
fracture sites in senile osteoporosis	• **femoral neck,** • *proximal humerus,* • *pelvis*
secondary causes of osteoporosis	• *endocrine disorders:* e.g., * Cushing's, * hyperthyroidism, * primary HPTH, * hypogonadism, • *drugs*; e.g., * heparin, * corticosteroids, • *genetic disorders:* e.g., * osteogenesis imperfecta (♦ defect in type I collagen synthesis), * sickle cell disease, • *renal failure:* osteoporosis due to * chronic metabolic acidosis, * secondary HPTH, • *immobilization*, • *lack of gravity:* common in space travel, • *malignancy:* PTH-like peptide
risk factors for developing osteoporosis	• *smoking*, • *sedentary lifestyle*, • *estrogen deficiency*, • *weight loss syndromes*
clinical findings in osteoporosis	• **pathologic fractures,** • *bone pain,* • *reduced height,* • *Dowager's cervical hump*
radiographic findings in osteoporosis	• **osteopenia:** third metacarpal bone good index, • *trabecular stress lines:* best noted in femoral neck/lateral spine radiographs, • *cortical thinning*, • *prominent vertebral endplates*, • *"codfish" appearance of vertebrae:* biconcavity of vertebrae

Table 11–3. CALCIUM/PHOSPHORUS DISORDERS AND METABOLIC BONE DISEASE *Continued*

Most Common...	Answer and Explanation
lab test to diagnose osteoporosis	• **dual-photon absorptiometry:** * noninvasive test that measures bone density at the distal radius, • *quantitative CT*
lab tests that measure bone turnover	• *osteocalcin:* released from increased osteoclastic resorption of bone, • *pyridinium collagen cross-links:* constituent of bone collagen released with bone resorption, • *serum calcium/phosphorus, alkaline phosphatase:* normal
recommendations for prevention of postmenopausal osteoporosis	• **estrogen with/without progestin:** * estrogen inhibits bone resorption (reduces fracture risk by 50%), * estrogen reduces risk of CAD by 50% (maintains high HDL levels), * progestin protects against endometrial cancer (risk of 0.1%/y), * progestin unnecessary if uterus is absent, • *exercise:* * weight-bearing types, * swimming is not recommended as a substitute, • *calcium 1000/1500 mg/d:* * former dose for women with adequate estrogen, * latter dose for those lacking estrogen, • *vitamin D 400 U/d*
drugs used in Rx of established osteoporosis	• **estrogen,** • *exercise,* • *vitamin D:* as above, • *calcium:* as above, • *other drugs inhibiting bone resorption:* * **bisphosphonates** (orally administered alendronate most often used), * calcitonin (♦ analgesic effect, ♦ best for axial skeleton, ♦ good for high turnover states), • *fluoride:* * *not* recommended, * inadequate mineralization of new bone matrix, * accumulates in non-mineralized bone, * increases mineralization in vertebrae at the expense of appendicular skeleton
cause of osteoporosis in men	*low testosterone levels:* occurs later in men owing to a greater skeletal mass than women
fracture site for osteoporosis in men	*hip*
causes of osteomalacia	*refer to Table 9–11*

Table continued on following page

Table 11–3. CALCIUM/PHOSPHORUS DISORDERS AND METABOLIC BONE DISEASE *Continued*

Most Common...	Answer and Explanation
benign cause of a markedly elevated alkaline phosphatase in an elderly man	*Paget's disease of bone* (osteitis deformans)
cause of Paget's disease of bone	• **? slow virus disease:** targets osteoclasts, • *genetic predisposition*
phases of Paget's disease of bone	*osteoclastic → osteoblastic → sclerotic* [Bone formed after the osteoblastic phase is structurally weak mosaic bone.]
sites of predilection of Paget's disease	• **pelvis**, • *skull*, • *femur*, • *tibia*, • *spine*
clinical findings in Paget's disease	• **bone pain**, • *bone deformities:* * enlarged skull, * kyphosis, * bowed legs, • *pathologic fractures*, • *bone tumors*, • *high output cardiac failure:* mosaic bone is vascular, • *deafness:* bone enlargement, • *cranial nerve palsies/vascular compression:* bone enlargement
bone tumor in Paget's disease	*osteogenic sarcoma:* 1–3% risk
radiographic studies performed in Paget's disease	• **bone scan:** increased uptake, • *plain radiographs:* * ragged lytic areas, * fractures, * deformities
lab findings in Paget's disease	• **elevated alkaline phosphatase:** osteoblastic phase, • *increased urine excretion of pyridinium-collagen cross-links:* mainly in osteoclastic phase, • *increased urine hydroxyproline:* increased bone turnover, • *hypercalcemia:* if patient is immobilized
Rx of Paget's disease	• **bisphosphonates:** * IV pamidronate, * oral alendronate, • *calcitonin*

Table 11–3. CALCIUM/PHOSPHORUS DISORDERS AND METABOLIC BONE DISEASE *Continued*

Questions 1–7: The sets of options are followed by several numbered items. For each numbered item, select the **ONE** lettered option that is **MOST CLOSELY** associated with it. Each lettered option may be selected once, more than once, or not at all.

(A) Hypocalcemia/low PTH
(B) Hypocalcemia/high PTH
(C) Hypercalcemia/high PTH
(D) Hypercalcemia/low PTH
(E) Hypocalcemia/normal PTH
(F) Normocalcemia/High PTH

1. Patient with primary aldosteronism presents with tetany
2. Patient with previous history of thyroid cancer presents with tetany
3. Patient with breast cancer and lower lumbar pain
4. Patient with kwashiorkor has hypocalcemia and no signs of tetany
5. Patient has recurrent calcium stones and peptic ulcer disease
6. Patient with hypomagnesemia has tetany
7. Patient with chronic renal failure

Answers: 1. (F), 2. (A), 3. (D), 4. (E), 5. (C), 6. (A), 7. (B): Primary aldosteronism (1) is associated with metabolic alkalosis. Alkalosis increases negative charges on albumin. This leads to binding of some of the ionized calcium to albumin, thereby reducing the total calcium (tetany), without increasing PTH without reducing the total calcium (tetany). Since surgery is the Rx of choice for thyroid cancer (2) and the patient has tetany, primary hypoparathyroidism is likely (choice F). A patient with previous low serum calcium, low PTH, **choice A**. A patient with breast cancer (3) who has bone pain most likely has hypercalcemia due to bone metastasis. Hypercalcemia lowers the serum PTH. This is an example of malignancy-induced hypercalcemia (**choice D**). Kwashiorkor (4) is characterized by a low protein intake, hence hypo-albuminemia occurs. This automatically lowers the total serum calcium (40% of calcium is bound to albumin) without altering the ionized calcium, hence serum PTH is normal (**choice E**). A patient with recurrent calcium oxalate stones and an increased PTH is most likely has (5) PUD and most likely has primary HPTH, therefore hypercalcemia and an increased PTH is likely (**choice C**). Hypomagnesemia (6) inhibits the release of PTH and its target organ effect on cAMP, producing hypoparathyroidism with a low serum calcium and PTH (**choice A**). Chronic renal failure produces hypovitaminosis D with subsequent hypocalcemia and elevation of PTH (secondary) HPTH, **choice B**).

AD = autosomal dominant, ATP = adenosine triphosphate, CAD = coronary artery disease, cAMP = cyclic adenosine monophosphate, CNS = central nervous system, CRF = chronic renal failure, CT = computed tomography, DKA = diabetic ketoacidosis, FHH = familial hypocalciuric hypercalcemia, GI = gastrointestinal, HDL = high density lipoprotein, HPTH = hyperparathyroidism, HTLV-1 = human T cell lymphotropic virus, HTN = hypertension, IL-1 = interleukin 1, IV = intravenous, MCC = most common cause, OAF = osteoclast activating factor, PFK = phosphofructokinase, PTH = parathormone, PUD = peptic ulcer disease, RBC = red blood cell, Rx = treatment, S/S = signs and symptoms, SXD = sex-linked dominant, US = ultrasonography.

Table 11–4. ADRENAL DISORDERS, MULTIPLE ENDOCRINE NEOPLASIA, AND POLYENDOCRINOPATHY SYNDROMES

Most Common...	Answer and Explanation
hormones synthesized in zona glomerulosa	• *aldosterone:* * ATII activates 18-OHase enzyme, which converts corticosterone into aldosterone, * see Table 3–3 questions on adrenal steroids, • *weak mineralocorticoids:* * deoxycorticosterone, * corticosterone
hormones synthesized in zona fasciculata/ reticularis	• *glucocorticoids,* • *17-ketosteroids:* * DHEA, * androstenedione, • *testosterone:* synthesized from androstenedione via an oxidoreductase reaction [ACTH stimulates the zona fasciculata/reticularis. The urine for 17-hydroxycorticoids measures 11-deoxycortisol and cortisol byproducts.]
cause of Cushing's syndrome	*exogenous administration of glucocorticoids*
pathologic causes of Cushing's syndrome	• **pituitary:** * Cushing's disease, * 60% of cases, • *adrenal:* * 25%, * functioning adenoma most common, • *ectopic Cushing's:* * 15%, * SCC of lung (50%), * endocrine tumors (♦ 35%, ♦ thymic carcinoid, ♦ medullary carcinoma of thyroid)
S/S of cortisol excess in Cushing's syndrome	• **central obesity:** * moon facies (75%), * buffalo hump, * truncal obesity, • *violaceous striae:* * 65%, * structurally weakened vessels are prominent in stretch marks, • *glucose intolerance:* 65%, • *proximal muscle weakness:* * 60%, * muscle breakdown, • *plethoric face:* * 60%, * stimulation of erythropoiesis, • *easy bruising:* * 40%, * vessel instability from weakened collagen, • *osteoporosis:* 40%

Table 11–4. ADRENAL DISORDERS, MULTIPLE ENDOCRINE NEOPLASIA, AND POLYENDOCRINOPATHY SYNDROMES *Continued*

Most Common...	Answer and Explanation
S/S of weak mineralocorticoid excess	• **weight gain:** * 90%, * salt/water retention, • *diastolic HTN:* 75%, • *hypokalemic metabolic alkalosis:* 15%
S/S of androgen excess	• **hirsutism:** * 65%, * increase in 17-KS, • *menstrual dysfunction:* 60%, • *acne:* 40%
type of Cushing's syndrome with hyperpigmentation	*ectopic Cushing's*
type of Cushing's syndrome with virilization	*adrenal Cushing's:* usually a carcinoma
screening tests for Cushing's syndrome	**24-h urine for free (unbound) cortisol:** * increased in >97%, * excess cortisol not bound to transcortin is excreted, • *1 mg low-dose dexamethasone suppression test:* * dexamethasone is a cortisol analogue, * no suppression of cortisol, * 13–25% FP rate (e.g., ♦ obesity, ♦ chronic disease, ♦ depression), • *loss of diurnal cortisol rhythm:* * useless test, * high in AM/PM, * normally high in AM and low in PM
confirmatory tests for Cushing's syndrome	**8 mg high-dose dexamethasone suppression test:** * cortisol suppression in pituitary Cushing's (partially autonomous), * no suppression in adrenal/ectopic Cushing's, • *plasma ACTH:* * lowest in adrenal Cushing's, * highest in ectopic Cushing's, * "normal" to increased in pituitary Cushing's
localizing tests for Cushing's syndrome	*CT/MRI sella first, then abdominal cavity if sella study is negative:* * normal sella in >50% pituitary Cushing's, * venous petrosal sinus sampling in equivocal pituitary Cushing's
Rx of pituitary Cushing's	*surgery*
Rx of adrenal Cushing's	• *unilateral adrenalectomy:* adenoma, • *unilateral adrenalectomy + o,p'-DDD:* carcinoma

Table continued on following page

Table 11–4. ADRENAL DISORDERS, MULTIPLE ENDOCRINE NEOPLASIA, AND POLYENDOCRINOPATHY SYNDROMES *Continued*

Most Common...	Answer and Explanation
Rx of ectopic Cushing's	• **surgical removal of tumor if operable,** • *block steroid synthesis if inoperable:* * ketoconazole, * metyrapone, * somatostatin analogue
cause of Nelson's syndrome	*bilateral adrenalectomy in a patient who has an underlying pituitary adenoma:* * drop in cortisol post-adrenalectomy causes further enlargement of pre-existing pituitary adenoma, * headache, * hyperpigmentation (excessive ACTH)
mineralocorticoid excess states	*see Table 5–4 discussions of primary aldosteronism, Bartter's syndrome, Liddle's syndrome*
adrenal medulla tumor in adults	*pheochromocytoma:* ~90% are * benign rather than malignant (usually familial type), * found in adults rather than children, * located in adrenal medulla rather than extra-adrenal sites, * sporadic rather than familial, * unilateral rather than bilateral (usually MEN IIa/IIb)
extra-adrenal sites of pheochromocytoma	• **abdominal cavity,** • *bladder,* • *organ of Zuckerkandl,* • *posterior mediastinum*
pheochromocytoma associations	• **MEN IIa/IIb,** • *von Hippel-Lindau disease,* • *neurofibromatosis*
S/S of a pheochromocytoma	• **diastolic HTN:** * 95%, * sustained (20%), * sustained with paroxysms (50%), * paroxysmal (25%), * resistant to standard Rx, • *headache:* 85%, • *palpitations:* 65%, • *drenching sweats:* 65%, • *abdominal pain:* ileus, • *postural hypotension,* • *chest pain:* subendocardial ischemia
screening tests to diagnose pheochromocytoma	• **24-h urine for metanephrine:** best test, • *24-h urine for VMA,* • *free catecholamines,* • *plasma catecholamines:* * levels >2000 ng/mL diagnostic, * <500 ng/mL excludes Dx, • *provocative tests:* * performed when plasma catecholamines between 500 and 2000 ng/mL, * glucagon or histamine are used
pheochromocytoma sites if epinephrine is secreted	• **adrenal medulla,** • *organ of Zuckerkandl* [These sites contain *N*-methyltransferase, which converts NOR into EPI. Other sites lack

Table 11–4. ADRENAL DISORDERS, MULTIPLE ENDOCRINE NEOPLASIA, AND POLYENDOCRINOPATHY SYNDROMES *Continued*

Most Common...	Answer and Explanation
Continued	this enzyme and only have an increase in NOR metabolites.]
ancillary lab findings in pheochromocytoma	• **neutrophilic leukocytosis:** decreased adhesion molecule synthesis (release of marginating pool), • *hyperglycemia:* * increased glycogenolysis, * enhanced gluconeogenesis
confirmatory tests to diagnose pheochromocytoma	*usually unnecessary:* if indicated, the clonidine suppression test is employed
radiographic studies to diagnose pheochromocytomas	• **MRI,** • *CT*
additional screening tests in patients with pheochromocytoma	• *MEN IIa/IIb:* screen for RET proto-oncogene, • *von Hippel-Lindau disease:* DNA testing to localize abnormal suppressor gene on chromosome 3
Rx of pheochromocytoma	*surgical excision:* * α-adrenergic blocking agents (e.g., phenoxybenzamine) are used preoperatively to control HTN, * after HTN control, beta-blockers control tachycardia
Rx of hypertensive crisis in pheochromocytoma	*phentolamine:* alpha-blocker
cause of acute adrenal insufficiency (adrenal crisis)	• **abrupt glucocorticoid withdrawal,** • *bilateral adrenal hemorrhage:* * **meningococcemia,** * trauma, * anticoagulation, • *Rx of primary hypopituitarism with thyroid hormone replacement before glucocorticoid replacement*
clinical findings of acute adrenal insufficiency	• **hypovolemic shock:** out of proportion to intercurrent illness, • *hyponatremia,* • *hyperkalemia,* • *prerenal azotemia,* • *abdominal pain,* • *eosinophilia:* loss of glucocorticoids, • *hypercalcemia:* volume depletion, • *fasting hypoglycemia:* reduced gluconeogenesis
causes of chronic primary adrenal insufficiency (Addison's disease)	• **autoimmune destruction:** Addison's disease, • *TB:* * most common global cause, * adrenal calcifications, • *histoplasmosis,* • *bilateral adrenal hemorrhage:* see above, • *AIDS:* disseminated CMV, • *drugs:* * ketoco-

Table continued on following page

**Table 11–4. ADRENAL DISORDERS, MULTIPLE
ENDOCRINE NEOPLASIA, AND POLYENDOCRINOPATHY
SYNDROMES** *Continued*

Most Common...	Answer and Explanation
Continued	nazole, * aminoglutemide, • *adrenoleukodystrophy:* * SXR, * high levels of very long chain fatty acids, • *adrenogenital syndrome:* * MCC in children, * see Table 3–3, • *metastasis:* lung cancer MCC
S/S of Addison's disease	• **weakness/weight loss:** 100%, • *hyperpigmentation:* * 95%, * due to MSH-like activity of increased ACTH, * sites: ♦ buccal mucosa, ♦ scars, ♦ nipples, • *orthostatic hypotension:* hypoaldosteronism
lab findings in Addison's disease	• **hyponatremia:** 90%, • *hyperkalemia:* * 65%, * cannot excrete K^+, • *normal AG metabolic acidosis:* cannot excrete H^+ ions, • *prerenal azotemia:* volume depletion, • *fasting hypoglycemia:* reduced gluconeogenesis, • *high plasma ACTH:* loss of negative feedback, • *hypercalcemia:* volume depletion, • *anti-adrenal antibodies:* ~50%, • *no cortisol response to short or prolonged ACTH stimulation,* • *hematologic abnormalities:* * due to hypocortisolism, * eosinophilia, * lymphocytosis, * neutropenia
Rx of Addison's disease	• *hydrocortisone:* treat glucocorticoid deficiency, • *fludrocortisone:* treat mineralocorticoid deficiency, • *increase salt intake*
lab distinctions between primary/ secondary hypocortisolism	• *serum Na^+:* more severe in primary vs secondary, • *serum K^+:* * hyperkalemia in primary, * no significant change in secondary, • *plasma ACTH:* * high in primary, * low in secondary, • *prolonged ACTH stimulation:* * no response in primary, * eventual response in secondary
cause of Waterhouse-Friderichsen syndrome	*disseminated meningococcemia (Neisseria meningitidis):* leads to * DIC, * bilateral adrenal hemorrhage, * shock, * death
disorders in MEN I syndrome (AD, Wermer's syndrome)	• **primary HPTH:** * 80%, * hypercalcemia, * bilateral parathyroid hyperplasia > adenomas, • *pancreatic islet cell tumor:* * 75%, * **usually ZE,** * insulinoma, • *pituitary adenoma:* * 60%, * usually nonfunctional, • *PUD*

Table 11–4. ADRENAL DISORDERS, MULTIPLE ENDOCRINE NEOPLASIA, AND POLYENDOCRINOPATHY SYNDROMES *Continued*

Most Common...	Answer and Explanation
disorders in MEN IIa syndrome (Sipple's syndrome)	• **medullary carcinoma of thyroid:** * >90%, * multicentric, * calcitonin increased, • *primary HPTH:* * 50%, * hypercalcemia, * adenoma/hyperplasia, • *pheochromocytoma:* * 20–35%, * usually bilateral [Screen family members for * RET mutations (>98% sensitivity), * medullary carcinoma (stimulation tests, total thyroidectomy if positive screen), * pheochromocytoma.]
disorders in MEN IIb syndrome	• **mucosal neuromas:** * >90%, * lips acromegaloid, * macroglossia, * *medullary carcinoma:* 80%, • *pheochromocytoma:* 60% [Screen family members as discussed for MEN IIa.]
tumors secreting ectopic hormones	*see Table 4–1*
dominant disorders in polyglandular deficiency type I	• **Addison's disease,** • *primary hypoparathyroidism,* • *mucocutaneous candidiasis* [AR inheritance. Mean age of onset is 12 y. No HLA association.]
dominant disorders in polyglandular deficiency type II	• **Addison's disease,** • *autoimmune thyroid disease,* • *type I-insulin dependent DM* [AD inheritance. Association with HLA DR3/DR4 haplotype. Mean age of onset is 24 y.]
endocrine tumors	*see Table 9–9*

Question: Which of the following clinical and/or lab abnormalities is a consistent feature in pheochromocytoma, pituitary Cushing's syndrome, and primary aldosteronism? **SELECT 1**
(A) Hypokalemia
(B) Hyperglycemia
(C) Diastolic hypertension
(D) Metabolic alkalosis
(E) Neutrophilic leukocytosis

Answer: (C): Hypokalemia and metabolic alkalosis are noted in both primary aldosteronism and pituitary Cushing's syndrome, owing to the increase in mineralocorticoids (aldosterone in the former and weak mineralocorticoids in the latter, **choices A and D are incorrect**). Hyperglycemia is present in pheochromocytoma and pituitary Cushing's syndrome (**choice B is incorrect**). The hyperkalemia in primary aldosteronism has an inhibitory effect on insulin release. Neutrophilic leukocytosis is noted in pheochromocytoma and pituitary Cushing's syndrome (**choice E is incorrect**).

ACTH = adrenocorticotropic hormone, AD = autosomal dominant, AG = anion gap, AIDS = acquired immunodeficiency syndrome, AR = autosomal recessive, ATII = angiotensin II, CMV = cytomegalovirus, CT = computed tomography, DHEA = dehydroepiandrosterone, DIC = disseminated intravascular coagulation, DM = diabetes mellitus, Dx = diagnosis, EPI = epinephrine, FP = false positive, HLA = human leukocyte antigen, HTN = hypertension, HPTH = hyperparathyroidism, 17-KS = 17-ketosteroid, MCC = most common cause, MEN = multiple endocrine neoplasia, MRI = magnetic resonance imaging, MSH = melanocyte-stimulating hormone, NOR = norepinephrine, PUD = peptic ulcer disease, SCC = small cell carcinoma, Rx = treatment, S/S = signs and symptoms, SXR = sex-linked recessive, TB = tuberculosis, ZE = Zollinger-Ellison syndrome.

Table 11–5. DIABETES MELLITUS, HYPOGLYCEMIA

Most Common...	Answer and Explanation
classification scheme for DM	• **primary DM:** * type I (10–20%), * **type II** (80–90%, * subtypes: ♦ obese [80%], ♦ non-obese, maturity onset type), • *secondary DM:* * pancreatic disease (e.g., CF), * drugs (e.g., glucocorticoids, pentamidine, thiazides, streptozotocin, α-interferon), * endocrine disease (e.g., pheochromocytoma), * genetic disease (e.g., hemochromatosis, myotonic dystrophy), * insulin-receptor deficiency (acanthosis nigricans), * infections (congenital rubella, CMV), • *impaired glucose tolerance,* • *gestational DM*
differences between type I and II DM	• *age:* * I: <20 yrs old, * II: >30 yrs old, • *body habitus:* * I: thin, * II: obese, • *pathogenesis:* * I: absolute insulin lack, * II: ♦ relative insulin deficiency, ♦ insulin resistance (receptor deficiency, post-receptor defect), • *HLA relationships:* * I: Dr3/Dr4, * II: none, • *family history:* * I: none, * II: multifactorial inheritance, • *concordance rate:* * I, 50%, * II: ~100%, • *ketoacidosis:* * I: yes, II: no, • *Rx:* * I: insulin dependent, * II: ♦ diet, ♦ oral drugs, ♦ insulin in some cases
antibodies noted in type I	• **anti-islet cell antibodies:** * directed against glutamic acid decarboxylase, * marker rather than cause of β-islet cell deficiency, • *anti-insulin antibodies:* present before insulin Rx, • *autoantibodies against tyrosine phosphatases* [One or more of the above antibodies are present in 85–90%. There is a strong HLA relationship with presence of antibodies.]

Table 11–5. DIABETES MELLITUS, HYPOGLYCEMIA
Continued

Most Common...	Answer and Explanation
agents associated with β-islet cell destruction in type I	• **viruses:** * coxsackie B, * mumps, * EBV, * rubella, • *autoimmune destruction:* * cytotoxic T cells, * "insulitis," • *environmental factors:* * drugs (see above), * exposure of infants to bovine albumin
factors increasing insulin resistance in type II DM	• *pre-receptor:* anti-insulin antibodies, • *receptor:* * down-regulation of insulin receptors due to obesity/hyperinsulinemia, * antibodies against insulin receptors, • *post-receptor:* * defects in glycogen synthesis, * tyrosine kinase abnormalities, * problems with GLUT-4 translocation to cell membrane (adipose, muscle) to bind glucose
effect of obesity on glucose metabolism	*down-regulation of insulin receptor synthesis:* underscores role of diet in Rx of type II DM
clinical features of MODY	• *AD:* three genetic loci (chromosomes 7, **12**, 20), • *mild hyperglycemia:* impaired glucose stimulation of insulin release, • *resistance to ketosis*
clinical features of syndrome X	• **hyperinsulinemia:** genetic defect producing insulin resistance, • *hyperglycemia,* • *hyperlipidemia:* * increased VLDL due to increased insulin, * increased atherosclerosis risk, • *obesity:* exacerbates insulin resistance by down-regulating insulin receptor synthesis, • *HTN:* * Na^+ retention, * ? role of hyperinsulinemia
pathologic processes in DM	• **NEG:** * glucose combines with amino groups in basement membranes, Hb, LDL, * advanced glycosylation products produced: ♦ enhance atherosclerosis, ♦ increase vessel permeability, ♦ produce oxidized LDL, • *osmotic damage:* aldose reductase in Schwann cells, lens, pericytes around retinal vessels convert glucose into sorbitol (osmotically active) leading to cell damage
diseases where DM is MCC	• *peripheral neuropathy,* • *nontraumatic leg amputation,* • *blindness:* true for persons aged 30–65 y old, • *chronic renal disease,* • *multiple cranial nerve palsies*

Table continued on following page

Table 11–5. DIABETES MELLITUS, HYPOGLYCEMIA
Continued

Most Common...	Answer and Explanation
clinical presentation of type I DM	• **abrupt-onset polyuria, polydipsia, polyphagia, unexplained weight loss,** • *nocturia,* • *volume depletion,* • *DKA,* • *coma*
clinical presentation of type II DM	• **insidious onset,** • *recurrent blurry vision:* * alteration of lens refraction by sorbitol, * constant changing of glasses, • *recurrent infections:* * bacterial, * *Candida,* • *target organ disease:* e.g., * nephropathy, * retinopathy, * neuropathy, * AMI, • *pruritus,* • *HNKC,* • *reactive hypoglycemia*
complication of type I DM	*insulin-induced hypoglycemia:* * 10–25% have severe hypoglycemia at least once a year, * hypoglycemia occurs in type II DM patients taking long-acting sulfonylureas
S/S of insulin-induced hypoglycemia	• **sympathetic signs:** * sweating, * tachycardia, * palpitations, * tremulousness, • *parasympathetic signs:* * nausea, * hunger, • *others:* * focal neurologic deficits, * mental confusion, * coma
complications in hypoglycemia	• **irreversible brain damage,** • *seizures,* • *induce cardiac arrhythmias*
Rx of hypoglycemia	• **candy bar,** • *glucagon injection:* eventually lose glucose response to glucagon, • *infusion of 50% glucose in comatose patients*
precipitating causes of DKA	• **medical illness,** • *omission of insulin,* • *unknown*
clinical presentation of DKA	• **N/V,** • *abdominal pain:* * acute pancreatitis from increased TG, * decreased splanchnic blood flow from increased TG, • *severe volume depletion:* * hypotension, * decreased skin turgor, • *eruptive xanthoma:* * hyperchylomicronemia syndrome, * see Table 5–2, • *lipemia retinalis:* * hyperchylomicronemia syndrome, * blurry vision, • *coma*
causes of hyperglycemia in DKA	• **increased gluconeogenesis:** glucagon effect, • *increased glycogenolysis:* * glucagon, * catecholamines
cause of lipolysis in DKA	*activation of hormone-sensitive lipase in adipose:* * glucagon, * catecholamines [FAs/glycerol released. Glycerol is used as a substrate for gluconeogenesis. FAs are β-oxidized.]

Table 11–5. DIABETES MELLITUS, HYPOGLYCEMIA
Continued

Most Common...	Answer and Explanation
cause of ketoacidosis in DKA	*β-oxidation of FAs:* increased formation of acetyl CoA → liver converts into AcAc, acetone, β-OHB
cause of an increase in VLDL and chylomicrons in DKA	*decreased capillary lipoprotein lipase activity owing to insulin deficiency* [Insulin normally activates capillary lipoprotein lipase to remove FAs/glycerol from chylomicrons and VLDL. Glycerol enters hepatocytes and is used to synthesize more VLDL. FAs enter adipose to combine with glycerol-3 phosphate to synthesize TG. Hormone sensitive lipase is inhibited to keep TG in the adipose.]
cause of volume depletion in DKA	*osmotic diuresis from glucosuria with loss of water, sodium, and potassium* [~6 liters of hypotonic salt solution are lost when patients present with DKA. Volume repletion with crystalloids is the most important initial step in management.]
lab findings in DKA	• **hyperglycemia/hyperketonemia:** glucose ranges from 250–1000 mg/dL, • *dilutional hyponatremia:* * glucose draws water out of ICF, * see Table 10–2, • *hyperkalemia:* * transcellular shift due to increased H^+ ions, * patient actually has ~300–500 mEq loss K^+ depletion due to osmotic diuresis, * see Table 10–2, • *increased AG metabolic acidosis:* * ketoacidosis, * lactic acidosis, * see Table 10–2, • *prerenal azotemia:* volume depletion, • *hypophosphatemia:* may occur when insulin is infused and phosphate enters adipose/muscle to phosphorylate glucose
Rx of DKA	• **volume replacement with crystalloids:** * 0.9% normal saline or Ringer's lactate until volume deficit is corrected, * switch to 0.45% saline after volume restoration, • *monitor glucose/electrolytes/ABGs/serum ketones:* see above lab findings, • *insulin Rx:* * IV infusion of regular insulin, * add 5% dextrose in 0.45% saline when serum glucose reaches ~300 mg/dL, * maintain glucose 200–250 mg/dL, • *add K^+ to IV infusions:* insulin drives K^+ into cells and uncovers K^+ deficit, • *add potassium phosphate to IV infusions if*

Table continued on following page

Table 11–5. DIABETES MELLITUS, HYPOGLYCEMIA
Continued

Most Common...	Answer and Explanation
Continued	phosphate <1 mg/dL: avoid respiratory paralysis, • *infuse bicarbonate if arterial pH <7.1 until pH is 7.1* [Mortality in DKA is 5–10%.]
cause of false-negative ketone testing in DKA	*hypovolemic shock increases anaerobic metabolism and increases NADH+, which increases AcAc conversion into β-OHB:* * β-OHB is not detected with the standard nitroprusside reaction, * restoration of volume deficits reverses tissue hypoxia and conversion of β-OHB into AcAc (test becomes positive)
cause of normal AG metabolic acidosis in Rx of DKA	*infusion of normal saline:* * contains Cl⁻ ions but does not contain bicarbonate, * Cl⁻ ions bind with excess H+ ions producing hyperchloremic normal AG metabolic acidosis, * dilutional effect of normal saline on bicarbonate concentration
cause of HNKC	*type II DM:* enough insulin to prevent ketogenesis but not hyperglycemia
precipitating causes of HNKC	• **medical illness:** e.g., * AMI, * pancreatitis, • *drugs:* e.g., thiazides, • *surgery*
complications of HNKC	• *AMI,* • *CVA,* • *hypoglycemia:* too much insulin given
Rx of HNKC	*similar to DKA except less insulin is necessary* [Mortality is 20–50% since patients are older and have target organ disease.]
ADA recommendation for microalbuminuria screening in type I and II DM	• *annual screening of type I patients with DM for ≥5 y,* • *immediate annual screening of all type II DM patients:* due to insidious onset of disease [Ratio of a random urine albumin (mg/dL)/creatinine (nmol/L) ≤3.5/1 is normal, ≥10/1 is abnormal, 3.6–9.9 borderline.]
causes/Rx of diabetic nephropathy	*see Table 10–3 discussion*
ADA recommendation for ophthalmologic exam in type I and II DM	*annual dilated eye and visual exams* (ophthalmologist or optometrist) *in:* * all patients 10 y and older with type I DM for 3–5 y, * all type II DM patients at time of Dx, * all DM patients who present with visual findings
types of eye disease in DM	• **retinopathy,** • *impaired pupillary reaction,* • *cataracts:* osmotic damage, • *glaucoma:* * 6%, * open angle type

Table 11–5. DIABETES MELLITUS, HYPOGLYCEMIA
Continued

Most Common...	Answer and Explanation
types of retinopathy in DM	• *background diabetic retinopathy:* * microaneurysms (osmotic damage of pericytes weakens vessel), * hard exudates (increased vessel permeability), * retinal edema, * focal macular abnormalities, • *pre-proliferative:* * soft exudates (infarction), * more diffuse retinal edema/macular disease, • *proliferative:* * capillary proliferation, * retinal detachment, * vitreous hemorrhage [If retinopathy is present, nephropathy is present.]
Rx of diabetic retinopathy	• **strict glycemic control,** • *HTN control,* • *laser photocoagulation*
Rx of pupillary reaction abnormalities	*panretinal photocoagulation*
Rx of cataracts	*surgical removal*
neurologic disorders in DM	• **peripheral neuropathy,** • *autonomic neuropathy,* • *neuromuscular disease:* * symmetrical atrophy of intrinsic muscles of hand (similar to ALS), * weakness of pelvic girdle/anterior thigh, • *stroke:* * due to enhanced atherosclerosis, * poor control of HTN, • *cranial nerve palsies:* * MCC of multiple cranial nerve palsies, * IIIrd, IVth, VIth nerve ocular palsies are common, * VIIth nerve Bell's palsy
type of peripheral neuropathy in DM	*distal sensorimotor neuropathy:* 50% have potentially disabling neuropathy
clinical finding in peripheral neuropathy	• **sensory changes:** * numbness/tingling of feet, * burning foot syndrome (worse at night), • *pressure ulcers,* • *motor changes:* * muscle atrophy, * loss of distal reflexes
Rx of peripheral neuropathy	• **good glycemic control,** • *amitriptyline,* • *topical capsaicin cream*
causes of DM pressure ulcers on feet	*peripheral neuropathy:* * cannot feel pressure, * complicated by ischemia/infection
Rx of DM pressure ulcers	• **debridement,** • *antibiotics,* • *correct maldistribution of pressure on foot,* • *improve peripheral circulation*

Table continued on following page

Table 11–5. DIABETES MELLITUS, HYPOGLYCEMIA
Continued

Most Common...	Answer and Explanation
GI findings due to autonomic neuropathy in DM	• **constipation:** follows diarrhea, • *gastric hypomotility:* see Table 9–3, • *diarrhea:* * impaired sympathetic inhibition → hypermotility, * bacterial overgrowth
cardiovascular findings due to autonomic neuropathy in DM	• **initial sinus bradycardia leading to a persistent resting tachycardia:** less heart beat drop than expected with a Valsalva maneuver, • *orthostatic hypotension:* * impaired sympathetic vasoconstrictor response, * Rx with fludrocortisone, • *inability to sense cardiac pain:* silent AMI
musculoskeletal finding due to autonomic neuropathy in DM	*neuropathic joint:* * usually affects ankles/feet, * bilateral, * osteolysis of bone noted on radiograph
sudomotor findings due to autonomic neuropathy in DM	• *distal anhidrosis,* • *nocturnal truncal/facial sweating,* • *heat intolerance,* • *gustatory sweating,* • *increased risk for heat stroke,* • *enhances foot ulcers:* keeps skin moist
Rx of sudomotor findings in DM	*anticholinergic agents*
urogenital findings due to autonomic neuropathy in DM	• **impotence:** * male: 50% (absent testicular sensitivity), * female: 25% (vaginal dryness), • *retrograde ejaculation,* • *neurogenic bladder:* * susceptible to urinary retention, * LUT/UUT infection
cause of HTN in DM	*diabetic nephropathy*
Rx for HTN in DM	• **ACE inhibitor:** * reduce BP, * normalizes intraglomerular pressure, * reduces proteinuria, * danger of ARF if bilateral renal artery stenosis is present, • *calcium channel blocker:* * nicardipine or diltiazem, * avoid nifedipine, • *α-adrenergic antagonists,* • *thiazides:* * not recommended, * enhance glucose intolerance (hypokalemia inhibits insulin release), * cause hyperlipidemia (increased LDL/TG), • *β-blockers:* * not recommended, * block adrenergic symptoms of hypoglycemia (except for sweating), * produce hyperlipidemia

Table 11–5. DIABETES MELLITUS, HYPOGLYCEMIA
Continued

Most Common...	Answer and Explanation
skin findings in DM	• ***Candida* vulvovaginitis,** • *necrobiosis lipoidica diabeticorum:* * well demarcated yellow plaques over anterior surface of legs/dorsum of ankles, * female dominance, • *eruptive xanthomas:* high TG levels, • *lipoatrophy:* * atrophy at insulin injection sites, * impure insulin, • *lipohypertrophy:* increased fat synthesis at insulin injection sites
infections noted in DM	• **cutaneous infections:** * *Staphylococcus aureus* abscesses, * skin pyodermas, • *UTIs:* * cystitis, * pyelonephritis, • *malignant external otitis: Pseudomonas aeruginosa,* • *rhinocerebral mucormycosis:* * occurs in poorly controlled DM, * extension of *Mucor* from sinuses through cribriform plate into frontal lobe, • *emphysematous cholecystitis:* anaerobic infection (*Clostridium perfringens* >50%) with gas formation
lab criteria for Dx of DM	• *random plasma glucose ≥200 mg/dL + classic symptoms of DM:* * polyuria, * polydipsia, * unexplained weight loss, • *FPG ≥126 mg/dL,* • *2-h glucose post 75-g glucose challenge ≥200 mg/dL* [Any of the above three criteria is a presumptive Dx of DM. To confirm DM, one of the three criteria must be present on a subsequent day.]
use of fasting plasma glucose (FPG)	• *FPG <110 mg/dL:* * normal, * fasting defined as no caloric intake for at least 8 h, • *FPG ≥110 and <125:* impaired fasting glucose (IFG), • *FPG ≥126 mg/dL:* * provisional DM, * confirm on subsequent day with one of the previously described three criteria
use of OGTT	• *2-h 75-g postload glucose <140 mg/dL:* normal, • *2-h 75-g postload glucose ≥140 mg/dL and <200 mg/dL:* IGT, • *2-h 75-g postload glucose ≥200 mg/dL:* * provisional DM, * confirm with previously described three criteria
use of HbA$_{Ic}$ in diagnosis of DM	*not currently recommended for Dx of DM*

Table continued on following page

Table 11–5. DIABETES MELLITUS, HYPOGLYCEMIA
Continued

Most Common...	Answer and Explanation
general steps in managing type I DM	• **insulin Rx,** • *nutrition,* • *exercise,* • *patient education*
sources of insulin	• **human:** recombinant DNA, • *beef,* • *pork,* • *fish*
types of insulin	• *rapid-acting:* e.g., regular, • *intermediate-acting:* e.g., NPH, • *long-acting:* Ultralente, • *mixed insulin preparations:* e.g., regular + NPH
site used for SC injection	*abdomen*
types of insulin Rx regimens	• **split dose insulin mixtures:** * split doses of regular + NPH twice daily, * AM and PM, • *intensive insulin Rx:* * three injections including: ♦ regular + NPH in AM, ♦ regular to cover PM dinner and NPH at bedtime, * long-acting insulin for basal level throughout day plus insulin lispro (peaks 1–3 h) to cover each meal (♦ most physiologic, ♦ labor intensive), • *insulin pump*
method of evaluating 7 AM hyperglycemia in type I DM	*blood glucose at 3 AM*
cause/Rx of low 3 AM glucose and high 7 AM glucose	• *Somogyi effect:* hypoglycemia at 3 AM causes rebound release of counter-regulatory hormones (glucagon, catecholamines) with subsequent increase in glucose, • *Rx:* less NPH at dinner or bedtime
cause/Rx of high 3 AM glucose and high 7 AM glucose	• *waning effect,* • *Rx:* more NPH at dinner or bedtime
cause/Rx of normal 3 AM glucose and high 7 AM glucose	• *dawn effect:* GH release at 5 AM antagonizes insulin effect, • *Rx:* division of NPH dose between dinner and bedtime
cause/Rx of high lunch time glucose	• *insufficient regular insulin in AM,* • *Rx:* increase regular insulin at breakfast
cause/Rx of high glucose at dinner	• *insufficient NPH in AM,* • *Rx:* increase NPH at breakfast

Table 11–5. DIABETES MELLITUS, HYPOGLYCEMIA
Continued

Most Common...	Answer and Explanation
recommendation for fasting and pre-meal glucose	• *glucose 80–120 mg/dL:* * other authors recommend 70–105 mg/dL (greater danger of hypoglycemia), • *other:* additional action suggested if glucose <80 mg/dL or >140 mg/dL
recommendation for 2-h post-meal glucose	*80–120 mg/dL*
recommendation for bedtime glucose	• *glucose 100–140 mg/dL,* • *other:* additional action if glucose <100 mg/dL or >160 mg/dL
recommendation for 2–4 AM glucose	*70–105 mg/dL*
recommendation for HbA$_{IC}$%	• *HbA$_{1c}$ 6–7%,* • *other:* additional action suggested if HbA$_{1c}$ >8%
role of HbA$_{IC}$ in DM	*measure of glycemic control for last 4–8 wks*
benefits of intensive glycemic control in DM	*50–75% reduction in risk of development or progression of* (in decreasing order of benefit) *retinopathy, neuropathy, nephropathy*
recommendations for diabetics requiring surgery	• *operative care in major surgery:* insulin and glucose infusion to maintain glucose between 120 and 200 mg/dL, • *operative care in minor surgery in stable diabetic:* * withhold AM dose of insulin or oral agent, * measure glucose q 2–4 h and adjust glucose levels with SC regular insulin, * resume original insulin or oral Rx after surgery, • *postoperative care after major surgery:* * continue insulin/glucose infusion, * begin SC regular insulin when patient is stabilized, * check glucose q 2–4 h
dietary recommendations for DM	*standard Step 1 or 2 cholesterol lowering diet* (see Table 5–2)
primary goals of Rx for diabetics with no previous Hx of CHD	• *LDL <130 mg/dL,* • *raise HDL to >35 mg/dL in men and >45 mg/dL in women,* • *TG <400 mg/dL*
primary goals of Rx for diabetics with previous Hx of CHD	• *LDL ≤100 mg/dL,* • *raise HDL to >35 mg/dL in men and >45 mg/dL in women,* • *TG <400 mg/dL*

Table continued on following page

Table 11–5. DIABETES MELLITUS, HYPOGLYCEMIA
Continued

Most Common...	Answer and Explanation
recommendations for artificial sweeteners in DM	• *aspartame:* * Nutrasweet, * aspartic acid + phenylalanine, * acceptable in DM, • *saccharin:* safe in DM, • *sorbitol-containing foods:* risk not established, • *fructose sweeteners:* * best to avoid in DM, * raises LDL
recommendations for alcohol ingestion in DM	*limited intake:* promotes * fasting hypoglycemia, * lactic acidosis, * β-OHB ketoacidosis
recommendations for insulin adjustment in prolonged exercise	*reduction in insulin* [Tissues utilize glucose in exercise. Less insulin is required. Danger of hypoglycemia in exercise. Patients should monitor glycemic response to exercise and adjust insulin dose accordingly.]
recommendations for insulin adjustment in severe illness	*patients often need more insulin when sick:* may have to use a sliding scale approach with regular insulin for good glycemic control
Rx for type II DM	• *glycemic control,* • *weight reduction,* • *exercise*
MOA of sulfonylureas in Rx of type II DM	• **sulfonylureas:** * e.g., glyburide, glipizide, • *MOA:* stimulate insulin secretion by remaining β-islet cells
MOA of biguanides in Rx of type II DM	• *biguanides:* e.g., * metformin, • *MOA:* enhance insulin effect on liver/peripheral tissue, * reduce gluconeogenesis, * danger of lactic acidosis if patient has liver disease, renal disease, alcohol abuse
MOA of α-glucosidase inhibitor	• *α-glucosidase inhibitor:* e.g., * acarbose, • *MOA:* interferes with disaccharide/complex CHO digestion, * reduces postprandial hyperglycemia
MOA of thiazolidinedione	• *thiazolidinedione:* e.g., troglitazone, • *MOA:* enhances peripheral uptake of insulin
side-effects of chlorpropamide	• **enhances ADH activity leading to SIADH,** • *Antabuse-like effect*
use of insulin in type II DM	• *first line Rx in non-obese types, pregnancy,* • *second line Rx in those failing diet + oral agents* (single and in combination)

Table 11–5. DIABETES MELLITUS, HYPOGLYCEMIA
Continued

Most Common...	Answer and Explanation
method of patient monitoring of glucose	*SMBG:* * type I DM, SMBG 3–4 times/d, * type II DM, optimal frequency unknown but should be sufficient to maintain glucose goals, * SMBG measures the whole blood glucose
method of converting whole blood glucose values into plasma glucose	*plasma glucose = whole blood glucose value x 1.10*
COD in DM	• **AMI**, • *stroke,* • *renal failure*
complications associated with impaired glucose tolerance (IGT)	• **syndrome X:** see above, • *macrovascular complications:* e.g., * AMI, * PVD, • ~30% develop DM within 10 y*
lab findings in IGT	• *FPG ≥110 mg/dL but <126 mg/dL,* • *2-h glucose post 75 g glucose load ≥140 mg/dL but <200 mg/dL*
clinical findings in GDM	• *glucose intolerance develops during pregnancy:* * ~4% of pregnancies, * develops between 24th and 28th week, * intolerance due to anti-insulin activity of hPL, estrogen, progesterone, • *glucose levels normalize after pregnancy,* • *left untreated, it increases perinatal morbidity/mortality,* • *increased rate of cesarean delivery,* • *increased incidence maternal HTN,* • *increased risk for DM:* 60% develop type II DM in 15 y [The normal fasting glucose in pregnancy is 60–80 mg/dL.]
fetal abnormalities associated with GDM	• **RDS:** * increased insulin in fetus in response to maternal hyperglycemia decreases fetal surfactant synthesis, * increased risk with cesarean delivery, • *complete transposition of great vessels,* • *open neural tube defects,* • *neonatal polycythemia,* • *macrosomia,* • *neonatal hypoglycemia,* • *neonatal hypocalcemia*
screening test used for GDM in pregnancy	*50 g glucose challenge between 24th and 28th week:* * glucose ≥140 mg/dL after 1 h is a positive test, * confirmed with a 3-h OGTT using 100 g of glucose

Table continued on following page

Table 11–5. DIABETES MELLITUS, HYPOGLYCEMIA
Continued

Most Common...	Answer and Explanation
lab values used for 3-h OGTT to confirm GDM	*any two of the following four plasma glucose values:* * fasting glucose ≥105 mg/dL, * 1-h glucose ≥190 mg/dL, * 2-h glucose ≥165 mg/dL, * 3-h glucose ≥145 mg/dL
Rx of GDM	• *SMBG,* • *monitor urine ketones,* • *ADA diet,* • *snacks to avoid hypoglycemia,* • *insulin if glycemic goals not maintained by diet*
glycemic goals to maintain in GDM	• *FPG 60–90 mg/dL,* • *pre-meal glucose 60–105 mg/dL,* • *1-h post-meal glucose 70–140 mg/dL,* • *2-h post-meal glucose 60–120 mg/dL,* • *bedtime glucose 60–120 mg/dL,* • *2 AM–4 AM glucose 60–100 mg/dL*
types of hypoglycemia	• **fed state:** * normal fed state has a rising insulin/falling glucagon, * increase in glycolysis, glycogen synthesis, • *fasting:* normal fasting state has a rising glucagon/falling insulin, increase in gluconeogenesis, glycogenolysis
S/S of fed state hypoglycemia	• *sweating,* • *tremor,* • *anxiety,* • *palpitations,* • *weakness,* • *hunger* [Note that the symptoms are adrenergic. Symptoms usually begin 1–5 h after eating. Beta-blockers mask these symptoms except sweating.]
S/S of fasting state hypoglycemia	• *headache,* • *dizziness,* • *altered mentation,* • *visual disturbances,* • *motor disturbances,* • *seizures,* • *coma* [S/S due to neuroglycopenia. Brain primarily uses glucose in fasting state. Symptoms occur when there is a gradual decline in glucose to levels <45 mg/dL.]
causes of fed state hypoglycemia	• **insulin-dependent DM:** sulfonylurea-related hypoglycemia is less common, • *alimentary hypoglycemia:* e.g., * dumping syndrome (post-Billroth II operation), * post vagotomy/pyloroplasty, • *IGT:* excessive insulin released for glucose absorbed, • *idiopathic postprandial syndrome*
mechanism of alimentary hypoglycemia	*rapid entry of glucose load into small bowel with rapid increase in plasma glucose and inappropriately large increase in insulin release:* symptomatic hypoglycemia develops in 1–2 h after eating

Table 11–5. DIABETES MELLITUS, HYPOGLYCEMIA
Continued

Most Common...	Answer and Explanation
clinical findings in idiopathic postprandial syndrome	*lack of energy, mental dullness, chronic anxiety:* S/S rarely accompanied by hypoglycemia
causes of fasting hypoglycemia	• **alcohol:** * pyruvate converted into lactate by increase in NADH in alcohol metabolism, * decreased gluconeogenesis, • *renal failure:* kidney is a site of gluconeogenesis, • *sepsis,* • *malnutrition,* • *primary hypothyroidism,* • *liver disease:* * decreased gluconeogenesis, * glycogen depletion, • *insulinoma:* see Table 9–9, • *hypopituitarism:* decreased GH, TSH, cortisol, • *secretion of insulin-like factor in HCC or mesenchymal tumors*
test to confirm fasting hypoglycemia	*prolonged fast:* must satisfy Whipple's triad: * symptoms, * hypoglycemia, * symptoms relieved by glucose
islet cell tumors	*see Table 9–9*

Question: Which of the following characterize the clinical and laboratory features of DKA? **SELECT 3**
  (A) Dilutional hyponatremia
  (B) Normal AG metabolic acidosis
  (C) Hyperphosphatemia
  (D) Prerenal azotemia
  (E) Volume expansion
  (F) Hypokalemia after insulin Rx

Answers: (A), (D), (F): Hyponatremia is commonly present due to the osmotic effect of glucose drawing water into the ECF from the ICF (**choice A**). Normal AG metabolic acidosis only occurs after Rx with 0.9% saline, which contains Cl⁻ ions but does not contain bicarbonate. Hence, bicarbonate is diluted and the excess Cl⁻ combines with H⁺ ions. Normally, DKA has an increased AG due to AcAc, β-OHB, and lactate anions (**choice B is incorrect**). Hyperphosphatemia is more likely to occur in DKA. Hypophosphatemia is secondary to insulin Rx, which drives glucose, phosphate (phosphorylates glucose, **choice C is incorrect**), and K⁺ into the cells, the latter resulting in hypokalemia (**choice F**). Hyperkalemia is commonly present early in DKA owing to transcellular shift of H⁺ into cells for buffering and K⁺ moving out of cells to maintain electroneutrality. In reality, patients are K⁺ deficient from osmotic diuresis. Insulin Rx uncovers the deficiency when glucose is driven into adipose and muscle. Prerenal azotemia (**choice D**) is common owing to volume depletion (**choice E is incorrect**) and increased proximal tubule reabsorption of urea.

ABGs = arterial blood gases, AcAc = acetoacetic acid, ACE = angiotensin converting enzyme, AD = autosomal dominant, ADA = American Diabetes Association, ADH = antidiuretic hormone, AG = anion gap, ALS = amyotropic lateral sclerosis, AMI = acute myocardial infarction, ARF = acute renal failure, β-OHB = beta-hydroxybutyric acid, BP = blood pressure, CF = cystic fibrosis, CHD = coronary heart disease, Cl^- = chloride ions, CMV = cytomegalovirus, CoA = coenzyme A, COD = cause of death, CVA = cerebrovascular accident, DKA = diabetic ketoacidosis, DM = diabetes mellitus, Dx = diagnosis, EBV = Epstein-Barr virus, ECF = extracellular fluid, FAs = fatty acids, FPG = fasting plasma glucose, GDM = gestational diabetes mellitus, GH = growth hormone, GI = gastrointestinal, GLUT = glucose transport unit, H^+ = hydrogen ions, $HbAI_c$ = hemoglobin A_{1c}, HCC = hepatocellular carcinoma, HDL = high density lipoprotein, HLA = human leukocyte antigen, HNKC = hyperosmotic non-ketotic coma, hPL = human placental lactogen, HTN = hypertension, ICF = intracellular fluid, IFG = impaired fasting glucose, IGT = impaired glucose tolerance, IV = intravenous, K^+ = potassium ions, LDL = low density lipoprotein, LUT = lower urinary tract, MCC = most common cause, MOA = mechanism of action, MODY = maturity-onset diabetes of youth, $NADH^+$ = nicotinamide adenine dehydrogenase (reduced), NEG = non-enzymatic glycosylation, NPH = neutral protamine Hagedorn, N/V = nausea and vomiting, OGTT = oral glucose tolerance test, PVD = peripheral vascular disease, RDS = respiratory distress syndrome, Rx = treatment, SIADH = syndrome of inappropriate antidiuretic hormone, SMBG = self-monitoring of blood glucose, S/S = signs and symptoms, TG = triglyceride, TSH = thyroid stimulating hormone, UTIs = urinary tract infections, UUT = upper urinary tract, VLDL = very low density lipoproteins.

Table 11–6. FEMALE ENDOCRINE DISORDERS AND GYNECOMASTIA

Most Common...	Answer and Explanation
cells evaluated in a cervical Pap smear	• *superficial squamous cells:* estrogen primed, • *intermediate squamous cells:* progesterone primed, • *parabasal cells:* unstimulated squamous cells, • *ECCs*
gold standard of an adequate cervical Pap smear	*presence of ECCs:* ECCs indicate that the junction of endocervix with cervix has been sampled, * junction is primary site for dysplasia/cancer
method of evaluating hormonal status in a cervical Pap smear	*100-cell count of superficial, intermediate, and parabasal cells:* called the maturation index (MI)

**Table 11–6. FEMALE ENDOCRINE DISORDERS AND
GYNECOMASTIA** *Continued*

Most Common...	Answer and Explanation
MI of a non-pregnant, pregnant, and women without estrogen stimulation	• *non-pregnant:* * superficial 70%, * intermediate 30%, * parabasal 0%, • *pregnant:* 100% intermediate, • *women without estrogen:* predominantly parabasal cells (atrophic smear)
MI expected in a woman with a granulosa cell tumor of ovary	*100% superficial squamous cells:* granulosa cells produce excess estrogen
order of events leading to menarche	• *breast development:* thelarche, • *growth spurt,* • *pubic hair,* • *axillary hair,* • *menarche*
hormones involved in proliferative/secretory phases of menstrual cycle	• *estrogen:* proliferative phase with gland hyperplasia, • *progesterone:* secretory phase with gland tortuosity and secretion
clinical evidence of ovulation	• **rise in basal body temperature of 0.6° F:** progesterone effect, • *ferning of cervical mucus,* • *mittelschmerz:* blood from ruptured follicle causes localized peritoneal irritation
hormonal effects of estrogen during menstrual cycle	• *negative feedback on FSH,* • *positive feedback on LH:* midcycle estrogen surge increases LH leading to ovulation on day 14
hormonal effects of estrogen/progesterone during menstrual cycle	*see Table 11–1*
location for fertilization	*ampulla of fallopian tube:* requires ~5–6 d to implant in endometrial mucosa (~day 21)
hormone maintaining the corpus luteum in pregnancy	*β-hCG:* * LH analogue that keeps corpus luteum synthesizing 17-OHP for 8–10 wks, * corpus luteum involutes after 8–10 wks, * placenta synthesizes progesterone, * bleeding may occur with low 17-OHP
source of estradiol	*aromatization of testosterone synthesized in theca interna:* aromatase is in granulosa cells
source of estriol	• **metabolite of estradiol,** • *primary estrogen of pregnancy*

Table continued on following page

Table 11–6. FEMALE ENDOCRINE DISORDERS AND GYNECOMASTIA *Continued*

Most Common...	Answer and Explanation
source of androgens in women	• *testosterone:* * 50% from peripheral conversion of androstenedione in adipose, * 25% from ovary, * 25% from adrenal cortex, • *androstenedione:* * 50% from ovary, * 50% from adrenal cortex, • *DHEA-S:* 95% from adrenal cortex
binding protein for estrogen/testosterone	*SHBG:* * greater affinity for testosterone than estrogen, * estrogen "amplifier"
cause of increased liver synthesis of SHBG	*estrogen*
effect of an increase in SHBG	*lowers free testosterone levels*
causes of a decrease in SHBG	• *androgens,* • *obesity,* • *hypothyroidism*
effect of a decrease in SHBG	*increases free testosterone levels:* potential for hirsutism
effects of combination birth control pills on menstrual cycle	• *estrogen inhibits FSH,* • *low baseline levels of estrogen prevent estrogen surge, leading to LH surge,* • *progestin arrests proliferative phase and inhibits LH,* • *cervical mucus hostile to sperm,* • *alters fallopian tube motility*
S/S/lab findings of menopause	• **secondary amenorrhea,** • *hot flushes,* • *decreased vaginal secretions,* • *night sweats*
lab findings in menopause	• **high FSH,** • *low estradiol*
cause of DUB between menarche and 20 y of age	*anovulatory cycles* [DUB is bleeding due to hormone imbalance rather than organic causes. In anovulatory DUB, estrogen is increased. Estrogen increases glandular tissue, which sloughs off due to poor support.]
ovulatory causes of DUB	• *irregular shedding of endometrium,* • *inadequate luteal phase*
types of amenorrhea	• *primary:* * menarche absent by 16 y of age in presence of normal secondary sex characteristics, * menarche absent by age 14 in female without secondary sex characteristics, •

Table 11–6. FEMALE ENDOCRINE DISORDERS AND GYNECOMASTIA *Continued*

Most Common...	Answer and Explanation
Continued	*secondary:* * absence of menses for a time greater than three previous cycle intervals, * absence of menses for 6 mths [Amenorrhea may be physiologic (e.g., constitutional delay, pregnancy) or pathologic.]
classification scheme of amenorrhea	• *hypogonadotropic hypogonadism:* * hypothalamic/pituitary origin, * low FSH/LH, * low estradiol, • *hypergonadotropic hypogonadism:* * primary ovarian origin, * high FSH/LH, * low estradiol, • *end-organ disease:* * normal gonadotropins, * normal estradiol, * anatomic defect
causes of primary amenorrhea	• **gonadal dysgenesis:** 45%, • *constitutional delay:* 20%, • *end-organ disease:* * 15%, * müllerian agenesis (Rokitansky-Kuster-Hauser syndrome), * imperforate hymen, • *hypothalamic/pituitary dysfunction:* e.g., * craniopharyngioma, * weight loss syndrome, * Kallmann's syndrome
cause of primary amenorrhea associated with anosmia/color blindness	*Kallmann's syndrome:* see Table 11–1
approach to primary amenorrhea	• **β-hCG:** R/O pregnancy, • *evaluate secondary sex characteristics:* * if normal: consider constitutional delay, end-organ problem, * if delayed, consider gonadal dysgenesis, • *serum gonadotropins:* * low in hypothalamic/pituitary disease, * high in gonadal dysgenesis, • *pelvic exam:* R/O end-organ problems, • *serum testosterone level in male range:* consider testicular feminization, • *karyotype if testicular feminization or gonadal dysgenesis is suspect*
physiologic cause of secondary amenorrhea	*pregnancy:* always order a β-hCG

Table continued on following page

Table 11–6. FEMALE ENDOCRINE DISORDERS AND GYNECOMASTIA *Continued*

Most Common...	Answer and Explanation
pathologic causes of secondary amenorrhea	• **hypothalamic dysfunction:** * 40%, * hyperprolactinemia, * stress, * weight loss syndrome, • *POS:* 30%, • *pituitary dysfunction:* * 20%, * prolactinoma, * hypopituitarism, • *ovarian failure:* * 10%, * **menopause,** * autoimmune, * radiation, * cyclophosphamide, • *end-organ:* Asherman's syndrome (repeated D/C removes stratum basalis)
tests to evaluate secondary amenorrhea	• **β-hCG:** R/O pregnancy, • *progesterone challenge,* • *gonadotropin/estradiol levels,* • *serum testosterone,* • *serum DHEA-S,* • *serum prolactin,* • *serum TSH*
use of progesterone challenge in secondary amenorrhea	• *absence of bleeding after progesterone:* * hypothalamic/pituitary, * ovarian, * end-organ problem, • *bleeding:* normal hypothalamic/pituitary/outflow tract
use of gonadotropins/ estradiol in secondary amenorrhea	• *low FSH/low estradiol:* hypothalamic/pituitary disorder, • *high FSH/low estradiol:* ovarian problem, • *normal FSH/normal estradiol:* end-organ problem, • *LH/FSH ratio >2/1:* POS
use of serum testosterone in secondary amenorrhea	*increased levels suggest an ovarian problem:* e.g., * POS, * androgen secreting tumor
use of serum DHEA-S in secondary amenorrhea	*increased levels suggest an adrenal cortex abnormality:* e.g., * Cushing's syndrome, * late-manifestation type of 21-OHase deficiency
use of serum prolactin in secondary amenorrhea	*R/O hyperprolactinemia:* e.g., * prolactinoma, * drugs, * primary hypothyroidism [See Table 11–1]
use of serum TSH in secondary amenorrhea	• **R/O primary hypothyroidism:** * high TSH, * high TRH increases prolactin, which inhibits GnRH, • *R/O secondary hypothyroidism:* low TSH
difference between hirsutism and virilization	• *hirsutism:* * excess hair in normal hair-bearing areas, * no male secondary sex characteristics, • *virilization:* * hirsutism + male secondary sex characteristics, * clitoromegaly is diagnostic

Table 11–6. FEMALE ENDOCRINE DISORDERS AND
GYNECOMASTIA *Continued*

Most Common...	Answer and Explanation
ovarian-testosterone producing causes of hirsutism	• **idiopathic hirsutism,** • *POS,* • *hyperthecosis:* * associated with acanthosis nigricans, * resistance to insulin
ovarian tumors with increased androgen production	*Sertoli-Leydig cell tumor:* alias * androblastoma, * arrhenoblastoma, • *Leydig cell tumor:* alias hilar cell tumor [Serum testosterone >200 ng/dL.]
adrenal–DHEA-S producing causes of hirsutism	• **late-onset 21-OHase deficiency:** * see Table 3–3, * increased 17-OHP, • *hyperprolactinemia:* stimulates adrenal production of DHEA-S, • *pituitary Cushing's,* • *adrenal carcinoma*
drugs associated with hirsutism	• **progestins,** • *minoxidil,* • *anabolic steroids*
endocrine causes of hirsutism	• **primary hypothyroidism,** • *hyperprolactinemia:* see above
cause of POS	*excessive pituitary release of LH* [Excess LH leads to increased synthesis of ovarian androgens (hirsutism). Androgens are aromatized into estrogens (endometrial hyperplasia). Estrogen has a negative feedback on FSH and positive feedback on LH, which continues the cycle.]
ovarian findings in POS	*enlarged ovaries with subcortical cysts:* * 70%, * suppression of FSH leads to follicle degeneration
S/S of POS	**menstrual irregularities:** * ~90%, * oligomenorrhea, • *hirsutism:* ~70%, • *infertility:* ~75%, • *obesity:* 50%
lab findings in POS	• **LH/FSH ratio >2/1:** ~75%, • *increased androstenedione,* • *increased testosterone:* * ~70%, * <200 ng/dL, • *increased estrone:* weak estrogen, • *hyperinsulinism,* • *hyperprolactinemia*
causes of virilization	• *ovarian:* * Sertoli-Leydig cell, * Leydig cell tumors, • *adrenal:* * Cushing's syndrome, * adrenogenital syndrome

Table continued on following page

Table 11–6. FEMALE ENDOCRINE DISORDERS AND GYNECOMASTIA *Continued*

Most Common...	Answer and Explanation
drugs used to treat hirsutism	• **spironolactone:** * blocks hair follicle androgen receptors, * blocks androgen production, • *birth control pills:* * blocks LH, * increases SHBG, which decreases T levels, * Rx for idiopathic hirsutism and POS, • *dexamethasone:* * blocks ACTH, * Rx for late-onset 21-OHase deficiency
disorder of the male breast	*gynecomastia:* * benign proliferation of glandular component of male breast, * unilateral or bilateral depending on breast sensitivity to estrogen
sources of estrogen in males	• **peripheral aromatization of androgens:** * 85%, * testosterone → estradiol, * androstenedione → estrone, • *Leydig cells:* 15%
mechanisms of gynecomastia (GYN)	• **increased free estrogen,** • *decrease in endogenous free androgens:* estrogen unopposed, • *defects in androgen receptors:* estrogen unopposed
causes of increased free estrogen	• **aromatization of 17-KS to estrogen in liver disease,** • *conversion of estrone to estradiol:* * 17-KS reductase, * estradiol is most potent estrogen and estrone the weakest, • *decreased liver metabolism of estrogen,* • *drug displacement from SHBG:* e.g., * spironolactone, * ketoconazole, • *drugs with estrogen activity:* e.g., * DES, * digitoxin (activates estrogen receptors)
causes of decreased free androgens	• **old age,** • *increased SHBG:* hyperestrinism, • *drugs:* e.g., * leuprolide, * spironolactone/ketoconazole (inhibit testosterone synthesis), • *primary hypogonadism:* testicular disease, • *secondary hypogonadism:* hypothalamic/pituitary dysfunction, • *genetic diseases:* e.g., Klinefelter's syndrome
causes of androgen receptor defects	• **drugs:** e.g., * flutamide, * spironolactone, • *genetic diseases:* e.g., testicular feminization
drugs of abuse causing GYN	• **alcohol,** • *marijuana,* • *amphetamines,* • *heroin*

Table 11–6. FEMALE ENDOCRINE DISORDERS AND GYNECOMASTIA *Continued*

Most Common...	Answer and Explanation
time frames when GYN is normal	*newborn:* * 60–90%, * transplacental passage of estrogen, • *puberty:* * unilateral or bilateral, * peak ages 13–14, • *old age:* 50–80 y olds
tests to evaluate GYN	• *serum hCG,* • *serum FSH/LH,* • *serum testosterone* (T), • *serum estradiol* (E$_2$)
cause of GYN if above studies are normal	*idiopathic gynecomastia*
cause of GYN if hCG is high	*testicular cancer with trophoblastic component:* hCG is an LH analogue that stimulates breast tissue
cause of GYN when LH is high and T low	*primary testicular dysfunction:* e.g., * Klinefelter's syndrome, * see Table 10–5
cause of GYN when FSH/LH and T are low	• **secondary hypogonadism,** • *prolactinoma,* • *androgen/estrogen producing tumor:* * testes, * adrenal
cause of GYN when LH and T are high	*androgen receptor insensitivity*
cause of GYN when E$_2$ is high	*estrogen-producing tumor in testes or adrenal gland*
overall causes of pathologic gynecomastia in decreasing frequency	• **idiopathic,** • *drugs,* • *cirrhosis,* • *primary hypogonadism,* • *testicular tumors,* • *secondary hypogonadism,* • *hyperthyroidism:* increased breast sensitivity to estrogens, • *renal disease*

Table continued on following page

Table 11–6. FEMALE ENDOCRINE DISORDERS AND
GYNECOMASTIA *Continued*

Questions 1–5: The sets of options are followed by several numbered items. For each numbered item, select the **ONE** lettered option that is **MOST CLOSELY** associated with it. Each lettered option may be selected once, more than once, or not at all.

(A) Normal FSH/LH/no withdrawal bleeding post-progesterone
(B) High FSH/LH/no withdrawal bleeding post-progesterone
(C) Low FSH/LH/no withdrawal bleeding post-progesterone
(D) High LH/Low FSH/high free T
(E) Normal FSH/LH, withdrawal bleeding post-progesterone

1. 16-y-old female with primary amenorrhea, normal secondary sex characteristics, normal pelvic exam
2. 22-y-old woman with obesity, hirsutism, oligomenorrhea
3. 28-y-old woman with secondary amenorrhea, normal secondary sex characteristics, normal pelvic exam, history of repeated D/Cs for DUB
4. 25-y-old woman with anorexia nervosa and secondary amenorrhea
5. 16-y-old female with poor secondary sex characteristics, decreased stature, webbed neck

Answers: 1. (E), 2. (D), 3. (A), 4. (C), 5. (B): Patient (1) has constitutional delay of puberty owing to normal gonadotropins and bleeding post-progesterone challenge **(choice E)**. Patient (2) has POS with a high LH/low FSH and increased free T **(choice D)**. Patient (3) has Asherman's syndrome due to loss of stratum basalis from repeated D/Cs **(choice A)**. Patient (4) with anorexia nervosa has secondary hypogonadism due to inhibition of GnRH release from weight loss **(choice C)**. Patient (5) has Turner's syndrome with primary ovarian failure **(choice B)**.

ACTH = adrenocorticotropic hormone, DES = diethylstilbestrol, DHEA-S = dehydroepiandrosterone-sulfate, D/C = dilatation and curettage, DHT = dihydrotestosterone, DUB = dysfunctional uterine bleeding, E_2 = estradiol, ECCs = endocervical cells, FSH = follicle stimulating hormone, GnRH = gonadotropin-releasing hormone, GYN = gynecomastia, β-hCG = human chorionic gonadotropin, 17-KS = 17-ketosteroids, LH = luteinizing hormone, MI = maturation index, 21-OHase = 21-hydroxylase, 17-OHP = 17-hydroxyprogesterone, POS = polycystic ovarian syndrome, R/O = rule out, Rx = treatment, SHBG = sex hormone-binding protein, S/S = signs and symptoms, T = testosterone, TRH = thyrotropin releasing hormone, TSH = thyroid stimulating hormone.

CHAPTER

RHEUMATOLOGY

CONTENTS

Table 12–1. SYNOVIAL FLUID ANALYSIS, JOINT DISORDERS

Most Common...	Answer and Explanation
routine SF tests	• *cell count* (<200 WBCs/μL) *and differential*, • *culture*, • *crystal analysis*, • *mucin clot test*
monoclinic SF crystals	• **MSU**, • *CPP* [Monoclinic crystals are needle-shaped. Without special polarization, MSU is indistinguishable from CPP.]
triclinic crystal	*CPP* [Triclinic crystals are rhomboid and represent CPP crystals.]
appearance of MSU crystals when aligned parallel to slow axis of compensator	*yellow monoclinic crystal* [Background of the slide turns red with red filter in place. Crystals are yellow/blue depending on orientation with slow axis of compensator. If crystal is yellow when parallel to slow axis, it defines negative birefringence and MSU.]
appearance of CPP crystal when aligned parallel to slow axis of compensator	*blue monoclinic or triclinic crystal:* if crystal is blue when parallel to slow axis, it defines positive birefringence and CPP
test evaluating SF viscosity	*mucin clot test:* * acid added to SF clots hyaluronic acid (SF lubricant), * poor clot reflects deficient hyaluronic acid and joint inflammation

Table continued on following page

Table 12–1. **SYNOVIAL FLUID ANALYSIS, JOINT DISORDERS** *Continued*

Most Common...	Answer and Explanation
S/S of joint disease	• **arthralgia:** general term for joint pain, • *arthritis:* pain associated with * joint swelling, * tenderness, * warmth, * e.g., RA, • *morning stiffness:* e.g., * RA, * SLE, * polymyalgia rheumatica, • *abnormal mobility:* damage to ligaments/joint capsule, • *swelling:* * increased joint fluid, * e.g., exudate, blood, • *joint crepitus:* * crackling feeling when moving joint, * e.g., OA
classification of joint disorders	• **group I:** noninflammatory, • *group II:* inflammatory, • *group III:* septic, • *group IV:* * hemorrhagic, * e.g., trauma, hemophilia
noninflammatory joint diseases	• **OA,** • *neuropathic joint*
disabling joint disease	*OA:* * female dominant disease, * progressive and disabling degeneration of articular cartilage
predisposing cause of OA	*abnormal load placed on a weight-bearing joint:* increased pressure produces * ischemia, * FRs, * destruction of articular cartilage
joints involved in OA	• **weight-bearing joints:** * hip, * knee, • *hands:* * DIP/PIP joints, * genetic predisposition, • *vertebral column:* see below
vertebral findings in OA	• *anterolateral spinous osteophytes* ("spurs"), • *degenerative disc disease,* • *narrow joint space,* • *compression neuropathies,* • *spondylolysis:* * posterior neural arch defect, * bilateral spondylolysis causes subluxation of one vertebra over another (spondylolisthesis)
secondary causes of OA	• **trauma:** * usually isolated joint, * e.g., meniscus tear, • *Legg-Perthes:* aseptic necrosis of femoral head in young boys, • *obesity,* • *hemochromatosis:* * 50%, * chondrocalcinosis with pseudogout, • *Wilson's disease:* 50%, • *ochronosis:* see below
clinical findings in ochronosis	• *AR disease:* deficient homogentisic acid oxidase, • *calcified intervertebral discs at multiple levels,* • *association with pseudogout,* • *grayish-brown scleral pigmentation,* • *urine turns black after light exposure*

Table 12–1. SYNOVIAL FLUID ANALYSIS, JOINT DISORDERS *Continued*

Most Common...	Answer and Explanation
sites rarely involved by primary OA	• *shoulders,* • *MCP joints,* • *ulnar side of wrist*
site for primary isolated OA	*DIP joint*
S/S of OA	• **arthralgia,** • *joint stiffness:* <15 m, • *Heberden's node of DIP joint:* osteophyte, • *Bouchard's node of PIP joint:* osteophyte, • *compression neuropathies*
radiographic findings in OA	• **narrow joint space:** wearing down of articular cartilage, • *osteophytes:* reactive bone formation at joint margins, • *subchondral bone cysts,* • *dense subchondral bone*
Rx of OA	• **pain relievers:** e.g., * acetaminophen, * NSAIDs (some believe this may worsen OA), • *weight loss,* • *protect joints from overuse,* • *? glucosamine salts + chondroitin sulfates,* • *surgery*
causes of a neuropathic (Charcot) joint	• **DM:** targets tarsometatarsal joint, • *syringomyelia:* * shoulder, * elbow, * wrist joint, • *tabes dorsalis:* * hip, * knee, * ankle
mechanism of joint disease in neuropathic joint	*combination of insensitivity to pain* (neuropathy) *and ischemia*
infectious complication of neuropathic joint	*osteomyelitis:* infection spreads from skin ulceration to bone
clinical findings of diabetic osteopathy	• *neuroarthropathy,* • *osteopenia of distal metacarpals/proximal phalanges,* • *osteolysis causing juxta-articular cortical defects,* • *increased osteomyelitis risk*
predisposing factors for developing RA	• *HLA Dr4:* 60–70%, • *infection:* e.g., * **EBV,** * rubella, * parvovirus, • *autoimmunity against immunoglobulins,* • *unknown genetic factors* [RA occurs between 30 and 50 y of age. More common in women than men.]
mechanism of destruction of articular cartilage in RA	*chronic synovitis with pannus formation:* * hyperplastic synovial tissue destroys articular cartilage and underlying bone (erosions), * reactive fibrosis causes joint fusion (ankylosis)

Table continued on following page

Table 12–1. SYNOVIAL FLUID ANALYSIS, JOINT DISORDERS *Continued*

Most Common...	Answer and Explanation
cytokine released into joint in RA	*tumor necrosis factor-α*
antibody synthesized by synovial tissue lymphocytes in RA	*rheumatoid factor:* * RF in 70%, * IgM antibody against IgG, * forms ICs with itself by binding to Fc components of IgG, * ICs activate complement system producing C5a, which attracts neutrophils into joint
cell type that phagocytoses RF to form a ragocyte in SF	*neutrophil*
joints involved in RF	• **symmetric involvement of second/third MCP/PIP joints:** * >85%, * ulnar deviation, * morning stiffness, * carpal tunnel syndrome, • *knees:* 80%, • *ankles:* 80%, • *elbows:* 50%, • *hips:* 50%, • *shoulders:* * AC joint, * 50%, • *cervical spine:* 40%, • *TMJ:* 30%
lung diseases in RA	• **chronic pleuritis:** * 40%, * usually asymptomatic, • *rheumatoid nodules,* • *diffuse ILD,* • *Caplan's syndrome:* see below, • *pseudochylous effusions:* see below
clinical/lab findings in pseudochylous effusions in RA	• *usually asymptomatic,* • *milky-white exudate with neutrophils/cholesterol-laden macrophages,* • *low PF glucose:* * 10–50 mg/dL, * selective pleural block of glucose
hematologic diseases in RA	• **ACD,** • *iron deficiency:* from PUD, • *warm AIHA,* • *Felty's syndrome:* see below
clinical findings with cervical spine disease in RA	• **atlantoaxial joint instability:** subluxation when patient looks down, • *danger of vertebrobasilar insufficiency:* * ataxia, * limb weakness, * tetraplegia
cause of a popliteal (Baker's) cyst in RA	*posterior outpouching of joint space from high intra-articular pressure:* * US diagnostic, * differentiate from popliteal artery aneurysm
complication of a popliteal cyst	*rupture into calf muscle:* * resembles acute thrombophlebitis, * e.g., fever, neutrophilic leukocytosis, ecchymoses around the ankle
type of tenosynovitis in RA	*finger flexor/extensor tendon sheaths:* * swelling between joints, * palpable grating in flexor tendon sheaths with digit movement

Table 12–1. SYNOVIAL FLUID ANALYSIS, JOINT
DISORDERS *Continued*

Most Common...	Answer and Explanation
cause of hand paresthesias in RA	*carpal tunnel syndrome:* * RA second to pregnancy as MCC, * median nerve compressed in transverse carpal ligament
clinical findings in carpal tunnel syndrome	• **thumb, index, second finger, third finger, radial side of fourth finger are painful, numb, or have paresthesias,** • *thenar atrophy,* • *positive Tinel's sign:* pain with tapping over median nerve, • *positive Phalen's sign:* symptoms with forced wrist flexion
locations for rheumatoid nodules	• **extensor aspect of forearm,** • *lungs,* • *heart* [Occur in 20–35% of those with high RF titers. Ulceration/infection may occur.]
location for rheumatoid vasculitis	*malleoli of lower extremities:* * IC small vessel vasculitis with palpable purpura/ulceration, * high RF titers, * deforming RA, * digital nail fold infarcts
clinical appearance of "swan neck" deformity in RA	• *flexion of DIP joint,* • *extension of PIP joint*
clinical appearance of boutonniere deformity in RA	• *hyperextension of DIP joint,* • *flexion of PIP joint*
ocular findings in RA	• **keratoconjunctivitis sicca:** * dry eyes, * "feels like sand in my eyes," * autoimmune destruction of lacrimal glands, * Sjögren's syndrome, • *episcleritis/scleritis:* blindness
cardiac findings in RA	• **pericarditis:** * 40–50%, * constrictive type, • *aortitis:* RA vasculitis and high titered RF
syndromes associated with RA	• **Sjögren's syndrome (SS),** • *Caplan's syndrome,* • *Felty's syndrome*
clinical findings in SS	• **keratoconjunctivitis sicca:** * dry eyes, * enlarged lacrimal glands, • *xerostomia:* * dry mouth, * "I can't swallow dry crackers," * salivary gland enlargement, * dental caries, • *arthritis:* usually RA, • *type I distal RTA:* * 20%, * due to interstitial nephritis, • *ILD,* • *predisposition for NHL/Waldenström's macroglobulinemia* [Eye/mouth findings due to autoimmune destruction of lacrimal/minor salivary glands by CD$_4$ T helper cells.]

Table continued on following page

Table 12–1. SYNOVIAL FLUID ANALYSIS, JOINT DISORDERS *Continued*

Most Common...	Answer and Explanation
lab findings in SS	• **positive RF:** 75–90%, • *anti-SS-A/Ro antibodies: 70–80%,* • *positive serum ANA:* 50–80%, • *anti-SS-B/La antibodies:* * 50–70%, * more specific for SS than other disorders
confirmatory test for SS	*lip biopsy of minor salivary glands:* lymphocyte destruction of glands
clinical findings of Caplan's syndrome	*CWP + large cavitating rheumatoid nodules located along the periphery of the lungs:* see Table 6–6
clinical findings of Felty's syndrome	• **RA,** • *splenomegaly,* • *leukopenia:* * <3500 cells/μL, * marrow maturation arrest of granulocytes, * other cytopenias possible, • *high RF titers*
lab findings in RA	• **positive RF:** 70–90%, • *positive serum ANA:* ~30%, • *ACD,* • *normal to high serum C3:* low SF C3, • *high ESR:* disease activity marker, • *eosinophilia:* * 30%, * accompanies RA vasculitis, * ? marker of gold Rx sensitivity, • *cryoglobulinemia,* • *hypergammaglobulinemia*
radiographic findings in RA	• **symmetric narrowing of joint space,** • *periarticular osteoporosis,* • *bone erosions at joint margins*
natural history of RA	• **cyclic disease with flares/remissions,** • *progressive disabling disease:* 10–20%, • *shorter life-span than normal*
initial first-line Rx of RA	*NSAIDs:* glucocorticoids may be used to preserve function
disease-modifying (second line) drugs used in RA	• **methotrexate,** • *hydroxychloroquine:* danger of pigmentary retinitis, • *gold salts:* * IM, * 60% response, * dermatitis, * proteinuria, • *penicillamine,* • *sulfasalazine:* danger of * neutropenia, * thrombocytopenia, • *azathioprine,* • *cyclophosphamide*
cause of seronegative RA in adults	*adult-onset Still's disease*
clinical findings in adult-onset Still's disease	• **spiking quotidian fever:** * >95%, * fever spike with return to normal temperature in 24 h, • *arthritis:* * 95%, * sites: wrist, shoulders, knees, hips, • *generalized lymphadenopathy:* ~70%, • *hepatosplenomegaly:* 50%, •

Table 12–1. SYNOVIAL FLUID ANALYSIS, JOINT
DISORDERS *Continued*

Most Common...	Answer and Explanation
Continued	*salmon-colored macular rash,* • *sore throat,* • *neutrophilic leukocytosis,* • *negative RF and serum ANA*
inheritance pattern in primary gout	*multifactorial inheritance*
causes of secondary gout	• **alcoholism,** • *chronic renal insufficiency,* • *lead nephropathy,* • *DM,* • *diuretics,* • *PRV*
primary causes of increased UA synthesis	• **obesity,** • *decrease in HGPRT,* • *increase in PRPP* [Uric acid is byproduct of purine metabolism. UA overproduction ~10% cases. 24-h urine UA >1000 mg.]
cause of hyperuricemia in primary/secondary gout	*decreased excretion of uric acid in kidneys:* * 90% of cases, 24-h urine UA <1000 mg
secondary causes of UA overproduction	• **Rx of cancer,** • *psoriasis:* increased skin turnover, • *sickle cell disease:* chronic hemolysis, • *MPD*
secondary causes of UA underexcretion	• **alcohol:** lactate/β-OHB compete with UA for proximal tubule excretion, • *DKA,* • *chronic renal insufficiency,* • *low-dose aspirin:* high-dose aspirin uricosuric, • *diuretics,* • *Pb nephropathy*
clinical presentation of acute gouty arthritis	**acute onset** (usually nocturnal) of **inflammation in first metatarsophalangeal joint:** * 50%, * called *podagra,* • *fever,* • *neutrophilic leukocytosis,* • *more common in men than women except after menopause*
factors precipitating acute gouty arthritis	• **alcohol,** • *trauma,* • *postoperative state,* • *post-cardiac transplantation:* * 25%, due to: * diuretics, * cyclosporine, • *AMI,* • *stroke,* • *fasting,* • *infection:* e.g., septic arthritis
cause of joint inflammation in acute gouty arthritis	*interaction of MSU with neutrophils:* causes release of leukocyte-derived chemotactic factor

Table continued on following page

Table 12–1. SYNOVIAL FLUID ANALYSIS, JOINT DISORDERS *Continued*

Most Common...	Answer and Explanation
lab test to confirm gout	*SF analysis:* * demonstrate negatively bire-fringent crystals, * hyperuricemia does not define gout, * UA usually >7.5 mg/dL, * ~20% have normal UA
Rx of acute gouty arthritis	• **NSAIDs:** indomethacin, • *intra-articular injection of corticosteroids,* • *colchicine:* * rarely used due to GI effects, * blocks release of leukocyte-derived chemotactic factor
clinical findings in interval gout	*usually asymptomatic:* UA crystals confined to vacuoles within SF neutrophils
clinical finding in chronic gout	*tophus formation:* * MSU deposits in tissue around joint (MC) and other sites, * develop ~10 y of disease in poorly controlled patients
complications of gout	*disabling arthritis, renal disease:* urate ne-phropathy
clinical disorders associated with gout	• *HTN,* • *obesity,* • *CHD,* • *chronic renal insufficiency*
dietary recommendations in gout	• *avoid foods high in purines:* * red meats, * seafood, • *avoid alcohol*
drugs used to lower UA during interval period	• **uricosuric drugs:** e.g., * **probenecid,** * sul-finpyrazone, * UA urine levels <1000 mg/d, • *drugs that decrease UA production:* e.g., * allopurinol (blocks xanthine oxidase), * UA urine levels >1000 mg/d
causes of CPPD	• **metabolic disease:** e.g., * primary HPTH, * hemochromatosis, * Wilson's disease, * och-ronosis, • *idiopathic,* • *genetic,* • *trauma*
S/S of CPPD (pseudogout)	• **chondrocalcinosis involving knee:** * arthri-tis with CPP crystals/linear deposits of CPP in articular cartilage, • *other joints:* * wrists, * elbows, * intervertebral discs, * ankles
Rx of CPPD	• **NSAIDs,** • *IV colchicine,* • *drain joint and inject corticosteroids in resistant cases*
seronegative (RF negative) spondyloarthropathy	*AS:* * inflammatory arthritis afflicting young men, * HLA B27 positive (>90%)

Table 12–1. SYNOVIAL FLUID ANALYSIS, JOINT DISORDERS *Continued*

Most Common...	Answer and Explanation
joints and other sites targeted in AS	• **sacroiliac joint,** • *vertebral column:* * "bamboo spine," • *other joints:* * shoulder, * hip, • *aorta:* aortitis with aortic insufficiency, • *uveal tract:* uveitis with blurry vision
S/S of AS	• **morning stiffness in sacroiliac joints:** improves with exercise, • *fever,* • *diminished anterior flexion:* eventual ILD, • *kyphoscoliosis,* • *aortic insufficiency,* • *visual problems,* • *Achilles' tendinitis*
Rx of AS	• **NSAIDs:** indomethacin, • *exercise*
S/S of Reiter's syndrome	• **urethritis:** *Chlamydia trachomatis,* • *dysentery: Shigella, Campylobacter, Yersinia,* • *conjunctivitis:* noninfectious, • *HLA B27 positive arthritis:* * 80%, * toes: "sausage" toe, • *mucocutaneous disease:* * balanitis, * aphthous ulcers in mouth, • *Achilles' tendinitis:* periostitis at tendon insertion, • *skin disease:* * keratoderma blennorrhagicum, * similar to psoriasis, • *cardiac conduction abnormalities,* • *aortitis*
cell of origin of Reiter's cell in SF	*macrophage that has phagocytosed a neutrophil*
Rx of Reiter's syndrome	• **NSAIDs,** • *Rx underlying infectious disease if present*
S/S of psoriatic arthritis	• **morning stiffness similar to RA:** symmetrical disease, • *sausage-shaped DIP joints* (finger to toe) *with nail pitting and erosive joint disease:* radiographs exhibit "pencil-in-cup" deformity, • *psoriatic spondylitis:* * HLA B27 positive 50–75%, * sacroiliac joint, * AS commonly present, • *severe skin disease:* precedes arthritis in 80%, • *hyperuricemia*
Rx of psoriatic arthritis	• **NSAIDs,** • *methotrexate,* • *gold*
IBD associated with HLA B27 positive arthritis	*UC:* next to anemia, HLA B27 positive arthritis (~75%) is second MC extraintestinal manifestation of IBD

Table continued on following page

Table 12–1. **SYNOVIAL FLUID ANALYSIS, JOINT DISORDERS** *Continued*

Most Common...	Answer and Explanation
infections associated with aseptic (reactive) HLA B27 positive arthritis	***Chlamydia trachomatis,*** • *Ureaplasma urealyticum,* • *Shigella flexneri,* • *Yersinia enterocolitica,* • *Salmonella,* • *Campylobacter jejuni* [~80% are HLA B27 positive. Arthritis is self-limited and nonerosive.]
cause of episodic destruction of cartilage in ears/ nose/upper airways + arthritis	*relapsing polychondritis*
nongonococcal cause of septic arthritis	*Staphylococcus aureus:* * hematogenous spread in elderly or immunocompromised patients, * gram-negative organisms (*Escherichia coli, Pseudomonas aeruginosa*) more likely in elderly
cause of septic arthritis in urban populations	*Neisseria gonorrhoeae:* * female/male ratio 3 : 1, * in women, it most commonly occurs during menses/pregnancy
S/S of disseminated gonorrhoeae	• **tenosynovitis:** * 60%, * sites: wrists, ankles, • *septic arthritis:* knee, • *dermatitis:* * pustules involving wrists, ankles [<50% have fever. <25% have GU symptoms. Culture all sites.]
complement deficiencies in disseminated gonococcemia	*C5–C9:* components are necessary for phagocytosis of the organisms
lab findings in GC septic arthritis	• *SF Gram stain:* positive in 25%, • *SF culture:* positive 30–50%, • *blood culture:* * positive in 40% with tenosynovitis, * negative in suppurative arthritis, • *culture of skin lesions:* positive in 40–60%
Rx of GC septic arthritis	*ceftriaxone*
cause of Lyme disease	*tick-transmitted* (*Ixodes dammini* in East/ Midwest, *Ixodes pacificus* in West) *Borrelia burgdorferi* (spirochete): white-tailed deer is animal reservoir for the organism

Table 12–1. SYNOVIAL FLUID ANALYSIS, JOINT DISORDERS *Continued*

Most Common...	Answer and Explanation
skin lesion in early Lyme disease	*erythema chronicum migrans:* * 50%, * red, expanding lesion with concentric circles emanating from site of the tick bite, * pathognomonic of Lyme disease. [Doxycycline is the Rx of choice at this stage of the disease.]
late manifestations of Lyme disease	• **arthritis:** 30–50%, • *CNS disease:* ~15%, • *cardiovascular disease:* ~5%*
musculoskeletal findings in Lyme disease	• *most commonly involves the knee,* • *may develop popliteal cysts that rupture,* • *obliterative endarteritis in synovial tissue,* • *disabling arthritis if left untreated*
neurologic findings in Lyme disease	• **bilateral Bell's palsy,** • *other cranial nerve palsies,* • *meningoencephalitis*
cardiovascular findings in Lyme disease	• **myocarditis/pericarditis,** • *heart blocks*
secondary infection transmitted by Ixodes	*babesiosis* [It is an intraerythrocytic protozoal disease due to *Babesia microti.*]
clinical findings in babesiosis	• *fever,* • *headache,* • *myalgia,* • *mild/moderate hemolytic anemia,* • *usually self-limited in patients with a spleen*
lab findings in babesiosis	• **blood smears with intraerythrocytic organisms,** • *serologic tests positive in 2–4 wks*
Rx of babesiosis	*clindamycin + quinine*
lab findings in Lyme disease	• *ELISA:* • screening test, * many FP test results, • requires 4–6 wks to become positive, • *Western blot assay:* confirmatory test, • *culture:* 60–70% sensitivity in biopsy specimens of ECM, • *silver stains of synovial biopsy positive in ~30%*
Rx of early and late stages of Lyme disease	*doxycycline and ceftriaxone, respectively*
viral diseases associated with arthritis	• *rubella:* particularly in adults, • *EBV,* • *HIV,* • *parvovirus B19:* mimics RA, • *mumps,* • *HBV/HCV:* serum sickness-like prodrome [In general, viral arthritis is nondestructive.]

Table continued on following page

Table 12–1. SYNOVIAL FLUID ANALYSIS, JOINT DISORDERS *Continued*

Most Common...	Answer and Explanation
types of rheumatologic disease in HIV	• **Reiter's syndrome:** * usually occurs with onset of HIV infection, * Achilles' tendinitis common, * conjunctivitis uncommon, * enteric infections MC initiating event, • *SLE-like syndrome,* • *Sjögren-like syndrome,* • *HIV vasculitis*

Questions 1–9: The set of options is followed by several numbered items. For each numbered item, select the ONE lettered option that is MOST CLOSELY associated with it. Each lettered option may be selected once, more than once, or not at all.

  (A) OA
  (B) RA
  (C) Gout
  (D) CPPD
  (E) AS
  (F) Reiter's syndrome
  (G) Psoriatic arthritis
  (H) Nongonococcal septic arthritis
  (I) Gonococcal septic arthritis
  (J) Lyme disease
  1. A 25-y-old man has Achilles' tendinitis and skin rash
  2. An afebrile 23-y-old woman has tenosynovitis in her left hand and a painful, hot right knee
  3. A 31-y-old woman with a recent history of an erythematous skin lesion now presents with bilateral Bell's palsy
  4. A 68-y-old man has right hip pain and radiographic findings in the femoral head of narrowing of the joint space, subchondral bone cysts, and osteophytes at the joint margin
  5. A 52-y-old man with hemochromatosis has a hot right knee, linear calcifications in the articular cartilage, and monoclinic crystals that are blue when aligned to the slow axis of the compensator
  6. A 45-y-old woman becomes dizzy and ataxic when looking down
  7. A 48-y-old man has swollen, sausage-shaped fingers with a "pencil-in-cup" radiographic appearance
  8. A 25-y-old man complains of low back pain when waking up in the morning and states that the pain resolves with exercise
  9. A 45-y-old febrile alcoholic presents with sudden onset of pain and swelling in the right first metatarsophalangeal joint

Answers: 1. (F), 2. (I), 3. (J), 4. (A), 5. (D), 6. (B), 7. (G), 8. (E), 9. (C): Patient (1) has clinical findings most consistent with Reiter's syndrome (Achilles' tendinitis, keratoderma blennorrhagicum, **choice F**). Patient (2) most likely has gonococcal septic arthritis with tenosynovitis and septic arthritis in the knee **(choice I)**. Patient (3) has a classic history for Lyme disease, mainly a skin rash (ECM) followed by bilateral Bell's palsy involving the VIIth nerve **(choice J)**. Patient (4) has OA involving the femoral head and the classic radiographic findings associated with wearing away of the articular cartilage **(choice A)**. Patient (5) has CPPD secondary to hemochromatosis. The SF findings are compatible with a positively birefringent crystal (blue and parallel to the slow axis of the compensator) consistent with pseudogout **(choice D)**. Patient (6) has vertebrobasilar insufficiency secondary to subluxation of the atlanto-axial joint. This is most commonly associated with cervical arthritis secondary to RA **(choice B)**. Patient (7) has the "pencil-in-cup" deformity of the digits that is noted in psoriatic arthritis **(choice G)**. Patient (8) has bilateral sacroiliitis that is worse in the AM and improves with exercise **(choice E)**. These findings are the initial presentation for AS. Patient (9) has a classic history of acute gouty arthritis involving the big toe **(choice C)**. SF would exhibit monoclinic crystals that are negatively birefringent (yellow when parallel to the slow axis of the compensator).

AC = acromioclavicular joint, ACD = anemia of chronic disease, AIHA = autoimmune hemolytic anemia, AMI = acute myocardial infarction, ANA = antinuclear antibody, AR = autosomal recessive, AS = ankylosing spondylitis, β-OHB = beta-hydroxybutyrate, CHD = coronary heart disease, CNS = central nervous system, CPP = calcium pyrophosphate, CPPD = calcium pyrophosphate dihydrate crystal deposition arthropathy, CWP = coal worker's pneumoconiosis, DIP = distal interphalangeal joint, DKA = diabetic ketoacidosis, DM = diabetes mellitus, ELISA = enzyme-linked immunosorbent assay, EBV = Epstein-Barr virus, ECM = erythema chronicum migrans, ESR = erythrocyte sedimentation rate, FP = false-positive, FR = free radical, GC = gonococcus, GI = gastrointestinal, GU = genitourinary, HBV = hepatitis B virus, HCV = hepatitis C virus, HGPRT = hypoxanthine-guanine phosphoribosyltransferase, HIV = human immunodeficiency virus, HLA = human leukocyte antigen, HPTH = hyperparathyroidism, HTN = hypertension, IBD = inflammatory bowel disease, ICs = immunocomplexes, Ig = immunoglobulin, ILD = interstitial lung disease, IV = intravenous, MC = most common, MCC = most common cause, MCP = metacarpophalangeal joint, MPD = myeloproliferative disease, MSU = monosodium urate, NHL = non-Hodgkin's lymphoma, NSAIDs = nonsteroidal anti-inflammatory drugs, OA = osteoarthritis, Pb = lead, PF = pleural fluid, PIP = proximal interphalangeal joint, PRPP = 5-phospho-α-D-ribosyl-1-pyrophosphate, PRV = polycythemia rubra vera, PUD = peptic ulcer disease, RA = rheumatoid arthritis, RF = rheumatoid factor, RTA = renal tubular acidosis, Rx = treatment, SF = synovial fluid, SLE = systemic lupus erythematosus, SS = Sjögren's syndrome, S/S = signs and symptoms, TMJ = temporomandibular joint, UA = uric acid, UC = ulcerative colitis, US = ultrasonography; WBC = white blood cell.

Table 12–2. AUTOIMMUNE DISORDERS

Most Common...	Answer and Explanation
organ-specific AD	• **Hashimoto's thyroiditis,** • *Addison's disease:* see Table 11–4, • *PA:* see Table 8–5
systemic AD	*RA:* see Table 12–1
test used to screen for ADs	*serum ANA:* antibodies detected are against * DNA (double- and single-stranded), * histones, * acidic proteins (anti-Sm, anti-RNP), * nucleolar antigens
serum ANA pattern	*speckled:* present in: * SLE, * PSS (due to anti-Scl antibody), * MCTD (due to anti-RNP), * SS (due to anti-SS-A [Ro], -SS-B [La]), * RA
cause of a rim pattern on a serum ANA	*SLE with anti-dsDNA:* marker for renal disease
causes of a homogeneous ANA pattern	• **SLE,** • *drug-induced SLE,* • *MCTD,* • *PSS* [This is the second most common ANA pattern.]
cause of a nucleolar ANA pattern	*PSS* [This is the least common ANA pattern.]
cause of a centromere ANA pattern	*CREST syndrome*
cause of a positive LE prep	*SLE:* * 70–90%, * LE cell is a neutrophil that has phagocytosed DNA altered by anti-DNA antibodies, * not pathognomonic of SLE, * *tart cell* is monocyte with phagocytosed DNA
mechanisms implicated in SLE	• *polyclonal activation of B lymphocytes:* decrease in CD_8-suppressor T cells, • *increased conversion of estradiol to a metabolite with sustained estrogen activity,* • *? type C oncornavirus infection in HLA B8, -Dr2, -Dr3 patient* [8:1 female:male ratio. Common in African and Native Americans.]
presentation of SLE	*arthritis/arthralgia:* * 95%, * similar to RA (symmetrical, morning stiffness), * absence of joint deformity/erosions
cutaneous findings in SLE	• **butterfly rash,** • *alopecia,* • *nail fold infarctions* [See Table 14–1.]
cardiovascular finding in SLE	• **fibrinous pericarditis with effusion,** • *Libman-Sacks endocarditis:* see Table 5–9, • *myocarditis,* • *arrhythmias*

Table 12–2. AUTOIMMUNE DISORDERS *Continued*

Most Common...	Answer and Explanation
pulmonary findings in SLE	• **pleuritis with pleural effusion,** • *interstitial fibrosis*
hematologic findings in SLE	• **ACD,** • *warm AIHA,* • *autoimmune thrombocytopenia,* • *autoimmune neutropenia, autoimmune lymphopenia,* • *generalized lymphadenopathy*
coagulation disorder in SLE	*anti-phospholipid syndrome* (APL): see Table 8–14
renal disease associated with SLE	*diffuse proliferative GN:* nephrotic or nephritic [see Table 10–3.]
CNS findings in SLE	• **psychosis,** • *seizures,* • *defects in cognitive function*
clinical findings in pregnancy in SLE	• **SLE worsens,** • *spontaneous abortions:* APL syndrome, • *complete heart block in newborn:* • transplacental transfer of anti-Ro antibodies, * mother is usually HLA B8/Dr3 positive, • *autoimmune cytopenias in newborn:* transplacental passage of IgG
lab findings in SLE	• **positive serum ANA:** 99–100%, • *antidsDNA:* * 70%, * confirmatory test, • *antissDNA:* * 60–100%, *anti-Sm:* * 30%, * confirmatory test, • *anti-SS-A* (Ro): 30%, • *low C3:* * 40–70%, * sign of active disease, • *FP syphilis serology:* * 25%, * due to anticardiolipin antibodies, • *low C2:* familial deficiency, • *positive RF,* • *proteinuria, hematuria, RBC casts:* renal disease
Rx of SLE	• **systemic corticosteroids:** * autoimmune hematologic problems, * organ involvement, • NSAIDs: arthritis, • *hydroxychloroquine:* * rash, * arthritis
COD in SLE	• **renal disease,** • **infection:** due to steroids/immunosuppressive Rx, • *CNS disease*
findings more often associated with drug-induced SLE than systemic SLE	• **elevated anti-histone antibodies:** 95%, • *sex ratio ~ equal:* older population, • *lower incidence of renal, CNS, skin involvement,* • *absence of anti-dsDNA/anti-Sm antibodies,* • *normal complement levels,* • *reversible disease with D/C of drug*
drugs causing SLE	• **procainamide:** 15–25%, • *hydralazine:* 5%

Table continued on following page

Table 12–2. AUTOIMMUNE DISORDERS *Continued*

Most Common...	Answer and Explanation
types of systemic scleroderma	• **limited type:** 80%, * CREST syndrome, • *diffuse type:* * 20%, * PSS
cause of PSS/CREST syndrome	*small vessel vasculitis:* followed by excessive collagen deposition in interstitial tissue
initial sign of PSS/ CREST syndrome	• *Raynaud's phenomenon:* * 90%, * color changes from digital vasospasm/fibrosis
clinical findings in CREST syndrome	• <u>c</u>alcinosis cutis: subcutaneous calcification, • <u>R</u>aynaud's phenomenon: MC initial presentation, • <u>e</u>sophageal motility dysfunction, • <u>s</u>clerodactyly, • <u>t</u>elangiectasia
clinical findings in CREST syndrome that differ from PSS	• **anti-centromere antibody in 70–90% versus 10–20% in PSS,** • *skin tightening limited to hands/face:* no trunk involvement as in PSS, • *less renal involvement than PSS,* • *cor pulmonale more common than PSS,* • *better prognosis,* • *anti-Scl-70 antibodies in 10% versus 25–30% in PSS*
skin findings in PSS	• **Raynaud's phenomenon,** • *symmetric swelling/induration of fingers, toes:* proximal to MCP or MTP joints, • *sclerodactyly:* loss of finger pad substance, • *pursed lips/tight facial features,* • *subcutaneous calcifications,* • *telangiectasias over face, fingers, lips,* • *parchment-like skin over trunk*
GI findings in PSS	• **dysphagia for solids/liquids:** smooth muscle replaced by collagen, • *aperistalsis of esophagus/small bowel,* • *LES relaxation/reflux,* • *wide mouthed diverticula:* small intestine
kidney findings in PSS	• **vasculitis:** * hyperplastic arteriolosclerosis, * microangiopathic hemolytic anemia, • *IC GN,* • *malignant HTN,* • *ARF/CRF*
pulmonary findings in PSS	• *diffuse interstitial fibrosis:* * 70%, * diffusion capacity decreased when radiograph is normal
cardiac findings in PSS	• **conduction defects,** • *supraventricular arrhythmias,* • *left ventricular dysfunction* [Cardiac defects occur in 70% of cases.]

Table 12–2. AUTOIMMUNE DISORDERS *Continued*

Most Common...	Answer and Explanation
joint disease in PSS	• **symmetrical nondeforming arthritis,** • *bone resorption in distal tufts of digits*
lab findings in PSS	• **positive serum ANA:** 70–90%, • *anti-Scl-70 antibodies:* * anti-topoisomerase antibodies, * 25–30%, • *anticentromere antibodies:* 10–20%
Rx of PSS	D-*penicillamine*
COD in PSS	*respiratory failure:* secondary to ILD
disorder associated with ingestion of L-tryptophan	*eosinophilic myalgia syndrome*
clinical findings in eosinophilic myalgia syndrome	• **eosinophilia,** • *myositis,* • *indurated skin,* • *peripheral neuropathy*
acquired myopathy in adults	*polymyositis* (PM)
S/S of PM/DM	• **muscle weakness/atrophy,** • *purple-red discoloration/puffiness of eyelids:* heliotrope eyelids, • *increased incidence of lung cancer,* • *dysphagia for solids/liquids:* see Table 9–2, • *Gottron's patches over PIP joints*
lab findings in DM/PM	• **increased serum CK,** • *positive serum ANA:* 80–90%, • *positive anti-PM1:* ~50%, • *positive anti-Jo-1 antibody:* ~25%
confirmatory test in DM and PM	*muscle Bx:* lymphocytic infiltrate
Rx of PM/DM	*prednisone*
S/S of MCTD ("overlap syndrome")	*variable features of SLE, polymyositis, PSS, RA*
differences of MCTD with other AD diseases	• **anti-RNP antibodies:** 100%, • *low incidence of renal disease*

Table continued on following page

Table 12–2. AUTOIMMUNE DISORDERS *Continued*

Question: Which of the following distinguish SLE, PSS, and PM from each other? **SELECT 4**
- (A) Anti-dsDNA
- (B) Elevated serum CK
- (C) Positive serum ANA
- (D) Anti-Scl-70
- (E) Abnormal diffusion capacity
- (F) Autoimmune cytopenias
- (G) Normal serum complement

Answers: (A), (B), (D), (F): Anti-dsDNA **(choice A)** is present only in SLE. An elevated serum CK **(choice B)** is primarily increased in PM. A positive serum ANA is present in all of them **(choice C is incorrect)**. Anti-Scl-70 **(choice D)** is increased only in PSS. An abnormal diffusion capacity is seen in SLE and PSS **(choice E is incorrect)**. Autoimmune cytopenias **(choice F)** are primarily noted in SLE. Normal serum complement levels are present in PSS and PM, whereas low levels are characteristic of SLE **(choice G is incorrect)**.

ACD = anemia of chronic disease, AD = autoimmune disease, AIHA = autoimmune hemolytic anemia, ANA = antinuclear antibodies, APL = anti-phospholipid syndrome, anti-dsDNA = anti-double-stranded DNA, anti-RNP = anti-ribonucleoprotein, anti-Scl = anti-scleroderma antibody, anti-Sm = anti-Smith, ARF = acute renal failure, Bx = biopsy, CK = creatine kinase, CNS = central nervous system, COD = cause of death, CREST = calcinosis, Raynaud's, esophageal dysfunction, sclerodactyly, telangiectasia, CRF = chronic renal failure, D/C = discontinue, DM = dermatomyositis, FP = false-positive, GI = gastrointestinal, GN = glomerulonephritis, HLA = human leukocyte antigen, IC = immunocomplex, Ig = immunoglobulin, ILD = interstitial lung disease, LE = lupus erythematosus, LES = lower esophageal sphincter, MC = most common, MCP = metacarpophalangeal joint, MCTD = mixed connective tissue disease, MTP = metatarsophalangeal joint, NSAIDs = nonsteroidal anti-inflammatory drugs, PIP = proximal interphalangeal joint, PM = polymyositis, PSS = progressive systemic sclerosis, RA = rheumatoid arthritis, RBC = red blood cell, RF = rheumatoid factor, Rx = treatment, SLE = systemic lupus erythematosus, SS = Sjögren's syndrome, ss-DNA = single stranded DNA.

Table 12–3. VASCULITIS

Most Common...	Answer and Explanation
sign of small vessel vasculitis	*palpable purpura:* * e.g., HSP, * palpable purpura due to IC deposition (type III HSR) in post-capillary venules
clinical presentation for vasculitis involving muscular arteries	*vessel thrombosis with infarction:* e.g., PAN
clinical presentation for vasculitis involving elastic arteries	• **lack of a pulse:** e.g., Takayasu's giant cell arteritis involving subclavian artery, • *stroke,* • *blindness*
vasculitis in adults	*giant cell arteritis:* * temporal arteritis, * granulomatous vasculitis of temporal artery and extracranial vessels
presentation of giant cell arteritis	• **headache along the course of temporal artery,** • *jaw claudication,* • *polymyalgia rheumatica:* * 40–50%, * pain and morning stiffness, * normal serum CK, • *blindness:* arteritis of branches of ophthalmic/posterior ciliary arteries → ischemic optic neuritis
lab test to screen for temporal arteritis	*ESR:* * positive clinical Hx + increased ESR sufficient to begin Rx with corticosteroids (prevent permanent blindness), * temporal artery Bx confirms Dx
vasculitis in children	*Henoch-Schönlein purpura (HSP):* small vessel vasculitis of post-capillary venules
S/S of HSP	• **palpable purpura limited to buttocks/lower extremity,** • *abdominal pain*: sometimes GI bleed, • *hematuria with RBC casts*: GN, • *polyarthritis,* • *usually follows a URI,* • *IgA-C3 ICs deposit in small vessels*
Rx of HSP	*corticosteroids*
vasculitis associated with HBV	*polyarteritis nodosa* (PAN): * male dominant IC vasculitis of muscular arteries, * lesions are in different stages of development (acute/chronic), * ~30–40% HBsAg positive, * "nodosa" refers to focal aneurysm formation

Table continued on following page

Table 12-3. VASCULITIS *Continued*

Most Common...	Answer and Explanation
S/S of PAN	• **fever,** • **kidneys:** * 85%, * vasculitis/GN, * hematuria/RBC casts, • *coronary vessels:* * 75%, * thrombosis, * aneurysms, • *liver:* * 65%, * cystic duct artery calcification, • *GI tract:* * 50%, * bowel infarction, • *skin:* * >25%, * painful nodules with ulceration, * livedo reticularis, • *peripheral neuropathy,* • *lungs:* * not usually involved, * commonly involved in microscopic PAN
clinical associations of PAN	• **HBV,** • *cryoglobulinemia,* • *hairy cell leukemia,* • *MDS,* • *RA,* • *Sjögren's syndrome*
lab findings in PAN	• **p-ANCA:** * ~90%, * p refers to perinuclear staining, * involved in producing vasculitis, • *neutrophilic leukocytosis,* • *eosinophilia,* • *HBsAg positive,* • *thrombocytosis*
confirmatory tests for PAN	• **angiography,** • *Bx of tissue:* * peripheral nerve, * testicle, * muscle
Rx of PAN	*corticosteroids:* often combined with antimetabolites or cytotoxic drugs
COD in PAN	• **renal failure,** • *bowel infarction*
vasculitis associated with HCV	*cryoglobulinemia vasculitis*
clinical associations of type I cryoglobulinemia	• **multiple myeloma,** • *Waldenström's macroglobulinemia,* • *malignant lymphomas* [Type I disease monoclonal. No vasculitis.]
clinical association of type II cryoglobulinemia	*HCV:* * mixed monoclonal/polyclonal or pure polyclonal cryoglobulinemia, * necrotizing vasculitis, * IC deposition of cryoglobulins (reversible cold-precipitating IgM or IgM/IgG antibodies) and complement in skin/renal vessels (type I MPGN)
clinical findings in type II cryoglobulinemia	• **palpable purpura:** limited to lower extremities, • *urticaria,* • *skin ulcers,* • *progressive renal disease,* • *arthritis,* • *peripheral neuropathy*
Rx of cryoglobulinemia	• **corticosteroids,** • *immunosuppressive agents*
adult cause of palpable purpura	*Churg-Strauss vasculitis:* 60%

Table 12–3. VASCULITIS *Continued*

Most Common...	Answer and Explanation
S/S of Churg-Strauss vasculitis	• **recurrent asthma, allergic rhinitis, nasal polyps,** • *eosinophilia,* • *systemic vasculitis:* e.g., * pulmonary vessels, * kidneys, • *granulomatous vasculitis of small/medium arteries,* • *PAN variant*
lab findings in Churg-Strauss vasculitis	• **p-ANCA:** 70%, • *eosinophilia,* • *increased IgE*
Rx of Churg-Strauss vasculitis	*corticosteroids + cyclophosphamide*
vasculitis in young male smokers	*thromboangiitis obliterans* (TAO, Buerger's disease): * involves arteries/veins/nerves of digital vessels in upper/lower extremities, * vessels thrombose leading to gangrene often requiring amputation, * unlike Raynaud's, pulse is absent due to vessel thrombosis, not vasospasm
S/S of TAO	• **claudication of instep of foot,** • *loss of digits due to ischemic necrosis*
Rx of TAO	*stop smoking*
cause of pulseless disease	*Takayasu's arteritis:* * granulomatous vasculitis involving aortic arch vessels, * aneurysms may develop, * may involve ♦ aortic valve, ♦ coronary ostia, ♦ renal arteries (renovascular HTN), ♦ pulmonary vessels, * MC in Asian women <50 y old
S/S of Takayasu's arteritis	• **upper extremity claudication,** • *unequal blood pressures between upper/lower extremity:* opposite of coarctation, • *blindness,* • *strokes*
Rx of Takayasu's arteritis	*corticosteroids*
COD in Takayasu's arteritis	• **CHF,** • *CVA*
vasculitis producing a saddle nose deformity	*Wegener's granulomatosis* (WG): * necrotizing granulomatous vasculitis, * sites: ♦ upper/lower respiratory tract (sinuses, nose, lungs: nodular, central cavitating lesions), ♦ kidneys: focal segmental GN, * cartilage destroyed, leading to saddle nose deformity

Table continued on following page

Table 12–3. VASCULITIS *Continued*

Most Common...	Answer and Explanation
lab findings in WG	• **c-ANCA:** >90%, • *neutrophilic leukocytosis,* • *eosinophilia*
Rx of WG	*cyclophosphamide*
clinical/lab findings of microscopic PAN	• *targets elderly patients,* • *necrotizing vasculitis with few or no ICs,* • *clinical: * sinusitis, * cough, * hemoptysis,* • *GN,* • *lab: p-ANCA* (50%)

Questions: The set of options is followed by several numbered items. For each numbered item, select the **ONE** lettered option that is **MOST CLOSELY** associated with it. Each lettered option may be selected once, more than once, or not at all.

(A) Giant cell arteritis
(B) Takayasu's arteritis
(C) PAN
(D) Cryoglobulinemia vasculitis
(E) Churg-Strauss vasculitis
(F) Wegener's granulomatosis
(G) Thromboangiitis obliterans

1. Centrally located, thick-walled cavitating lesions in the lungs
2. Vasculitis in a man with chronic HBV
3. Vasculitis, urticaria, cutaneous ulcers in a patient with chronic HCV
4. Peripheral eosinophilia, bronchial asthma, and glomerulonephritis in a young woman
5. 65-y-old woman with jaw claudication, scalp tenderness, and diffuse arthralgias and myalgias
6. Male smoker with pain on the instep of the foot when walking
7. Young woman with dizziness and an absent radial pulse

Answers: 1. (F), **2.** (C), **3.** (D), **4.** (E), **5.** (A), **6.** (G), **7.** (B): Patient (1) has the classic lung lesion of Wegener's granulomatosis. It is an angiocentric lesion **(choice F).** Patient (2) has chronic HBV and a vasculitis most likely due to PAN, which forms immunocomplexes from HBsAg **(choice C).** Patient (3) has chronic HCV and cutaneous lesions that are consistent with type II cryoglobulinemia **(choice D).** Patient (4) has a history that is most compatible with Churg-Strauss vasculitis **(choice E).** Patient (5) is an elderly woman with giant cell arteritis and polymyalgia rheumatica **(choice A).** Patient (6) is a male smoker with TAO who has claudication leading to pain in the instep of the foot **(choice G).** Patient (7) has CNS signs and lack of a radial pulse consistent with Takayasu's arteritis **(choice B).**

ANCA = anti-neutrophil cytoplasmic antibodies, Bx = biopsy, CHF = congestive heart failure, CK = creatine kinase, CNS = central nervous system, COD = cause of death, CVA = cerebrovascular accident, Dx =

diagnosis, ESR = erythrocyte sedimentation rate, GI = gastrointestinal, GN = glomerulonephritis, HBsAg = hepatitis B surface antigen, HBV = hepatitis B virus, HCV = hepatitis C virus, HSP = Henoch-Schönlein purpura, HTN = hypertension, Hx = history, IC = immunocomplex, Ig = immunoglobulin, MC = most common, MDS = myelodysplastic syndrome, MPGN = membranoproliferative glomerulonephritis, PAN = polyarteritis nodosa, RA = rheumatoid arthritis, RBC = red blood cell, Rx = treatment, S/S = signs and symptoms, TAO = thromboangiitis obliterans, URI = upper respiratory infection, WG = Wegener's granulomatosis.

Table 12–4. SELECTED BONE AND CARTILAGE DISORDERS

Most Common...	Answer and Explanation
hereditary bone disease	*osteogenesis imperfecta:* AD/AR disease with defect in synthesis of type I collagen
S/S of osteogenesis imperfecta	• **pathologic fractures:** "brittle bone" disease, • *blue sclera,* • *deafness*
metabolic bone disease	*osteoporosis:* see Table 11–3
cause of osteomyelitis in young adults	*Staphylococcus aureus:* usually spreads to bone by the hematogenous route
site in bone targeted by osteomyelitis	*metaphysis:* richest blood supply
complications of osteomyelitis	• **draining sinus tracts,** • *nidus for septicemia,* • *squamous cancer in sinus tract,* • *amyloidosis*
type of osteomyelitis in sickle cell anemia	*Staphylococcus aureus: Salmonella,* though common in the setting of sickle cell disease, is not the MC overall osteomyelitis
method for diagnosing osteomyelitis	• **radionuclide bone scan:** more sensitive than plan radiographs, • *bone Bx with culture for confirmation*
cause of Pott's disease	*TB:* * TB involves vertebral column, * bone destruction/extension of inflammation along psoas muscle sheath
common sites for Pott's disease	• **lower thoracic vertebra,** • *lumbar vertebra*
bone lesion present in congenital syphilis	*osteochondritis:* associated with new bone formation around long bones leading to *saber shins* with forward bowing of tibia

Table continued on following page

Table 12–4. SELECTED BONE AND CARTILAGE DISORDERS *Continued*

Most Common...	Answer and Explanation
infection due to puncture wounds while wearing rubber footwear	*Pseudomonas aeruginosa osteomyelitis*
femoral fracture	*femoral neck fracture* [It most commonly occurs in the elderly male patient with osteoporosis. Compromises medial femoral circumflex artery.]
wrist bone fracture leading to aseptic necrosis	*scaphoid* (navicular) *fracture*
fracture associated with falling on the outstretched hand	*Colles' fracture of the distal radius* [It produces a "dinner fork" deformity of the proximal radial fragment, which is displaced upward and backward. Second most common fracture in osteoporosis in women.]
cause of pathologic fractures	*metastatic disease to bone* [Breast cancer is the most common cause of bone metastasis.]
site/cause of avascular (aseptic) necrosis of bone	• **femoral head:** femoral head fracture, • *steroids,* • *sickle cell disease,* • *osteoporosis,* • *Legg-Perthes disease*
osteochondrosis	*Legg-Perthes disease involving the femoral head.* [Osteochondrosis refers to aseptic necrosis of ossification centers. Legg-Perthes is more common in boys between 3–10 years of age and presents with a painless limp. OA is a common sequela.]
test used to identify aseptic necrosis	• **MRI:** exhibits increased density in the area of involvement, • *plain radiograph:* increased density from reactive bone formation
S/S of Albright's syndrome	• **polyostotic fibrous dysplasia:** benign bone disease, • *cafe-au-lait pigmentation,* • *precocious puberty* (usually in females)
cancer associated with hypertrophic osteoarthropathy	*primary lung cancer* [Hypertrophic osteoarthropathy refers to periosteal inflammation with new bone formation and arthritis. It may or may not be associated with clubbing of the fingers.]

Table 12–4. SELECTED BONE AND CARTILAGE DISORDERS *Continued*

Most Common...	Answer and Explanation
benign bone tumor producing nocturnal pain relieved by aspirin	*osteoid osteoma* [It involves the cortical aspect of the proximal femur. It has a radiolucent nidus surrounded by dense sclerotic bone.]
primary bone tumors in order of increasing age	• *Ewing's sarcoma:* first and second decade, • *osteogenic sarcoma:* 10–25 years old, • *chondrosarcoma:* >30 years old, • *multiple myeloma:* >50 years old
primary malignant bone tumors in descending order of frequency	• **multiple myeloma,** • *osteogenic sarcoma,* • *chondrosarcoma,* • *Ewing's sarcoma,* • *giant cell tumor of bone*
malignancy of bone	*metastatic breast cancer*
benign bone tumor	*osteochondroma:* * benign cartilaginous tumor arising as outgrowth from metaphysis, * capped by benign proliferating cartilage
bone tumors arising in epiphysis	• **giant cell tumor:** female dominant tumor arising in distal end of femur/proximal tibia, • *chondroblastoma:* * benign cartilaginous tumor, * "popcorn appearance" on radiograph
classic radiographic findings in osteogenic sarcoma	• **"sunburst appearance":** calcified malignant osteoid in soft tissue surrounding tumor, • *Codman's triangle:* periosteum elevated due to tumor infiltrating out of metaphysis into soft tissue
classic radiographic finding in Ewing's sarcoma	concentric *"onion skin layering":* * due to new bone formation around primary tumor, * usually in tibia or flat bones of pelvis
location of an osteogenic sarcoma	*distal femur or proximal tibia*
risk factors for an osteogenic sarcoma	• **radiation,** • *Paget's disease,* • *inactivation of Rb suppressor gene on chromosome 13*
bone tumor associated with Gardner's polyposis syndrome	*osteoma:* * benign tumor * most commonly located in the ♦ **sinuses,** ♦ jaws, ♦ facial bones
primary bone tumor located in vertebra	*osteoblastoma:* "giant osteoid osteoma"

Table continued on following page

636 MOST COMMONS IN MEDICINE

Table 12–4. SELECTED BONE AND CARTILAGE DISORDERS *Continued*

Most Common...	Answer and Explanation
malignant cartilaginous tumor	*chondrosarcoma:* most often located in **pelvis** and *upper end of femur*
risk factors for chondrosarcoma	• **multiple osteochondromas:** * osteochondromatosis, * AD disease, • *Ollier's disease:* * multiple enchondromas, * arise in medullary cavity

Question: Which of the following bone disorders are more common in patients over 30 years of age? **SELECT 3**
- (A) Osteochondroma
- (B) Multiple myeloma
- (C) Chondrosarcoma
- (D) Legg-Perthes disease
- (E) Giant cell tumor
- (F) Osteoid osteoma
- (G) Ewing's sarcoma
- (H) Paget's disease
- (I) Osteogenic sarcoma

Answers: (B), (C), (H): Multiple myeloma **(choice B)**, chondrosarcoma **(choice C)**, and Paget's disease **(choice H)** are more common in patients >30 years of age. Osteochondroma, Legg-Perthes disease, giant cell tumor, osteoid osteoma, Ewing's sarcoma, and osteogenic sarcoma are more common in a younger age-bracket **(choices A, D, E, F, G, I are incorrect).**

AD = autosomal dominant, AR = autosomal recessive, MC = most common, MRI = magnetic resonance imaging, OA = osteoarthritis, S/S = signs and symptoms, TB = tuberculosis.

Table 12–5. SELECTED MUSCLE AND SOFT TISSUE DISORDERS

Most Common...	Answer and Explanation
symptom of muscle disease	*weakness*
causes of muscle weakness	• **UMN or LMN disease:** e.g., ALS, • *defects in neuromuscular synapse:* e.g., MG, • *primary muscle disease:* e.g., DMD
causes of neurogenic atrophy	• **axonal degeneration:** e.g., distal sensorimotor peripheral neuropathy in DM, • *destruction of motor neuron:* e.g., * polio

Table 12–5. SELECTED MUSCLE AND SOFT TISSUE DISORDERS *Continued*

Most Common...	Answer and Explanation
adult MD	*myotonic dystrophy:* AD disease with a triplet repeat defect
S/S of myotonic dystrophy	• **inability to relax muscles:** myotonia, • *facial weakness,* • *frontal balding,* • *cataracts,* • *testicular atrophy,* • *cardiac disease*
infectious causes of myositis	• **viral:** e.g., * coxsackievirus, * influenza, • *bacterial: Clostridium perfringens,* • *parasitic:* * *Toxoplasma gondii,* * *Taenia solium,* * *Trichinella spiralis*
drugs causing myositis	• **alcohol,** • *clofibrate,* • L-*tryptophan,* • *penicillamine*
acid-base causes of myositis	• **hypokalemia,** • *hypophosphatemia*
cause of MG	*autoantibodies against ACh receptor:* type II HSR
antibody source in MG	*B cells in germinal follicles within thymus*
S/S of MG	• **ptosis,** • *muscle weakness that worsens with exercise,* • *diplopia,* • *respiratory failure*
thymus findings in MG	• **B cell hyperplasia:** 85%, • *thymoma:* 15%
initial lab tests performed in MG	• **Tensilon test:** * edrophonium, * blocks acetylcholinesterase, * ACh increased in synapse, which improves muscle strength, • *measuring serum autoantibodies:* ~85–90%, • *EMG*
Rx of MG	• **acetylcholinesterase inhibitors:** e.g., pyridostigmine, • *corticosteroids,* • *thymectomy*
cause of botulism	*Clostridium botulinum:* * ingestion of preformed toxins (food poisoning) in adults, * bowel colonization with subsequent toxin formation in infants (via honey in milk)
site of action of botulinum toxin	*blocks release of ACh:* * descending paralysis, * pupils dilated
drug blocking ACh release	*aminoglycosides*

Table continued on following page

**Table 12–5. SELECTED MUSCLE AND SOFT
TISSUE DISORDERS** *Continued*

Most Common...	Answer and Explanation
fibromatosis	*Dupuytren's contracture:* * fibromatosis is non-neoplastic proliferation of connective tissue, * Dupuytren's contracture involves the palmar fascia and causes contraction of 4th/ 5th fingers, * common in alcoholics
fibromatosis associated with Gardner's polyposis syndrome	*desmoid tumor:* usually occurs in anterior abdominal wall
fibromatosis associated with methysergide	*retroperitoneal fibrosis:* often leads to hydronephrosis
benign soft tissue tumor	*lipoma:* arises from adipose cells
benign soft tissue tumor in GI tract	*leiomyoma:* most commonly located in the stomach
benign soft tissue tumor of heart in adults	*myxoma:* most commonly occurs in left atrium
risk factors for producing sarcomas	• **ionizing radiation:** e.g., * malignant fibrous histiocytoma, * osteogenic sarcoma, • *genetic predisposition:* e.g., neurofibrosarcoma in neurofibromatosis
sarcoma in adults	• **malignant fibrous histiocytoma,** • *liposarcoma:* second MC

Table 12–5. SELECTED MUSCLE AND SOFT TISSUE DISORDERS *Continued*

Question: Which of the following disorders is associated with normal muscle strength? SELECT 3
- (A) Polymyositis
- (B) Parkinson's disease
- (C) MG
- (D) Hypokalemia
- (E) Myotonic dystrophy
- (F) Primary hypothyroidism
- (G) Hypophosphatemia
- (H) Polymyalgia rheumatica
- (I) Sensory polyneuropathy

Answers: (B), (H), (I): Polymyositis, unlike polymyalgia rheumatica **(choice H)**, is associated with muscle weakness **(choice A is incorrect)**. Parkinson's disease **(choice B)** is associated with muscle rigidity leading to bradykinesia, which is misinterpreted by the patient as representing muscle weakness. MG, hypokalemia, myotonic dystrophy, and primary hypothyroidism are all associated with muscle weakness **(choices C, D, E, and F are incorrect)**. Sensory neuropathy **(choice I)** is not associated with muscle weakness; however, if axon damage occurs, the muscle will undergo atrophy.

ACh = acetylcholine, AD = autosomal dominant, ALS = amyotropic lateral sclerosis, DM = diabetes mellitus, DMD = Duchenne's muscular dystrophy, GI = gastrointestinal, HSR = hypersensitivity reaction, LMN = lower motor neuron, MC = most common, MD = muscular dystrophy, MG = myasthenia gravis, S/S = signs and symptoms, UMN = upper motor neuron.

CLINICAL IMMUNOLOGY

CONTENTS

Table 13–1. HEREDITARY AND ACQUIRED IMMUNODEFICIENCIES, COMPLEMENT SYSTEM TESTS

Most Common...	Answer and Explanation
B cell functions	• *Ig synthesis,* • *defense against encapsulated organisms,* • *neutralization of bacterial and chemical toxins,* • *mucosal defense against pathogens and pollens:* e.g., secretory IgA
T cell functions	• *defense against intracellular pathogens,* • *DRH reactions,* • *regulation of B lymphocytes:* CD_8 suppressor T cells, • *lymphokine production:* e.g., IL-2
lymphocyte in PB	CD_4 *helper T cells:* * T cells 60% of PB lymphocytes, * ratio of CD_4/CD_8 T cells 2/1
causes of reversal of CD_4/CD_8 T cell ratio	• **AIDS,** • *EBV*
B cell tests	• Ig concentration, • *marker studies:* mature versus immature B cell, • *presence of isohemagglutinins:* e.g., anti-A-IgM antibody in blood group B individual, • *B cell count:* 10–20% of PB lymphocytes, • *B cell mitogen stimulation:* * functional test, * mitogens: ♦ staphylococcal A antigen, ♦ pokeweed, • *lymph node Bx:* * B cells located in germinal follicles, * plasma cells indicate antigenic stimulation of B cells
T cell tests	• *T cell count:* flow cytometry, • *marker studies:* identify T cell subsets— * CD_4 helper cells, * CD_8 cytotoxic/suppressor cells, * TdT (indicates immature T cell), • *mitogen stimu-*

Table continued on following page

**Table 13–1. HEREDITARY AND ACQUIRED
IMMUNODEFICIENCIES, COMPLEMENT SYSTEM TESTS**
Continued

Most Common...	Answer and Explanation
Continued	lation: mitogens— * PHA, * ConA, • *intradermal skin testing with common antigens:* * functional T cell test, * antigens— ♦ streptokinase/streptodornase, ♦ *Candida* (most cost effective test), ♦ mumps antigens, ♦ no skin reaction indicates anergy, • *lymph node Bx:* T cells in paracortical areas
cytokine secreted by macrophages	*IL-1:* * augments immune response, * responsible for fever production
cytokines secreted by CD_4 helper T cells	• *IL-2:* T lymphocyte activator, • *γ-IF:* * antiviral, * antitumor, * enhances CD_8 T/NK cells
cytokine that augments allergic reactions	*IL-4:* * helps stimulate IgE synthesis, * helps develop CD_4 TH_2 subsets involved in type I hypersensitivity reactions
cytokine that augments hematopoiesis	*IL-3:* stimulates pluripotential stem cell
predisposing causes of ID	• **infections:** e.g., AIDS, • *prematurity,* • *autoimmune disease:* e.g., SLE, • *lymphoproliferative disease:* e.g., CLL, • *immunosuppressive therapy:* e.g., corticosteroids
complications associated with ID	• **infections:** * defense against encapsulated pathogens (♦ B cell dysfunction, ♦ e.g., *Streptococcus pneumoniae*), * defense against intracellular pathogens (♦ T cell dysfunction, ♦ e.g., TB, fungi, viruses), • *leukemia/lymphoma,* • *autoimmune disease*
genetic ID	*IgA deficiency:* * occurs in 1 : 500, * intrinsic defect in differentiation of B cells committed to synthesizing IgA
complications in IgA deficiency	• **sinopulmonary disease,** • *diarrhea:* giardiasis, • *allergies,* • *autoimmune disease,* • *anaphylactic reaction if infused with blood products containing IgA:* * patients develop anti-IgA antibodies, * must use washed RBC products or plasma from IgA deficient patients

Table 13–1. HEREDITARY AND ACQUIRED
IMMUNODEFICIENCIES, COMPLEMENT SYSTEM TESTS
Continued

Most Common...	Answer and Explanation
cause of ID in CVID	*mature B cell maturation defect into plasma cells:* occurs in 15–35-y-old age bracket
S/S in CVID	• **sinopulmonary disease,** • *diarrhea:* giardiasis, • *malabsorption:* due to celiac disease or lactose intolerance, • e.g., *autoimmune disease* * celiac disease, * PA, • *panhypogammaglobulinemia*
Rx of CVID	*IV gamma globulin*
ID associated with IgG_2/IgG_4 subclass deficiency	*IgA deficiency*
S/S of IgG_2/IgG_4 subset deficiency	• *recurrent sinusitis,* • *recurrent otitis media,* • *bronchopulmonary infections*
immunologic complication associated with blood transfusion in T cell deficient patients	*graft-versus-host reaction:* donor T cells attack recipient
infection associated with blood transfusion in T cell deficiency patients	*CMV:* * CMV in donor lymphocytes, * donor transfusions are irradiated prior to transfusion to prevent GVH and CMV
complement factors measured to identify classical/alternative pathway dysfunction	• *classical pathway dysfunction:* * C2, * C4, • *alternative pathway dysfunction:* factor B, • *both pathways:* C3
test to assess functional activity of complement system	CH_{50} *total hemolytic complement assay:* * tests complement system's ability to lyse sheep RBCs coated with rabbit IgG antibodies against sheep RBC antigens, * low values indicate low complement levels
cause of complement deficiency	*complement consumption in immunocomplex disease*
clinical findings in C1 esterase inhibitor deficiency	• *AD disease:* also called hereditary angioedema, • *recurrent swelling of face and/or oropharynx,* • *most often precipitated by den-*

Table continued on following page

Table 13-1. HEREDITARY AND ACQUIRED
IMMUNODEFICIENCIES, COMPLEMENT SYSTEM TESTS
Continued

Most Common...	Answer and Explanation
Continued	*tal work and oral mucosal trauma,* • *cramps and diarrhea, absence of pruritus:* unlike urticarial reactions, • *no response to epinephrine*
mechanism of angioedema in C1 esterase inhibitor deficiency	*increased production of C2-derived kinins:* increase vessel permeability causing edema to develop in deep soft tissue
screening tests for hereditary angioedema	• **C4 levels:** low, • *C2:* low, • *C3:* normal, • *enzyme assay:* confirmatory test
Rx of hereditary angioedema	*androgens*
COD in hereditary angioedema	*laryngeal edema*
complement deficiencies in disseminated gonococcemia	*C5–C9 deficiency:* components necessary for phagocytosis of *Neisseria gonorrhoeae*

Question: Which of the following are expected in a patient with AIDS? **SELECT 2**
   (A) Low CD₄ helper T cell count
   (B) Skin reaction to *Candida*
   (C) Low Ig levels
   (D) Absent germinal follicles
   (E) Abnormal PHA mitogen assay

Answers: (A), (E): The CD₄ T helper cell count **(choice A)** is always <200 cells/μL in AIDS, since the virus infects and destroys these cells. Skin reactions to common antigens are weak to absent (anergy), since these reactions require normal T cell function **(choice B is incorrect).** The total Ig levels are increased in AIDS patients owing to polyclonal stimulation of B cells by EBV and CMV **(choice C is incorrect).** Germinal follicles are present in AIDS patients owing to EBV and CMV stimulation of B cells **(choice D is incorrect).** Dendritic cells within the follicle house the HIV during the early asymptomatic stage. The functional PHA mitogen assay **(choice E)** is abnormal owing to deficiency of CD₄ T helper cells.

AD = autosomal dominant, AIDS = acquired immunodeficiency syndrome, Bx = biopsy, CLL = chronic lymphocytic leukemia, CMV = cytomegalovirus, COD = cause of death, ConA = concanavalin A, CVID = common variable immunodeficiency, DRH = delayed reaction hypersensitivity, EBV = Epstein-Barr virus, GVH = graft-versus-host reaction, HIV = human immunodeficiency virus, ID = immunodeficiency, IF = interferon, Ig = immunoglobulin, IL = interleukin, IV = intravenous, NK = natural killer, PA = pernicious anemia, PB = peripheral blood, PHA = phytohemagglutinin, RBC = red blood cell, Rx = treatment, SLE = systemic lupus erythematosus, S/S = signs and symptoms, TB = tuberculosis.

Table 13–2. ACQUIRED IMMUNODEFICIENCY SYNDROME

Most Common...	Answer and Explanation
acquired immunodeficiency (ID) in the United States	*AIDS*
etiologic agent of AIDS in the United States	*human immunodeficiency virus* (HIV)-1: * RNA retrovirus, * HIV-2 is MCC of AIDS in Western and Central America
COD in black males and women between 25 and 44 y of age	*AIDS:* accidents (usually motor vehicle) are now the most common COD in white males in this age bracket
racial groups with AIDS	• **whites 47%,** • *African-Americans* 35%, • *Hispanics* 18%, • *Asians* <1%, • *American Indians* <1%
steps in HIV infection	• *attachment of virus to CD_4 T helper cell:* * gp 120 is viral envelope protein that attaches to CD_4 molecule, * requires a co-receptor for fusion to host cell membrane, • *reverse transcriptase produces proviral DNA,* • *proviral DNA integrated into host DNA:* requires viral integrase, • *viral mRNA produced codes for polyprotein,* • *polyprotein cleavage by viral proteases,* • *small proteins assembled into virions at host cell membrane,* • *budding of virions off the host cell membrane*
cells other than CD_4 T helper cells infected by HIV	• **monocytes/macrophages,** • *dendritic cells,* • *astrocytes,* • *microglial cells:* CNS macrophage
protein surrounding viral genomic RNA	*p24 core protein:* increased in serum at two times: the initial infection and when the patient develops AIDS

Table continued on following page

Table 13–2. ACQUIRED IMMUNODEFICIENCY SYNDROME *Continued*

Most Common...	Answer and Explanation
cell lysed by HIV	*CD₄ T helper cell*
reservoir cell for viral replication	*monocyte lineage cells:* * macrophage, * dendritic cells, * viruses replicate in these cells without killing them
body fluids containing the virus	• **blood:** most infective body fluid, • *saliva,* • *semen,* • *amniotic fluid,* • *breast milk:* breast feeding contraindicated, • *spinal fluid,* • *urine,* • *tears,* • *bronchoalveolar lavage material*
mode of transmission of HIV in United States	*intimate sexual contact between homosexual men:* blood is second most common mode (IVDU and sharing needles)
mode of transmission of HIV worldwide	*heterosexual transmission*
modes of sexual transmission of HIV in United States in descending order	• **receptive anal intercourse between men,** • *vaginal intercourse male to female:* female mucosa has more surface area for exposure to infected semen, • *female to male*
mode of transmission of HIV in women	*heterosexual transmission in minority females who are IV drug abusers:* * sharing contaminated needles, * vaginal intercourse with HIV-positive males
mechanism of transmission by anal intercourse	*direct inoculation into blood from mucosal trauma or an open wound:* e.g., * syphilitic chancre, * proctitis
blood product containing virus	*whole blood/packed red blood cells:* 1:676,000 risk of transmission per unit
mode of transmission of HIV in health care workers	*accidental needle stick:* 0.3% risk
Rx recommended after needle stick from patient with HIV	• *AZT,* • *lamivudine:* prevents seroconversion in ~80%, • *high-risk exposures:* * deep punctures, * patients with advanced disease and high viral loads, * add protease inhibitor
mode of transmission in children	*vertical transmission* (mother to fetus) *from an infected mother* (90%): most cases are transplacental, followed by breast feeding and blood contamination during delivery

Table 13–2. ACQUIRED IMMUNODEFICIENCY
SYNDROME *Continued*

Most Common...	Answer and Explanation
Rx of pregnant women who are HIV-positive	*AZT:* reduced newborn rate of developing AIDS from ~25–30% to 7.6%
antibody detected by EIA	*anti-gp 120 antibody:* * EIA sensitivity 99.5–99.8%, * poor specificity (low prevalence of HIV in general population), * EIA is usually positive in 4–8 wks
cause of an FP EIA	*autoimmune disease*
test performed if the EIA is indeterminate or positive	*Western blot assay:* * positive test is p24 and gp41 antibodies and either gp120 or gp160 antibodies, * combined positive predictive value of positive EIA/Western blot is 99.5%
recommendations for EIA if person is exposed to HIV-positive patient	*EIA at time of exposure → 6 wks → 3 mths → 6 mths*
tests performed to screen for HIV in blood banks	• *EIA for HIV-1/HIV-2,* • *p24 capture assay*
test used to monitor current immune status of HIV-positive patient	*CD_4 T helper cell count:* e.g., count <200 cells/μL implies an increased risk for PCP
test to monitor viral burden in HIV-positive patient	*HIV RNA by PCR*
immunologic abnormalities in AIDS	• *lymphopenia:* low CD_4 T helper count, • *hypergammaglobulinemia:* polyclonal stimulation of B cells by EBV/CMV, • *anergy to skin testing,* • *decreased T cell mitogen blastogenesis,* • *decreased cytokine production,* • *dysfunctional NK cells,* • *increased p24 antigens,* • CD_4/CD_8 *ratio <1*
PPD skin test value considered positive for TB in HIV-positive patient	*>5 mm induration:* set for highest sensitivity owing to skin anergy
S/S of acute retroviral syndrome	• **fever:** 98%, • *generalized lymphadenopathy:* 75%, • *pharyngitis:* 70%, • *rash:* 60%, •

Table continued on following page

Table 13–2. ACQUIRED IMMUNODEFICIENCY SYNDROME *Continued*

Most Common...	Answer and Explanation
Continued	*myalgia:* 60%, • *headache:* 35% [Above usually occur 3–6 wks after exposure.]
phase following acute HIV syndrome	*asymptomatic, clinically latent phase:* viral replication occurs in dendritic cells in lymph nodes
phase following asymptomatic latent phase	*early symptomatic phase:* * non-AIDS defining infections, * lymphadenopathy, * hematologic abnormalities
non-AIDS defining infections in early symptomatic phase	• **oral thrush,** • *hairy leukoplakia:* EBV tongue infection, • *recurrent herpes simplex/herpes genitalis,* • *condyloma acuminatum:* HPV, • *shingles: herpes zoster,* • *molluscum contagiosum:* poxvirus
hematologic abnormality in early symptomatic phase	*thrombocytopenia:* possible mechanisms include * immunocomplex destruction (type III HSR), * antibodies against platelet antigens (type II HSR)
infections/ malignancy encountered with CD₄ T helper count 200–500 cells/μL	• **hairy leukoplakia/oral candidiasis,** • *TB,* • *mucocutaneous KS,* • *recurrent bacterial pneumonia:* * *Streptococcus pneumoniae,* * *Haemophilus influenzae*
infections/ malignancy encountered with CD₄ T helper count 100–200 cells/μL	• **PCP,** • *HSV,* • *disseminated histoplasmosis,* • *visceral KS*
infections/ malignancy encountered with CD₄ T helper count <100 cells/μL	• **disseminated MAI:** usually <75 cells/μL, • *Candida esophagitis,* • *CMV retinitis/esophagitis,* • *Toxoplasma encephalitis,* • *Cryptosporidiosis:* diarrhea, • *Cryptococcal meningitis,* • *CNS lymphoma*
AIDS-defining conditions: HIV-positive plus	• **CD₄** T helper cell count <200 cells/μL, • *specific malignancies:* see below, • *specific infections:* e.g., Pneumocystis carinii pneumonia
AIDS-defining malignancies	• **KS,** • *Burkitt's lymphoma,* • *invasive cervical cancer,* • *primary CNS lymphoma*

Table 13–2. ACQUIRED IMMUNODEFICIENCY
SYNDROME *Continued*

Most Common...	Answer and Explanation
AIDS-defining opportunistic bacterial infections	• **MAI:** disseminated/extrapulmonary, • *Mycobacterium kansasii:* disseminated/intrapulmonary, • *Mycobacterium tuberculosis:* any site, • *recurrent pneumonia:* usually *Streptococcus pneumoniae*, • *Salmonella* septicemia
AIDS-defining opportunistic fungal infections	• **P. carinii pneumonia,** • *candidiasis:* * airways, * esophagus, • *coccidioidomycosis:* disseminated/extrapulmonary, • *cryptococcosis:* extrapulmonary, • *histoplasmosis:* disseminated/extrapulmonary
systemic fungal infection in AIDS	*candidiasis*
CNS systemic fungal infection	*cryptococcosis:* meningitis
opportunistic viral infections in AIDS	• **CMV:** * CMV retinitis with visual loss, * biliary tract disease, * diarrhea, • *herpes simplex:* * PUD, * esophagitis, * bronchitis/pneumonia, * diarrhea, * proctitis, • *HIV-related encephalopathy:* AIDS dementia, • *HIV-related wasting syndrome,* • *PML:* papovavirus
opportunistic parasitic viral infections in AIDS	• **CNS toxoplasmosis,** • *cryptosporidiosis:* chronic intestinal >1 month, • *isosporiasis:* chronic intestinal >1 month
target organ involved in AIDS	*lungs:* * PCP, * *S. pneumoniae* pneumonia
cause of fever, night sweats, weight loss in AIDS	*disseminated MAI*
cause of lymphoid interstitial pneumonia in AIDS	*EBV*
fungal organisms involving GI tract in AIDS	• ***Candida:*** * mouth, * esophagus, • *Histoplasma:* colon
viruses associated with GI disease in AIDS	• **CMV:** * esophagus, * colon, * biliary tract, • *HSV:* * esophagus, * colon, * anus, • *adenovirus:* colon

Table continued on following page

Table 13–2. ACQUIRED IMMUNODEFICIENCY
SYNDROME *Continued*

Most Common...	Answer and Explanation
protozoans that are acid-fast positive and a cause of diarrhea in AIDS	• *Cryptosporidium:* * biliary tract, * Rx with paromomycin, • *Isospora*
infectious cause of Whipple's-like syndrome in AIDS	*MAI:* infect macrophages in lamina propria of small bowel, which in turn block off lymphatic drainage from the intestinal cell
cause of anal squamous cancer in AIDS	*HPV:* related to anal intercourse
cause of viral hepatitis in AIDS	*HBV*
electrolyte abnormality in AIDS	*hyponatremia:* SIADH
cause of KS	*herpesvirus 8*
disease that simulates KS in AIDS	*bacillary angiomatosis due to Bartonella henselae*
cutaneous lesion in AIDS	*KS:* vascular malignancy
lymphoma in AIDS	*B cell immunoblastic lymphoma:* high grade
lymphoma in AIDS related to EBV	*Burkitt's lymphoma*
cause of primary CNS lymphoma	*HIV in association with EBV*
extranodal site for lymphoma in AIDS	*CNS*
drug-induced cause of marrow suppression in AIDS	*AZT*
nutritional cause of anemia in AIDS	B_{12} *deficiency*
cause of neutropenia in AIDS	*marrow suppression from AZT*

Table 13–2. ACQUIRED IMMUNODEFICIENCY
SYNDROME *Continued*

Most Common...	Answer and Explanation
renal disease in AIDS	*focal segmental glomerulosclerosis:* nephrotic syndrome
drugs producing nephrotoxic damage in AIDS	• *amphotericin:* Rx of systemic fungal infections, • *pentamidine:* Rx of PCP, • *foscarnet:* Rx of disseminated CMV
cause of weight loss of >10%, fever, chronic diarrhea >1 mth, and fatigue	*HIV-related wasting syndrome:* one of the top three causes of death in AIDS
source of entry of HIV into CNS	*monocytes*
reservoir cell for HIV in CNS	*microglial cell:* CNS macrophage
HIV-related CNS disease	*HIV encephalopathy:* 60%
S/S of HIV encephalopathy	• **cognitive deficits,** • *motor impairment,* • *neurologic deficits,* • *behavioral impairment*
type of HIV-related spinal cord lesion	*vacuolar myelopathy:* * 20–30%, * similar to B$_{12}$ deficiency (subacute combined degeneration)
HIV-related peripheral neuropathy	*ascending paralysis:* similar to Guillain-Barré syndrome
causes of space-occupying lesions in CNS in AIDS	• **toxoplasmosis,** • *primary CNS lymphoma*
cause of focal epileptic seizures in AIDS	*toxoplasmosis*
cause of blindness in AIDS	*CMV retinitis*
Rx of CMV retinitis	*ganciclovir:* foscarnet is used if the patient is resistant to ganciclovir
initial drug regimen used in Rx of HIV	*two nucleoside analogues* (e.g., AZT, 3TC) + *one protease inhibitor* (e.g., indinavir)

Table continued on following page

**Table 13–2. ACQUIRED IMMUNODEFICIENCY
SYNDROME** *Continued*

Most Common...	Answer and Explanation
tests to monitor Rx of HIV	• **HIV RNA by PCR:** monitors viral burden during Rx, * performed q 3–6 mths, • *CD₄T helper count:* * immune status, * prophylaxis marker, * performed q 3–6 mths
MOA of nucleoside drugs	*block reverse transcriptase*
MOA of protease inhibitors	*suppress HIV replication by blocking protein processing later in the HIV cycle*
MOA of nonnucleoside reverse transcriptase inhibitors	*noncompetitively inhibit reverse transcriptase:* e.g., nevirapine
side effects of AZT	• *headache,* • *insomnia,* • *GI intolerance,* • *bone marrow suppression:* * macrocytic anemia unrelated to B₁₂ deficiency, * neutropenia, * anemia, • *proximal muscle disease,* • *dark blue nails*
side effects of didanosine	• *pancreatitis,* • *hepatitis,* • *peripheral neuropathy*
side effects of lamivudine (3TC)	• *rash,* • *peripheral neuropathy,* • *bone marrow toxicity*
protease inhibitor associated with renal stones	*indinavir*
side effect of non-nucleoside reverse transcriptase inhibitors	*rash*
CD₄ helper T cell count for prophylaxis against PCP	*<200 cells/μL:* Rx with TMP/SMX
CD₄ helper T cell count for prophylaxis against toxoplasmosis	*<100 cells/μL:* * also requires IgG antibody elevation, * Rx with TMP/SMX
CD₄ helper T cell count for prophylaxis against MAI	*<50–100 cells/μL:* Rx with azithromycin

Table 13–2. ACQUIRED IMMUNODEFICIENCY
SYNDROME Continued

Most Common...	Answer and Explanation
indication for prophylaxis against *M. tuberculosis*	*PPD reaction >5 mm:* Rx with INH + pyridoxine
recommendations to prevent AIDS	• **abstinence,** • *latex condoms with nonoxynol-9 viral spermicide*
immunizations recommended in HIV-positive patients	• *Salk* (killed) *vaccine:* live vaccine not recommended, • *HBV,* • *influenza,* • *Hib,* • *Pneumococcal vaccine*
live viral vaccine permitted in HIV-positive patients	*measles/mumps/rubella:* natural infection is worse than the potential infection from the vaccination
COD in AIDS	• **bacterial infection:** * *S. pneumoniae,* * disseminated *MAI,* • *wasting disease*

Question: Which of the following are AIDS-defining disorders? **SELECT 4**
  (A) Oral thrush
  (B) Molluscum contagiosum
  (C) Burkitt's lymphoma
  (D) Wasting syndrome
  (E) Hairy leukoplakia
  (F) Thrombocytopenia
  (G) Recurrent pneumonia
  (H) Cervical dysplasia
  (I) Bacillary angiomatosis
  (J) Cryptosporidiosis

Answers: (C), (D), (G), (J): Oral thrush, molluscum contagiosum, hairy leukoplakia, and bacillary angiomatosis are pre-AIDS-defining conditions (**choices A, B, E, I are incorrect**). Cervical dysplasia is not AIDS-defining (**choice H is incorrect**), but invasive cervical cancer is an AIDS-defining lesion. Thrombocytopenia is not AIDS-defining but is the most common hematologic abnormality predating AIDS (**choice F is incorrect**). Burkitt's lymphoma (**choice C**), wasting syndrome (**choice D**), recurrent pneumonia (usually *S. pneumoniae,* **choice G**), and cryptosporidiosis (**choice J**) are AIDS-defining lesions.

AIDS = acquired immunodeficiency syndrome, AZT = azidothymidine, CMV = cytomegalovirus, CNS = central nervous system, COD = cause of death, EBV = Epstein-Barr virus, EIA = enzyme immunoassay, FP = false-positive, GI = gastrointestinal, HBV = hepatitis B virus, Hib = *Haemophilus influenzae* type B, HIV = human immunodeficiency virus, HPV = human papillomavirus, HSR = hypersensitivity reaction, HSV = herpes simplex virus, ID = immunodeficiency, INH = isoniazid, IVDU = intravenous drug use, KS = Kaposi's sarcoma, MAI = *Mycobacterium avium-intracellulare,* MCC = most common cause, MOA = mechanism of action, PCP = *Pneumocystis carinii* pneumonia, PCR = polymerase chain reaction, PML = progressive multifocal leukoencephalopathy, PPD = purified protein derivative, PUD = peptic ulcer disease, Rx = treatment, SIADH = syndrome of inappropriate antidiuretic hormone, S/S = signs and symptoms, TB = tuberculosis, 3TC = lamivudine, TMP/SMX = trimethoprim/sulfamethoxazole.

Table 13–3. HYPERSENSITIVITY DISORDERS

Most Common...	Answer and Explanation
effector cells and antibody involved in type I reactions	• *mast cell/basophils,* • *IgE,* respectively
T cell subtype involved in type I reactions	CD_4 TH_2: antigen presenting cells (macrophage/dendritic cells in skin) present allergens to TH_2 subclass cells, with subsequent release of IL-4 that causes B cells to switch from IgM to IgE synthesis
causes of mast cell/basophil degranulation (release reaction) in type I reactions	• **cross-bridging of IgE antibodies by pollens,** • *food allergens:* e.g., peanuts, • *anaphylatoxins:* e.g., * C3a, * C5a, • *temperature changes:* reason for pruritus in PRV after taking warm baths/showers, • *pressure,* • *drugs:* e.g., penicillin
preformed chemicals released with mast cell/basophil degranulation	• **histamine,** • *eosinophil/neutrophil chemotactic factors,* • *heparin,* • *proteases*
secondary mediators released from activated mast cells/basophils	• *prostaglandins,* • *leukotrienes,* • *PAF* [Synthesis occurs directly after the release reaction. Chemicals enhance inflammatory reaction.]
term to describe an allergic individual	*atopic*
signs of type I reactions involving skin	• **atopic dermatitis:** * eczema, * rash involving ♦ face, ♦ intertriginous areas, ♦ extensor/flexor surfaces, • *urticaria*
signs of allergic rhinitis	• **pale boggy nasal mucosa,** • *allergic shiner,* • *allergic nasal crease,* • *allergic polyps*
S/S of allergic conjunctivitis	• **itchy eyes,** • *conjunctival redness,* • *tearing,* • *normal vision*

Table 13–3. HYPERSENSITIVITY DISORDERS *Continued*

Most Common...	Answer and Explanation
COD due to a venomous bite	*bee sting with an anaphylactic reaction:* type I HSR
COD in anaphylaxis	• **laryngeal obstruction by edema,** • *cardiovascular collapse*
initial Rx for anaphylactic reaction	*SC administration of 0.3–0.5 mL aqueous epinephrine 1 : 1000*
causes of food allergy	• **peanuts,** • **shellfish,** • **true nuts,** • *eggs,* • *milk,* • *soybean,* • *wheat*
stinging insect allergies	• **bees:** honeybee venom does not cross-react with vespid venom, • *vespids:* * yellow jackets, * wasps, * hornets
food allergies associated with latex allergy	*allergic reactions to bananas, avocado, kiwifruit*
drugs causing type I HSR	• **penicillin,** • *cephalosporins*
test to measure total IgE concentration	*PRIST:* * paper-based radioimmunosorbent test, * insensitive test, * high IgE 30–40%
skin test to evaluate type I HSR	*prick (scratch) skin testing:* * best all-around test for type I HSR, * positive test is a wheal/flare reaction, * in general, ~15% have positive skin tests
allergens tested by prick testing	• **pollens,** • *dust mite,* • *bee/vespid:* not necessary if patient already has known skin reactions, • *food*
serum test to measure specific IgE antibodies	*RAST:* * radioallergosorbent test, * not as sensitive/more expensive than scratch testing
test to R/O food allergies	*eliminate suspected food from diet and record changes*
PB finding in type I HSR	*eosinophilia*
screening test for allergic rhinitis	*nasal smear for eosinophils*
Rx for allergic rhinitis	• **antihistamines,** • *decongestants,* • avoid offending allergens: e.g., cats, • *intranasal*

Table continued on following page

Table 13–3. HYPERSENSITIVITY DISORDERS *Continued*

Most Common...	Answer and Explanation
Continued	corticosteroids, • *environmental modification for dust mites:* e.g., * encase bedding, * D/C house humidifier, * run dehumidifier, * wash bedding in hot water
recommendations for bee/vespid allergies	• **patient awareness:** * do not walk barefoot, * avoid cosmetics/outdoor maintenance, • *carry epinephrine,* • *immunotherapy*
uses of immunotherapy	• **allergic rhinitis,** • *bee/vespid allergy*
mediators of type II reactions	• **antibodies,** • *complement,* • *NK cells,* • *macrophages,* • *eosinophils*
type II HSR with autoantibodies against receptors	• **Graves' disease:** IgG thyroid stimulating antibodies against TSH receptor, • *myasthenia gravis:* IgG antibodies against Ach receptors
test to identify IgG and/or C3 on RBCs	*Coombs' test:* detects IgG and/or C3 on RBC surface (direct Coombs') or antibodies causing hemolysis in serum (indirect Coombs')
mediators of type III HSR	• *antigens,* • *antibodies:* * IgG, * IgM, * complement fixing antibodies, • *neutrophils,* • *macrophages,* • *complement* [The above mediators are involved in the formation of ICs and their pathogenicity.]
mechanism of tissue damage in type III HSR	*IC activation of complement system:* * C5a attracts neutrophils to tissue with ICs (e.g., small vessels, synovium, glomerulus), * C3a/C5a are anaphylatoxins → release histamine → increased vessel permeability/vasodilatation of arterioles
disorders associated with type III HSR	• **small vessel vasculitis:** e.g., HSP, • *GN:* e.g., SLE, • *arthritis:* e.g., RA, • *serum sickness:* e.g., Rx of rattlesnake envenomation with horse serum, • *hematologic cytopenias:* e.g., drug-induced AIHA
term applied to localized type III HSR	*Arthus reaction*

Table 13–3. HYPERSENSITIVITY DISORDERS *Continued*

Most Common...	Answer and Explanation
site of an Arthus reaction	*lungs:* e.g., farmer's lung: antigen is thermophilic actinomycetes + antibodies + complement
tests to evaluate type III HSR	• **complement levels:** low owing to consumption, • *IC assays:* e.g., * Raji cell assay, * C1q binding assay, • *IF:* e.g., detects IC deposition
mediators of type IV HSR	• *CD$_4$ T helper cells,* • *CD$_8$ cytotoxic T cells,* • *macrophages,* • *dendritic cells in skin:* Langerhans cells, • *antigens,* • *microbial pathogens:* e.g., TB [Type IV HSR does not involve antibodies (cellular immunity).]
types of type IV HSR	• **DRH:** e.g., * granulomatous disease, * allergic contact dermatitis, * certain autoimmune diseases, * certain skin test reactions (e.g., PPD, skin tests to evaluate T cell function), • *CD$_8$ cytotoxicity:* see below
test to document allergic contact dermatitis	*patch test:* suspected irritant is placed on a patch and applied to uninvolved skin for 48 h to evaluate whether an eczematous reaction to the irritant occurs
cell types involved in granulomas (e.g., TB)	• *macrophage,* • *CD$_4$ helper T cells:* * TH$_1$ subclass helper T cells are formed when macrophages secrete IL-12 after interacting with CD$_4$ helper T cells, * this subclass retains memory of antigen exposure, • *epithelioid cells:* γ-IF activated macrophages, • *multinucleated giant cells:* * fused macrophages, * marker of a granuloma
functions of CD$_8$ cytotoxic T cells in type IV HSR	• *kill tumor cells,* • *kill virally infected cells:* e.g., HBV, • *transplant rejection:* e.g., acute rejection [CD$_8$ T cells interact with class I antigens on target cells. Neoplastic/virally infected cells have altered class I antigens to which cytotoxic T cells react by secreting perforins that destroy the cell.]

Table continued on following page

Table 13–3. HYPERSENSITIVITY DISORDERS *Continued*

Question: Which of the following diseases are examples of type II hypersensitivity? **SELECT 4**
- (A) Goodpasture's syndrome
- (B) Serum sickness
- (C) PAN
- (D) Graves' disease
- (E) Poison ivy
- (F) AIHA due to penicillin
- (G) ABO hemolytic transfusion reaction
- (H) Hereditary angioedema

Answers: (A), (D), (F), (G): Goodpasture's syndrome (**choice A**, antibodies directed against basement membranes), Graves' disease (**choice D**, IgG antibody directed against TSH receptor), AIHA due to penicillin (**choice F**, IgG antibody directed against drug attached to RBC membrane), and an ABO hemolytic transfusion reaction (**choice G**, IgM antibodies directed against ABO antigens on donor RBCs) are all examples of type II reactions. Serum sickness and PAN are type III reactions involving immunocomplexes (**choices B and C are incorrect**). Poison ivy is a type IV reaction (**choice E is incorrect**). Hereditary angioedema is not a hypersensitivity reaction (**choice H is incorrect**). It is due to a deficiency of C1 esterase inhibitor, leading to activation of complement components C4 and C2.

Ach = acetylcholine, AIHA = autoimmune hemolytic anemia, COD = cause of death, D/C = discontinue, DRH = delayed reaction hypersensitivity, GN = glomerulonephritis, HBV = hepatitis B virus, HSP = Henoch-Schönlein purpura, HSR = hypersensitivity reaction, ICs = immunocomplexes, γ-IF = interferon, Ig = immunoglobulin, IL = interleukin, NK = natural killer, PAF = platelet activating factor, PAN = polyarteritis nodosa, PB = peripheral blood, PPD = purified protein derivative, PRV = polycythemia rubra vera, RA = rheumatoid arthritis, RAST = radioallergosorbent test, RBC = red blood cell, R/O = rule out, Rx = treatment, SLE = systemic lupus erythematosus, TB = tuberculosis, TSH = thyroid-stimulating hormone.

14

DERMATOLOGY

CONTENTS

Table 14–1. BENIGN NONINFECTIOUS SKIN DISORDERS

Most Common...	Answer and Explanation
skin diseases seen in clinical practice	• **superficial dermatophyte infections,** • *acne vulgaris,* • *seborrheic dermatitis*
uses of Wood's lamp in noninfectious disease	• **detect hypopigmented areas:** e.g., * vitiligo, * ash leaf macule in tuberous sclerosis, • *urine in PCT fluoresces coral red*
uses for direct IF of skin biopsies	• **autoimmune bullous diseases:** e.g., * bullous pemphigoid, * pemphigus vulgaris, * DH, • *discoid lupus,* • *SLE*
test for allergic contact dermatitis	*patch test:* see Table 13–3
epidermal layer involved in hyperkeratosis	*stratum corneum:* * anucleate cells with keratin, * increased thickness produces a scaly appearance called hyperkeratosis
appearance of a macule	*flat lesion:* e.g., * café-au-lait, * vitiligo, * junctional nevus
appearance of a papule	*peaked or dome-shaped lesion:* e.g., lichen planus
appearance of a nodule	*elevated, dome-shaped lesion that may or may not ulcerate:* e.g., BCC
appearance of a plaque	*flattened, elevated area often associated with scaling/erythema:* e.g., psoriasis
appearance of a vesicle	*fluid-filled blister* <5 mm: e.g., * varicella, * HSV

Table continued on following page

Table 14–1. BENIGN NONINFECTIOUS SKIN DISORDERS
Continued

Most Common...	Answer and Explanation
appearance of a bulla	*fluid-filled blister >5 mm:* e.g., bullous pemphigoid
appearance of a pustule	*blister filled with exudate:* e.g., folliculitis
inherited disorder of keratinization	*ichthyosis vulgaris:* AD disorder with prevalence of 1:250
clinical findings in ichthyosis vulgaris	• *hyperkeratotic, dry skin,* • *locations:* * palms, * soles, * extensor areas (not flexural), • *50% have atopic history*
acquired causes of ichthyosis	• *nutritional disorders:* * essential FA deficiency, * vitamin A deficiency, * kwashiorkor (flaky paint dermatitis), * pellagra (niacin deficiency), • *malignancy:* * NHL, * HD, * mycosis fungoides, * leukemia
skin changes in elderly	• *extrinsic:* related to UV light, • *intrinsic:* age-dependent
extrinsic changes in aging skin	• **solar lentigo:** * "liver spots", * brown, raised lesions on sun-exposed areas, * increased melanocytes/melanin synthesis, • *abnormal keratinocyte maturation:* produces dry skin (keratosis), • *solar elastosis:* * abnormal elastic fibers, * yellowish, chicken foot wrinkles in sun-exposed areas, • *freckles,* • *senile purpura:* * UV damage to perivascular fibroblasts, * develop in areas exposed to trauma (e.g., dorsum of hand), • *comedones on face:* * UV light destruction, * perifollicular elastic tissue causes dilatation
intrinsic changes in aging skin	• *decreased adhesion of keratinocytes:* causes dry skin (xerosis), • *decreased number of hair follicles, sweat glands:* predisposed to heat stroke, • *decreased thickness of epidermis/flattening of rete ridges,* • *decreased dermal collagen/elastic tissue,* • *reduced subcutaneous fat:* e.g., over dorsum of hands
skin disorder in elderly	*xerosis:* * dry skin with pruritus, * see above
term applied to skin inflammation	*dermatitis*

Table 14–1. BENIGN NONINFECTIOUS SKIN DISORDERS
Continued

Most Common...	Answer and Explanation
dermatitis	*eczema*
types of eczema	• **acute,** • *subacute,* • *chronic*
appearance of acute eczema	*weeping, erythematous rash with vesicle formation*
Rx of acute eczema	*application of:* * colloidal oatmeal, * sodium bicarbonate, * saline
appearance of subacute eczema	*erythematous rash with beginning hyperkeratosis*
clinical finding in eczema	*pruritus*
Rx of subacute eczema	*topical high potency corticosteroid*
appearance of chronic eczema	*thickened, dry, hyperkeratotic skin* (lichenification): due to constant scratching
Rx of chronic eczema	*highest potency topical corticosteroids under occlusive dressings*
cause of atopic dermatitis	*genetic predisposition for type I, IgE-mediated HSR:* allergic family Hx (atopic)
cause of pruritus in atopic dermatitis	*lower itch threshold than normal*
locations for atopic dermatitis	*cheeks, trunk, extensor surfaces in infants:* moves to flexor creases after 3 y of age
microbial pathogens complicating atopic dermatitis	• ***Staphylococcus aureus,*** • *HSV:* eczema herpeticum, • *molluscum contagiosum,* • *HPV:* wart
types of contact dermatitis (CD)	• **irritant contact dermatitis,** • *allergic CD,* • *contact photodermatitis,* • *contact urticaria*
type IV contact allergens	• **poison ivy,** • *nickel*
clinical findings in irritant contact dermatitis	• *nonimmunologic skin reaction,* • *local toxic effect from exposure to an antigen or irritating substance:* e.g., * detergent, * shampoo
mechanism for allergic contact dermatitis	*type IV CMI:* e.g., * poison ivy, * reaction to nickel, * reaction to certain chemicals

Table continued on following page

Table 14–1. BENIGN NONINFECTIOUS SKIN DISORDERS
Continued

Most Common...	Answer and Explanation
sensitizing agent causing allergic CD in jewelry	*nickel sulfate*
sensitizing agent causing allergic CD in sunscreen lotion	*PABA*
sensitizing agent causing allergic CD in hair dyes	*paraphenylenediamine*
sensitizing agent causing allergic CD in cosmetics	*formaldehyde*
sensitizing agent causing allergic CD in contact lens fluid	*thimerosal*
sensitizing agent causing allergic CD in rubber wear	*thiuram*
sensitizing agent causing allergic CD in construction workers	*potassium dichromate:* present in * cement, * leather, * paints
mechanism of contact urticaria	• **type I, IgE-mediated HSR,** • *nonimmunologic reaction*
mechanism of contact photodermatitis	*type IV CMI secondary to UVB light:* rash develops on * face, * V of neck, * dorsum of hands/forearms
drugs producing a contact photodermatitis	• **tetracycline:** phototoxic reaction resembles sunburn, • *PABA,* • *sulfonamides,* • *thiazides,* • *phenothiazines,* • *griseofulvin,* • *NSAIDs*
cause of chronic photodermatitis	*polymorphous light eruption* (PLE)
clinical finding in PLE	• *family Hx:* common in American Indians, • *rash begins with sun exposure and lessens over time as exposure increases,* • *lesions:* erythematous macules/papules/vesicles/bullae

Table 14–1. BENIGN NONINFECTIOUS SKIN DISORDERS
Continued

Most Common...	Answer and Explanation
Rx of PLE	*sunscreen*
clinical findings in pompholyx (dyshidrotic eczema)	• **recurrent vesicles along lateral border of fingers** (~80%), **palms, soles,** • *prickly sensation precedes onset of vesicles,* • *dystrophic nails,* • *Rx with topical steroids*
type of eczema confused with tinea corporis	*nummular eczema:* * coin-like, scaly lesions on extensor surfaces of lower extremity in 55–65-y-old, * possible HSR against *Staphylococcus aureus*
mechanism of lichen simplex chronicus (neurodermatitis)	*self-perpetuating "itch that rashes":* * most do not consider this a disease, * psychosomatic overtones in most patients
sites for lichen simplex chronicus	• *nape of neck,* • *wrists,* • *antecubital fossa,* • *forearms*
Rx of lichen simplex chronicus	*topical corticosteroids*
topical drugs with greatest risk for skin sensitization	• **neomycin,** • *diphenhydramine,* • *benzocaine*
skin lesion noted in acute sarcoidosis	*small, violaceous papules on eyelids, side of nose, neck: 20–35%*
skin lesion noted in chronic sarcoidosis	*nodular rash over trunk:* noncaseating granulomas are present in Bx
cause of toxic epidermal necrolysis (TEN)	*drugs:* * 80%, * diffuse erythematous rash develops ~1–3 wks post-drug, * rash followed by diffuse sloughing of skin, * mortality ranges from 25–70%
drugs associated with TEN	• **barbiturates,** • *sulfonamides,* • *ampicillin,* • *NSAIDs*
types of skin reactions produced by drugs	• **maculopapular rashes,** • *urticaria,* • *fixed drug eruption,* • *erythema multiforme*
type of drug producing anaphylactic shock	β-*lactam antibiotics*
drugs producing rashes	• **amoxicillin,** • *TMP/SMX,* • *ampicillin,* • *cephalosporins*

Table continued on following page

Table 14–1. BENIGN NONINFECTIOUS SKIN DISORDERS
Continued

Most Common...	Answer and Explanation
drug producing slate-gray discoloration of sun-exposed skin	• **chloroquine,** • *chlorpromazine*
drug producing slate-blue skin discoloration	*amiodarone*
drugs producing yellow pigmentation	*antimalarials:* * quinacrine, * sclera not yellow
drugs producing morbilliform eruptions	• **penicillin,** • *ampicillin,* • *cephalosporins*
drugs producing fixed drug eruptions	• **phenolphthalein:** laxatives, • *barbiturates,* • *salicylates,* • *oral contraceptives*
sites for fixed drug eruptions	• *genital region:* * glans penis, * scrotum, • *face* [Lesions are hyperpigmented.]
location/appearance of actinic (solar) keratosis	• **face,** • *hands,* • *forearms*
appearance of actinic (solar) keratosis	*erythematous to gray-white scaly lesions*
cause of actinic (solar) keratosis	*UVB light*
complications of actinic (solar) keratosis	• **squamous carcinoma in situ:** Bowen's disease, • *invasive squamous carcinoma*
Rx of actinic keratosis	• **liquid nitrogen,** • *5-fluorouracil cream*
appearance of lichen planus	• **pruritic purple papules on wrists, lower back, scalp,** • *leukoplakic, net-like lesion on buccal mucosa called Wickham's stria* [Trauma to skin causes lesions to develop at trauma site (Koebner's reaction).]
systemic infection associated with lichen planus	*HCV*

Table 14–1. BENIGN NONINFECTIOUS SKIN DISORDERS
Continued

Most Common...	Answer and Explanation
Rx of lichen planus	*topical steroids*
cause of lupus pernio	*sarcoidosis:* purplish plaques develop on nose, ears, lips, face
causes of psoriasis	• **genetic:** * HLA Cw6, * multifactorial inheritance, • *environmental factors:* * physical injury, * infection (streptococcal pharyngitis), * withdrawal from steroids
types of psoriasis	• **plaque type,** • *guttate,* • *pustular*
appearance of psoriatic plaques	*raised, well-demarcated, flat, salmon-colored plaques covered by silver-white scales:* when plaques picked off, pinpoint areas of bleeding (Auspitz sign)
sites for psoriasis	• **scalp,** • *elbows,* • *knees,* • *trunk* [Develop in areas of pressure/trauma (Koebner's reaction).]
nail finding in psoriasis	*pitting*
drugs exacerbating psoriasis	• *beta-blockers,* • *lithium,* • *antimalarials*
Rx of psoriasis	• **topical steroid creams,** • *UBV light + coal tar,* • *UVA light + psoralen,* • *methotrexate for disseminated disease*
type of psoriasis exacerbated by systemic corticosteroids	*pustular psoriasis*
clinical findings in pityriasis rosea	• **initial, pruritic oval-shaped, pink patch on trunk:** "herald patch", • *patch followed in 1–2 wks by papular rash in "Christmas tree" distribution on trunk* [~50% of patients are women. The rash occurs in spring/fall.]
Rx of pityriasis rosea	*UVB light*
trace metal deficiency producing vesiculobullous lesions	*zinc deficiency:* * lesions develop on the acral portions of extremities and around the mouth, * see Table 9–12
autoimmune bullous skin diseases	• **bullous pemphigoid,** • *pemphigus vulgaris*

Table continued on following page

Table 14–1. BENIGN NONINFECTIOUS SKIN DISORDERS
Continued

Most Common...	Answer and Explanation
cause of pemphigus vulgaris	*IgG antibodies/C3 directed against intercellular attachments between keratinocytes above basal cell layer* (type II HSR): * flaccid bullae develop above basal cells, * bullae contain acantholytic keratinocytes (lost attachments to each other)
locations for pemphigus vulgaris	• **oral mucosa,** • *skin:* lesions separate easily from basal layer (Nikolsky sign)
direct IF findings in pemphigus vulgaris	*IgG + C3 deposited in intercellular areas of epidermis:* antibodies against intercellular bridges also present in serum
Rx of pemphigus vulgaris	*corticosteroids:* * dapsone, * azathioprine, or * cyclophosphamide often used in severe cases
COD in pemphigus vulgaris	*Staphylococcus aureus sepsis*
cause of bullous pemphigoid	*IgG antibodies against basement membrane* (type II HSR): * subepidermal bullae, * no acantholytic cells, * contain eosinophils, * no Nikolsky sign, * serum antibodies ~70%
direct IF findings in bullous pemphigoid	*IgG + C3 along basement membrane*
drugs causing acquired bullous pemphigoid	• **D-penicillamine,** • *tetracycline,* • *captopril*
Rx of bullous pemphigoid	*corticosteroids*
clinical findings of DH	• *pruritic papules/vesicles,* • *sites:* * elbows, * knees, * buttocks, • *IgA anti-reticulin/IgA anti-endomysial antibodies in 70%*
direct IF findings in DH	*Deposition of IgA complexes at tips of dermal papilla:* subepidermal vesicles filled with neutrophils
clinical associations of DH	• **celiac disease:** autoimmune disease with antibodies against gluten (gliadin fraction), • *thyroid disease*
Rx of DH	• *gluten-free diet,* • *dapsone*

Table 14–1. BENIGN NONINFECTIOUS SKIN DISORDERS
Continued

Most Common...	Answer and Explanation
clinical findings in erythema multiforme (EM)	• *immunologic reaction targeting skin/mucous membranes,* • *lesions:* * bull's eye (like target cells), * vesicles, * bullae, * plaques, • *sites:* * palms/soles, * extensor surfaces, * lips, * buccal mucosa (Stevens Johnson syndrome)
drugs associated with EM	• **phenytoin,** • *barbiturates,* • *sulfonamides,* • *penicillin*
infections associated with EM	• **HSV,** • *Mycoplasma pneumoniae,* • *Yersinia enterocolitica,* • *Histoplasma capsulatum*
Rx of EM	• *systemic corticosteroids for oral lesions,* • *? use of corticosteroids for EM in other areas*
cause of pustular dermatitis	*acne vulgaris*
types of acne vulgaris	• **noninflammatory:** * closed (whiteheads), * open (blackheads) comedones, • *inflammatory:* * papules/pustules, * nodules, * cysts
mechanisms producing acne vulgaris	• *abnormal keratinization of follicular epithelium:* obstructs follicle, • *increased androgen-induced sebum formation,* • *bacterial lipase:* * produced by gram-positive anaerobe *Propionibacterium acnes,* * irritating fatty acids cause inflammation
inciting agents predisposing to acne vulgaris	• **hormones: e.g.,** * testosterone, * progesterone, * corticosteroids, • *lithium,* • *bromides,* • *occupational factors:* e.g., grease
role of dietary factors in acne vulgaris	*none:* e.g., chocolate and nuts are not associated with acne
Rx of noninflammatory acne vulgaris	• *topical tretinoin:* skin peeling agent, • *benzoyl peroxide:* * comedolytic agent, * kills *P. acnes,* * peeling agent
Rx of inflammatory type of acne vulgaris	*as above plus topical or systemic antibiotics:* * tetracycline, * erythromycin
Rx of cystic acne vulgaris	• **isotretinoin:** * synthetic retinoic acid, * improves keratinization, * decreases sebum production, * decreases inflammation, • *systemic antibiotics*

Table continued on following page

Table 14–1. BENIGN NONINFECTIOUS SKIN DISORDERS
Continued

Most Common...	Answer and Explanation
complications associated with isotretinoin	• **teratogenic:** * pregnancy test prior to starting drug, * place on BCPs, • *liver toxicity:* elevates LFTs, • *pseudotumor cerebri:* high intracerebral pressure, • *nail dystrophy,* • *leukopenia,* • *hyperlipidemia:* high TG/CH
clinical findings in acne rosacea	• *inflammation of facial pilosebaceous units:* pustules, • *rhinophyma:* sebaceous gland hyperplasia, • *flushing of cheeks,* • *telangiectasias:* reddened facial appearance
Rx of acne rosacea	*systemic antibiotics:* e.g., * tetracycline, * erythromycin
types of urticaria	• **type I, IgE-mediated HSR:** e.g., foods (peanuts, shellfish), • *cholinergic:* * urticaria with hot showers, * lesions on upper thorax/neck, * shaped like a pencil eraser, • *solar urticaria:* * papules/plaques appear minutes after UV exposure, * painful/pruritic, • *infections:* e.g., serum sickness syndrome in HBV, • *biting insects:* * e.g., fleas, gnats, * papular urticaria, • *drugs:* e.g., * aspirin, * penicillin, * codeine/morphine, * radiographic contrast media, • *chronic:* most are idiopathic, • *cold urticaria:* risk of cold water drowning due to shock
mediators of urticaria	• **histamine,** • *bradykinin,* • *leukotrienes,* • *prostaglandins,* • *PAF*
time-frame for urticaria due to type I HSR	*minutes to hours:* IgE-mediated histamine release from mast cells
time-frame for urticaria due to type III reactions	1–3 wks
drugs causing type III reactions	• **β-lactam antibiotics,** • *sulfonamides,* • *cholecystogram dyes*
S/S of type III drug reactions	• *serum sickness-like:* * **urticaria,** * erythema along sides of palms/soles, • *fever,* • *arthralgia*
mechanism for nonimmunologic drug-induced urticaria	*direct stimulation of histamine release from mast cells without IgE:* e.g., * codeine/morphine, * radiographic contrast media

Table 14–1. BENIGN NONINFECTIOUS SKIN DISORDERS
Continued

Most Common...	Answer and Explanation
sign of chronic urticaria	*dermatographism:* can write on skin and produce urticaria
drug aggravating existing urticaria	*aspirin*
mechanism of angioedema	*diffuse swelling of skin due to edema in deep subcutaneous tissue:* e.g., * C1 esterase inhibitor deficiency (see Table 13–3), * ACE inhibitors (due to bradykinin release)
cause of "red man" syndrome	*IV vancomycin:* redness due to histamine release
clinical findings in urticaria pigmentosum	• *pigmented macules/papules when scratched lead to urticaria:* * Darier's sign (urticaria when scratched), * histamine release from underlying mast cells, • *Dx by skin Bx and staining mast cells*
cause of cutaneous changes in SLE	*DNA-anti-DNA ICs against BM:* * IC deposits along BM (basis of band test), * direct IF test on skin Bx, * involved/uninvolved skin has positive band in SLE (only involved skin with discoid lupus)
benign skin lesion simulating a well-differentiated SCC	*keratoacanthoma:* * develops rapidly in a few months, * crateriform appearance, * normally regresses with scarring
clinical findings in erythema nodosum	*painful, raised nodule on anterior aspect of the shins:* localized inflammation of SC fat
inciting agents associated with erythema nodosum	• **infections:** e.g., **streptococcal pharyngitis,** * coccidioidomycosis, * histoplasmosis, * *TB,* * *Yersinia enterocolitica,* • *sarcoidosis,* • *UC,* • *drugs:* * **BCPs,** * sulfonamides
clinical findings in Lofgren's syndrome	• *fever,* • *arthralgias,* • *uveitis,* • *bilateral hilar adenopathy,* • *erythema nodosum* [These are the classic findings in acute sarcoidosis.]
Rx of erythema nodosum	• **Rx underlying disease,** • *NSAIDs*
types of pigmentation disorders	• *leukoderma:* * depigmentation, * mechanism: ♦ melanocyte loss, ♦ decreased melanin synthesis, • *melanoderma:* * hyperpigmentation, * mechanism: ♦ increased melanocytes, ♦ increased melanin synthesis

Table continued on following page

Table 14–1. BENIGN NONINFECTIOUS SKIN DISORDERS
Continued

Most Common...	Answer and Explanation
cause of generalized hypopigmentation	*albinism:* * AR disease, * absent tyrosinase, * melanocytes present
drugs decreasing melanin synthesis	• **topical corticosteroids,** • *antimalarials*
cause of vitiligo	*autoimmune melanocyte destruction:* * well-demarcated depigmentation skin/hair, * majority appear before 20 y old
clinical associations with vitiligo	• **Hashimoto's thyroiditis,** • *autoimmune hypoparathyroidism,* • *type I DM,* • *PA*
Rx of vitiligo	*UVA light + 8-methoxypsoralen*
cause of chloasma	*pregnancy:* hyperpigmentation produces pregnancy mask on face
appearance of seborrheic keratosis	*raised, pigmented lesion with a "stuck on" appearance:* commonly occur in middle age
sites for seborrheic keratosis	• **face,** • *trunk*
Rx of seborrheic keratosis	• **cryotherapy,** • *curetting*
appearance of acanthosis nigricans	*pigmented, verrucoid lesion commonly located in axilla and other intertriginous areas*
benign tumor of melanocytes	*nevocellular nevus:* neural crest origin
order of histologic development of nevocellular nevi	• *junctional nevus:* * young child, * macule, • *compound nevus:* * older child, * raised, pigmented, • *intradermal nevus:* puberty/adult
porphyrias in United States	**PCT:** * **acquired disease,** * AD disease, • *AIP:* * AD disease
porphyria with skin involvement	*PCT*
enzyme deficiency in PCT	*uroporphyrinogen decarboxylase:* catalyzes conversion of uroporphyrinogen III into coproporphyrinogen III
clinical findings in PCT	• **bullous skin lesions develop after light exposure:** porphyrins in skin are light sensitive, • *hypertrichosis:* vellus type hair, • *fragile skin,* • *wine-red color of urine*

Table 14–1. BENIGN NONINFECTIOUS SKIN DISORDERS
Continued

Most Common...	Answer and Explanation
precipitating causes of PCT	• **alcohol,** • *toxins:* * chlorinated phenols, * hexachlorobenzene, • *estrogen:* exacerbated in pregnancy, • *iron overload,* • *HCV*
lab findings in PCT	• **increased urine uroporphyrin I:** -ogen compounds are colorless and must be oxidized to have color, • *normal porphobilinogen levels,* • *low uroporphyrinogen decarboxylase*
Rx of PCT	• **phlebotomy:** lower iron levels, • *avoid precipitating causes:* * UV light, * alcohol, • *small doses of hydroxychloroquine*
enzyme deficiency in AIP	*uroporphyrinogen synthase:* * catalyzes conversion of PBG into uroporphyrinogen III, * heme has a negative feedback on ALA synthase, * decreased heme (e.g., drug metabolism) precipitates an acute attack by enhancing ALA synthase activity
clinical findings in AIP	• **sudden onset of colicky abdominal pain:** * often misinterpreted as surgical abdomen, * "bellyful of scars", • *neurologic problems:* * neuropathies, * dementia, • *precipitated by drugs enhancing liver cytochrome system:* * e.g., alcohol, barbiturates, * drug metabolism decreases heme
lab findings in AIP	• **increased urine PBG:** * colorless at first, * turns color with exposure to light (porphobilin formed), * called "window sill test", • *increased urine δ ALA,* • *low enzyme activity in asymptomatic periods:* confirmatory test
Rx of AIP	• **avoid drugs enhancing cytochrome system,** • *heme infusions:* inhibit ALA synthase
phases of hair growth in succession	• *anagen phase:* * development of new shaft of hair from hair bulb, * hair length determined in this stage, • *catagen phase:* * regression of growth site of hair shaft, * resting phase, • *telogen phase:* * regression of hair-producing elements of hair follicle, * followed by anagen phase [Hair growth is usually *asynchronous,* hence only a small percentage of hair is lost at any point in time.]

Table continued on following page

Table 14–1. BENIGN NONINFECTIOUS SKIN DISORDERS
Continued

Most Common...	Answer and Explanation
cause of massive hair loss	• **postpartum,** • *BCP,* • *stress* [Estrogen causes synchronous hair growth, by causing all hairs to enter resting phase at once. In the telogen phase, all hairs fall out at once, hence the term telogen effluvium for the hair loss.]
mechanism of hair loss in cancer patients Rx with radiochemotherapy	*inhibition of anagen phase when cells in hair bulb are dividing:* called anagen effluvium
hair loss pattern in males	*symmetrical loss of hair from vertex and crown of scalp*
drugs causing an increase in hair growth	• **minoxidil,** • *finasteride:* * 5 α-reductase inhibitor, * drug side-effect, * decreases DHT, * increases testosterone causing hair growth
clinical findings in alopecia areata	• **hairless areas on scalp,** • *scattered short, underdeveloped hairs on areas of baldness,* • *nail pitting:* 10%
areas of nail involved with disease	• *lunula:* * white half-mooned shape area proximal to cuticle, * underlying nail bed is partially keratinized (white color), • *nail plate:* * composed of layers of keratinized and fused cells, * attached to nail bed except distally where it separates from hyponych-ium, • *nail matrix:* * beneath lunula, * origin of nail plate
diseases causing nail changes	• **psoriasis:** * >80%, * pitting, • *lichen planus:* * 10%, * vertical ridges (depressions/ bulges), * thinning of nail plate
acquired cause of koilonychia (spoon nails)	*iron deficiency*
cause of splinter hemorrhages in nails	• **IE:** IC vasculitis, • *trichinosis,* • *vasculitis:* e.g., * RA, * TAO, • *trauma,* • *psoriasis*
cause of yellow nail syndrome	*syndrome of:* * unexplained ankle lymphe-dema and recurrent pleural effusions, * dys-trophic yellow nails [The first two changes often precede nail changes. Associated with bronchiectasis, thyroid disease, malignancy.]

Table 14–1. BENIGN NONINFECTIOUS SKIN DISORDERS
Continued

Most Common...	Answer and Explanation
cause of Terry nails	*cirrhosis:* * nail plates (particularly thumb and index fingers) are a uniform opaque white color that extends up to a few millimeters of distal border of nail, which still retains its pink color, * unknown etiology
cause of Beau's nails	*systemic illness causing temporary regression of nail growth:* nail with transverse furrow extending from nail matrix and progressing proximal until it is pared off
cause of Mees' lines	• **arsenic poisoning**, • *systemic illness of any kind:* * transverse white lines in nail plate that extend proximally until they are pared off, * may represent a type of Beau's lines
cause of Muercke's nails	*nephrotic syndrome:* * nails have paired, transverse white bands of pallor in nail bed (not nail plate), * white lines represent localized edema in vascular nail bed compressing vessels, * bands resolve when albumin levels normalize
cause of striate white transverse lines in nail plate	*SLE:* 25%
cause of a red lunula	• **cardiac failure**, • *RA*
cause of a blue lunula	*Wilson's disease*
cause of half and half nails	*chronic renal failure:* * proximal nail bed is white, * distal nail bed red, pink, or brown
cause of green nails	*Pseudomonas aeruginosa infection*
cause of a subungual hematoma	*trauma:* confused with acral lentiginous malignant melanoma (see Table 14–3)
cause of pyoderma gangrenosum	*unknown*
site for pyoderma gangrenosum	*lower extremities*
appearance of pyoderma gangrenosum	• *begins as a dermal pustule secondary to necrotizing vasculitis,* • *skin ulcerates,* • *ulcer margins are purple*

Table continued on following page

Table 14–1. BENIGN NONINFECTIOUS SKIN DISORDERS
Continued

Most Common...	Answer and Explanation
diseases associated with pyoderma gangrenosum	• UC, • *Crohn's disease,* • *RA,* • *myelogenous leukemia,* • *HIV*
Rx of pyoderma gangrenosum	*corticosteroids*
cause of pinch purpura	*cutaneous amyloidosis:* * amyloid in vessels weakens structural integrity, * MC in primary amyloidosis (see Table 8–10)
type of cutaneous amyloidosis	*lichen amyloidosis:* * pruritic flesh-colored to brown papular lesions, * located on shins
cause of dystrophic calcinosis cutis	• **PSS/CREST,** • *dermatomyositis* [Calcinosis cutis is calcification of subcutaneous tissue.]
cause of metastatic calcinosis	*primary HPTH:* * skin calcification presents as yellow to white hard nodules, * usually in proximity to large joints

Question: Which of the following are associated with urticarial reactions? **SELECT 5**
- (A) Sun exposure
- (B) Aspirin
- (C) HAV
- (D) PCT
- (E) Erythema nodosum
- (F) Cold temperature
- (G) C1 esterase inhibitor deficiency
- (H) Radiocontrast dyes
- (I) Peanuts
- (J) ACE inhibitors

Answers: (A), (B), (F), (H), (I): Sun exposure **(choice A)** is associated with solar urticaria. Aspirin **(choice B)** may be associated with urticarial reactions. HAV, unlike HBV, is not associated with an IC-mediated serum sickness-like prodrome **(choice C is incorrect)**. PCT is a bullous disorder associated with deposition of photosensitive porphyrins in the skin **(choice D is incorrect)**. Erythema nodosum is a type of fat necrosis **(choice E is incorrect)**. Cold temperature **(choice F)** may be associated with cold urticaria. C1 esterase inhibitor deficiency produces angioedema and not urticaria **(choice G is incorrect)**. Radiocontrast dyes **(choice H)** and peanuts **(choice I)** are common causes of urticarial reactions progressing into anaphylactoid reactions. ACE inhibitors produce angioedema and not urticaria **(choice J is incorrect)**.

ACE = angiotensin converting enzyme, AD = autosomal dominant, AIP = acute intermittent porphyria, ALA = aminolevulinic acid, AR =

autosomal recessive, BCC = basal cell carcinoma, BCPs = birth control pills, BM = basement membrane, Bx = biopsy, CD = contact dermatitis, CH = cholesterol, CMI = cell-mediated immunity, COD = cause of death, CREST = calcinosis, Raynaud's, esophageal motility dysfunction, sclerodactyly, telangiectasia, DM = diabetes mellitus, DH = dermatitis herpetiformis, DHT = dihydrotestosterone, Dx = diagnosis, EM = erythema multiforme, FA = fatty acid, HAV = hepatitis A virus, HBV = hepatitis B virus, HCV = hepatitis C virus, HD = Hodgkin's disease, HIV = human immunodeficiency virus, HLA = human leukocyte antigen, HPTH = hyperparathyroidism, HPV = human papillomavirus, HSR = hypersensitivity reaction, HSV = herpes simplex virus, Hx = history, IC = immunocomplex, IE = infective endocarditis, IF = immunofluorescent, Ig = immunoglobulin, MC = most common, NHL = non-Hodgkin's lymphoma, NSAIDs = nonsteroidal anti-inflammatory drugs, PA = pernicious anemia, PABA = para-aminobenzoic acid, PAF = platelet-activating factor, PBG = porphobilinogen, PCT = porphyria cutanea tarda, PLE = polymorphous light eruption, PSS = progressive systemic sclerosis, RA = rheumatoid arthritis, Rx = treatment, SC = subcutaneous, SLE = systemic lupus erythematosus, S/S = signs and symptoms, TAO = thromboangiitis obliterans, TB = tuberculosis, TEN = toxic epidermal necrolysis, TG = triglyceride, TMP/SMX = trimethoprim/sulfamethoxazole, UC = ulcerative colitis, UV = ultraviolet.

Table 14–2. INFECTIOUS SKIN DISORDERS

Most Common...	Answer and Explanation
infectious skin diseases in clinical practice	• **superficial dermatophyte infections,** • *seborrheic dermatitis*
initial test to identify superficial dermatophyte infections	*scraping of lesion followed by KOH digestion of keratin material, followed by microscopic examination for yeasts and hyphae*
uses of Wood's lamp (UVA or black light) in infectious disease	• **detect fluorescent metabolites in dermatophyte infections:** * *Microsporum species,* * *Malassezia furfur* in tinea versicolor (dull yellow), • *cutaneous bacterial infections:* * *Pseudomonas aeruginosa* (green color), * erythrasma (♦ *Corynebacterium minutissimum,* ♦ coral red color)
test to identify viral inclusions in vesicular lesions	*Tzanck preparation:* * scrapings taken from base of unroofed vesicle, * slide stained and examined for inclusions, * HSV I/II and varicella have intranuclear inclusions in multinucleated cells, * sensitivity 60% for HSV and 75% for varicella/zoster

Table continued on following page

Table 14–2. INFECTIOUS SKIN DISORDERS *Continued*

Most Common...	Answer and Explanation
types of warts	• **common:** * hands, * children, • *plantar:* * soles, * adolescents, • *genital:* anogenital area, • *flat:* * hands, * face
methods of transmitting warts	• **contact,** • *autoinoculation,* • *sexual transmission:* condyloma acuminatum
cause of warts	*HPV*
occupations associated with warts	*meat/fish handlers:* e.g., * butchers, * meat packing
cause of condyloma acuminatum	*HPV:* see Table 10–6
cause of molluscum contagiosum	*poxvirus:* * raised, flesh-colored, umbilicated papules filled with keratin containing viral particles, * common in AIDS
Rx of molluscum contagiosum	• **liquid nitrogen,** • *curettage*
skin findings in HSV-1	*see Table 9–2*
inciting agents for HSV-1	• **UVB exposure,** • *menses,* • *fever,* • *postviral infection* [HSV infects cutaneous neurons and spreads up to sensory ganglia where it remains latent.]
clinical findings in herpetic whitlow	• *painful HSV infection in soft tissue of finger,* • *transmitted by needle stick or traumatic implantation:* e.g., dentists
cause of genital herpes	*see Table 10–6*
appearance of varicella (chickenpox)	*macules, vesicles, pustules in different stages of development:* * begins on trunk and extends to extremities and face, * contagious from 4 d prior to onset of rash until all lesions crusted
complications associated with varicella	• **persistence into adult life:** *herpes zoster,* • *cerebellar inflammation:* self-limited, • *Reye's syndrome,* • *pneumonia*
clinical finding in herpes zoster (shingles)	• *dermatome pain 48 h prior to eruption of vesicular rash,* • *eruption of vesicles follows dermatome of sensory nerve:* virus is dormant

Table 14–2. INFECTIOUS SKIN DISORDERS *Continued*

Most Common...	Answer and Explanation
Continued	in sensory dorsal root ganglia, • *lasts 1–2 wks,* • *patients usually >50 y old,* • *may or may not be associated with an underlying malignancy,* • *pre-AIDS-defining lesion*
sites for herpes zoster	• **trunk,** • *face:* trigeminal distribution
site for Ramsay-Hunt syndrome	*herpes zoster involving sensory portion of cranial nerve VIII in outer external ear canal*
complications of herpes zoster	• **postherpetic neuralgia:** * pain after lesions have disappeared, * MC after trigeminal nerve involvement, • *ophthalmic zoster:* * ~10–15%, * patients >60 y old more susceptible (>50%), * resolves within a year
Rx of herpes zoster	• **acyclovir:** most effective prior to rash, • *systemic corticosteroids:* * reduce pain without worsening infection in immunocompetent patient, * should not be used in immunocompromised patient
rickettsial disease in the United States	*Rocky Mountain spotted fever:* * *Rickettsia rickettsii* transmitted by *Dermacentor andersoni* (also transmits Colorado tick fever)
clinical findings in RMSF	• **rash:** * 90%, * rash occurs between 2 and 6 d of fever, * begins on hands/wrists and soles/ankles and spreads centrally, * petechial lesions due to a vasculitis, • **fever, Hx of tick exposure:** all three present in 60–70%, • *GI complaints:* * N/V, * abdominal pain, • *CNS changes:* * headache, * convulsions, • *ARF,* • *hepatitis,* • *myositis,* • *noncardiogenic pulmonary edema*
lab findings in RMSF	• **serology:** * IF antibody, * CF, • *skin Bx with direct IF:* 75% sensitivity, • *Weil-Felix reactions:* * positive OX2, * positive OX19, * negative OXK, • *neutrophilic leukocytosis,* • *hyponatremia:* * 50%, * probable SIADH, • *hypoalbuminemia:* 30%, • *CSF findings:* * increased mononuclear cells/neutrophils, * high protein, * slightly low glucose, • *hematuria,* • *proteinuria*
Rx of RMSF	• **doxycycline,** • *chloramphenicol*

Table continued on following page

Table 14–2. INFECTIOUS SKIN DISORDERS *Continued*

Most Common...	Answer and Explanation
COD in RMSF	*pneumonitis with respiratory/cardiac failure:* mortality 20–70% if left untreated (better prognosis in a child than the elderly)
cause/transmission of ehrlichiosis	• *Ehrlichia chaffeensis:* * rickettsial-like organism, * intracellular parasite of leukocytes, • *tick-transmitted: Amblyomma americanum*
clinical findings in ehrlichiosis	• **fever,** • *Hx of tick bite,* • *rash less likely to occur than RMSF,* • *less common:* * ARF, * encephalopathy, * respiratory failure
lab Dx of ehrlichiosis	• **serum indirect IF antibody,** • *PCR*
tick-borne diseases in United States	• **rickettsia:** * RMSF, * ehrlichiosis, • *viruses:* Colorado tick fever, • *bacteria:* * *Lyme disease,* * *relapsing fever,* * *tularemia,* • *protozoa:* babesiosis
skin infections in which *Staphylococcus aureus* is primary pathogen	• *furuncles,* • *carbuncles,* • *bullous impetigo:* see below, • *hidradenitis suppurativa:* apocrine gland abscess, • *paronychial infections,* • *postoperative wound infections,* • *postpartum breast abscess*
cause of TSS	*toxin producing S. aureus:* * most frequent in tampon-wearing menstruating women, * may occur with occlusive dressings over wounds, * negative blood cultures
S/S of TSS	• **high fever,** *hypotension, diffuse red maculopapular rash with late desquamation of palms/soles:* 1–2 wks, • *pharyngitis/conjunctivitis/vaginal hyperemia,* • *mental confusion,* • *diarrhea*
lab findings in TSS	• *increased serum CK,* • *hypocalcemia,* • *hypophosphatemia,* • *elevated liver transaminases,* • *increased serum creatinine,* • *thrombocytopenia*
Rx of TSS	*nafcillin:* * TSS mortality due to *S. aureus* is <5%, * TSS mortality due to streptococcal disease is ~30%
cause of scalded skin syndrome	*toxin-producing S. aureus*
skin infection in AIDS	*folliculitis due to S. aureus*

Table 14–2. INFECTIOUS SKIN DISORDERS *Continued*

Most Common...	Answer and Explanation
cause of impetigo	*Streptococcus pyogenes:* * honey-colored and crusted lesions, * superinfection with *S. aureus* produces bullous lesions
Rx of impetigo	• *limited infection:* topical mupirocin, • *extensive infection:* dicloxacillin
microbial pathogen causing cellulitis with lymphangitis	*S. pyogenes:* produce hyaluronidase, which spreads infection in subcutaneous tissue
cause of erysipelas	*S. pyogenes:* * raised, red, hot cellulitis ("brawny edema"), * favors facial area, * septicemia is common
Rx of erysipelas	*penicillin V*
cause of necrotizing fasciitis	*polymicrobial:* * *S. pyogenes* ("flesh-eating bacteria"), * *Bacteroides fragilis,* * *Clostridium* species, * *S. aureus*
clinical findings of necrotizing fasciitis	• **severe, painful, cellulitis with systemic toxicity,** • *nerve destruction,* • *thrombosis of microcirculation*
Rx of necrotizing fasciitis	• *surgical exploration/débridement,* • *broad-spectrum antibiotics*
sites for pressure ulcers	• **sacrum,** * *greater trochanter,* • *ischial tuberosity,* • *calcaneus,* • *lateral malleolus*
risk factors for pressure ulcers	• **immobility,** • *urinary/fecal incontinence,* • *nutritional deficiency:* e.g., zinc
causes of pressure ulcers	• **pressure:** * tissue ischemia by compressing capillaries, * predisposes to ulceration, • *shearing force/friction:* e.g., * patient dragged across bed, * angulates/occludes subcutaneous vessels, • *moisture:* * tissue maceration, * urine is a common offender
complications of pressure ulcers	• **infection:** obtain culture from deep tissue, not surface of ulcer, • *osteomyelitis:* * suspect when wound does not heal, * bone Bx is gold standard for culture/diagnosis
Rx of pressure ulcers	• **rotate patient q 2 hs,** • *pressure-reducing mattresses,* • *débride dead tissue,* • *control urinary incontinence,* • *nutritional support,* • *antibiotics for infections*

Table continued on following page

Table 14–2. INFECTIOUS SKIN DISORDERS *Continued*

Most Common...	Answer and Explanation
cause of scarlet fever	*group A Streptococcus:* gram-positive coccus that produces an erythrogenic toxin
S/S of scarlet fever	• **pharyngitis,** • *fever,* • *white strawberry tongue followed by strawberry tongue,* • *red, maculopapular, blanching rash that begins on trunk and limbs and resolves with desquamation,* • *petechiae in skin folds:* Pastia's lines, • *circumoral pallor*
complications associated with scarlet fever	• **post-streptococcal GN,** • *rheumatic fever*
Rx of scarlet fever	*IM benzathine penicillin*
cause of hand crippling worldwide	*leprosy*
cause of fish handler's disease	*Erysipelothrix rhusiopathiae:* * Gram + bacillus, * also called erysipeloid
clinical findings of erysipeloid	• **localized, painless purplish skin rash:** usually fingers, • *no systemic signs,* • *no lymphadenopathy*
Rx of erysipeloid	*penicillin G or ampicillin*
clinical findings of cutaneous diphtheria	*usually a secondary infection of neglected wound: Corynebacterium diphtheriae* is a Gram + bacillus
Rx of cutaneous diphtheria	*erythromycin*
clinical findings of *Arcanobacterium* (formerly *Corynebacterium) hemolyticus*	• **pharyngitis,** • *scarlatiniform rash:* MC on extremities
Rx of *A. hemolyticus*	*erythromycin*
cause of erythrasma	*Corynebacterium minutissimum*
clinical findings in erythrasma	• *patchy, pruritic red intertriginous rash,* • *Wood's lamp reveals coral red fluorescence*
Rx of erythrasma	*erythromycin*

Table 14–2. INFECTIOUS SKIN DISORDERS *Continued*

Most Common...	Answer and Explanation
cause of tetanus in United States	• **IVDU,** • *puncture wounds in nonimmunized people* [See Table 2–2 for tetanus Rx in clean/dirty wounds, immunized and nonimmunized.]
organisms associated with human bites	• ***Eikenella corrodens*** • *viridans streptococcus,* • *Staphylococcus epidermidis,* • *Corynebacterium* spp, • *S. aureus,* • *Bacteroides* spp, • *Peptostreptococcus* spp
organism associated with cat bites	*Pasteurella multocida*
organisms associated with dog bites	• ***viridans streptococci,*** • *Pasteurella multocida*
initial Rx of bites	• **cleaning:** * quaternary ammonium compounds, * water, • *irrigation,* • *débridement*
bites requiring antimicrobial prophylaxis	• **human bites:** most serious bite, • *cat bites:* tenosynovitis, • *high-risk dog bites:* e.g., * hand, * puncture wounds, * bites older than 6–12 h, • *wild animals:* * bats, * raccoons, * skunks
antibiotic prophylaxis recommended for human, cat, dog, wild animal bites	*amoxicillin/clavulanate*
animals causing rabies in United States	• **skunks,** • *raccoons,* • *fox,* • *bats* [See Table 2–2 for Rx of rabies.]
cause of myonecrosis	*Clostridium perfringens:* gram-positive bacillus
cutaneous findings associated with *C. perfringens*	• **sudden pain/edema in wound site,** • *prostration,* • *foul-smelling bloody brown serous discharge,* • *discolored skin/soft tissue,* • *crepitance in tissue due to gas*
Rx of *C. perfringens* myonecrosis	• *débridement,* • *clindamycin + penicillin G,* • *hyperbaric oxygen*
type of anthrax in the United States	• **cutaneous:** 90–95%, • *pulmonary,* • *oral/ oropharyngeal,* • *GI* [*Bacillus anthracis* is a spore-forming gram-positive bacillus.]

Table continued on following page

Table 14–2. INFECTIOUS SKIN DISORDERS *Continued*

Most Common...	Answer and Explanation
occupations as risk factors for developing anthrax	• **veterinarians/farmers,** • *wool workers,* • *tanners* [Inoculation of the organism is through broken skin or inhalation.]
cutaneous findings in anthrax	• **"malignant pustule" at inoculation site:** black scab with central area of necrosis, • *fever and systemic signs*
Rx of cutaneous anthrax	*IV penicillin G:* * mortality 20% in untreated cases, * pulmonary anthrax has 100% mortality (used in germ warfare)
infection associated with sulfur granules	*Actinomyces israelii:* * gram-positive filamentous bacteria (present in sulfur granule draining from sinus tract), * see Table 9–2
filamentous bacteria associated with mycetomas	*Nocardia asteroides:* * partially acid-fast, gram-positive filamentous bacteria, * filamentous bacteria and true fungi (see below) may cause mycetomas
cause of malignant external otitis	*Pseudomonas aeruginosa:* primarily occurs in poorly controlled DM
Rx of malignant external otitis	*imipenem cilastatin + anti-pseudomonal β-lactamase*
cause of ecthyma gangrenosum	*Pseudomonas aeruginosa bacteremia:* hemorrhagic vesicles with central necrosis due to vessel thrombosis by bacteria
cause of hot tub folliculitis	*Pseudomonas aeruginosa:* * improper chlorination of water, * self-limited
types of tularemia	• **ulceroglandular:** 75%, • *glandular,* • *oculoglandular:* * *Francisella tularensis* is a gram-negative bacillus, * rabbits MC reservoir
clinical findings in cutaneous tularemia	• *Hx of arthropod bite* (e.g., deer fly, tick) *or dressing out rabbits,* • *papular lesion develops at inoculation site,* • *papule ulcerates,* • *lymph nodes draining bite site exhibit granulomatous inflammation,* • *infection may spread systemically*
lab Dx	• **serologic tests,** • *culture:* difficult
Rx of tularemia	*streptomycin or gentamicin*

Table 14–2. INFECTIOUS SKIN DISORDERS *Continued*

Most Common...	Answer and Explanation
cause of rat bite fever	• ***Spirillum minus,*** • *Streptobacillus monili-formis* [Both are gram-negative spirochetal bacilli. Infection occurs from rat bites, usually in slum areas.]
clinical findings of rat bite fever	• *rat bite wound resolves,* • *in a few weeks, bite site becomes swollen, painful, dusky purplish color,* • *systemic signs,* • maculopapular rash, • *arthralgia/myalgia* (very severe with *Streptobacillus*), • *relapsing pattern of disease is characteristic,* • *mortality rate 10% if left untreated*
lab Dx of rat bite fever	• *dark field of aspirates of skin lesions reveals spirochetes,* • *serologic tests*
Rx of rat bite fever	*procaine penicillin G*
cause of leptospirosis	*Leptospira interrogans:* * tightly wound spirochete, * best visualized with dark field (resembles a shepherd's crook), * dogs are most important reservoir in United States, * dogs shed infected urine into soil/water, * organisms enter abraded skin
people at risk for leptospirosis	• *farmers,* • *veterinarians,* • *people swimming in infected ponds*
clinical findings of leptospirosis	• *biphasic:* septicemic phase followed by immune phase, • *septicemic phase:* * fever, * flu-like syndrome, * anicteric hepatitis (if severe hepatitis, renal failure, jaundice, it is called *Weil's disease*), * hemorrhagic rash (organisms infect endothelial cells), * conjunctivitis/photophobia, * oliguria (interstitial nephritis), * meningitis, • *immune phase:* * antibodies develop, * organisms plentiful in urine
lab Dx of leptospirosis	• **identify organisms in urine by dark field,** • *serologic tests,* • *culture*
Rx of leptospirosis	*penicillin G*
cause of lupus vulgaris	• *Mycobacterium tuberculosis:* may predispose to SCC
cause of scrofula in adults/children	• *Mycobacterium tuberculosis:* adults, • *Mycobacterium scrofulaceum:* children

Table continued on following page

Table 14–2. INFECTIOUS SKIN DISORDERS *Continued*

Most Common...	Answer and Explanation
clinical findings of scrofula	• **nontender cervical lymphadenitis,** • *usually afebrile,* • *may drain to skin surface from underlying lymph node*
Rx of scrofula	• *adults:* Rx as *M. tuberculosis* for 9 mths, • *children:* * surgical drainage, * anti-TB Rx not necessary
atypical *Mycobacteria* associated with skin/ soft tissue infections	• *Mycobacterium fortuitum,* • *Mycobacterium chelonei*
clinical associations of *M. fortuitum/ M. chelonei*	• *sternal osteomyelitis:* complication of cardiac surgery, • *abscesses,* • *puncture wounds,* • *septic arthritis*
Rx of *M. fortuitum/ M. chelonei* infections	• *surgical drainage,* • *antibiotics:* e.g., clarithromycin
cause of swimming pool granulomas	*Mycobacterium marinum:* nodular skin lesions in areas of abrasion
Rx of *Mycobacterium marinum*	*doxycycline*
cause of leprosy (*Mycobacterium leprae*)	• **droplet infection,** • *direct contact*
areas leprosy occurs in United States	• *Texas,* • *Louisiana,* • *Florida,* • *California,* • *Hawaii*
types of leprosy	• **borderline,** • *tuberculoid,* • *lepromatous,* • *indeterminate*
clinical findings in borderline leprosy	• **neural involvement precedes cutaneous:** sensory/motor destruction of nerves, • *cutaneous lesions:* * flat, depigmented macule, * raised plaque (partial loss of sensation)
clinical findings in tuberculoid leprosy	• *intact cellular immunity:* * positive lepromin skin test, * no viable organisms, • *cutaneous lesions:* * flat, depigmented macule, * raised plaque (partial loss of sensation), • *thickening/swelling of nerves next to skin lesions,* • *bilateral ulnar neuropathy is pathognomonic,* • *autoamputation of digits*

Table 14–2. INFECTIOUS SKIN DISORDERS *Continued*

Most Common...	Answer and Explanation
clinical findings in lepromatous leprosy	• **stiffness in nose:** * first sign, * ulcers in nose, * saddle nose deformity, • *lack of cellular immunity:* * negative lepromin skin test, * numerous organisms, • *cutaneous lesions:* * macules/papules/nodules (skin lesions favor cooler locations), * may be depigmented, * distort tissue (leonine facies), • *nerve involvement late,* • *orchitis,* • *blindness*
clinical findings in indeterminate leprosy	• **hypopigmented macules,** • *loss of cutaneous sensation in skin lesions*
Rx of leprosy	• **dapsone,** • *clofazimine,* • *rifampin*
types of reactive leprosy	• **lepra reaction:** frequents all types of leprosy, • *erythema nodosum leprosum:* primarily in lepromatous type
clinical findings of lepra reaction	• **skin lesions become more erythematous and warm:** skin lesions are not erythema nodosum, • *skin ulceration,* • *nerve involvement increases,* • *nerve paralysis:* e.g., * ulnar nerve, * facial nerve, • *increased cellular immunity*
clinical findings in erythema nodosum leprosum	• **crops of painful erythematous nodules appear/disappear:** * IC disease, * skin vasculitis, * skin ulceration, • *GN,* • *arthritis*
Rx of erythema nodosum leprosum	• **thalidomide,** • *corticosteroids*
skin presentations of cutaneous candidiasis	• **oral thrush:** wipes off with blood at base, • *perlèche:* fissuring at angles of mouth, • *intertrigo:* creamy exudates in body folds, • *paronychia:* red proximal/lateral nail fold
cause of onychomycosis in patients with autoimmune hypoparathyroidism	*Candida albicans*
cause of dandruff	*Malassezia furfur:* * dandruff better called seborrheic dermatitis, * superficial dermatophyte infection involving stratum corneum
sites for seborrheic dermatitis	• **scalp,** • *eyelid margin,* • *bridge of nose,* • *face,* • *body folds*

Table continued on following page

Table 14–2. INFECTIOUS SKIN DISORDERS *Continued*

Most Common...	Answer and Explanation
clinical disorders associated with seborrheic dermatitis	• **AIDS:** often disseminated, • *Parkinson's disease*
Rx of seborrheic dermatitis	• *selenium or coal tar preparations for scalp,* • *topical hydrocortisone for face*
dermatophyte associated with skin infections	*Trichophyton rubrum*
cause of tinea capitis	*Trichophyton tonsurans:* * 75–90%, * infects inner hair shaft (hair breaks off, producing black dot appearance), * negative Wood's lamp, * common in African-American children
method of transmission of tinea capitis	*airborne spores:* 30% carrier rate for tinea capitis without symptomatic lesions
complications associated with tinea capitis	• *impetigo like lesions,* • *kerions:* tender, solid masses exuding pus, • *cervical lymphadenitis*
cause of tinea capitis with a positive Wood's lamp	*Microsporum canis:* * infects outer hair shaft, * positive Wood's lamp test
Rx of tinea capitis	• **oral griseofulvin,** • *itraconazole for T. tonsurans*
cause of favus	*Trichophyton schoenleinii:* * invades hair shaft, * Wood's lamp positive
cause of tinea corporis	*Trichophyton rubrum:* superficial dermatophyte skin infection
appearance of tinea corporis	*circular, pruritic lesions with pale center and red, crusted leading edge:* sample leading edge for KOH study
Rx of tinea corporis	• **imidazole compounds:** interferes with ergosterol in fungal cell membranes, • *oral griseofulvin:* blocks cell division by interfering with spindle formation in G2
cause of onychomycosis	*Trichophyton rubrum*
cause of tinea pedis	*Trichophyton rubrum*

Table 14–2. INFECTIOUS SKIN DISORDERS *Continued*

Most Common...	Answer and Explanation
cause of a dermatophytid reaction	*superficial dermatophyte infection at a distant site:* * inflammatory reactions occur at a distant site from another dermatophyte infection (e.g., tinea pedis), * in tinea pedis, lesions may appear as a dermatitis on palm
clinical findings in black/white Piedra	*fungus attaches to hair shaft without any skin manifestations:* * black Piedra due to *Piedraia hortae,* * white Piedra due to *Trichosporon beigelii*
cause of tinea versicolor	*M. furfur:* superficial dermatophyte infects stratum corneum
appearance of tinea versicolor	*uneven areas of both hyper- and hypopigmented scaly papules on trunk:* * hypopigmentation due to dicarboxylic acid (blocks tyrosinase activity in melanocytes), * hyperpigmentation is inflammatory response
KOH appearance of *M. furfur*	*"spaghetti (hyphae) and meatballs (yeasts)"*
Rx of tinea versicolor	• **selenium sulfide,** • *ketoconazole shampoo*
cause of chromoblastomycosis	*traumatic implantation of pigmented fungus (e.g., Fonsecaea pedrosoi) into subcutaneous tissue:* * usually introduced by a splinter, * verrucoid lesion is resistant to Rx
cause of sporotrichosis	*traumatic implantation of Sporothrix schenckii:* usually a thorn prick in a rose gardener
clinical findings in sporotrichosis	*draining lymphocutaneous nodules from initial inoculation site*
Rx of sporotrichosis	*oral potassium iodide*
cause of mycetomas in the United States	*Pseudallescheria boydii*
clinical findings in mycetomas	• *deep infection of skin/subcutaneous tissue,* • *usually develop on the foot from traumatic implantation,* • *nodules develop that drain purulent material containing colored granules:* red, black, yellow, white, • *causes disfigurement, often requiring amputation*
Rx of mycetoma due to *P. boydii*	*surgery + itraconazole*

Table continued on following page

Table 14–2. INFECTIOUS SKIN DISORDERS *Continued*

Most Common...	Answer and Explanation
clinical findings in fire ant bites	• *sharp, painful bite,* • *wheal/flare reaction:* type I HSR, • *vesiculation/skin necrosis follow*
site for hematogenous spread of *Coccidioides immitis*	*skin:* * warty papules/plaques/nodules, * risk for hematogenous spread greatest in Filipinos > African-Americans > whites
skin findings in histoplasmosis	• *acute disease:* erythema nodosum, • *chronic disease:* * mucocutaneous lesions with verrucoid appearance simulating SCC, * organisms in macrophages
skin findings in blastomycosis	*crusted verrucous plaques with central clearing:* * skin involved in 40–80%, * sites: face, hands, arms
cause of cutaneous larva migrans ("creeping eruption")	*larva of Ancyclostoma braziliense* (cat/dog hookworm) or *Ancyclostoma caninum* (dog hookworm)
clinical findings in cutaneous larva migrans	*intensely pruritic serpiginous burrows located on soles, back, thighs, buttocks:* * commonly transmitted in sand boxes where cats/dogs urinate, * PB eosinophilia
Rx of cutaneous larva migrans	• **albendazole,** • *10% topical thiabendazole*
cause of cutaneous leishmaniasis in the United States	*Leishmania mexicana complex* [It is transmitted by sandflies of the genus *Phlebotomus* or by direct contact. It is endemic in south central Texas.]
skin finding of cutaneous leishmaniasis	• *initially, a pruritic red papule with a serous exudate that ulcerates,* • *may disseminate in anergic or hypersensitive patient*
lab Dx of cutaneous leishmaniasis	• **aspiration of skin lesions/identify organisms in macrophages,** • *Montenegro skin test*
Rx of cutaneous leishmaniasis	*sodium stibogluconate*
clinical findings in chigger bites	• *chiggers are mites:* small red dot on skin, • *intensely pruritic, well-demarcated erythematous lesions,* • *Rx:* topical anti-pruritic agents

Table 14–2. INFECTIOUS SKIN DISORDERS *Continued*

Most Common...	Answer and Explanation
clinical findings produced by human itch mite (scabies)	• *Sarcoptes scabiei:* mite, • *female mites bore into stratum corneum:* burrows between fingers, flexor surface of wrist, around nipples, axilla, scrotal area, glans penis, • *spares head/neck,* • *scrape burrow with blade and identify organism:* best method of Dx
Rx of scabies	• **permethrin cream,** • *lindane*
types of pediculosis	• **pediculosis capitis:** * nits (eggs) in hair, * nonpruritic papular bites, • *pediculosis corporis:* * clothes louse, * not found on skin but live in clothing, * eggs located in body creases, • *pediculosis pubis:* * "crabs", * *Phthirus pubis,* * lives in pubic hairs
Rx of pediculosis	*benzene hexachloride*

Question: A diabetic patient presents with a foul-smelling, brownish-red serous discharge exuding from a pressure ulcer on the right foot. The skin bordering the ulcer is discolored and crepitance is palpated in the subcutaneous tissue. What would you expect a Gram stain of material aspirated from deep in the ulcer to reveal? **SELECT 1**

- (A) Gram-positive cocci in clusters
- (B) Gram-negative cocci
- (C) Thin gram-negative rods
- (D) Thick gram-positive rods
- (E) Gram-positive cocci in chains

Answer: (D): The patient has an anaerobic infection most likely due to *Clostridium perfringens,* a thick gram-positive rod **(choice D)**. Although these types of wound infections are usually painful, diabetics do not complain of pain owing to peripheral neuropathy, hence infections can extend into muscle and bone before they are discovered. *Staphylococcus aureus* is the most common cause of skin infections in diabetics; however, the infection described in this case with foul-smelling exudate and gas in the subcutaneous tissue is clearly due to *Clostridium perfringens* **(choice A is incorrect)**. Gram-negative cocci would not be expected to produce skin infections **(choice B is incorrect)**. Thin gram-negative rods could be *Pseudomonas aeruginosa,* but the infection characteristics are not typical for ecthyma gangrenosum **(choice C is incorrect)**. Gram-positive rods in chains representing *Streptococcus pyogenes* is an unlikely cause of this wound infection, since *Streptococci* characteristically produce cellulitis and do not produce gas **(choice E is incorrect)**.

AIDS = acquired immunodeficiency virus, ARF = acute renal failure, Bx = biopsy, CF = complement fixation, CK = creatine kinase, CNS = central nervous system, COD = cause of death, CSF = cerebrospinal fluid, DM = diabetes mellitus, Dx = diagnosis, GI = gastrointestinal,

GN = glomerulonephritis, HPV = human papillomavirus, HSR = hyper-sensitivity reaction, HSV = herpes simplex virus, Hx = history, IC = immunocomplex, IF = immunofluorescence, IM = intramuscular, IV = intravenous, IVDU = intravenous drug user, KOH = potassium hydrox-ide, MC = most common, N/V = nausea and vomiting, PB = peripheral blood, PCR = polymerase chain reaction, RMSF = Rocky mountain spotted fever, Rx = treatment, SCC = squamous cell carcinoma, SIADH = syndrome of inappropriate antidiuretic hormone, S/S = signs and symptoms, TSS = toxic shock syndrome, UV = ultraviolet.

Table 14–3. MALIGNANT SKIN DISORDERS/ CUTANEOUS MANIFESTATIONS OF SYSTEMIC DISEASE

Most Common...	Answer and Explanation
skin cancers	• **BCC:** invade but do not metastasize, • *SCC,* • *malignant melanoma*
predisposing causes of non-melanoma skin cancers	• **UVB,** • *radiation,* • *arsenic exposure,* • *xeroderma pigmentosum,* • *basal cell nevus syndrome:* * AD, * BCCs develop at early age, • *chronic draining ulcers,* • *third-degree burn sites,* • *topical exposure to tar or soot*
appearance of a BCC	• **noduloulcerative:** * raised, translucent to pearly lesion with telangiectatic vessels on wall, * ulcerated center, • *superficial spreading:* plaque-like lesion that spreads out later-ally, • *morpheaform:* * resemble a scar, * most aggressive BCC
locations for BCC	• **inner aspect of nose,** • *periorbital area,* • *upper lip*
Rx of BCC	• **excision:** * noduloulcerative, * morphea-form, • *cryosurgery:* all types except mor-pheaform, • *Mohs' surgery:* * serial excisions with frozen sections of margins, * very expen-sive
skin cancer in African-Americans	*SCC*
causes of SCC of skin other than UVB light	• **immunosuppression:** MC cancer of immu-nosuppression, • *chronic draining sinuses,* • *keloids in third-degree burns,* • *arsenic poi-soning,* • *radiation therapy*
appearance/locations of SCC	• *appearance:* * nodular, * ulcer, * nodulo-ulcerative, • *locations:* sun (lower lip, hands) and non-sun exposed areas [Most SCCs are preceded by actinic (solar) keratosis. Mucosal lesions may metastasize.]

Table 14–3. MALIGNANT SKIN DISORDERS/
CUTANEOUS MANIFESTATIONS OF SYSTEMIC DISEASE
Continued

Most Common...	Answer and Explanation
Rx of SCC	*similar to BCC*
COD due to skin disease	*malignant melanoma*
nevus with potential for melanoma	*dysplastic nevus:* * >5 mm, * irregular borders, * irregular melanin distribution
types of melanoma	• **SSM:** * lower extremities, * back, • *nodular melanoma,* • *LMM:* face of elderly patients, • *ALM:* * under nails, * soles, * palms
melanoma in African-Americans	*acral lentiginous melanoma*
risk factors for melanoma	• **severe sunburn at early age,** • *dysplastic nevi,* • first-degree relative with melanoma, • xeroderma pigmentosum, • familial atypical mole-dysplastic nevus syndrome* (AD), • *fair skin,* • HIV positive, • tanning beds
natural history of an SSM and LMM	• *radial growth phase:* * tumor spreads along epidermis or within superficial dermis, * non-metastatic in this phase, • *vertical growth phase:* * after variable time period, melanoma enters vertical growth phase, * invasion into reticular dermis, * risk for metastasis
natural history of nodular/acral lentiginous melanomas	*lack a radial growth phase:* * only have a vertical growth phase, * poor prognosis
clinical findings suggesting melanoma	• **increase in size,** • *irregular borders,* • *color variation,* • *ulceration*
factors affecting prognosis of a melanoma	*tumor thickness:* * **Breslow** system directly measures level of invasion, * invasion <0.76 mm has 100% 5-y survival, * invasion >1.7 mm has metastatic potential, * invasion >3 mm has 46% 5-y survival, * *Clark system* divides skin into levels I–V, * level I is intraepidermal, * level II is invasion into papillary dermis, * level III is melanoma filling papillary dermis and pushing (not infiltrating) reticular dermis, * level IV is invasion into reticular dermis, * level V is invasion into subcutaneous fat

Table continued on following page

**Table 14–3. MALIGNANT SKIN DISORDERS/
CUTANEOUS MANIFESTATIONS OF SYSTEMIC DISEASE**
Continued

Most Common...	Answer and Explanation
site of metastasis for melanoma	*regional lymph nodes:* * ~40% 5-y survival if only lymph nodes are involved, * 5-y survival drops to 5% with extranodal involvement
initial Rx of melanoma	*total excision*
Rx after a Dx of melanoma is confirmed	*re-excision of excision site:* * in situ lesions require a margin of 0.5 cm around excision site (includes subcutaneous fat), * lesions <1 mm in thickness require a 1.0 cm margin
recommendation to prevent malignant melanoma	*sun screen >15:* particularly in children and adolescents
malignancies involving the nail	• **SCC,** • *melanoma,* • *BCC*
mesenchymal tumor of skin	*acrochordon* (skin tag): * flesh-colored to dark brown pedunculated lesions, * bag-like polyps called fibroepithelial polyps, * sites: neck, back, axilla, groin, * relationships: ♦ DM, ♦ pregnancy, ♦ obesity, ♦ menopause
cancers metastatic to skin in a woman	• **breast,** • *colon,* • *malignant melanoma*
cancers metastatic to skin in a man	• **lung,** • *colon,* • *malignant melanoma*
cancers metastatic to scalp	• **breast,** • *lung,* • *kidney*
cancer associated with Leser-Trélat sign	*gastric adenocarcinoma:* Leser-Trélat sign is a sudden outcropping of seborrheic keratoses
systemic associations of acanthosis nigricans	• *gastric adenocarcinoma:* * 60%, * skin lesion occurs suddenly, * remits when cancer remits, * returns when cancer returns, • *insulin receptor deficiency,* • *Cushing's syndrome,* • *acromegaly,* • *hirsutism with hyperthecosis*
cancer associated with necrolytic migratory erythema	*glucagonoma:* see Table 9–9

**Table 14–3. MALIGNANT SKIN DISORDERS/
CUTANEOUS MANIFESTATIONS OF SYSTEMIC DISEASE**
Continued

Most Common...	Answer and Explanation
cancers associated with superficial migratory thrombophlebitis	• **pancreatic adenocarcinoma,** • *lung cancer* [Called Trousseau's sign. Erythematous skin lesions (arms/legs, abdomen) overlie thrombosed cutaneous veins.]
cancer associated with Paget's disease of nipple	*intraductal or infiltrating ductal carcinoma:* nipple has an eczematous-appearing rash due to epidermal invasion by breast cancer
cancer associated with Sweet's syndrome	*myelogenous leukemia:* see Table 8–8
cancer associated with Gardner's syndrome	*colorectal cancer:* see Table 9–5
cancers associated with Cowden's syndrome	*thyroid and breast cancer:* * AD, * additional findings: ♦ KAs, ♦ acral keratosis, ♦ facial papules, ♦ soft tissue tumors, ♦ FCC
disorders associated with pseudoxanthoma elasticum	• *AMI,* • *stroke,* • *GI bleeding,* • *retinal angioid streaks:* * AD/AR, * elastic tissue degeneration, * yellow plaques with "plucked chicken" appearance (skin folds/back of neck)
causes of Sister Mary Joseph sign	*metastatic cancer to umbilicus:* * **stomach,** * colon, * ovary, * pancreas
disorders associated with hereditary hemorrhagic telangiectasia	see Table 8–12
cancer associated with Torres' syndrome	*colorectal:* * usually low-grade, * additional findings: ♦ multiple sebaceous tumors, ♦ MEN IIb, ♦ KAs
skin manifestations of CRF	• **pruritus:** cause unknown, • *yellow discoloration:* ? β-carotenemia, • *hyperpigmentation palms/soles:* decreased metabolism of MSH
cancer associated with acquired ichthyosis	• **Hodgkin's disease,** • *NHL,* • *multiple myeloma,* • *MF*

Table continued on following page

**Table 14–3. MALIGNANT SKIN DISORDERS/
CUTANEOUS MANIFESTATIONS OF SYSTEMIC DISEASE**
Continued

Most Common...	Answer and Explanation
findings in LEOPARD syndrome (AD disorder)	• *L = lentigines:* flat, pigmented, macules, • *E = ECG abnormalities:* conduction defects, • *O = ocular hypertelorism,* • *P = pulmonic stenosis,* • *A = abnormal genitalia:* * cryptorchidism, * hypospadias, • *R = retarded growth, rib anomalies:* pectus excavatum, • *D = deafness:* sensorineural
findings in NAME syndrome (AD disorder)	• *N = nevi,* • *A = atrial myxoma,* • *M = mucocutaneous myxomas,* • *E = ephelides:* freckles
findings in LAMB syndrome	• *L = lentigines:* * face, * vulva, • *A = atrial myxoma,* • *M = mucocutaneous myxomas,* • *B = blue nevi*
disorder associated with erythema marginatum	*acute rheumatic fever:* see Table 5–9
disorder associated with erythema chronicum migrans	*Lyme disease:* see Table 12–1
disorder associated with erythema nodosum	*group A streptococcal pharyngitis:* see Table 14–1
disorder associated with erythema multiforme	*HSV:* see Table 14–1

Table 14–3. MALIGNANT SKIN DISORDERS/
CUTANEOUS MANIFESTATIONS OF SYSTEMIC DISEASE
Continued

Question: A 54-y-old African-American man with CNS alterations has multiple space-occupying CNS lesions. A biopsy reveals metastatic malignant melanoma. Which of the following sites is the most likely primary site for the malignant melanoma? **SELECT 1**
- (A) Eye
- (B) CNS
- (C) Back
- (D) Face
- (E) Nails

Answer: (E): Acral lentiginous malignant melanomas are the most common type of malignant melanoma in African-Americans. These tumors only have a vertical growth phase and occur under nails **(choice E)** and on the palms and soles. Malignant melanomas are the most common malignant tumor of the eye in adults; however, this would be an unlikely primary site **(choice A is incorrect)**. The other sites listed, CNS, back (common site for SSM), and face (common site for LMM) are very unlikely sites for a primary malignant melanoma in an African-American **(choices B, C, and D are incorrect)**.

AD = autosomal dominant, ALM = acral lentiginous melanoma, AMI = acute myocardial infarction, AR = autosomal recessive, BCC = basal cell carcinoma, CNS = central nervous system, COD = cause of death, CRF = chronic renal failure, DM = diabetes mellitus, Dx = diagnosis, ECG = electrocardiogram, FCC = fibrocystic change, GI = gastrointestinal, HIV = human immunodeficiency virus, KA = keratoacanthoma, LAMB = lentigines, atrial myxoma, mucocutaneous myxomas, blue nevi, LEOPARD = lentigines, ECG abnormalities, ocular hypertelorism, pulmonic stenosis, retarded growth, deafness, LMM = lentigo malignant melanoma, MC = most common, MEN = multiple endocrine neoplasia, MF = mycosis fungoides, MSH = melanocyte stimulating hormone, NAME = nevi, atrial myxoma, mucocutaneous myxomas, ephelides, NHL = non-Hodgkin's lymphoma, Rx = treatment, SCC = squamous cell carcinoma, SSM = superficial spreading melanoma, UVB = ultraviolet light B.

CHAPTER

15

NEUROLOGY

CONTENTS

Table 15–1. OVERVIEW OF NEUROLOGIC EXAM, TESTS USED IN NEUROLOGY

Most Common...	Answer and Explanation
neurologic symptoms encountered	• **backache/headache,** • *dizziness,* • *syncope,* • *mental status abnormalities,* • *movement disorders*
elements of neurologic exam	• *state of consciousness:* * awake, * lethargic, * comatose, • *mental status/higher cortical functions,* • *gait/station,* • *cranial nerves,* • *motor evaluation,* • *sensory evaluation:* primary/cortical sensations, • *coordination:* * finger to nose, * heel to shin, * abnormal movements/tremor, • *vascular system:* bruits
elements of mental status exam	• *orientation:* * person, * place, * time, • *memory:* * immediate, * recent, * long-term, • *language:* ? aphasia problems, • *intellect:* *

Table continued on following page

Table 15–1. OVERVIEW OF NEUROLOGIC EXAM, TESTS USED IN NEUROLOGY *Continued*

Most Common...	Answer and Explanation
Continued	proverb interpretation, * recognizing similarities/differences, • *thought,* • *mood:* e.g., * euphoric, * angry
gait/station tests	• *normal walking,* • *tandem walking,* • *toe walking:* checks S1, • *heel walking:* checks L5, • *squat and rise:* checks pelvic girdle muscles, • *hop on each foot*
gait abnormalities	• *hemiparesis:* * circumduction of leg with knee stiff, * arm flexed and adducted, * decreased arm swing, • *spastic paraparesis:* * stiff, slow gait, * knees straight or slightly flexed, * scissored gait with hip adduction, • *waddling gait:* pelvic girdle muscle weakness, • *Parkinson's type gait:* * short steps, * trouble stopping, * wide turns, * decreased arm movements, • *steppage gait:* * feet lifted high/slap to ground, * common peroneal nerve injury, • *cerebellar gait:* * broad-based gait, * problems with tandem walking, * lurching/staggering
tests of olfactory nerve (CN I)	*smell:* * aromatic oil, * diminished in smokers/allergies, * anosmia (absence of smell) may be normal in elderly, * see Table 15–3 for pathologic conditions causing anosmia
tests of optic nerve (CN II)	• *visual acuity:* see Table 15–3, • *visual field:* see Table 15–3 for pathologic conditions, • *eye/fundus:* see Table 15–9 for pathologic conditions [CN II is afferent limb of pupillary light reflex. Visual acuity should be 20/20 in each eye. A pinhole in a card corrects refraction errors.]
tests of oculomotor nerve (CN III)	• *pupil reactivity:* * efferent limb of pupillary light reflex, * constricts pupil (parasympathetic), * accommodates (contracts ciliary muscle to thicken lens/increase refractive power), * converges (eyes focus on near object due to medial rectus contraction), * ~15% normal people have unequal pupil size (anisocoria), • *check for ptosis:* levator palpebrae, • *check extraocular movements:* CN III innervates all eye muscles except lateral rectus, superior oblique [In general, CN III

Table 15–1. OVERVIEW OF NEUROLOGIC EXAM, TESTS
USED IN NEUROLOGY *Continued*

Most Common...	Answer and Explanation
Continued	constricts the pupil, moves the eye, accommodates, and converges. See Table 15–3 for pathologic disorders.]
functions of eye muscles innervated by CN III	• *medial rectus:* adduction, • *superior rectus:* elevation of abducted eye, • *inferior rectus:* depression of abducted eye, • *inferior oblique:* elevation of adducted eye
clinical disorders involving CN III	• **transtentorial herniation compressing CN III:** * fixed, dilated pupil (first change), * ptosis of eye (second change), * affected eye looks "down and out" (patient cannot elevate or adduct eye), * diplopia, * paralysis of accommodation (cycloplegia), • *CNS aneurysms compress CN III:* headache + above findings, • *diabetic oculomotor palsy:* * vasculopathic palsy, * above findings except intact pupillary constriction, • *lid stare:* * hyperthyroidism, * sympathetic overactivity of levator palpebrae
tests of trochlear nerve (CN IV)	*movement of superior oblique:* depression of adducted eye
clinical disorder involving CN IV	*trauma resulting in paralysis:* * vertical diplopia when looking down, * eye slightly elevated and patient cannot depress eye in adduction, * head tilting toward damaged side
tests of trigeminal nerve (CN V) motor function	• *masseter and temporal muscles:* clench jaw and palpate, • *pterygoid muscles:* * open/close jaw, * jaw deviates to side of weakened pterygoid
tests of trigeminal nerve (CN V) sensory function	*check for pain, light touch, temperature sensation in all three divisions:* * ophthalmic, * maxillary, * mandibular
tests of trigeminal nerve (CN V) reflexes	• *corneal reflex:* * afferent limb CN V, * efferent limb CN VII, • *jaw jerk:* * mandibular reflex, * CN V controls afferent/efferent limbs, * pseudobulbar palsy if hyperactive
clinical disorders involving CN V	• trigeminal neuralgia: see Table 15–3, • *compression of CN V:* * e.g., acoustic neuroma in cerebellopontine angle, * clinical findings: ♦ hemianesthesia of face/mucous membranes of mouth/nasal cavities, ♦ loss of corneal reflex,

Table continued on following page

Table 15–1. OVERVIEW OF NEUROLOGIC EXAM, TESTS USED IN NEUROLOGY *Continued*

Most Common...	Answer and Explanation
Continued	♦ hypoacusis (paralysis of tensor tympani muscle), ♦ paralysis of muscles of mastication, ♦ jaw deviated to side of lesion (paralysis of pterygoid muscle)
test of abducens nerve (CN VI)	*abducts eye*
clinical disorder involving CN VI	*paralysis due to:* * trauma, * meningitis, * subarachnoid hemorrhage, * transtentorial herniation, * clinical findings: ♦ convergent strabismus with inability to abduct eye, ♦ horizontal diplopia
cause of bilateral CN VI palsy	*increased intracranial pressure*
tests of facial nerve (CN VII)	• *motor:* innervates: * orbicular oris/oculi (purse lips, close eye), * buccinator (blow out cheek/hold air), * frontalis (crease forehead muscles), • *taste:* anterior two-thirds of tongue, • *lacrimation,* • *salivation,* • *sensation external ear,* • *efferent limb corneal reflex*
clinical findings in Bell's palsy	• *LMN* (peripheral) *lesion,* • *etiology:* * **idiopathic,** * HSV, * Lyme disease (commonly bilateral), * malignant parotid gland tumor, • *ipsilateral paralysis of upper/lower facial muscles:* * face droops, * flattened nasolabial fold, • *cannot close eyes,* • *loss buccinator tone,* • *loss corneal reflex,* • *hyperacusis:* CN VII innervates stapedius muscle, • *diminished tearing,* • *sensory sparing*
clinical findings in supranuclear facial palsy	• *UMN lesion,* • *etiology:* stroke involving internal capsule, • *contralateral paralysis of lower face muscles with sparing of upper face muscles,* • *normal opening/closing of eye,* • *normal corneal reflex*
causes of bilateral Bell's palsy	• **Lyme disease,** • *Guillain-Barré syndrome*
tests of vestibular nerve (CN VIII)	• *cochlear division* (hearing): * Weber/Rinne test, * normal Weber: no lateralization to either ear, * normal Rinne: air conduction > bone conduction, • *vestibular division* (balance/equilibrium): * caloric testing, * Dix-Hallpike test (test for positional vertigo/nystagmus)

**Table 15–1. OVERVIEW OF NEUROLOGIC EXAM, TESTS
USED IN NEUROLOGY** *Continued*

Most Common...	Answer and Explanation
clinical disorders associated with vestibular nerve	• *disequilibrium,* • *vertigo,* • *nystagmus:* see Table 15–3
clinical disorder associated with cochlear nerve	• **sensorineural hearing loss,** • *tinnitus:* e.g., * acoustic neuroma, * see Table 15–3
tests of glossopharyngeal nerve (CN IX)	• *taste:* posterior one-third of tongue, • *gag reflex:* * CN IX afferent limb, * CN X efferent limb, • *test sensation of pharynx, soft palate, tonsils, back of tongue:* also mediated by CN X
clinical disorders affecting CN IX	• **glossopharyngeal neuralgia:** see Table 15–3, • *syncope:* * hypersensitive carotid sinus, * CN IX mediates input into carotid sinus
tests of vagus nerve (CN X)	• *test phonation:* * ask patient to say "ah," * palate should rise in midline, • *test sensation of soft palate/pharyngeal wall,* • *gag reflex:* CN X efferent limb, • *cough reflex:* * CN X afferent/efferent limb, * CN X innervates muscles of larynx, pharynx, • *oculocardiac reflex:* * pressure on eye should slow heart rate, * CN V afferent limb, * CN X efferent limb, • *carotid sinus reflex:* * pressure should slow heart rate, * afferent limb CN IX, * efferent limb CN X
clinical disorders involving CN X	• *bulbar palsy:* * LMN, * muscle weakness/ atrophy, * e.g., * ALS, * polio, • *pseudobulbar palsy:* * UMN, * weakness/spasticity, * e.g., large frontal lobe tumors, • *aortic aneurysms compress CN X:* hoarseness, • *parasympathetic dysfunction of CN X:* * bradycardia if nerve irritated, * tachycardia if nerve destroyed, * gastroparesis
clinical signs of CN X damage	• *loss of gag reflex,* • *loss of cough reflex:* lack of sensation in pharynx, larynx, • *hoarseness:* unilateral vocal cord paralysis, • *aphonia:* bilateral vocal cord paralysis, • *nasal speech:* weakness of soft palate, • *loss of taste,* • *dysphagia for solids/liquids*
tests of spinoaccessory nerve (CN XI)	• *test sternocleidomastoid muscle:* turn head against resistance, • *test trapezius muscle:* shrug shoulders

Table continued on following page

Table 15–1. OVERVIEW OF NEUROLOGIC EXAM, TESTS USED IN NEUROLOGY *Continued*

Most Common...	Answer and Explanation
clinical disorders associated with CN XI	• *paralysis of sternocleidomastoid or trapezius,* • *paralysis of larynx:* cranial root must be damaged
test of hypoglossal nerve (CN XII)	*test tongue movement:* innervates intrinsic/extrinsic tongue muscles
clinical disorder associated with CN XII	• *bulbar palsy:* * LMN, * e.g., ALS, polio, • *pseudobulbar palsy:* * UMN, * e.g., stroke
clinical findings of CN XII disease	*tongue deviation to side of weakness:* particularly in LMN disease
tests evaluating the sensory system	• *primary sensations:* * light touch, * pinprick/pain (STT), * temperature (STT), * vibratory sensation (♦ posterior column function, ♦ 128 Hz tuning fork), * proprioception (♦ position sense, ♦ Romberg test, ♦ posterior column function), • *cortical sensations:* * two-point discrimination (parietal lobe function), * graphesthesia (♦ trace numbers on palm, ♦ parietal lobe function), * stereognosis (recognize objects placed in hand) [Important sensory dermatomes include: * thumb: C6, * nipple: T4, * umbilicus: T10, * sole of foot: L5.]
elements of motor system evaluation	• *muscle observation,* • *evaluate muscle tone,* • *evaluate muscle power,* • *evaluate reflexes*
clinical findings noted on muscle observation	• *muscle atrophy:* * sign of LMN disease, * axonal degeneration, * muscle disuse, • *muscle fasciculations:* * sign of LMN disease, * may be normal after exercise or stressed/fatigued individuals, • *adventitious movements:* e.g., * chorea, * tremor, * myoclonus
clinical findings noted on examination of muscle tone	• *decreased tone, floppy muscles:* sign of LMN disease, • *spasticity:* * increased muscle tone, * sign of UMN disease, * e.g., claspknife reflex (increased resistance to passive movement of flexed arm followed by reflex relaxation), • *rigidity:* * increased tone throughout range of motion (cogwheel effect), * sign of extrapyramidal disease, e.g., * Par-

Table 15–1. OVERVIEW OF NEUROLOGIC EXAM, TESTS USED IN NEUROLOGY *Continued*

Most Common...	Answer and Explanation
Continued	kinson's disease, • *paratonia:* * patient resists flexion with extension or extension with flexion, * sign of diffuse cerebral dysfunction
clinical findings indicating muscle weakness	• *arm drift when hands are extended in front of body and maintained for 30–45 s,* • *inability to rise up out of chair or climb stairs:* proximal muscle weakness, • *inability to walk on the heels or toes:* distal muscle weakness, • *impaired fine movements of hands*
reflexes tested	• *DTRs,* • *abnormal reflexes,* • *superficial reflexes*
tendon reflexes	• *biceps:* C5–6, • *supinator:* C5–6, • *triceps:* C6–7, • *patellar:* L3–4, • *Achilles:* S1–2
superficial reflexes	• *abdominal:* * upper T8–9, * lower T10–11, • *cremasteric:* L1–2, • *bulbocavernous:* S3–4
abnormal reflexes	• *Babinski:* * extensor plantar sign, * indicates corticospinal tract disease, • *frontal release signs:* * snout, * suck, * palmomental, * forced grasping
cerebellar tests	• *finger-to-nose/heel-to-shin:* dysfunction is called dysmetria (undershoots/overshoots goal), • *rebound test:* * flex arm hard/let go, * poor rebound is for antagonist muscles not to check active rebound movement of arm, • *rapid alternating movements of hands/feet:* * cerebellar dysfunction, * called dysdiadochokinesis, • *walk normally and in tandem:* dysfunction is called ataxia, • *check for tremor:* intention tremor (tremor with voluntary movement) noted in cerebellar dysfunction
S/S of cerebral cortex disorders	• *alterations in consciousness:* arousal, • *alterations in cognition,* • *focal neurologic symptoms:* * single limb, * single neurologic symptom (numbness or weakness), • *dominant hemisphere dysfunction:* * speech, * language, • *nondominant hemisphere dysfunction:* * visual/spatial deficits, * contralateral neglect, * confusion, • *visual system disorders:* homonymous deficits

Table continued on following page

Table 15–1. OVERVIEW OF NEUROLOGIC EXAM, TESTS USED IN NEUROLOGY *Continued*

Most Common...	Answer and Explanation
S/S of subcortical disorders	• *weakness/numbness involving more than one limb,* • *visual system disorders:* homonymous deficits
S/S of basal ganglia disorders	*movement disorders:* e.g., * rigidity, * tremor, * chorea
S/S of thalamus disorders	*unilateral sensory alterations*
S/S of hypothalamus disorders	• *autonomic nervous system dysfunction,* • *temperature abnormalities,* • *fluid disturbances:* related to ADH, • *satiety alterations,* • *sleep disorders*
S/S of brain stem disorders	• *ocular motility dysfunction,* • *diplopia,* • *nystagmus:* * vertical (cervicomedullary junction lesion), * horizontal, * rotary, • *cranial nerve palsies:* ipsilateral, • *crossed syndromes:* long-tract signs contralateral, • *MLF dysfunction:* * internuclear ophthalmoplegia, * 1 1/2 syndrome, • *vertigo,* • *ataxia,* • *dysphagia*
S/S of cerebellar dysfunction	• *ipsilateral ataxia involving arm/leg:* cerebellar hemisphere dysfunction, • *gait ataxia with sparing of arms, speech, eye motility:* anterior superior vermis dysfunction, • *equilibrium/ walking alterations but finger-to-nose/heel-to-shin intact:* flocculonodular lobe dysfunction
S/S of spinal cord dysfunction	• *bladder incontinence/saddle anesthesia:* conus medullaris disorder, • *muscle fasciculations/atrophy:* anterior horn cell disorder, • *pain/temperature alterations:* crossed spinothalamic tract dysfunction, • *proprioception, DTR abnormalities:* posterior column dysfunction, • *spasticity:* lateral corticospinal tract dysfunction, • *radicular pain:* extramedullary disorder, • *painless, nonlocalizable signs with sacral sparing:* intramedullary cord dysfunction
S/S of PNS disorders	• *sharp, lancinating nerve root pain with dermatome localization:* pain exacerbated by coughing/straining, • *nerve root pain with myotome localization:* e.g., C5–C6 pain to deltoid/biceps, • *muscle weakness,* • *absent DTRs*

Table 15–1. OVERVIEW OF NEUROLOGIC EXAM, TESTS USED IN NEUROLOGY *Continued*

Most Common...	Answer and Explanation
neurologic S/S considered normal in elderly	• *intrinsic muscle atrophy of hand,* • *decreased ankle reflexes,* • *decreased vibratory sensation in legs,* • *decreased visual pursuit movements,* • *impaired upward gaze,* • *difficulty with tandem gait,* • *difficulty with balancing on one leg,* • *slowing of rapid alternating movements,* • *otosclerosis,* • *presbycusis,* • *cataracts,* • *decreased smell/taste sensation,* • *presbyopia:* * problems with close focus, * decreased lens flexibility
indications for a lumbar puncture	• **R/O meningitis,** • *R/O metastases to meninges,* • *R/O demyelinating disease:* e.g., * MS, * Guillain-Barré, • *increased intracranial pressure suspected but CT/MRI normal,* • *intrathecal Rx,* • *Dx/Rx pseudotumor cerebri:* high CSF pressure, • *infectious diseases:* e.g., * AIDS, * Lyme disease, * syphilis, • *paraneoplastic syndromes:* e.g., measure Hu/Yo antibodies to diagnose cerebellar degeneration
routine tests performed on CSF	• *clarity,* • *cell count/differential,* • *glucose,* • *protein,* • *Gram stain,* • *bacterial culture*
cause of a bloody CSF tap	*iatrogenic:* absence of pink supranate after centrifugation of tubes and drop in RBC count in successive tubes indicates a nonpathologic cause of blood in CSF
cause of yellow colored CSF (xanthochromia)	• **pathologic bleed in CNS:** * yellow color is bilirubin pigment, * occurs 4 h post bleed, • *high CSF protein:* e.g., * MS, * TB, * normal CSF protein = 15–45 mg/dL
causes of increased CSF protein	• **CNS inflammation:** increased vessel permeability, • *synthesis of IgG by plasma cells in CNS:* e.g., MS [gamma-globulins are normally <12% of total CSF protein. TB has high CSF protein that forms a pellicle when left in a refrigerator overnight.]
tests to identify cause of elevated CSF gamma-globulin to R/O demyelination	• **oligoclonal bands on CSF high resolution electrophoresis:** * multiple small bands in gamma-globulin region, * indicate demyelination, * sensitivity of ~80%/specificity 99% for MS, • *IgG index:* * CSF IgG/serum IgG ÷ CSF albumin/serum albumin, * normal 0.3–

Table continued on following page

Table 15–1. OVERVIEW OF NEUROLOGIC EXAM, TESTS USED IN NEUROLOGY *Continued*

Most Common...	Answer and Explanation
Continued	0.6, * most sensitive of all ratio tests, • *CSF IgG/serum albumin ratio:* * albumin is synthesized in liver and not CNS, * ratio <25% indicates increased vessel permeability and leakage of albumin + gamma-globulins into CNS, * increased ratio indicates CNS synthesis of IgG, • *IgG synthesis rate:* * measures synthesis rate of B cells in CSF, * normal −9.9 to +3.3 mg/d
cause of a low CSF glucose (hypoglycorrhachia)	• **bacterial meningitis,** • *fungal meningitis,* • *metastatic disease to meninges,* • *sarcoidosis involving meninges,* • *some types of viral meningitis:* e.g., mumps, • *subarachnoid hemorrhage:* used up by RBCs in glycolysis, • *amebic meningoencephalitis,* • *peripheral blood hypoglycemia* [CSF glucose is ~60% of serum glucose. Normal CSF glucose = 40–70 mg/dL. Glucose may remain low after 2 wks even though infection is eradicated (due to CSF block in glucose transport).]
disorders with a normal CSF glucose	• *viral meningitis/encephalitis,* • *cerebral abscess,* • *neurosyphilis,* • *degenerative diseases,* • *demyelinating diseases*
WBC response in CSF in viral versus bacterial meningitis	• *viral:* * initially a neutrophilic response, * switches to lymphocyte response in 24–48 h, • *bacterial:* * neutrophilic response, * TB has a mononuclear response [The normal CSF WBC count = 0–5 mononuclear cells/μL. Neutrophils are not normal in adult CSF.]
lab test on CSF to detect bacterial/ fungal pathogens	*Gram stain of cytocentrifuged specimen:* * sensitivity CSF Gram stain = ~60–90%, * positive CSF cultures in 85–90%, * blood cultures positive in most cases (MC route of infection is hematogenous)
latex agglutination tests available on CSF	• *pneumococcus,* • *meningococcus,* • *Haemophilus influenzae type B,* • *group B streptococcus,* • *Escherichia coli,* • *Cryptococcus neoformans* [Sensitivity LA tests = 85–90%. India ink test for *C. neoformans* sensitivity = 50–60%. Sensitivity of culture is same as LA tests. PCR of CSF available for *Listeria monocytogenes* and *Neisseria meningitidis.*]

Table 15–1. OVERVIEW OF NEUROLOGIC EXAM, TESTS USED IN NEUROLOGY *Continued*

Most Common...	Answer and Explanation
tests to diagnose neurosyphilis	• **CSF VDRL:** * sensitivity = ~55%, * cannot use RPR on CSF, • *CSF FTA-ABS:* * usually not recommended, * does not distinguish active from old infection, • *increased CSF cell count:* mononuclear cells, • *increased CSF protein,* • *normal CSF glucose,* • *oligoclonal bands:* 75%
differences between serum and CSF	• *protein:* CSF < serum, • *glucose:* CSF 60% of serum level, • *chloride:* CSF > serum, • *cell count:* CSF 0–5 cells/µL (no neutrophils)
uses of EEG	• **Dx of epilepsy:** * factors enhancing diagnostic yield: ♦ hyperventilation, ♦ sleep deprivation, ♦ photic stimulation, * normal EEG does not R/O epilepsy, * specific for petit mal, • *differentiates seizures from metabolic encephalopathy,* • *localizes brain disorders,* • *Dx of brain death:* EEG isoelectric for 30 m
types of evoked potentials (EP)	• *visual EP:* * optic nerve and cerebral visual pathway integrity, * excellent for optic neuritis in MS, • *brain stem auditory EP:* * auditory pathways, * excellent for acoustic neuromas, brain stem disease, • *somatosensory EP:* * central sensory pathways, * excellent for lower brain stem/spinal cord disease
use of nerve conduction velocity	*distinguish demyelination* (slows conduction without affecting amplitude) *from axonal degeneration* (reduction in amplitude) *of peripheral nerves*
use of neurotransmission tests	• **Dx of MG,** • *Dx of Eaton-Lambert syndrome,* • *Dx of botulism*
uses of EMG	*distinguishes neuropathies* (* demyelination, * axonal degeneration) *from myopathies* (* inflammatory, * metabolic, * LMN disease)
CNS disorders where CT has greater sensitivity than MRI	• **Dx of parenchymatous intracranial hemorrhage in first 72 h,** • *initial test in acute stroke,* • *Dx of subarachnoid hemorrhage,* • *Dx of acute brain contusions,* • *Dx of disk disease:* nerve entrapment in intervertebral disk disease in cervical/thoracic areas, • *meningiomas,* • *brain stem gliomas*

Table continued on following page

Table 15–1. OVERVIEW OF NEUROLOGIC EXAM, TESTS USED IN NEUROLOGY *Continued*

Most Common...	Answer and Explanation
CNS disorders where MRI has greater sensitivity than CT	• *CNS tumors:* * primary, * metastatic, • *aneurysms/AVM,* • *inflammatory lesions,* • *demyelination:* white matter lesions, • *atrophy/hydrocephalus,* • *sellar tumors,* • *posterior fossa lesions,* • *acoustic neuroma,* • *spinal cord lesions,* • *lumbar disk disease,* • *multi-infarct dementia:* CT is equal to MRI in Alzheimer's disease
uses of CNS angiograms that are superior to CT/MRI	• **aneurysms/AVM,** • *CNS vasculitis*
use of carotid duplex ultrasonography	*extracranial carotid artery stenosis:* not useful in intracranial stenosis

Question: Diplopia plus pupillary abnormalities characterize which of the following cranial nerve palsies? SELECT 1

- (A) CN II
- (B) CN III
- (C) CN IV
- (D) CN V
- (E) CN VI
- (F) CN VII
- (G) CN VIII
- (H) CN IX
- (I) CN X

Answer: (B): Diplopia occurs when one or more of the extraocular muscles are weakened. CN II is the optic nerve, which does not innervate any of the extraocular muscles. Defects in visual acuity are the primary abnormality **(choice A is incorrect).** CN III **(choice B),** the oculomotor nerve, innervates four muscles (medial rectus, superior rectus, inferior rectus, inferior oblique). It also carries the parasympathetic nerve, hence injury to the nerve may result in mydriasis. CN IV, the trochlear nerve, innervates the superior oblique and produces a vertical diplopia when injured **(choice C is incorrect).** CN V, the trigeminal nerve, is primarily involved in facial sensation **(choice D is incorrect).** CN VI, the abducens nerve, innervates the lateral rectus muscle. A horizontal diplopia occurs when it is injured **(choice E is incorrect).** CN VII, the facial nerve, is primarily involved with the facial muscles **(choice F is incorrect).** CN VIII, the vestibular/cochlear nerve, produces problems with disequilibrium and hearing, respectively **(choice G is incorrect).** CN IX, the glossopharyngeal nerve, and CN X, the vagus nerve, primarily innervate muscles in the tongue, palate, larynx, and upper pharynx **(choices H and I are incorrect).**

ADH = antidiuretic hormone, AIDS = acquired immunodeficiency syndrome, ALS = amyotrophic lateral sclerosis, AVM = arteriovenous malformation, C = cervical, CN = cranial nerve, CNS = central nervous system, CSF = cerebrospinal fluid, CT = computed tomography, DTR = deep tendon reflex, Dx = diagnosis, EEG = electroencephalogram, EMG = electromyography, EP = evoked potential, FTA-ABS = fluorescent treponema antibody absorption, HSV = herpes simplex virus, Hz = Hertz, Ig = immunoglobulin, LA = latex agglutination, L = lumbar, LMN = lower motor neuron, MC = most common, MG = myasthenia gravis, MLF = medial longitudinal fasciculus, MRI = magnetic resonance imaging, MS = multiple sclerosis, PCR = polymerase chain reaction, PNS = peripheral nervous system, RBC = red blood cell, R/O = rule out, RPR = rapid plasma reagin, Rx = treatment, S = sacral, S/S = signs and symptoms, STT = spinothalamic tract, T = thoracic, TB = tuberculosis, UMN = upper motor neuron, VDRL = Venereal Disease Research Laboratory, WBC = white blood cell.

Table 15–2. DISORDERS OF CONSCIOUSNESS AND HIGHER BRAIN FUNCTION

Most Common...	Answer and Explanation
S/S of cerebral cortex dysfunction	• **defects in cognition, consciousness:** cerebral cortex, • *defects in speech/language:* dominant hemisphere, • *visual-spatial defects, confusion, neglect of contralateral side of body:* nondominant hemisphere defects, • *focal neurologic symptoms involving single limb:* * numbness (sensory system), * weakness (motor system) involve cerebral cortex, • *numbness in more than one limb:* subcortical defect, • *movement disorders:* basal ganglia defect, • *unilateral sensory abnormalities:* thalamus defect, • *temperature, food, water regulation:* hypothalamus defect, • *defects in sleep, endocrine, cardiovascular function, autonomic regulation:* hypothalamus, • *visual defects:* cortical/subcortical defects
location in hypothalamus controlling circadian rhythms/REM/non-REM cycles	• *suprachiasmatic nucleus:* circadian rhythms within 24-h day, • *pontomesencephalic area:* e.g., * locus ceruleus, * dorsal raphe, * certain cholinergic nuclei control sequencing of REM and non-REM sleep
stages of sleep	• *non-REM:* * stage 1 (♦ lightest/shortest stage of sleep, ♦ ψ-waves), * stage 2 (♦ longest stage of sleep, ♦ sleep spindles and K complexes), * stages 3–4 (♦ slow wave sleep, ♦ δ-waves, ♦ most relaxed phase of sleep, ♦ gradually

Table continued on following page

Table 15–2. DISORDERS OF CONSCIOUSNESS AND HIGHER BRAIN FUNCTION *Continued*

Most Common...	Answer and Explanation
Continued	disappears after 40, ♦ stage associated with sleepwalking, night terror, bedwetting), • *REM sleep:* * occurs q 90 m during last third of night, * increased pulse, respiration, BP, nocturnal penile/clitoral erections, * dreams, * remains throughout life
neurotransmitters involved in sleep	• *serotonin:* * derived from tryptophan, * produces sleep, • *norepinephrine:* drugs stimulating noradrenergic neurons reduce REM sleep, • *ACh:* increases REM sleep, • *dopamine:* * drugs blocking dopamine increase time sleeping, * drugs increasing dopamine increase wakefulness
sleep changes in major depression	• *REM sleep occurs at beginning of sleep,* • *more time spent in REM sleep,* • *increased central cholinergic activity*
sleep changes in Alzheimer's disease	• *decreased cholinergic neurons in basal forebrain:* decreased ACh, • *reduced slow wave sleep:* stages 3–4 non-REM sleep, • *reduced REM sleep*
sleep disorder	*insomnia:* * problem in falling/staying asleep that occurs three times/wk for at least 1 month, * sleepiness during day
Rx of insomnia	• **reassurance/behavioral modification,** • *short-acting benzodiazepines,* • *tricyclics:* helpful in insomnia associated with depression
causes of hypersomnia	• **sleep apnea:** see Table 6–3, • *narcolepsy:* * AD disease, * specific DQB10602 haplotype, • *Kleine-Levin syndrome:* hypersomnolence + hyperphagia, • *premenstrual period,* • *depression* [Hypersomnia is sleep behavior consistently >25–30% of norm for that person.]
S/S of narcolepsy	• **sleep attacks:** sudden onset of REM sleep during times of wakefulness, • *cataplexy:* surprise/emotion leads to abrupt muscular hypotonia, • *hypnagogic hallucinations:* intense dream-like experiences that occur just as one falls asleep, • *sleep paralysis:* sense that one cannot move when awakening from sleep [The above may be normal to lesser degrees but are exaggerated in narcolepsy.]

Table 15–2. DISORDERS OF CONSCIOUSNESS AND HIGHER BRAIN FUNCTION *Continued*

Most Common...	Answer and Explanation
Rx of narcolepsy	*methylphenidate*
sites responsible for staying awake	• *cerebral hemispheres,* • *reticular activating system*
primary disturbances of arousal	• *stupor:* * psychologic unresponsiveness, * response only to vigorous external stimulation, • *coma:* * unarousable state, * eyes closed, * no evidence of awareness of inner thoughts or outer events
mechanisms for stupor/coma	• **supratentorial lesions involving posterior ventromedial diencephalon:** * **central/uncal herniation,** * invasion/destruction of posterior VMD, • *subtentorial lesions compressing/ damaging upper pontine midbrain reticular formation:* e.g., pontine/cerebellar bleed, • *metabolic/diffuse lesions:* e.g., * drugs/poisons, * myxedema coma, * liver failure, * hypo/hypernatremia, * meningitis, * hypoglycemia
causes of sudden acute coma	• **self-induced drug poisoning,** • *brain trauma,* • acute intracranial bleed, • *hypoglycemia,* • *meningitis*
clinical findings of supratentorial mass lesions	• **focal cerebral signs:** e.g., * headache on side of lesion, * aphasia, * contralateral hemiparesis, • *dysfunction moves front to back:* focal motor → bilateral motor → stupor/coma, • *dysfunction localized to a single or adjacent anatomic level,* • *absence of brain stem signs unless herniation occurs:* see below
clinical findings of central transtentorial herniation	• *midline diencephalon displaced caudally toward and through tentorial notch against the midbrain,* • *early decline in arousal,* • *pupils small, equal, and reactive,* • *bilateral UMN signs,* • *decerebrate early*
clinical findings of uncal transtentorial herniation	• *temporal fossa lesion herniates uncus over edge of ipsilateral tentorium,* • *compression of CN III:* * **unilateral mydriasis** (earliest finding), * ptosis, • late decline in arousal and decerebrate state: see below

Table continued on following page

**Table 15–2. DISORDERS OF CONSCIOUSNESS AND
HIGHER BRAIN FUNCTION** *Continued*

Most Common...	Answer and Explanation
cause of decerebrate state	*upper brain stem injury:* e.g., * brain stem infarction, * pontine/posterior fossa bleed, * tumor, * metabolic encephalopathy (♦ hepatic encephalopathy, ♦ hypoglycemia), * brain stem compression secondary to increased intracranial pressure
clinical findings in decerebrate state	• *arms adducted/extended,* • *wrists pronated/ fingers flexed,* • *extension of both legs with plantar flexion of feet* [It is an abnormal extensor response.]
neurologic test to establish whether brain stem is intact	*oculocephalic test* (doll's eyes): * performed by quickly turning the head laterally or vertically, * eyes should move conjugately in opposite direction of head movement if brain stem is intact, * absence of all eye movements indicates bilateral pontine lesion, * eye deviation toward side of hemiparesis indicates a contralateral pontine lesion, * eye deviation away from the side of hemiparesis indicates a contralateral frontal lobe lesion
cause of decorticate state	*damage to one or both corticospinal tracts:* e.g., * CVA, * head injury, * brain abscess, * brain tumor
clinical findings in decorticate state	• *adduction/flexion of arms up to chest,* • *wrists/fingers flexed on chest,* • *legs extended and internally rotated with plantar flexion of feet* [It is an abnormal flexor response.]
clinical findings of subtentorial lesions	• *compression of reticular activating system,* • *upper CN palsies,* • *sudden onset of coma:* brain stem dysfunction may precede coma, • *absent caloric responses:* see below, • *pupil abnormalities:* * pinpoint: pons, * fixed: midbrain, * irregular and/or unequal: midbrain-pontine, • *cerebellar dysfunction,* • *bilateral motor dysfunction*
clinical findings of metabolic/diffuse lesions	• *stupor/coma often preceded or replaced by delirium:* see below, • *commonly noted in elderly patients on multiple drugs admitted to medical/surgical units,* • *symmetric motor signs,* • *moderate hypothermia,* • *bilateral asterixis/myoclonus,* • *multiple anatomic levels involved,* • *preserved sensory function,* • *preserved pupillary function*

Table 15–2. DISORDERS OF CONSCIOUSNESS AND HIGHER BRAIN FUNCTION *Continued*

Most Common...	Answer and Explanation
uses of Glasgow Coma Scale (GCS)	• *quantitate level of consciousness,* • *quantitate severity of head injury*
parameters in GCS	• *eye-opening response:* scale of E1 (no response) to E4 (eyes open and blinking), • *verbal response:* scale of V1 (no verbal response at all) to V5 (oriented to person, place, time, etc.), • *best motor response:* * scale of M1 (no movement at all) to M6 (obeys verbal commands, moves limbs spontaneously), * best motor score is taken from any extremity even though worse responses may be present in other extremities
definition of coma according to GCS	• *unable to open eye,* • *unable to follow commands,* • *unable to utter words*
drugs associated with delirium	• *sedative/hypnotics,* • *NSAIDs,* • *beta blockers,* • *antipsychotic agents,* • *anticholinergic agents*
S/S of delirium	• **clouding of consciousness/lack of awareness of environment,** • *worse at night/early morning,* • *lack orientation to time and place:* not person, • *coarse tremor,* • *breathing alterations:* e.g., hyperpnea, • *visual hallucinations*
S/S of psychogenic coma	• *resist passive opening of eyelids, when eyelids raised,* • *eyelids shut abruptly when released,* • *brisk pupillary reactions,* • *normal caloric studies:* quick nystagmus, • *normal EEG,* • *no pathologic reflexes,* • *associations:* * severe depression, * catatonia of schizophrenia, * hysteria, * malingering
clinical findings of vegetative state	• **absent cognitive activity,** • *preservation of sleep-wake cycles,* • *primitive motor responses*
clinical findings of locked-in state	• **paralysis of communication and facial movements with retained consciousness:** bilateral ventral pontine lesions (e.g., pontine bleed, central pontine myelinolysis), • *quadriplegic:* damage to corticospinal tracts, • *reticular activating system intact:* conscious, • *can communicate by blinking eyelids:* supranuclear ocular motor pathways intact

Table continued on following page

Table 15–2. DISORDERS OF CONSCIOUSNESS AND HIGHER BRAIN FUNCTION *Continued*

Most Common...	Answer and Explanation
criteria used to define brain death	• **permanent loss of all essential brain functions:** * **no cerebral or brain stem function,** * e.g., ♦ no response to noxious stimuli, ♦ fixed pupils, ♦ apneic off ventilator, • *isoelectric EEG for 30 m,* • *known structural or irreversible systemic metabolic cause*
Rx of coma	• **intubate/oxygenate,** • *hyperventilate:* respiratory alkalosis vasoconstricts CNS vessels, • *IV thiamine,* • *IV glucose,* • *consider naloxone,* • *obtain emergency brain scan,* • *increase serum osmolality with mannitol,* • *treat specific cause if known*
causes of syncope	• **brief dysfunction of vasodepressor cardiovascular reflexes,** • *primary cardiovascular disease,* • *orthostatic hypotension*
mechanisms of syncope	• **impaired right heart filling:** e.g., * reflex abnormalities with venodilation, * hypovolemia, * Valsalva maneuver, • *global impaired cardiac output:* e.g., * vagal sinus arrest due to carotid sinus sensitivity, * intrinsic cardiac disease, such as AMI, aortic stenosis, hypertrophic cardiomyopathy
location for language deficits	*left hemisphere* (95%) *in general population:* * left-handed people (15% of population) primarily use left hemisphere, * tend to have some language function in both hemispheres (aphasia uncommon)
clinical findings in expressive aphasia	• **defect in expressing speech:** * halting, * nonfluent, • *good comprehension,* • *lesion in Broca's area in left inferior posterior frontal lobe,* • *right hemiparesis involving arm/face often present*
clinical findings in receptive aphasia	• **defect in speech comprehension,** • *speech abundant, fluent, semantic nonsense,* • *defect in Wernicke's area in superior-lateral posterior temporal lobe,* • *no other localizing signs usually present*
clinical findings in conduction aphasia	• **cannot comprehend or repeat phrases,** • *defect close to but not in primary speech area,* • *no other localizing signs usually present*

Table 15–2. DISORDERS OF CONSCIOUSNESS AND HIGHER BRAIN FUNCTION *Continued*

Most Common...	Answer and Explanation
clinical findings in global aphasia	• **loss of all major aspects of speech:** expressive/receptive aphasia, • *large defect in frontotemporal area of brain*, • *right hemiparesis/hemiplegia usually present*
clinical findings in mutism	*inability to speak or make sounds:* * acute defect in left pre-Broca area, * bilateral frontal lobe damage, * locked-in-state (see below)
clinical findings in dysarthria	• **inability to articulate speech clearly,** • *associated with bulbar/pseudobulbar palsy or lesions in vocal cord apparatus*
clinical findings in apraxia	• **loss of ability to perform learned motor functions despite absence of motor or sensory deficits,** • *signifies deep lesions in one or both parietal lobes*
clinical findings in agnosia	• **inability to recognize a complex sensory stimulus** (e.g., * visual recognition of familiar object, * tactile recognition of familiar object [astereognosis], * significance of sounds) **or body part** (e.g., * finger, * face) **in spite of normal elemental perceptions and language,** • *signifies large defects in parieto-occipital or posterior-temporal areas*
clinical findings in frontal lobe injury	• *distal contralateral spastic weakness of lower face/arm*, • *expressive aphasia:* dominant hemisphere, • *mutism*, • *sucking, groping, grasping reflexes*, • *emotional outbursts*, • *inappropriate social behavior*
clinical findings in parietal lobe injury of dominant (left) hemisphere	• **general:** problems with * language, * speech, * calculation, • *Gerstmann's syndrome:* * right/left disorientation, * dyscalculia (inability to do math problems), * dysgraphia (difficulty in writing), * body part agnosia (e.g., inability to recognize fingers), * right hemianopia, * contralateral loss of tactile discrimination (♦ astereognosis, ♦ contralateral sensory neglect), • *constructional apraxia:* cannot draw simple objects

Table continued on following page

**Table 15–2. DISORDERS OF CONSCIOUSNESS AND
HIGHER BRAIN FUNCTION** *Continued*

Most Common...	Answer and Explanation
clinical findings in parietal lobe injury of nondominant (right) hemisphere	• **general:** loss of * spatial perception and * nonverbal ideation, • *left-sided hemineglect,* • *constructional apraxia,* • *dressing apraxia,* • *anosognosia:* denial of a neurologic defect, • *topographic memory loss:* unable to negotiate familiar surroundings
memory disorders	• **dementia:** e.g., Alzheimer's disease, • *aging,* • *transient global amnesia* (TGA), • *psychogenic amnesia,* • *Korsakoff's syndrome*
site for memory formation and retrieval	• **hippocampal area of temporal lobe,** • *thalamus:* paramedian areas, • *mammillary bodies*
clinical findings in TGA	• *patients >65 y old,* • *acute onset of amnesia for time, place, past memory* (retrograde) *lasting 3–12 h,* • *vascular insufficiency to hippocampal/thalamic areas*
clinical findings in psychogenic amnesia	• *amnesia greatest for past emotional events,* • *mixture of recent/remote memory loss related to certain events,* • *absence of antegrade amnesia:* new memories laid down after a particular time/event, • *they do not ask questions about their amnesia*
clinical findings in organic causes of amnesia	• *recent memory is worse than remote,* • *antegrade and retrograde* (memories extending back from particular event) *amnesia equally dysfunctional,* • *repeatedly ask questions about their amnesia,* • *can recall emotionally important events*
causes of dementia	• **Alzheimer's disease (AD):** 50–70%, • *multi-infarct dementia:* 15–25%, • *combination of AD + multi-infarct dementia:* 15%, • *communicating hydrocephalus,* • *AIDS dementia,* • *pseudodementia associated with depression,* • *genetic disease:* e.g., * HD, * Wilson's disease, * AIP, • *infections:* e.g., * HIV, * neurosyphilis, * chronic fungal infections, * C-J disease, • *alcohol abuse,* • B_{12} *deficiency,* • *primary hypothyroidism,* • *chronic subdural hematoma* [Dementia is more common with advancing age.]
cause of Binswanger's dementia	*multiple subcortical white mater infarcts/demyelination:* due to hypertensive small vessel

Table 15–2. DISORDERS OF CONSCIOUSNESS AND HIGHER BRAIN FUNCTION *Continued*

Most Common...	Answer and Explanation
Continued	disease (hyaline arteriolosclerosis) involving perforating arterioles
infectious cause of dementia	*AIDS*
potentially reversible types of dementia	• **pseudodementia secondary to depression,** • *hypo/hyperthyroidism,* • *primary* HPTH, • *toxic agents:* e.g., * Pb, * alcohol, * pesticides, • *nutritional deficiencies:* e.g., * B$_{12}$, * niacin, * thiamine, • *normal pressure hydrocephalus,* • *subdural hematoma,* • *intracranial mass lesions,* • *advanced Parkinson's disease*
clinical findings associated with dementia	• **memory loss,** • *defects in:* * judgment, * abstract thinking, * orientation (days → years → months → place), * learning new material, * attention, * recognition/production of speech, • *behavioral changes:* e.g., * delusions, * paranoia, * agitation, * hallucinations, • *loss of social amenities:* usually occurs late in AD but early in frontal lobe disease, intracranial mass lesions, alcohol-drug dementia, • *sensorimotor disturbances:* * absent in AD, * present in ♦ multi-infarct dementia, ♦ hydrocephalic dementia, • *gait abnormalities:* present in hydrocephalic dementia
pathologic defects associated with AD	• **senile (neuritic) plaques:** * extracellular deposits of amyloid β-protein + glial processes, * positive silver stain, • *neurofibrillary tangles:* abnormal form of microtubule-associated protein (tau) located in cytoplasm of neuron cells, • *granulovacuolar degeneration:* * circular clear zones with granules, * located in hippocampus neurons, • *symmetric atrophy:* neuronal loss: * frontal/temporal/parietal lobes, * hippocampal cortex, * amygdala, * nucleus basalis of Meynert, • *damage to ascending cholinergic and norepinephrine regulating pathways*
factors predisposing to AD	• *genetic* factors: * ~25% have affected relatives, * rarely autosomal dominant, • *low ACh levels:* important in learning, • *reduced choline acetyltransferase levels,* • *aluminum toxicity,* • *severe past head injury*

Table continued on following page

Table 15–2. DISORDERS OF CONSCIOUSNESS AND HIGHER BRAIN FUNCTION *Continued*

Most Common...	Answer and Explanation
role of chromosome 21 in AD	*chromosome produces amyloid β-protein:* * toxic to neurons, * present in senile plaques, * association with Down syndrome and familial early onset-AD
role of chromosome 19 in AD	*chromosome contains apo gene E, allele ε4:* * gene produces a protein with high affinity for amyloid β-protein, * 50% risk for AD at ~65–68 y old if homozygous for E, allele ε4, * 50% with single allele develop AD ~73–74 y old, * associated with familial late-onset AD
role of chromosome 14 in AD	*chromosome produces tau-microtubule-associated proteins in neurofibrillary tangles*
method of Dx of AD	• *Hx,* • *cognitive exams,* • *postmortem:* confirmatory test
Rx of AD	• *tacrine:* * centrally acting acetylcholinesterase inhibitor of ACh metabolism, * delays cognitive decline in AD, * liver toxicity, • *donepezil:* * acetylcholinesterase inhibitor, * no significant liver abnormalities
COD in AD	• **respiratory infection,** • *intercurrent illness*
clinical findings in multi-infarct dementia	• *successive large/small strokes in deep subcortical nuclei of cerebral cortex,* • *association with:* * DM, * HTN, * hyperlipidemia, • *stepwise progression of dementia,* • *lack social amenities:* disheveled, • *UMN abnormalities common,* • *aphasia,* • *multiple bright spots with MRI*
clinical findings in communicating hydrocephalus dementia (normal pressure hydrocephalus)	• *may follow head trauma, infection, intracranial bleeds,* • *problem with absorption of CSF out of subarachnoid space,* • *shuffling, wide-based gait,* • *urinary incontinence,* • *bilateral UMN dysfunction in legs > arms:* positive Babinski, • *ataxic/spastic gait,* • *dilated ventricles noted on CT/MRI,* • *normal CSF pressure in most*

Table 15–2. DISORDERS OF CONSCIOUSNESS AND HIGHER BRAIN FUNCTION *Continued*

Most Common...	Answer and Explanation
clinical findings of dementia associated with Parkinson's disease	• *present in advanced disease* (20–40%) *in patients* >65 *y old,* • *depression commonly present,* • *resembles AD in clinical progression,* • *dopamine may improve cognitive function*
clinical findings in Pick's disease	• *earlier age of onset than AD:* fifth or sixth decade, • *neuronal degeneration in frontal lobes and temporal lobes:* posterior two-thirds of first temporal gyrus spared, • *associated with behavioral/personality changes*
clinical findings in Creutzfeldt-Jakob disease	• *earlier onset than AD:* sixth decade, • *transmission:* * slow virus disease due to prions (♦ subviral transmissible agent, ♦ extracellular protein with no nucleic acid), * health hazard for those working with brains, * "mad cow" disease (improperly cooked beef), * corneal transplants, • *myoclonic jerks/seizures,* • *rapidly progressive to vegetative state:* death in 1 y
clinical findings in HD	• *AD disease with a late-onset of dementia:* 30–40 y old, • *triplet repeat of CAG on chromosome 4:* detect triplet repeats with PCR, • *reduced levels of GABA, ACh, ATII,* • *clinical:* * dementia, * chorea, * extrapyramidal signs, * absence of sensory/UMN disease, • *loss of social amenities:* e.g., * eccentric behavior, * sexually hyperactive, * very irritable, • *depression/suicide common,* • *MRI shows atrophy of caudate/putamen*
clinical findings of Wilson's disease	*see Table 9–8*
tests recommended in evaluation of dementia	• *CBC,* • *syphilis serology,* • *serum TSH,* • *serum B_{12},* • *serum calcium, glucose, BUN,* • *MRI,* • *HIV serology:* selected cases

Table continued on following page

Table 15–2. DISORDERS OF CONSCIOUSNESS AND HIGHER BRAIN FUNCTION *Continued*

Question: Which of the following characterize AD rather than multi-infarct dementia? **SELECT 2**

(A) UMN abnormalities
(B) Chromosome defects
(C) Focal neurologic deficits
(D) Progressive dementia
(E) Association with DM and HTN
(F) Common in adult Down syndrome patients

Answers: (B), (F): UMN and focal neurologic deficits commonly occur in multi-infarct dementia and are absent in most cases of AD **(choices A and C are incorrect)**. AD, in some cases, is associated with chromosome defects **(choice B)** and is universal in adult Down syndrome patients **(choice F)** at an early age. Progressive dementia characterizes both disorders **(choice D is incorrect)**. Multi-infarct dementia is associated with DM and HTN **(choice E is incorrect)**.

ACh = acetylcholine, AD = Alzheimer's disease, AIDS = acquired immunodeficiency syndrome, AIP = acute intermittent porphyria, AMI = acute myocardial infarction, ATII = angiotensin II, BP = blood pressure, BUN = blood urea nitrogen, CBC = complete blood cell count, CN = cranial nerve, CNS = central nervous system, COD = cause of death, CSF = cerebrospinal fluid, CT = computed tomography, CVA = cerebrovascular accident, DM = diabetes mellitus, Dx = diagnosis, EEG = electroencephalogram, GABA = γ-aminobutyric acid, GCS = Glasgow Coma Scale, HD = Huntington's disease, HPTH = hyperparathyroidism, HTN = hypertension, HIV = human immunodeficiency virus, Hx = history, IV = intravenous, MRI = magnetic resonance imaging, NSAIDs = nonsteroidal anti-inflammatory drugs, Pb = lead, PCR = polymerase chain reaction, REM = rapid eye movement, Rx = treatment, S/S = signs and symptoms, TGA = transient global amnesia, TSH = thyroid stimulating hormone, UMN = upper motor neuron, VMD = ventromedial diencephalon.

Table 15–3. DISORDERS OF MOOD AND BEHAVIOR, ALCOHOL-RELATED NEUROLOGIC DISORDERS, AND DISORDERS OF SENSORY FUNCTION

Most Common...	Answer and Explanation
major psychoses	• **affective disorders:** * **depression,** * mania, * bipolar state, • *schizophrenia*
major neuroses	*anxiety disorders*

Table 15–3. DISORDERS OF MOOD AND BEHAVIOR, ALCOHOL-RELATED NEUROLOGIC DISORDERS, AND DISORDERS OF SENSORY FUNCTION *Continued*

Most Common...	Answer and Explanation
neurotransmitters involved in mood disorders	• **norepinephrine/serotonin:** decreased, • *dopamine:* * decreased in depression, * increased in mania, • *high ACh levels,* • *reduced platelet monoamine oxidase activity*
clinical findings of depression	• **depressed mood:** * hallmark of depression, * often unable to cry, • *sleep disturbances:* * 80%, * early AM awakening, * insomnia, • *loss of appetite/weight loss,* • *low self-esteem/ hopelessness,* • *suicidal ideation:* * ~65%, * risk of suicide increases when patient begins to feel better, • *cannot concentrate/impaired thinking,* • *hypochondriacal:* * constipation, * muscle aches/pains, * headache, • *apathy,* • *behavior better in PM than AM,* • *psychomotor retardation:* * common in elderly, * confused with dementia, • *absence of sensorimotor signs,* • *normal cognitive tests*
precipitating events leading to depression	• **early loss of parent/loss of spouse,** • *loss of job,* • *established physical illness:* e.g., * MS, * ALS, * hypothyroidism, • *drugs:* alcohol
Rx of depression	• **serotonin-reuptake inhibitors:** e.g., * fluoxetine, * paroxetine, * sertraline, * side effects: ♦ headache, ♦ insomnia, • *tricyclics:* e.g., * amitriptyline, * anticholinergic effects common, • *MAO inhibitors:* e.g., * phenelzine, * side effects: ♦ orthostatic hypotension, ♦ sexual dysfunction, ♦ insomnia, • *trazodone:* similar to tricyclics
clinical findings in mania	• **euphoric:** * manic episodes come abruptly, * may last up to 3 mths, • *extreme self-confidence,* • *racing thoughts/fast speech,* • *restless/irritable,* • *energetic,* • *impaired judgment when manic,* • *sudden changes in mood,* • *anger,* • *grandiose ideas:* often overspend, • *bipolar if swing from highs to low,* • *occurs equally in men and women:* strong genetic basis, • *hypomania:* milder degrees of mania which do not cause same degree of impairment as mania

Table continued on following page

**Table 15–3. DISORDERS OF MOOD AND BEHAVIOR,
ALCOHOL-RELATED NEUROLOGIC DISORDERS, AND
DISORDERS OF SENSORY FUNCTION** *Continued*

Most Common...	Answer and Explanation
disorders that mimic mania	• **corticosteroids,** • *thyrotoxicosis,* • *limbic system disease*
Rx of mania	• **lithium,** • *anticonvulsants:* * **valproate** (most often used if patients cannot tolerate lithium), * carbamazepine, * clonazepam
side effects of lithium	• **polyuria:** acquired nephrogenic DI, • *leuko-cytosis:* decreases neutrophil adhesion, • *acne,* • *weight gain,* • *hypothyroidism,* • *inter-stitial nephritis,* • *teratogenic:* ASD, • *low therapeutic index:* must be carefully moni-tored
clinical findings in schizophrenia	• **dysfunction in form/thought:** * neologisms (make up words), * word salad (incoherent words/phrases), * loose associations (move from one subject to next), * echolalia (repeat words over and over and over), • *deteriora-tion in psychosocial functioning:* * bizarre be-havior, * avoid social activities, * interest in religion/cults, * flat affect, • *delusions:* * false belief not shared by others, e.g., * controlled by outside forces, • *hallucinations:* * false sensory perception, e.g., * auditory, * often religious themes, • *usually oriented to place and time,* • *cognitive functions intact,* • *no gender difference:* strong genetic basis, • *hy-peractive dopaminergic system,* • *physical findings:* excessive blinking, • *CT/MRI:* en-larged lateral and third ventricles with over-lying cortical atrophy
Rx of schizophrenia	*neuroleptic drugs:* e.g., * phenothiazine, * clozapine (fewer extrapyramidal signs)
side effects of neuroleptic drugs	• **extrapyramidal signs:** e.g., * tremor, * rigid-ity, * muscle spasms, * more frequent in men than women and in young than old patients, • *tardive dyskinesia:* * writhing and jerking of trunk/extremities, * orolingual facial move-ments (tongue darks in/out), * may be irre-versible even with D/C of drug, * more com-mon in women/elderly patients

Table 15–3. DISORDERS OF MOOD AND BEHAVIOR, ALCOHOL-RELATED NEUROLOGIC DISORDERS, AND DISORDERS OF SENSORY FUNCTION *Continued*

Most Common...	Answer and Explanation
clinical findings in anxiety disorders	• **constant feeling of fear/anxiety,** • *phobias:* e.g., * agoraphobia (fear of being alone or in public places), * claustrophobia (fear of closed spaces), * fear of objects, • *panic attacks:* feelings of impending doom, • *physical findings:* * MVP, * diarrhea, * tachycardia, * mydriasis, * dizziness, * urinary urgency
Rx of anxiety disorders	• *phobias:* * behavioral therapy, * MAO inhibitors, * beta blockers (particularly if MVP is present), • *generalized anxiety:* * relaxation therapy, * benzodiazepines, • *panic disorder:* * imipramine
neurologic abnormalities in alcoholics	• **Wernicke-Korsakoff syndrome:** thiamine deficiency, • *optic neuropathy:* * reduced visual acuity, * central/paracentral scotomas (area of depressed vision in visual field), • *cerebral atrophy with dementia,* • *cerebellar degeneration,* • *central pontine myelinolysis:* see Table 10–2, • *distal sensorimotor peripheral neuropathy:* * axonal degeneration involving small pain/temperature fibers, * burning pain, * loss of DTRs, • *alcoholic myopathy:* * sudden acute rhabdomyolysis complicated by myoglobinuria/polyuric renal failure, * chronic myopathy with proximal muscle weakness
S/S of Wernicke-Korsakoff syndrome	• *Wernicke's syndrome:* * confusion, * ataxia, * nystagmus, * external ophthalmoplegia, * multiple cranial nerve palsies, * peripheral neuropathy, * tachycardia, * often precipitated by infusion of glucose-containing electrolyte solutions (♦ uses up remaining thiamine as pyruvate is converted into acetyl CoA, ♦ always administer IV thiamine before infusing glucose), • *Korsakoff's syndrome:* * targets limbic system, * inability to form new memories (antegrade amnesia) or recall old ones (retrograde amnesia), * confabulation
S/S of cerebellar degeneration	• *loss of Purkinje cells in anterior and superior cerebellar vermis,* • *broad-based, stiff-legged ataxia,* • *uncoordinated upper extremities,* • *nystagmus*

Table continued on following page

Table 15–3. DISORDERS OF MOOD AND BEHAVIOR, ALCOHOL-RELATED NEUROLOGIC DISORDERS, AND DISORDERS OF SENSORY FUNCTION *Continued*

Most Common...	Answer and Explanation
temporal/ pathogenetic classification of pain	• *temporal:* * acute (<3 months), * chronic (>3 months), • *pathogenesis:* * structural (e.g., ♦ RA, ♦ metastatic cancer), * delusional (e.g., schizophrenia), * psychophysiologic (♦ pain persists after structural defect is corrected, e.g., ♦ repair of herniated disk)
mechanisms of pain	• *somatic,* • *visceral,* • *neuropathic,* • *referred*
characteristics of somatic pain	• *due to activation of peripheral receptors and somatic efferent nerves without direct injury to nerves,* • *well localized,* • *intermittent,* • *sharp or dull,* • *can be controlled with nonopioid/opioid analgesics, anesthetic blocks*
characteristics of visceral pain	• *due to activation of visceral nociceptive receptors and efferent nerves,* • *deep, aching pain, cramping sensation,* • *may refer to cutaneous sites,* • *can be controlled with nonopioid/opioid analgesics, anesthetic blocks*
characteristics of neuropathic pain	• *due to injury to peripheral receptors, nerves, CNS,* • *burning pain that often occurs in an area of sensory loss:* e.g., postherpetic neuralgia, • *does not respond as well to analgesics*
characteristics of referred pain	*perceived at site distant* (often same dermatome/myotome) *from area of injury:* e.g., * cholecystitis → right scapula, * AMI → medial aspect left arm, jaw
types of headaches	• **tension-type:** e.g., * common tension headache, * TMJ, • *vascular:* e.g., * migraine/ migraine variants, * cluster, • *cranial neuralgias:* e.g., trigeminal neuralgia, • *intracranial disorders:* e.g., * increased intracranial pressure, * tumors, • *extracranial disorders:* e.g., * sinusitis, * cervical OA, * optic neuritis
clinical findings of tension-type headaches	• **steady, usually nonpulsatile aching pain often in a "band-like distribution" around scalp,** • *worsens as day progresses,* • *stress-related,* • *often daily occurrence,* • *tender*

**Table 15–3. DISORDERS OF MOOD AND BEHAVIOR,
ALCOHOL-RELATED NEUROLOGIC DISORDERS, AND
DISORDERS OF SENSORY FUNCTION** *Continued*

Most Common...	Answer and Explanation
Continued	posterior cervical/temporalis/masseter muscles, • *women > men*, • *may be associated with dizziness/facial pain:* chronic depression, • *rarely interrupts sleep*, • *often overlaps with migraine headaches*
Rx of tension-type headache	• **NSAIDs**, • *antidepressants*
clinical findings in classical migraine headaches	• *precipitating factors:* * exercise, * menses, * food (♦ MSG, ♦ methylxanthines), * alcohol, * bright lights, • *headache preceded by aura:* * due to VC, * photophobia/flashing lights, * N/V, * hemisensory/paretic findings, * aphasia, • *unilateral parietotemporal headache:* * due to VD, * neurologic symptoms usually (not always) disappear before onset, * usually lasts up to 30 m (can be longer)
Rx of classical migraines	• *symptomatic:* * ergots, * sumatriptan, * narcotics, * antinauseous agents (metoclopramide), • *prophylactic:* * ergots, * beta blockers, * amitriptyline, * methysergide (♦ serotonin inhibitor, ♦ danger of retroperitoneal fibrosis/interstitial fibrosis in lungs), * NSAIDs
clinical findings in cluster headaches	• *more common in men*, • *headache:* * severe, sharp, stabbing, unilateral orbital, supraorbital, or temporal pain, * lasts from 15 min up to 1–3 h, * no aura, * 50% occur during sleep, • *attack frequency:* * occur once every other day up to 8 per d, * cluster over 1–3 mths (usually at same time), • *ipsilateral findings:* * lacrimation, * nasal stuffiness/rhinorrhea, * conjunctival irritation, * ptosis/miosis/eyelid edema, * facial sweating
Rx of cluster headaches	• *symptomatic:* * O_2, * dihydroergotamine, * sumatriptan, • *prophylactic:* * **calcium channel blockers** (verapamil), * methysergide, * lithium, * ergotamine (best if attacks are nocturnal), * verapamil + lithium (chronic cluster headaches)

Table continued on following page

**Table 15–3. DISORDERS OF MOOD AND BEHAVIOR,
ALCOHOL-RELATED NEUROLOGIC DISORDERS, AND
DISORDERS OF SENSORY FUNCTION** *Continued*

Most Common...	Answer and Explanation
causes of intracranial headaches	• **meningitis:** * generalized, * throbbing, * nuchal rigidity, • *subarachnoid hemorrhage:* see Table 15–5, • *brain tumor:* * most frequent presenting symptom, * occur just after waking up in AM, * lateralize to side of tumor if supratentorial location, * lateralize to orbit or neck if posterior fossa location, • *pituitary tumor,* • *pseudotumor cerebri:* benign intracranial HTN, • *high-pressure hydrocephalus*
causes of extracranial headaches	• **sinusitis,** • *dental pain:* e.g., periapical abscess, • *aural pain:* e.g., otitis media, • *ocular pain:* e.g., * glaucoma, * optic neuritis, * refraction errors, * eye muscle imbalance, * uveitis
clinical findings in trigeminal neuralgia	• *precipitating factors:* * **chewing,** * large artery compressing nerve in elderly patients, • *sudden onset of paroxysmal, lancinating pain in maxillary/mandibular division lasting a few seconds and then repeating itself,* • *trigger point usually present,* • *always on same side:* if varies from side to side, consider MS, • *rarely occurs at night,* • *commonly spontaneously remits*
Rx of trigeminal neuralgia	• **carbamazepine,** • *phenytoin,* • *baclofen,* • *block of gasserian ganglion*
clinical findings in glossopharyngeal neuralgia	• *swallowing precipitates attack:* similar pain as in trigeminal neuralgia, • *unilateral pain in posterolateral pharynx/neck/radiates to ear,* • *syncope may occur*
Rx of glossopharyngeal neuralgia	*carbamazepine*
mechanisms of neck/back pain	• **paraspinal muscles:** spasm, • *ligament strains:* * anterior/posterior longitudinal ligaments, e.g., * cervical arthritis in RA, • *facet disease:* * articular cartilage, * capsule, e.g., * OA, * spondylolisthesis, • *nerve root irritation:* e.g., intervertebral disk disease with nerve root compression

Table 15–3. DISORDERS OF MOOD AND BEHAVIOR, ALCOHOL-RELATED NEUROLOGIC DISORDERS, AND DISORDERS OF SENSORY FUNCTION *Continued*

Most Common...	Answer and Explanation
clinical findings in causalgia	• *mechanism:* * injury to peripheral nerve (e.g., ♦ median nerve, ♦ sciatic nerve), • *severe burning pain following nerve injury,* • *sympathetic nervous system dysfunction:* * vasomotor instability (VD with warm, dry skin) → VC (edema, cyanosis, cool skin), * hypo/hyperhidrosis, * atrophy of skin/subcutaneous tissue, * muscle atrophy
clinical findings in reflex sympathetic dystrophy (RSD)	• *similar to causalgia except no Hx of nerve injury,* • *may follow a visceral illness:* e.g., AMI
Rx of causalgia, RSD	• *local anesthetic infiltration into areas of pain,* • *sympathetic ganglion block*
pathologic causes of anosmia	• **URI with rhinitis/allergic rhinitis,** • *Kallmann's syndrome:* * AD, * color blindness, * absent GnRH causing hypogonadism,* • *basilar skull fracture,* • *olfactory groove meningioma,* • *tumors at base of frontal lobes,* • *miscellaneous:* * MS, * Parkinson's disease, * nasal sprays, * CRF, * hepatic failure
pathologic causes of dysgeusia	• **smoking,** • *advanced age,* • *Bell's palsy,* • *zinc deficiency,* • *B_{12}/folate deficiency,* • *hypothyroidism,* • *infection:* e.g., * URI, * influenza,* • *cancer,* • *CRF,* • *liver failure* [Dysgeusia refers to an inability to taste.]
disorders affecting visual acuity	• *retinal disorders:* e.g., * central retinal artery embolism, * diabetic retinopathy,* • *optic nerve disorders:* e.g., optic neuritis,* • *chiasm disorders:* e.g., * craniopharyngioma, * lesions posterior to chiasm do not affect visual acuity*
disorders affecting visual fields	• *defects in one eye:* * globe, * retina, * prechiasmal optic nerve disorders,* • *bilateral defects:* lesions at or posterior to optic chiasm,* • *bitemporal field cuts:* chiasm lesions,* • *papilledema:* enlarged blind spot

Table continued on following page

Table 15–3. DISORDERS OF MOOD AND BEHAVIOR, ALCOHOL-RELATED NEUROLOGIC DISORDERS, AND DISORDERS OF SENSORY FUNCTION *Continued*

Most Common...	Answer and Explanation
terms applied to visual field defects	• *homonymous:* * right visual field: temporal half of right eye/nasal half of left eye, * left visual field: temporal half of left eye/nasal half of right eye, • *hemianopia:* impairment of nearly half of visual field, • *quadrantanopia:* smaller impairment involving only a quarter of visual field
cause of a unilateral loss of vision	*damage to retina or optic nerve proximal to the chiasm* (schematic: loss of vision in left eye) Left Right
cause of left/right inferior quadrantanopia	* *left:* right parietal lobe lesion, * *right:* left parietal lobe lesion (schematic: right inferior quadrantanopia) Left Right
cause of superior bitemporal quadrantanopia	*inferior chiasmal lesion:* e.g., pituitary adenoma Left Right
cause of a visual field defect with macular sparing	*posterior cerebral artery infarct with sparing of tips of occipital lobes* Left Right
cause of an enlarged blind spot (scotoma)	*increased intracranial pressure* Left Right
cause of cortical blindness	*bilateral damage to the visual radiation or occipital lobe:* e.g., * basilar artery insufficiency, * hypertensive encephalopathy

**Table 15–3. DISORDERS OF MOOD AND BEHAVIOR,
ALCOHOL-RELATED NEUROLOGIC DISORDERS, AND
DISORDERS OF SENSORY FUNCTION** *Continued*

Most Common...	Answer and Explanation
S/S of cortical blindness	• *normal funduscopic exam,* • *normal pupillary light reflexes,* • *patient often unaware of blindness*
causes of sudden unilateral loss of vision	• **optic neuritis,** • *amaurosis fugax,* • *central retinal artery occlusion,* • *central retinal vein occlusion*
causes of optic neuritis	• **demyelinating disease:** e.g., MS (75%), • *infection:* e.g, * measles, * mumps, * VZ, * syphilis, * TB, • *SLE,* • *methyl alcohol poisoning:* converted into formic acid
S/S in optic neuritis	• *retro-orbital pain when moving eyes,* • *globe tenderness to palpation,* • *flame hemorrhages around disk vessels/swollen optic disk:* only if neuritis is located at nerve head, not retrobulbar location
Rx of optic neuritis in MS	*intravenous methylprednisolone*
cause of amaurosis fugax	• **retinal embolus of atheromatous plaque material:** * Hollenhorst plaque, * often visible on retinal exam, **from the ipsilateral carotid artery,** • *type of TIA*
S/S in amaurosis fugax	• **described as curtain passing vertically across visual field followed in few minutes by curtain moving up and restoring vision,** • *less correlation with impending stroke than other types of TIAs*
causes of central retinal artery occlusion	• **embolization of plaque material from ipsilateral carotid or ophthalmic artery,** • *giant cell temporal arteritis,* • *APL syndrome*
S/S in central retinal artery occlusion	• **sudden, painless, complete loss of vision in one eye,** • *most commonly elderly patients with carotid artery stenosis,* • *pallor of optic disk,* • *"boxcar" segmentation of blood in retinal veins:* sign of stasis, • *cherry red fovea,* • *retinal edema,* • *bloodless, constricted arterioles*
causes of central retinal vein occlusion	• **hypercoagulable state:** e.g., * PRV, * APL syndrome, * protein C or S deficiency, • *essential HTN,* • *DM,* • *glaucoma,* • *hyperlipidemia:* serum TG > 1000 mg/dL

Table continued on following page

Table 15–3. DISORDERS OF MOOD AND BEHAVIOR, ALCOHOL-RELATED NEUROLOGIC DISORDERS, AND DISORDERS OF SENSORY FUNCTION *Continued*

Most Common...	Answer and Explanation
S/S of central retinal vein occlusion	• **sudden, painless, unilateral loss of vision,** • **swelling of optic disk,** • *"blood and thunder" appearance of retina from hemorrhages,* • *cotton wool exudates:* microinfarctions, • *engorged retinal veins*
types of glaucoma	• **chronic open-angle glaucoma:** * 90% of all cases, * decreased rate of aqueous outflow into canal of Schlemm, • *acute* (angle-closure) *glaucoma:* narrow anterior chamber angle
S/S of a chronic open-angle glaucoma	• **increased intraocular pressure,** • *usually asymptomatic in early phases,* • *bilateral aching eyes,* • *common in African-Americans,* • *pathologic cupping of optic disks,* • *optic atrophy,* • *nyctalopia,* • *gradual loss of peripheral vision leading to tunnel vision and blindness*
Rx of chronic open-angle glaucoma	• **β-adrenergic blocking agents:** e.g., timolol, • cholinergic agonist: e.g., *pilocarpine,* • *adrenergic agonist:* e.g., *epinephrine,* • *oral/topical carbonic anhydrase inhibitor*
S/S of acute angle glaucoma	• **rapid increase in intraocular pressure,** • *severe pain,* • *photophobia,* • *blurry vision:* blue or red halos around lights, • *red eye,* • *steamy cornea,* • *pupil fixed in mid-dilated position,* • *pupil nonreactive to light,* • *precipitated by:* * mydriatic agent, * uveitis, * lens dislocation
Rx of acute angle glaucoma	• **laser iridectomy,** • *carbonic anhydrase inhibitor,* • *pilocarpine*
causes of optic atrophy	• **optic neuritis,** • *glaucoma,* • *methyl alcohol poisoning*
S/S of optic nerve atrophy	• *visual field/color vision defects,* • *night blindness,* • *sluggish pupillary reactions,* • *decreased visual acuity,* • *extreme pallor of disk with sharply defined borders,* • *vessels normal:* not visible if due to increased intracranial pressure, • *visible physiologic cup:* not visible if due to increased intracranial pressure

Table 15–3. DISORDERS OF MOOD AND BEHAVIOR, ALCOHOL-RELATED NEUROLOGIC DISORDERS, AND DISORDERS OF SENSORY FUNCTION *Continued*

Most Common...	Answer and Explanation
causes of uveitis	• **sarcoidosis:** usually bilateral, • *AIDS:* CMV, • *ankylosing spondylitis,* • *juvenile RA,* • *ulcerative colitis,* • *TB,* • *trauma* [Uveitis is inflammation of uveal tract: iris, ciliary body, choroid.]
S/S of uveitis	• *pain,* • *blurry vision,* • *photophobia,* • *miotic pupil,* • *poor light reflex,* • *circumcorneal ciliary body vascular congestion,* • *normal to low intraocular pressure,* • *cornea usually clear,* • *synechia* (adhesions) *between iris and anterior lens capsule*
Rx of uveitis	• **topical corticosteroids** (anterior uveitis)/ **systemic corticosteroids** (posterior uveitis), • *Rx infection if present*
causes of retinal detachment	• **cataract extraction,** • *myopia,* • *trauma* [Retina usually detaches in superior temporal area.]
S/S of retinal detachment	• **blurred vision in eye progressively becomes worse:** "curtain came over my eye," • *retina hanging in vitreous,* • *no conjunctival redness,* • *no pain*
Rx of retinal detachment	*laser photocoagulation*
causes of vitreous hemorrhage	• **DM retinopathy,** • *retinal tears,* • *macular degeneration,* • *trauma,* • *blood dyscrasias:* e.g., * sickle cell disease, * Hb SC disease, • *retinal vein thrombosis*
cause of permanent visual loss in elderly	*macular degeneration:* * age-related, * ? relationship with cigarette smoking, * family Hx [Macula located lateral to optic disk. Normally light red. Central darker spot that reflects light (fovea centralis).]
S/S of macular degeneration	*gradual* (atrophic type) *or abrupt* (exudative type), *progressive bilateral* (atrophic type) *or sequential* (exudative type) *visual loss* (central visual loss): disruption of Bruch's membrane in retina responsible for permanent visual loss

Table continued on following page

**Table 15–3. DISORDERS OF MOOD AND BEHAVIOR,
ALCOHOL-RELATED NEUROLOGIC DISORDERS, AND
DISORDERS OF SENSORY FUNCTION** *Continued*

Most Common...	Answer and Explanation
Rx of macular degeneration	• *no specific Rx,* • *zinc supplements may be useful*
cause of blindness in AIDS	*CMV retinitis:* usually occurs when CD_4 T helper cell count <50 cells/μL
S/S of CMV retinitis	• **cotton wool exudates,** • *retinal hemorrhages,* • *visual disturbances when optic nerve involved or retinal detachment*
Rx of CMV retinitis	• **ganciclovir,** • *foscarnet if ganciclovir is not improving the condition*
causes of miotic (small, constricted) pupils	• **old age,** • *Horner's syndrome,* • *Argyll Robertson pupil,* • *barbiturates,* • *pontine hemorrhage,* • *opiate:* e.g., * heroin, * morphine, • *alcohol,* • *glutethimide,* • *pilocarpine drops,* • *sympathetic paralysis*
causes of mydriatic (dilated) pupils	• **anxiety,** • *parasympathetic paralysis:* e.g., uncal herniation, • *Adie's pupil,* • *amphetamines,* • *cocaine,* • *psychedelics:* e.g., * LSD, * phencyclidine, * scopolamine, • *cerebral death,* • *mydriatic drops:* e.g., atropine, • *childhood*
causes of anisocoria	• **normal finding in 15% of population,** • *CN III palsy,* • *Horner's syndrome* [Anisocoria refers to unequal pupil diameters.]
causes of Argyll Robertson pupil	• **tertiary syphilis,** • *DM*
signs of Argyll Robertson pupil	• *absence of miotic reaction to direct/consensual light,* • *pupils constrict to near stimulus:* accommodate, • *miotic, irregular pupil,* • *pupil does not dilate with atropine or painful stimulation in other parts of body*
cause of Marcus Gunn pupil	*retrobulbar optic neuritis:* lesion in afferent limb of pupillary light reflex
signs of Marcus Gunn pupil	*using the swinging flashlight test* (move light quickly from eye to eye): * light in normal eye causes pupillary constriction in both normal and abnormal eye, * light quickly moved to abnormal eye produces mydriasis

**Table 15–3. DISORDERS OF MOOD AND BEHAVIOR,
ALCOHOL-RELATED NEUROLOGIC DISORDERS, AND
DISORDERS OF SENSORY FUNCTION** *Continued*

Most Common...	Answer and Explanation
cause of Adie's tonic pupil	• **young patients with normally mydriatic pupils,** • *iris dysfunction from trauma,* • *topical mydriatics,* • *benztropine*
signs of Adie's tonic pupil	• *sluggish response to both direct/consensual light and accommodation,* • *unilateral or bilateral,* • *tonic pupil dilates with atropine* [Adie's syndrome is an accompanying absence of DTRs.]
cause of Horner's syndrome	*primary SCC of lung involving superior sulcus:* destruction of superior cervical sympathetic ganglion
signs of Horner's syndrome	*triad of:* * ipsilateral miosis, * anhidrosis, * ptosis
pupil signs in subtentorial lesions	• *pinpoint:* lesion in pons, • *fixed:* lesion in tectum of midbrain, • *irregular and/or unequal:* lesion in midbrain-pontine
pupil signs in metabolic encephalopathy/ diencephalic damage	*small, reactive pupils*
symptoms of ocular muscle weakness	• **blurry vision,** • *diplopia:* double vision
causes of horizontal diplopia	• **lateral rectus palsy:** CN VI, • *medial rectus palsy:* CN III [See Table 15–1.]
causes of vertical diplopia	• **CN III-related palsies:** * superior/inferior rectus, * inferior oblique, • *CN IV-related palsy:* superior oblique [See Table 15–1.]
cause of progressive diplopia	*compressive lesion:* e.g., tumor
cause of sudden diplopia	*vascular lesion:* e.g., infarction
cause of intermittent diplopia that occurs later in the day	*MG:* see Table 12–5
causes of acute (<48 h) bilateral ophthalmoplegia	• **brain stem stroke,** • *Wernicke's syndrome,* • *botulism:* see Table 12–5, • *MG:* see Table 12–5, • *Guillain-Barré*

Table continued on following page

Table 15–3. DISORDERS OF MOOD AND BEHAVIOR, ALCOHOL-RELATED NEUROLOGIC DISORDERS, AND DISORDERS OF SENSORY FUNCTION *Continued*

Most Common...	Answer and Explanation
causes of acute (<48 h) unilateral ophthalmoplegia	• **uncal herniation:** I compression, • *DM: ** CN III (pupil spared), * CN VI palsy), • *MG*
sites responsible for voluntary/tracking conjugate eye movement	*supranuclear pathways* [The pathway descends from the forebrain to the MLF in the brain stem. The MLF connects the CN III nucleus (MR [adducts]) with the CN VI nucleus (LR [abducts]) in the brain stem. The CN VI nucleus has a pathway connecting with the PPRF (lateral gaze center) on the same side of the brain stem. The MLF crosses in the midbrain and connects the CN III nucleus on one side with the pathway connecting the CN VI nucleus with the PPRF on the contralateral side. LR = lateral rectus, MR = medial rectus, PPRF = pontine paramedian reticular formation When the patient is asked to look right, the signal to the left CN III nucleus causes the left eye to adduct right and the signal to CN VI on the right causes abduction of the right eye. When the patient is asked to look left, the signal to the CN III nucleus on the right causes adduction of the right eye to the left and the signal to CN VI on the left to abduct the left eye. Therefore, with lesions involving the MLF, the MR is paralyzed (remains stationary) on attempted lateral gaze, while the

Table 15–3. DISORDERS OF MOOD AND BEHAVIOR, ALCOHOL-RELATED NEUROLOGIC DISORDERS, AND DISORDERS OF SENSORY FUNCTION *Continued*

Most Common...	Answer and Explanation
Continued	LR is intact. Furthermore, the abducting eye exhibits horizontal nystagmus. Hence, with a lesion in the left MLF **(lesion A, unilateral INO)**, conjugate gaze to the left is intact, but conjugate gaze to the right is paralyzed (right eye abducts and has horizontal nystagmus but left eye remains stationary). A lesion in the right MLF **(lesion B)**, allows conjugate gaze to the right, but conjugate gaze to the left is paralyzed (left eye can abduct, but the right eye remains stationary). A lesion involving both A and B is called **bilateral INO**. As expected, both left and right conjugate gaze are paralyzed. If one of the CN VI nuclei is destroyed and bilateral INO is present, it is called the 1 1/2 syndrome. For example if CN VI on the left is destroyed and a bilateral INO is also present, the left eye cannot abduct when the patient looks to the left, but the right can abduct, since the nucleus is intact. Since the ability to converge both eyes (both eyes adduct) comes from a different pathway originating from the superior colliculus, in all the above lesions, the ability to converge the eyes is left intact.]
cause of unilateral INO	*ischemic damage in the brain stem affecting MLF:* see above discussion
cause of bilateral internuclear ophthalmoplegia	*MS:* pathognomonic for MS
causes of strabismus	• **nonparalytic:** * intrinsic imbalance of muscle tone, * usually congenital, • *paralytic:* e.g., * CN III/IV/VI palsies, * MG [Strabismus is an involuntary deviation of the eyes from their normal physiologic position.]
complications associated with strabismus	• **headache,** • *diplopia,* • *amblyopia:* * suppression of vision in one eye to prevent diplopia leads to permanent reduction of vision, * more likely to occur in children with strabismus
symptoms of auditory dysfunction	• **hearing loss:** * **conductive,** * sensorineural, • *tinnitus:* ringing in ears

Table continued on following page

Table 15–3. DISORDERS OF MOOD AND BEHAVIOR, ALCOHOL-RELATED NEUROLOGIC DISORDERS, AND DISORDERS OF SENSORY FUNCTION *Continued*

Most Common...	Answer and Explanation
sites involved in conductive hearing loss	• **external ear canal,** • *middle ear*
causes of conductive hearing loss	• **impacted cerumen in outer ear canal,** • *fluid in middle ear,* • *otosclerosis:* MCC in elderly
cause of conductive hearing loss in the elderly	*otosclerosis:* * fixation of middle ear ossicles, * strong AD history
clinical findings in conductive hearing loss	• **Weber test lateralizes to affected ear and bone conduction > air conduction** (Rinne's test), • *affected ear feels full,* • *equal loss of all hearing frequencies,* • *well-preserved speech discrimination*
sites involved in sensorineural hearing loss	• **cochlea,** • *auditory nerve:* CN VIII
causes of sensorineural hearing loss	• **presbycuis:** degeneration of hairs in cochlea, • *noise trauma,* • *infection:* * viral, * bacterial, • *drugs:* e.g., * aminoglycosides (destroy cochlear hair cells), * salicylates, * diuretics, * cisplatin, • *Meniere's disease:* see below, • *acoustic neuroma*
clinical findings in sensorineural hearing loss	• **Weber test lateralizes to normal ear** (contralateral ear is affected) **and air conduction > bone conduction in both normal and affected ear,** • *low tones heard better than high tones,* • *cannot hear consonants owing to high frequency loss:* loss of speech discrimination, • *cannot hear well in noisy environments,* • *recruitment:* small increases in intensity of sound cause discomfort
cause of Meniere's disease	• **endolymphatic HTN:** hydrops, • *loss of cochlear hairs*
S/S of Meniere's disease	• **fluctuating, unilateral (75%), low-frequency sensorineural hearing loss,** • *recurrent episodes of vertigo,* • *tinnitus:* low-pitch roaring, • *sense of fullness in affected ear*

Table 15–3. DISORDERS OF MOOD AND BEHAVIOR, ALCOHOL-RELATED NEUROLOGIC DISORDERS, AND DISORDERS OF SENSORY FUNCTION Continued

Most Common...	Answer and Explanation
Rx of Meniere's disease	• **diuretics,** • *carbonic anhydrase inhibitors,* • *low salt diet,* • *surgical decompression of excess endolymph*
clinical findings of an acoustic neuroma	• **unilateral progressive sensorineural hearing loss,** • *tinnitus,* • *sensory changes in face:* trigeminal nerve irritation from large cerebellopontine angle tumor, • *abnormal corneal reflex:* loss of CN V afferent component, • *ataxia,* • *increased association with neurofibromatosis,* • *MRI locates lesion,* • *auditory EP useful in equivocal cases* [They are benign tumors derived from Schwann cells. Involve VIIIth nerve. Surgery Rx of choice.]
types of tinnitus	• **subjective:** abnormal discharge in auditory system not heard by examiner, • *objective:* patient hears real sound also heard by examiner with a stethoscope
causes of tinnitus	• **impacted cerumen,** • *otosclerosis:* roaring sound, • *severe HTN,* • *severe anemia:* increased blood flow, • *patent eustachian tube:* * normally closed, * tinnitus corresponds with breathing, • *Meniere's disease:* loud roars or clangings, • *vascular disorders:* * glomus jugulare (♦ reddish-blue mass behind tympanic membrane, ♦ pulsatile sound), * carotid artery stenosis, * compression of vertebral artery from osteophytes in cervical OA, • *post-traumatic:* e.g., gunshot, • *drugs:* e.g., * salicylates, * quinidine, * quinine, * indomethacin, • *raised intracranial pressure:* compression of jugular vein obliterates the sound
causes of dizziness	• **anxiety/hyperventilation,** • *eyes:* * eye muscle imbalance, * refractive error, • *vestibular disease,* • *carotid sinus syndrome,* • *hypotension:* * orthostatic, * arrhythmias, * AS, • *viral labyrinthitis,* • *impaired proprioception:* e.g., PA, • *basilar artery insufficiency*
S/S of dizziness	• *lightheadedness,* • *dysequilibrium when standing,* • *unsteadiness when walking*

Table continued on following page

Table 15–3. DISORDERS OF MOOD AND BEHAVIOR, ALCOHOL-RELATED NEUROLOGIC DISORDERS, AND DISORDERS OF SENSORY FUNCTION *Continued*

Most Common...	Answer and Explanation
symptom and sign of vestibular disease	• *symptom:* * vertigo, in which the patient or surroundings are whirling in a continuous direction, * symptoms related to vertigo include ♦ N/V (not seen in dizziness), ♦ imbalance/ataxia, ♦ past pointing, • *sign:* nystagmus: ♦ rhythmic to and fro involuntary oscillations of eyes, ♦ horizontal, ♦ vertical, ♦ rotary types
mechanisms causing vertigo	• **physiologic:** e.g., * motion sickness, * heights, * visual (roller coaster ride), * neck hyperextension, • *peripheral causes involving vestibular system:* * semicircular canals, * otolithic apparatus, • *central causes:* * brain stem, * cerebellum, * CN VIII
pathologic causes of vertigo	• **benign positional vertigo,** • *Meniere's disease,* • *viral labyrinthitis,* • *labyrinthine concussion after head trauma,* • *acoustic neuroma,* • *MS,* • *brain stem ischemia:* e.g., lateral medullary syndrome involving PICA, • *temporal lobe epilepsy,* • *cerebellar disorders:* e.g., * degenerative diseases, * tumors
tests to evaluate dizziness/vertigo	• *audiology,* • *ECG:* R/O arrhythmias, • *CBC:* R/O * anemia, * polycythemia, • *RPR,* • *glucose/electrolytes,* • *serum ANA:* if SLE suspected, • *MRI:* if acoustic neuroma or MS suspected, • *caloric testing:* * evaluate unconscious patients, * test vestibular function, * cold water irrigation causes nystagmus away from side of stimulation, * warm water causes nystagmus to side of stimulation, • *auditory EP:* R/O: * demyelinating disease, * acoustic neuroma
S/S of benign position vertigo	• **precipitated by head movements:** e.g., * first lying down in bed at night or arising in AM, * turning suddenly, • *not associated with tinnitus or sensorineural hearing loss:* key differentiating point from Meniere's disease, • *vertigo accompanied by nystagmus,* • *mechanism:* dislocation of utricular macular otoliths

Table 15–3. DISORDERS OF MOOD AND BEHAVIOR, ALCOHOL-RELATED NEUROLOGIC DISORDERS, AND DISORDERS OF SENSORY FUNCTION *Continued*

Most Common...	Answer and Explanation
Rx of BPV	• **positional maneuvers:** * reposition displaced otoliths, e.g., * move from sitting to lying down on side, • *antiemetics:* e.g., meclizine, • *vestibular suppressants:* e.g., diazepam
mechanisms of nystagmus	*dysfunction in:* * visual perceptual area, * vestibular system, * cerebellum, * labyrinthine proprioceptive influences from neck muscles, * reticular formation in pontine brain stem [Nystagmus is a type of supranuclear ocular palsy that is unrelated to problems in ocular muscles or cranial nerves III, IV, or VI.]
types of nystagmus	• **jerk nystagmus:** slow phase is away from visual object followed by a quick saccade (series of short jerks) back toward the target, • *pendular nystagmus:* slow, coarse, and equal in both directions, like the pendulum of a clock
types of jerk nystagmus	• **vestibular nystagmus:** * horizontal or rotary movement of eyes, * sign of vestibular disease, • *convergence-retraction nystagmus:* * upward gaze causes irregular jerking of eyes up into orbit, * indicates midbrain tegmental damage, • *downbeat nystagmus:* * downward gaze causes irregular downward jerking of eyes, * associated with lower medullary damage
types of pendular nystagmus	• **horizontal/pendular nystagmus:** * slow, steady oscillations of equal velocity around a center point, * causes: ♦ congenital, ♦ related to severe visual impairment (e.g., optic atrophy, albinism), ♦ sign of MS, • *vertical/seesaw nystagmus:* * rapid seesaw movement of both eyes (one rises, other is falling), * sign of optic chiasm disease

Table continued on following page

Table 15–3. DISORDERS OF MOOD AND BEHAVIOR, ALCOHOL-RELATED NEUROLOGIC DISORDERS, AND DISORDERS OF SENSORY FUNCTION *Continued*

Question: Which of the following are sensory disorders that are commonly seen in multiple sclerosis? **SELECT 4**
- (A) Bilateral INO
- (B) Vertigo
- (C) Amaurosis fugax
- (D) Unilateral loss of vision
- (E) Conductive hearing loss
- (F) Horner's syndrome
- (G) Adie's tonic pupil
- (H) Cortical blindness
- (I) Bitemporal hemianopia
- (J) Jerk nystagmus

Answers: (A), (B), (D), (J): Bilateral INO **(choice A)**, due to demyelination of both MLF tracts, is pathognomonic for MS. Acute attacks of vertigo **(choice B)** may be the first sign of MS. Amaurosis fugax is due to embolization of atheromatous plaque material from the internal carotid artery to the retinal artery leading to a temporary onset of unilateral blindness **(choice C is incorrect)**. A unilateral loss of vision **(choice D)** due to optic neuritis is a common presentation in MS. Conductive hearing loss is not a feature of MS, but sensorineural hearing loss may occur **(choice E is incorrect)**. Horner's syndrome is most often related to SCC of the lung infiltrating and destroying the cervical sympathetic ganglion **(choice F is incorrect)**. Adie's tonic pupil is usually seen in children with dilated eyes or as a sign of iris dysfunction from a previous injury **(choice G is incorrect)**. The Marcus Gunn pupil, however, is most often associated with retrobulbar optic neuritis in patients with MS. Cortical blindness is most often due to bilateral damage of the visual radiation or occipital lobe from HTN or basilar artery insufficiency **(choice H is incorrect)**. Bitemporal hemianopia is most often due to a lesion compressing the optic chiasm **(choice I is incorrect)**. Jerk nystagmus **(choice J)** is noted in MS. It tends to be intermittent.

ACh = acetylcholine, AD = autosomal dominant, AIDS = acquired immunodeficiency syndrome, ALS = amyotrophic lateral sclerosis, AMI = acute myocardial infarction, ANA = antinuclear antibody, APL = antiphospholipid syndrome, AS = aortic stenosis, ASD = atrial septal defect, BPV = benign positional vertigo, CBC = complete blood cell count, CMV = cytomegalovirus, CN = cranial nerve, CNS = central nervous system, CoA = coenzyme A, CRF = chronic renal failure, CT = computed tomography, D/C = discontinue, DI = diabetes insipidus, DM = diabetes mellitus, DTRs = deep tendon reflexes, ECG = electrocardiogram, EP = evoked potential, GnRH = gonadotropin releasing hormone, Hb = hemoglobin, HTN = hypertension, Hx = history, INO = internuclear ophthalmoplegia, LR = lateral rectus, LSD = lysergic acid diethylamide, MAO = monamine oxidase, MCC = most common cause, MG = myasthenia gravis, MLF = medial longitudinal fasciculus, MR =

medial rectus, MS = multiple sclerosis, MRI = magnetic resonance imaging, MSG = monosodium glutamate, MVP = mitral valve prolapse, NSAIDs = nonsteroidal anti-inflammatory drugs, N/V = nausea and vomiting, OA = osteoarthritis, PA = pernicious anemia, PICA = posterior inferior cerebellar artery, PPRF = pontine paramedian reticular formation, PRV = polycythemia rubra vera, RA = rheumatoid arthritis, R/O = rule out, RPR = rapid plasma reagin, RSD = reflex sympathetic dystrophy, Rx = treatment, SCC = squamous cell carcinoma, SLE = systemic lupus erythematosus, S/S = signs and symptoms, TB = tuberculosis, TG = triglyceride, TIA = transient ischemic attack, TMJ = temporomandibular joint, URI = upper respiratory infection, VC = vasoconstriction, VD = vasodilatation, VZ = varicella/zoster.

Table 15–4. DISORDERS OF MOTOR FUNCTION

Most Common...	Answer and Explanation
patterns of corticospinal tract neurologic/ muscular weakness	• *UMN*, • *LMN*
clinical findings in UMN disease	• *distal paresis/paralysis in major body part:* * weakness involves skilled movements, * paralysis never complete in face, • *minimal atrophy*: due to disuse, • *spasticity*, • *no muscle fasciculations*, • *increased DTRs*, • *positive Babinski's sign*
sites of hemiparesis in UMN lesions at cerebral level	• **hand/arm**, • *lower face*, • *foot/leg*, • *face/arm/leg*, • *face/hand/arm*
site of hemiparesis of arm/leg with sparing of face	*corticospinal tract between internal capsule and upper cervical cord*
clinical findings of LMN disease	• *proximal or distal paresis/paralysis*, • *prominent muscle atrophy*, • *muscle fasciculations present*, • *no spasticity*, • *decreased/absent DTRs*, • *no Babinski's reflex*
sites involved in LMN disease	• *motor nerve*, • *motor nerve root*, • *anterior horn cell*: no sensory dysfunction
type of weakness in basal ganglia disease	• *fatigue more than demonstrable muscle weakness*: * due to muscle rigidity, * difficulty in initiating/continuing muscle movement (called bradykinesia), • *no UMN/LMN signs*, • *slightly increased DTRs*, • *no Babinski's sign*

Table continued on following page

Table 15–4. DISORDERS OF MOTOR FUNCTION
Continued

Most Common...	Answer and Explanation
type of weakness in cerebellar disease	• *ipsilateral fatigue and/or sense of incomplete strength,* • *reduced muscle resistance to passive stretching,* • *hyperactive DTRs,* • *pendular swinging of knee jerk,* • *no Babinski's sign,* • *no muscle atrophy*
type of weakness in neuromuscular junction disease	• *MG*: see Table 12–5, • *Eaton-Lambert syndrome*: see Table 4–1
type of weakness in intrinsic muscle disease	• *usually progressive muscle weakness,* • *normal resistance to passive stretching,* • *tender muscles*: myositis, • *myotonia*: * failure to relax, * myotonic dystrophy, • *soft muscle*: hyperthyroidism, • *enlarged muscle*: pseudohypertrophy of MD, • *DTRs preserved until late in disease,* • *sensation intact*
types of movement	• **tremor** • *asterixis,* • *chorea,* • *ballism, dystonia,* • *athetosis,* • *dyskinesia,* • *myoclonus,* • *tics*
clinical findings in tremor	• **involuntary rhythmic oscillation,** • *resting and intention types*
causes of tremor	• **essential tremor**: * cerebellar and/or basal ganglia dysfunction, * genetic component, • *extrapyramidal disease*: e.g., * Parkinson's disease, * resting type, • *cerebellar disease*: intention type, • *drugs*: e.g., * alcohol withdrawal, * phenothiazines, * phenytoin, • *multiple sclerosis*: intention type, • *hyperthyroidism*: * fine intention tremor, • *metabolic encephalopathy*: e.g., * hepatic encephalopathy, * Wernicke's encephalopathy, Wilson's disease ("wing-flapping" and "pill-rolling" tremors), • *miscellaneous*: * alkalosis (intention), * hypoglycemia (intention)
clinical finding in essential tremor	• *posture-related*: * genetic component, * tremor begins with maintenance of posture, • *accentuated by voluntary movement/anxiety,* • *common in middle-age/elderly,* • *hands most often involved,* • *head/voice quivering*
Rx of essential tremor	• **alcohol,** • *beta-blockers,* • *benzodiazepines,* • *stereotaxic thalamotomy,* • *botulinum toxin*

Table 15–4. DISORDERS OF MOTOR FUNCTION
Continued

Most Common...	Answer and Explanation
clinical findings in asterixis	*irregularly flapping tremor involving distal extremities, tongue*: brief loss of muscle contraction in muscles controlling extension of involved extremity
clinical findings in chorea	*involuntary, rapid, nonrhythmic, nonrepetitive, jerky movements*
clinical findings in ballism	*repetitive, abrupt, wild-flinging movements*: infarct of contralateral subthalamic nucleus
clinical finding in dystonia	*bizarre, sustained or twisting movements affecting distal body parts*: e.g., torticollis
clinical finding in athetosis	*slow, proximally located writhing*
clinical findings in dyskinesia	*nonstereotyped fragmentary twitching*
clinical findings in myoclonus	*abrupt muscle contraction*
clinical findings associated with tics	*sudden repetitive, quick involuntary movement of specific muscle groups*: may involve * lip smacking, * tongue thrusting, * eyelid twitching, * chin protrusion
cause of Parkinson's disease	*defect in dopaminergic pathway connecting substantia nigra to striatum:* degeneration/depigmentation of substantia nigra/locus ceruleus neurons leading to depletion of dopamine (principal neurotransmitter of afferents in nigrostriatal tract involved in voluntary muscle movement)
S/S of Parkinson's disease	• **rigidity of muscles leading to cog-wheel rigidity in arm movements,** • **bradykinesia**: slow voluntary movement, • *resting tremor*: * initial symptom in 50–70%, * head tremor never occurs, * tremor in mouth, tongue, lips, jaw, • *stooped posture,* • *festinating gait*: shuffling, • *expressionless face,* • *decreased blinking rate,* • *small handwriting*: often unintelligible, • *slowed thinking,* • *dementia*: 25% in those developing Parkinson's disease after 60, • *extensive seborrheic dermatitis*

Table continued on following page

Table 15–3. DISORDERS OF MOTOR FUNCTION
Continued

Most Common...	Answer and Explanation
acquired cause of Parkinson's disease	• **drugs**: e.g., * phenothiazines, * MPTP (synthetic opioid used as DOA), * butyrophenones, • *CO*: globus pallidus necrosis, • *atherosclerosis*, • *postencephalitic*
Rx of Parkinson's disease	• **levodopa**: metabolic dopamine precursor + **carbidopa**: enhances levodopa by diminishing levodopa metabolism, • *bromocriptine*: dopamine agonist, • *pergolide*: dopamine agonist, • *anticholinergic agents*: for tremor, • *amantadine*: enhances synthesis, release, re-uptake of dopamine in surviving nigral neurons, • *selegiline*: selectively inhibits monoamine oxidase B (metabolizes dopamine), • *vitamin E*, • *transplanted fetal dopamine cells into caudate/putamen*, • *stereotactic thalamotomy/pallidotomy*, • *thalamic stimulation*
late complication of levodopa Rx in Parkinson's disease	*dopamine-induced dyskinesia*: uncontrollable movements of trunk and extremities
clinical findings in Shy-Drager syndrome	• *Parkinson's disease*, • *autonomic nervous system dysfunction*: orthostatic hypotension
cause of Huntington's disease (HD)	• *AD disease*: 100% penetrance, • *triplet repeats of CAG on chromosome 4*, • *low GABA, ACh, ATII in striatum*
S/S of HD	• *early dystonic posturing and rigidity*, • *late onset of chorea*: between 30 and 50 y, • *progressive muscle rigidity*, • *dementia*, • *lose social graces*, • *increased incidence of depression/suicide*
method for Dx of HD	• **MRI shows atrophy of putamen and caudate** (diagnostic finding) **and boxcar ventricles**: from cerebral atrophy and loss of tail of caudate, • *PCR detects triplet repeats*
focal dystonia	*spasmodic torticollis*: contraction of head/neck muscles with head turning to side
cause of tardive dyskinesia	*chronic ingestion of antidopaminergic antipsychotic drugs*: * e.g., phenothiazines, * supersensitivity of dopamine receptors of basal ganglia

Table 15–4. DISORDERS OF MOTOR FUNCTION
Continued

Most Common...	Answer and Explanation
clinical findings of tardive dyskinesia	• *abnormal, semirhythmic movements of the mouth*: * tongue darting, * chewing, * grimacing, • *trunk*: trunk flexing/extension, • *extremities*: * repetitive stepping of feet, * successive contraction of fingers/toes
Rx of tardive dyskinesia	*reserpine*
clinical features of Meige's syndrome	*dystonia of jaw/lower face*: * oromandibular dystonia, * confused with tardive dyskinesia
clinical findings in Tourette's syndrome	• *childhood onset*: ? AD disease, • *facial tics*: first sign, • *eventual involvement of limbs*: patient tries to control tics but they build up and are suddenly released, • *inappropriate vocalizations*, • *coprolalia*: * use of obscene language, * often related to feces/defecation, • *obsessive-compulsive tendencies*
Rx of Tourette's syndrome	• **haloperidol,** • *pimozide,* • *clonidine*
S/S of cerebellar disease	• *easy fatigability,* • *intention tremor,* • *gait ataxia*: wide-based, • *impaired rapid/alternating movements,* • *past-pointing,* • *under or over-shoot*: see Table 15–1, • *dysarthria,* • *nystagmus*: fast component to side of lesion
types of cerebellar degeneration	• **alcoholic thiamine deficiency,** • *hepatic encephalopathy,* • *paraneoplastic cerebellar degeneration*: * anti-Yo antibodies against Purkinje cells, * cancer associations: ovarian, breast, endometrial, • *early Creutzfeldt-Jakob disease,* • *olivopontocerebellar atrophy*: rare group of genetic disorders with olive atrophy
clinical findings in Friedreich's ataxia	• *AR/AD disease*: * chromosome 9 defect, * begins before 10 y of age, • *neuron degeneration in following tracts*: * posterior columns (position/vibratory sensation lost first), * spinocerebellar, * lateral corticospinal tracts, • *retinitis pigmentosum,* • *cardiac disease*: * conduction defects, * cardiomegaly, * heart failure, • *DM,* • *pes cavus deformity*
clinical findings in Wilson's disease	*see Table 9–8*

Table continued on following page

Table 15–4. DISORDERS OF MOTOR FUNCTION
Continued

Most Common...	Answer and Explanation
uses of botulinum toxin in movement disorders	• **blepharospasm**, • *cervical dystonia*, • *hemifacial spasm*
types of ALS	• **sporadic**: * Lou Gehrig's disease, * ? viral, * ? immunologic, • *familial*: * AD disease, * defect in zinc/copper binding SOD leading to FR damage to UMN/LMN
clinical findings in ALS	• *begins in middle to late life*, • *slightly more common in men*, • *initial complaints of cramps, weight loss, fasciculations*, • *bilateral LMN signs involving intrinsic muscles of the hands* (first site) *and forearms*, • *spastic UMN signs from nonspecific damage to corticospinal tract in lower extremities*, • *gait dysfunction*, • *oropharyngeal dysphagia for solids/ liquids*, • *respiratory muscle weakness*
COD in ALS	• **aspiration**, • *sepsis*
Rx of ALS	• *antioxidant cocktails*, • *riluzole*: for bulbar onset types

Question: Which of the following neurologic disorders are associated with muscle rigidity rather than muscle spasticity? **SELECT 3**
  (A) Friedreich's ataxia
  (B) Huntington's disease
  (C) B₁₂ deficiency
  (D) Parkinson's disease
  (E) Amyotropic lateral sclerosis
  (F) Lacunar strokes
  (G) Shy-Drager syndrome

Answers: (B), (D), (G). Muscle rigidity characterizes lesions involving the extrapyramidal system, whereas spasticity implies a UMN lesion. Therefore, muscle rigidity is associated with Huntington's disease **(choice B,** involves caudate, putamen), Parkinson's disease **(choice D,** involves substantia nigra connection to striatal system), and the Shy-Drager syndrome **(choice G,** Parkinson's disease plus autonomic system dysfunction). Disorders that target UMNs either directly or in combination with other lesions include Friedreich's ataxia **(choice A is incorrect,** involves the lateral corticospinal tract, spinocerebellar tract, and posterior columns), B₁₂ deficiency **(choice C is incorrect,** produces subacute combined degeneration with posterior column and lateral corticospinal tract disease), amyotrophic lateral sclerosis **(choice E is incorrect,** involves both UMNs and LMNs), and lacunar strokes **(choice F is incorrect,** often localizes to the internal capsule and produces a pure motor stroke).

ACh = acetylcholine, AD = autosomal dominant, ALS = amyotrophic lateral sclerosis, AR = automsomal recessive, ATII = angiotensin II, CO = carbon monoxide, COD = cause of death, DM = diabetes mellitus, DOA = drug of abuse, DTRs = deep tendon reflexes, Dx = diagnosis, FR = free radical, GABA = γ-aminobutyric acid, HD = Huntington's disease, LMN = lower motor neuron, MC = most common, MG = myasthenia gravis, MPTP = 1-methyl-4-phenyl-1,2,3,6-tetrahydroproline, PCR = polymerase chain reaction, Rx = treatment, SOD = superoxide dismutase, S/S = signs and symptoms, UMN = upper motor neuron.

Table 15–5. CENTRAL NERVOUS SYSTEM TRAUMA, CEREBROVASCULAR DISEASE

Most Common...	Answer and Explanation
sign following a cerebral concussion	*transient loss of consciousness with memory loss of events prior to or shortly after traumatic episode*: * most often caused by a nonpenetrating blunt impact, * temporary functional paralysis of neurons in reticular activating system
cause of a cerebral contusion	*acceleration-deceleration injuries*: superficial damage to brain
cause of coup/ contrecoup injury	*acceleration-deceleration injury causing contusion at impact site* (coup injury) *and at distant site from point of injury* (contrecoup injury): contrecoup worse than coup injury
sites for contrecoup injuries	*tips of frontal/temporal lobes*
cause of diffuse axonal injuries	*accleration/deceleration injuries*: * shearing of axons located in white mater tracts and/or brain stem
secondary brain injuries in diffuse axonal injury	• **cerebral edema**, • *hypoxic brain injury,* • *meningeal tears,* • *bleeding* [Occur several hours to a day or more after trauma.]
fractures producing rhinorrhea	• *orbital blow-out fracture,* • *basilar skull fractures in anterior cranial fossa*
clinical features of basilar skull fracture in anterior cranial fossa	• *fracture through cribriform plate of ethmoid bone*: not usually seen with radiograph, • *anosmia:* olfactory nerve rootlet transection, • *CSF leaks mixed with blood from one/both nostrils*: blood forms a ring with a clear center called "halo sign," • *subconjunctival hemorrhage,* • *periorbital hematoma*: "raccoon sign"

Table continued on following page

Table 15–5. CENTRAL NERVOUS SYSTEM TRAUMA, CEREBROVASCULAR DISEASE *Continued*

Most Common...	Answer and Explanation
clinical features of basilar skull fracture of middle cranial fossa	• *fracture through tegmen tympani of petrous portion of temporal bone*: * not seen by radiograph, * CT test of choice, • *hemotympanum* (blood in middle ear) *or ruptured membrane with otorrhea,* • *eardrum intact*: CSF moves through eustachian tube and out the nose (rhinorrhea), • *Battle's sign*: * bluish discoloration over mastoid bone, * rupture of mastoid emissary vein, • *peripheral CN VII paralysis*: * CN VII traverses temporal bone, * decreased flow of tears means injury is proximal to middle ear portion of CN VII
types of traumatic CNS bleeds	• **subdural hematoma**, • *epidural hematoma*
imaging technique used to initially identify subdural/ epidural hematomas	*CT scan*
cause of a subdural hematoma	• **blunt trauma to skull**, • *anticoagulation* [Blunt trauma causes fracture in 50% and tearing of bridging veins between dura and arachnoid membranes → venous clot over one/both convexities of brain. Elderly patients/alcoholics most at risk.]
CT finding in subdural hematoma	*high-density crescent-shaped collection of blood*
S/S of acute subdural hematoma	• **headache**, • *mydriasis*, • *fluctuating levels of consciousness*, • *mass effects*: * visual disturbances, * hemiparesis
S/S of chronic subdural hematoma	• **sustained, new headache**, • *confusion*, • *inattention*, • *dementia*, • hypersomnia, • *seizures*, • *coma* [Best diagnosed with MRI.]
Rx of subdural hematoma	*clot evacuation*
cause of epidural hematoma	*fracture of temporoparietal bone*: * fracture severs middle meningeal artery, * dura separated from periosteum by arterial blood, * ~30–50 mL accumulates over 4–8 h leading to increase in intracranial pressure

Table 15–5. CENTRAL NERVOUS SYSTEM TRAUMA, CEREBROVASCULAR DISEASE *Continued*

Most Common...	Answer and Explanation
CT finding of epidural hematoma	*high-density "lens-shaped" collection of blood with shift of brain contents*
S/S of epidural hematoma	• *immediate loss of consciousness followed by a lucid interval,* • *death by herniation in 5–6 h*
Rx of epidural hematoma	*surgical evacuation of blood clot*
acute post-traumatic problem of head injury	*delayed post-traumatic encephalopathy*: * occurs 15 m to 2 h after head injury, * patient develops N/V and becomes stuporous/obtunded, * cortical blindness (posterior cerebral artery compression) may occur from temporary uncal herniation, * most recover
subacute/chronic complications of head injury	• **chronic subdural hematoma**: see above, • *post-traumatic epilepsy*: * 50% chance with penetrating injuries, * 5% chance with closed injuries, * penetrating injuries prophylactically treated with phenytoin or carbamazepine, • *delayed dementia*: * 10× greater chance if patient has apo E ϵ4 on chromosome 14, * former boxers (dementia pugilistica), • *post-concussion syndrome*: * headache, * concentration difficulties, * irritable, * dizzy
CNS complications related to chronic ischemia	• **transient ischemic attack** (TIA), • *stroke,* • *watershed infarcts between two overlapping arterial supplies,* • *laminar necrosis of cerebral cortex*: leads to cerebral atrophy
mechanisms of ischemic CVA	• **thrombosis over atherosclerotic plaque at the carotid artery bifurcation** (MC site), **terminal branch of ICA, proximal or distal end of basilar artery, origin of MCA,** • *embolus from extracranial carotid artery to MCA,* • *embolus from heart*: particularly in presence of atrial fibrillation, • *dissecting aortic aneurysm involving carotid or vertebrobasilar system,* • *small vessel occlusive disease*: hyaline arteriolosclerosis due to HTN, DM, • *vessel thrombosis from hypercoagulable state/blood dyscrasia*: e.g., * PRV, * sickle cell anemia, * protein C/S deficiency, * APL syndrome, * SLE, • *illicit drugs*: e.g., cocaine

Table continued on following page

Table 15–5. CENTRAL NERVOUS SYSTEM TRAUMA, CEREBROVASCULAR DISEASE *Continued*

Most Common...	Answer and Explanation
risk factors for ischemic CVA	• **age**: * >45 in men, * >55 in women, • *family Hx of CAD/stroke,* • *smoking,* • *LDL ≥160 mg/dL,* • *HDL ≤40 mg/dL,* • *DM,* • *HTN,* • *oral contraceptives,* • *atrial fibrillation,* • *CHF,* • *anterior AMI with mural thrombus*
modifiable risk factors to prevent ischemic CVA	• **control HTN,** • *control DM,* • *stop smoking,* • *lose weight,* • *lower serum CH,* • *limit alcohol intake,* • *aspirin,* • *anticoagulation for atrial fibrillation*
site for TIAs	*cortical*
cause of TIA	*embolism from atherosclerotic plaque on ICA*
clinical manifestations of a TIA	• *neurologic deficits usually last <15 m,* • *~90% resolve in 24 h,* • *one-third progress to a stroke*: usually in same distribution as TIA, • *one-third have at least one more TIA,* • *one-third have no further problems,* • *amaurosis fugax*: see Table 15–3
types of strokes in descending order of frequency	• **atherosclerotic**: * 80%, * pale infarction, • *embolic*: hemorrhagic infarction, • *intracerebral*: HTN MC, • *subarachnoid*: ruptured berry aneurysm MC
S/S of left MCA CVA	• **contralateral hemiparesis/sensory changes in face/upper extremities**, • *expressive aphasia*: dominant hemisphere, • *acalculia,* • *alexia,* • *right hemianopia,* • *R/L disorientation,* • *head deviation to side of lesion*
S/S of right MCA CVA	• **contralateral hemiparesis/sensory changes in face/upper extremities**, • *right gaze preference,* • *hemineglect,* • *dressing apraxia,* • *anosognosia,* • *construction apraxia*
S/S of ACA CVA	*contralateral leg weakness/sensory loss*
S/S of PCA CVA	• **contralateral homonymous hemianopia**, • *superior quadrantanopia,* • *proximal branches to thalamus*: * memory loss, * sensorimotor hemiplegia
S/S of CVA at basilar artery junction with two PCAs	• **stupor/coma,** • *bilateral blindness,* • *amnesia,* • *hemiplegia/diplegia,* • *pupillary/oculomotor paralysis,* • *vertical gaze dysfunction*

Table 15–5. CENTRAL NERVOUS SYSTEM TRAUMA, CEREBROVASCULAR DISEASE *Continued*

Most Common...	Answer and Explanation
S/S of basilar artery occlusion	• **contralateral hemiparesis/sensory loss**, • *locked-in-state*: communicate with eyes or eyelids, • *ipsilateral bulbar/cerebellar signs*
S/S of vertebrobasilar CVA	• **ipsilateral sensory changes on face**, • **contralateral motor/sensory changes in trunk/ limbs**, • *vertigo*, • *ataxia*, • *diplopia*
clinical findings of PICA CVA (Wallenberg infarct)	• *usually secondary to vertebral artery disease*: involves lateral medullary plate, • *CN V ipsilateral face numbness*, • *contralateral body numbness*: spinothalamic tract, • *ipsilateral Horner's*: descending sympathetics, • *ipsilateral palate weakness with dysphagia for solids/liquids and decreased gag reflex*: nucleus ambiguus IX and X, • *hiccups*: nucleus solitarius, • *ipsilateral limb ataxia*: cerebellum/inferior cerebellar peduncle, • *N/V*: vestibular dysfunction
S/S of acute cerebellar infarction	• *ipsilateral headache*, • *vomiting*, • *vertigo*, • *CN VI/VII palsies*, • *inability to walk*, • *absence of long-tract signs*
causes of an embolic CVA	• **emboli originating from left heart**: * particularly in association with atrial fibrillation, * anterior/anterolateral AMI, * mechanical valves more prone to embolization than porcine valves, * 50% of atrial myxomas embolize, • *embolus from extracranial carotid artery to MCA*, • *embolus of vegetation from valvular disease in left heart*: * **rheumatic MV stenosis**, * MVP, * 15% of IE
steps in initial management of cerebral infarction	• **CT scan to determine if pale/hemorrhagic infarction**, • *tPA if onset symptoms <3 h and none of following are present* (partial list): * evidence of intracranial hemorrhage, * midline shift, * significant HTN present, * obtunded or comatose state, • *cardiac monitoring*: 30–40% prevalence CAD in patients with ischemic strokes, • *noninvasive assessment of the carotid arteries*
recommendation for asymptomatic or symptomatic ICA stenosis >60%	*carotid endarterectomy*

Table continued on following page

**Table 15–5. CENTRAL NERVOUS SYSTEM TRAUMA,
CEREBROVASCULAR DISEASE** *Continued*

Most Common...	Answer and Explanation
recommendation for symptomatic ICA stenosis 30–60%	*role of carotid endarterectomy under investigation*
recommendation for ICA stenosis <30%	• **aspirin**: 3% decrease in strokes over 3 y, • *ticlopidine if allergic to aspirin*: * 6% decrease in strokes over 3 y, * problem with neutropenia, * superior to aspirin, but more expensive, * clopidogrel does not have neutropenia effects of ticlopidine
recommendations for heparin/warfarin in atherosclerotic CVA	*controversial* [Use of anticoagulation individualized. Danger of creating/extending a hemorrhagic stroke. Evidence supports its use in evolving strokes and with minimal to mild ischemic lesions associated with clear arterial or cardiac sources of embolism.]
recommendation for stroke prevention in patients with mechanical prosthetic cardiac valves	*dipyramidole + warfarin*
causes of an intracerebral bleed	• **HTN**: * microaneurysms develop in lenticulostriate vessels (MCA branches) supplying basal ganglia (35–50% in putamen), * aneurysms rupture producing a hematoma, • *β-amyloid deposition in cerebral arteries*: mainly elderly patients, • *trauma*, • *anticoagulation*, • *rupture of berry aneurysm under pressure*
S/S of intracerebral bleed in basal ganglia/internal capsule	• *headache ipsilateral to bleed*, • *convulsions*, • *loss of consciousness*, • *contralateral hemiplegia*, • *eyes deviate to side of lesion* [Prognosis dependent on size/location of bleed.]
S/S of intracerebral bleed into thalamus	• *headache ipsi- or contralateral or both sides*, • *contralateral hemiparesis*, • *miotic pupils*, • *contralateral hemianopia*, • *contralateral hemisensory defect*, • *eyes deviate down and contralateral to lesion*, • *unconsciousness late occurrence*

Table 15–5. CENTRAL NERVOUS SYSTEM TRAUMA, CEREBROVASCULAR DISEASE *Continued*

Most Common...	Answer and Explanation
S/S of intracerebral bleed into pons	• *global headache followed quickly by coma,* • *noisy breathing,* • *vomiting,* • *gait loss,* • *quadriparesis,* • *pinpoint pupils,* • *ipsilateral gaze paralysis,* • *ocular bobbing*
S/S of intracerebral bleed into cerebellum	• *occipital headache ipsilateral to bleed,* • *ipsilateral facial weakness,* • *severe vomiting,* • *incoordination,* • *sensory changes occur late,* • *dysarthria,* • *paralysis of ipsilateral conjugate gaze,* • *stupor/coma*: * indicates brain stem compression, * late occurrence [Clot evacuation may be lifesaving.]
S/S of malignant HTN in the CNS	• **headache**: intracerebral edema, • *grade IV hypertensive retinopathy*: * papilledema, * hard/soft exudates, * hemorrhage [See Table 5–4.]
causes of subarachnoid hemorrhage	• **ruptured congenital berry** (saccular) **aneurysm**: * 80%, * usually located at junction of anterior communicating artery with ACA, * absence of internal elastica/smooth muscle in media, • *ruptured AVM,* • *rupture of fusiform aneurysm*: atherosclerotic, • *trauma*
risk factors for a subarachnoid hemorrhage	• **HTN**, • *APKD,* • *adult coarctation,* • *Marfan's disease,* • *Ehlers-Danlos disease,* • *previous Hx of berry aneurysm*: one-third have multiple aneurysms [All of these conditions increase risk for developing berry aneurysms.]
S/S of a subarachnoid hemorrhage	**sudden onset of severe occipital headache**: * 50% have sentinel bleed with a warning headache, * "worst headache I have ever had," • *N/V, loss of consciousness,* • *CN III deficits,* • *nuchal rigidity,* • *prognosis*: * depends on state of consciousness at initial presentation, * ~25% die from initial bleed, * additional 25–35% die from rebleed by end of year, * ~25% have permanent neurologic deficits
time-frame for vasospastic injury following subarachnoid hemorrhage	*4–14 d after bleed*: * vasospastic injury occurs in ~75%, * TXA_2 release from platelet in clot material contributes to vasospasm, * may produce further neurologic deficits

Table continued on following page

Table 15–5. CENTRAL NERVOUS SYSTEM TRAUMA, CEREBROVASCULAR DISEASE *Continued*

Most Common...	Answer and Explanation
complications associated with a subarachnoid bleed	• **rebleeding**: 20% rebleed within a 2-wk time-span, • *myocardial ischemia*: due to outpouring of catecholamines from reticular activating system, • *communicating hydrocephalus*: blockage of arachnoid granulations, • *SIADH,* • *seizures,* • *hyperglycemia*: catecholamine effect, • *delirium,* • *neutrophilic leukocytosis*: catecholamine effect
tests to document subarachnoid hemorrhage	• **CT within 24–48 h of bleed**: diagnostic in 90%, • *lumbar puncture if CT cannot identify blood,* • *cerebral angiography*: * confirmatory test, * FN rate 10–20%
Rx of ruptured berry aneurysm	• **surgical clipping**, • *nimodipine:* helps prevent vasospasm
symptomatic vascular anomaly in CNS	*AVM*: tangles of arteries directly connected to veins
complications associated with AVMs	• **subarachnoid bleeds**, • *focal epileptic seizures,* • *progressive neurologic deficits,* • *CT scan*: * diagnostic in ~85%, * MRI more sensitive than CT, * train track calcifications
diagnostic tests to identify AVMs	• **MRI**, • *CT,* • *angiography*: definitive test
cause of lacunar infarcts in the CNS	• **HTN,** • *DM* [Secondary to hyaline arteriolosclerosis/fibrinoid necrosis of penetrating subcortical/brain stem vessels. Sites: basal ganglia, internal capsule, pons, thalamus. Cognition not affected.]
S/S of lacunar infarcts in posterior limb of internal capsule	*pure motor hemiparesis*
S/S of lacunar infarcts in thalamus	*pure sensory stroke*
S/S of lacunar infarcts in pons	*ataxic hemiparesis*
S/S of lacunar infarcts in subthalamic nucleus	*hemiballismus*

Neurology   **755**

Table 15–5. CENTRAL NERVOUS SYSTEM TRAUMA, CEREBROVASCULAR DISEASE *Continued*

Most Common...	Answer and Explanation
S/S of lacunar infarcts in internal capsule + pons	• *clumsy hand,* • *dysarthria*

Question: Which of the following are most often associated with CNS hemorrhage? **SELECT 4**
  (A) Transient ischemic attack
  (B) Embolic stroke
  (C) Atherosclerotic stroke
  (D) Hypertensive stroke
  (E) Congenital berry aneurysm
  (F) Fusiform aneurysm
  (G) Watershed infarct
  (H) Fracture of temporoparietal bone
  (I) Cerebral concussion

Answers: (B), (D), (E), (H): Bleeds are not usually associated with transient ischemic attacks (**choice A is incorrect**), atherosclerotic strokes (**choice C is incorrect**, 20% may be hemorrhagic if reperfusion occurs), fusiform aneurysms (**choice F is incorrect**, usually atherosclerotic and rarely rupture), watershed infarcts (**choice G is incorrect,** junction of two overlapping blood supplies), and cerebral concussions (**choice I is incorrect,** no damage to the brain) are not associated with bleeding. Embolic strokes (**choice B**) produce a hemorrhagic infarction. Hypertensive strokes (**choice D**) produce an intracerebral bleed (hematoma). Fracture of the temporoparietal bone (**choice H**), is most often associated with an epidural hematoma, since the middle meningeal artery courses through the bone.

ACA = anterior cerebral artery, AMI = acute myocardial infarction, APL = antiphospholipid syndrome, APKD = adult polycystic kidney disease, AVM = arteriovenous malformation, CAD = coronary artery disease, CH = cholesterol, CHF = congestive heart failure, CN = cranial nerve, CNS = central nervous system, CSF = cerebrospinal fluid, CT = computed tomography, CVA = cerebrovascular accident, DM = diabetes mellitus, FN = false negative, HDL = high density lipoprotein, HTN = hypertension, Hx = history, ICA = internal carotid artery, IE = infective endocarditis, LDL = low density lipoprotein, MC = most common, MCA = middle cerebral artery, MRI = magnetic resonance imaging, MV = mitral valve, MVP = mitral valve prolapse, N/V = nausea and vomiting, PCA = posterior cerebral artery, PICA = posterior inferior cerebellar artery, PRV = polycythemia rubra vera, R/L = right/left, Rx = treatment, SIADH = syndrome of inappropriate antidiuretic hormone, SLE = systemic lupus erythematosus, S/S = signs and symptoms, TIA = transient ischemic attack, tPA = tissue plasminogen activator, TXA_2 = thromboxane A_2.

Table 15–6. EPILEPSY, ALTERED INTRACRANIAL PRESSURE, CENTRAL NERVOUS SYSTEM TUMORS

Most Common...	Answer and Explanation
differences between seizures and epilepsy	• *seizures:* * sudden electroclinical event associated with involuntary movements, altered awareness, or convulsions, * symptom of brain dysfunction, • *epilepsy:* * any disorder associated with recurrent seizures (e.g., meningioma), * always requires the presence of seizures, * not all seizures imply epilepsy (e.g., withdrawal from alcohol)
causes of epilepsy in children	• **idiopathic:** * 68%, * usually genetic, • *secondary:* in descending order: * **congenital,** * trauma, * infection, * vascular/neoplastic, * degenerative
causes of epilepsy in adults	• **idiopathic:** 55%, • *secondary:* in descending order: * **vascular,** * neoplastic, * trauma, * degenerative disease, * infection, * congenital
types of seizures	• **focal:** arise from one area of brain, • *generalized:* arise simultaneously from all areas of brain
general clinical findings in focal seizures	• *70% of adult seizures,* • *40% of childhood seizures,* • *usually related to anatomically localized lesions:* e.g., * scars, * AVM, * tumors, • *abnormal unilateral movements/sensations,* • *stereotypic behavioral patterns*
clinical findings in generalized seizures	• *bilateral motor abnormalities,* • *usually a brief loss of consciousness:* exception is myoclonic seizures, • *involve centrally located subcortical activating mechanisms*
cerebral sites that predispose to seizures	• **frontal lobes,** • *limbic system:* medial temporal lobes, • *diencephalic reticular formation,* • *occipital lobes*
seizure types in children in descending order	• **complex partial,** • *generalized tonic/clonic,* • *absence,* • *simple partial,* • *myoclonic*
seizure types in adults in descending order	• **complex partial,** • *generalized tonic/clonic,* • *simple partial,* • *myoclonic*
types of generalized seizures	• **tonic/clonic:** * grand mal seizure, * convulsive, • *absence:* staring, • *tonic,* • *clonic,* • *myoclonic:* brief jerks/twitches, • *atonic:* sudden loss of body tone

Table 15–6. EPILEPSY, ALTERED INTRACRANIAL PRESSURE, CENTRAL NERVOUS SYSTEM TUMORS
Continued

Most Common...	Answer and Explanation
clinical features of tonic/clonic seizures	• *little or no warning,* • *sudden loss of consciousness with falling,* • *tonic phase:* * stiffening of all muscle groups, * head extends back, * cry erupts when diaphragm contracts and forces air out, • *clonic phase:* rhythmic jerking of extremities, • *duration:* few minutes, • *post-ictal phase:* * flaccid relaxation, * snoring respirations, * frothing (increased salivation), * no responsiveness, * tongue biting, * incontinence, * injury
Rx of tonic-clonic seizures	• **carbamazepine,** • *valproate,* • *phenytoin,* • *phenobarbital* [Monotherapy is Rx of choice. All of the above drugs (except valproate) induce cytochrome P450 enzyme system, which reduces the effectiveness of oral contraceptives. Valproate is best for women on oral contraceptives.]
clinical features of absence (petit mal) seizures	• *begin from ages 2–12,* • *40% incidence of EEG abnormality in first-degree relatives,* • *staring spells:* * lasts 1–2 sec, * automatisms like blinking, * head droops, * sometimes arms jerk rhythmically, * patient unaware, * resumes previous activity, • *EEG:* * 3 Hz spike and slow wave complexes, * hyperventilation induces attacks, • *good cognitive prognosis,* • *50% develop tonic-clonic seizures by 20 y old*
Rx of absence seizures	• **ethosuximide,** • *valproic acid,* • *clonazepam*
clinical features of myoclonic seizures	• *begins late childhood/adolescence,* • *brief, bilaterally symmetric contraction of the muscles:* * usually face/upper extremities, * more common during drowsiness, • *associated with other seizure types,* • *EEG:* polyspike discharges
Rx of myoclonic seizures	• **valproic acid,** • *clonazepam*
types of partial (focal) seizures	• **complex partial,** • *simple partial* [Partial (focal) seizures imply structural damage to brain (exception: benign rolandic epilepsy).]

Table continued on following page

**Table 15–6. EPILEPSY, ALTERED INTRACRANIAL
PRESSURE, CENTRAL NERVOUS SYSTEM TUMORS**
Continued

Most Common...	Answer and Explanation
clinical findings of complex partial seizures	• *aura:* * dreamy feeling (parahippocampal area), * foul odor (♦ temporal lobe, ♦ uncinate fit), * déjà vu (♦ intense familiarity, ♦ parahippocampal/hippocampal area), * lip smacking, * epigastric rising, * borborygmi (automatisms located in insular, temporal-polar limbic system), * fragments of voices, phrases, songs (auditory association cortex), * aura occurs seconds before ictal phase, • *ictal phase:* * seizure lasts 30 sec to 2 min, * altered consciousness (amnestic of event), * focal motor activity (contralateral to focus), • *post-ictal phase:* * lasts from seconds to hours, * confusion, * lethargy, * sometimes psychotic behavior
clinical findings in primary motor (rolandic) partial complex seizures	• *classic jacksonian epileptic seizure,* • *rhythmic, clonic twitching beginning in contralateral thumb or corner of mouth →* • *usually spreads to produce adjacent movements from thumb to hand to arm to face:* sometimes spreads from face to hand → • *generalized convulsion →* • *post-ictal Todd's paralysis in some cases:* temporary limb paralysis
Rx of complex partial seizures	• **carbamazepine,** • *phenytoin,* • *valproic acid*
clinical findings in simple partial (focal) seizures	• **no change in mental status:** key distinction from complex partial seizure, • *restricted, focal motor activity:* e.g., hand jerking, • *usually caused by stroke/tumor in motor strip*
causes of status epilepticus	• **nonstructural:** * **drug withdrawal** (e.g., ♦ benzodiazepines, ♦ barbiturates, ♦ alcohol, ♦ cocaine), * drug intoxication (e.g., ♦ theophylline) * hypoglycemia, -calcemia, -natremia, • *underlying structural abnormality:* * **CNS infection,** * stroke [Status epilepticus is defined as >30 min of unconsciousness associated with continuous/intermittent generalized convulsive activity.]
Rx of status epilepticus	• **ABCs of CPR,** • *give IV glucose/thiamine* * *after thiamine,* • *IV diazepam or lorazepam*

Table 15–6. EPILEPSY, ALTERED INTRACRANIAL PRESSURE, CENTRAL NERVOUS SYSTEM TUMORS
Continued

Most Common...	Answer and Explanation
types of surgery for intractable epilepsy	• **anterior temporal lobe resections in complex partial seizures:** 70% cure, • *local resection epileptogenic foci,* • *corpus callosotomy in certain types of generalized seizures*
tests ordered in work-up of epilepsy	• **EEG:** with: * photic stimulation to R/O generalized seizures, * hyperventilation to R/O absence seizure, * sleep deprivation to R/O complex partial seizure, • *MRI*
differential to consider in seizure work-up	• **syncope,** • *cardiac arrhythmia,* • *TIA,* • *malingering,* • *movement disorder:* e.g., * tic, * chorea, • *drug-related*
distinctions between syncope and seizures	• **EEG:** * normal in syncope, * abnormal in seizure, • *consciousness:* * loss of consciousness during exercise in syncope of cardiac origin (e.g., prolonged QT interval syndrome), * sudden loss of consciousness during exercise <u>rarely due to seizure,</u> • *prodrome:* * swimming sensation in syncope, * aura/epigastric rise in seizure, • *body position:* * sitting/erect in syncope, * any position with seizure, • *motor activity:* * usually none with syncope, * usually present with seizure, • *pulse:* * slow/weak with syncope, * strong with seizure, • *appearance:* * pale/sweating with syncope, * flushed/salivating with seizure, • *post-ictal:* * oriented/nauseous in syncope, * confused/headache in seizure
anticonvulsant drugs with teratogenic effects in pregnancy	• **valproic acid:** neural tube defect, • *carbamazepine:* * neural tube defect, * fetal hemorrhage, • *primidone,* • *phenobarbital:* * fetal hemorrhage, • *phenytoin:* * fetal hemorrhage, * growth disturbances [Give mother folic acid to prevent neural tube defects/vitamin K to prevent fetal bleed.]
mechanism/uses/ side effects of carbamazepine	• *mechanism:* * blocks sodium channels in neurons, * decreases synaptic transmissions, • *uses:* * generalized tonic/clonic, * partial seizures, • *side-effects:* * SIADH, * neutropenia, * enhances cytochrome system

Table continued on following page

Table 15–6. EPILEPSY, ALTERED INTRACRANIAL PRESSURE, CENTRAL NERVOUS SYSTEM TUMORS
Continued

Most Common...	Answer and Explanation
mechanism/uses/ side effects of valproic acid	• *mechanism:* increases GABA levels, • *uses:* * generalized tonic-clonic, * absence, * partial seizures, * prevent seizures in women on birth control pills, • *side-effects:* * risk of neural tube defects, * alopecia, * hepatotoxicity
mechanism/uses/ side effects of phenytoin	• *mechanism:* blocks sodium channels, • *uses:* * generalized tonic-clonic, * partial seizures, • *side effects:* * teratogenic * gingival hyperplasia, * vertigo, * atypical lymphocytosis, * generalized lymphadenopathy, * hirsutism, * erythema multiforme, * enhances cytochrome system
mechanism/uses/ side effects of phenobarbital	• *mechanism:* binds to GABA-benzodiazepine receptor and prolongs opening of Cl⁻ channels, • *uses:* * most useful in pediatric epilepsy, * generalized tonic-clonic, * partial seizures, • *side effects:* * fetal hemorrhage in pregnancy, * skin disorders: ♦ erythema multiforme, ♦ fixed drug eruptions, ♦ toxic epidermal necrolysis, * enhances cytochrome system
mechanism/uses/ side effects of ethosuximide	• *mechanism:* blocks calcium channels, • *uses:* * absence, • *side effects:* dyspepsia
factors controlling intracranial pressure	• *CSF,* • *blood,* • *brain tissue* [An increase or decrease in one automatically impacts on other factors. Example: cerebral bleed compresses brain tissue → decreased CSF volume.]
factors controlling cerebral perfusion pressure	• *systolic blood pressure,* • *CSF pressure*
initial effect of decreased cerebral perfusion	*clouding of sensorium due to ischemia*
site for CSF synthesis	*choroid plexus in lateral ventricles* [CSF is an ultrafiltrate of plasma. CSF moves from lateral ventricles → third ventricle → duct of Sylvius → fourth ventricle → exit foramina of Luschka/Magendie → subarachnoid space.]

Table 15–6. EPILEPSY, ALTERED INTRACRANIAL PRESSURE, CENTRAL NERVOUS SYSTEM TUMORS
Continued

Most Common...	Answer and Explanation
site of resorption of CSF	*arachnoid granulations located along the summit of the brain:* CSF passes into dural venous sinuses → jugular venous system
effect of hypercapnia and hypocapnia on CSF pressure	• *hypercapnia* (respiratory acidosis): increases CSF pressure by increasing vessel permeability, • *hypocapnia* (respiratory alkalosis): decreases CSF pressure by vasoconstricting cerebral vessels, • *CSF pressure >200 mm Hg is pathologic:* called intracranial HTN
causes of intracranial hypertension	• **resistance to CSF flow:** * **tumor MC,** * aqueduct stenosis, * plugging of arachnoid villi (♦ blood in subarachnoid space, ♦ pus), * blockage of foramina of Luschka/Magendie, • *increased CSF production:* choroid plexus papilloma, • *increased dural sinus pressure:* * blocks CSF resorption, * e.g., ♦ sagittal sinus thrombosis, ♦ RHF, ♦ SVC syndrome
S/S of intracranial HTN	• **morning headache,** • *projectile vomiting without nausea,* • *visual disturbances,* • *papilledema,* • *sinus bradycardia,* • *HTN,* • *brain herniation syndromes:* see Table 15–2, • *noncardiogenic pulmonary edema*
cause of Cushing's reflex	*intracranial HTN*
signs of Cushing's reflex	• *HTN,* • *sinus bradycardia,* • *falling respiratory rate*
cause of intracranial hypotension	• **volume depletion,** • *leakage of CSF fluid post-lumbar puncture:* Rx with epidural patch using patient's blood
cause of intracranial HTN in absence of tumor/obstruction to CSF flow	*pseudotumor cerebri:* * secondary to decreased CSF resorption, * most commonly noted in young, obese females
conditions associated with pseudotumor cerebri	• **obesity,** • *hypervitaminosis A,* • *endocrine disease:* * Addison's disease, * Cushing's syndrome, • *drugs:* * tetracycline, * phenytoin, • *venous sinus thrombosis,* • *pregnancy,* • *prolonged corticosteroid Rx,* • *birth control pills,* • *head trauma*

Table continued on following page

Table 15–6. EPILEPSY, ALTERED INTRACRANIAL PRESSURE, CENTRAL NERVOUS SYSTEM TUMORS
Continued

Most Common...	Answer and Explanation
S/S of pseudotumor cerebri	• **headache,** • *papilledema,* • *visual disturbances:* * bilateral visual loss, * enlarged blind spot with visual field testing
method of diagnosing pseudotumor cerebri	• **normal CT/MRI,** • *increased CSF pressure:* * usually >300 mm Hg, * low CSF protein
Rx of pseudotumor cerebri	• **weight reduction,** • *drugs:* * steroids, * carbonic anhydrase inhibitor, * thiazides, • *CSF removal,* • *CSF shunting to peritoneal cavity,* • *optic nerve decompression if visual loss*
types of hydrocephalus	• **noncommunicating:** * obstructive, * CSF blocked in ventricles, • *communicating:* * nonobstructive, * open communication between ventricles/subarachnoid space, • *ex vacuo:* cerebral atrophy causes ventricles to enlarge
cause of hydrocephalus in adults	• **aqueductal stenosis:** * noncommunicating, * paralysis of upward gaze (Parinaud's syndrome), • *complication of subarachnoid hemorrhage:* communicating
method of diagnosing hydrocephalus	*MRI*
cause of normal pressure hydrocephalus	*chronic communicating hydrocephalus*
cause of acute hydrocephalus	• **CNS bleed:** e.g., * subarachnoid, * cerebellar, • *trauma,* • *colloid cyst third ventricle,* • *bacterial meningitis*
S/S of normal pressure hydrocephalus	• **dementia,** • *urinary incontinence,* • *shuffling gait,* • *bilateral UMN signs:* Babinski's sign, • *extrapyramidal signs may be present*
neurologic symptoms in patients with cancer	• **headache:** e.g., * metastasis, * hemorrhage, * drug effects, • *back pain:* * vertebral metastasis, * epidural metastasis, • *altered mental status:* metabolic encephalopathy MCC

**Table 15–6. EPILEPSY, ALTERED INTRACRANIAL
PRESSURE, CENTRAL NERVOUS SYSTEM TUMORS**
Continued

Most Common...	Answer and Explanation
neurologic complication of systemic cancer	*cerebral metastasis*
cancer metastatic to brain	• **lung,** • *breast,* • *colon,* • *malignant melanoma,* • *leukemia:* particularly ALL
CNS sites of metastasis	• **cerebral cortex,** • *cerebellum,* • *brain stem* [Most metastases are multiple and target the junction of gray/white matter or leptomeninges (particularly leukemia/lymphomas).]
cancers metastatic to vertebra/epidural space	• **breast,** • *lung,* • *prostate*
cancer involving nerve plexuses	*metastatic colorectal cancer*
cancers metastatic to the base of the skull	*head/neck cancers*
cancer with most neurologic complications	*metastatic malignant melanoma*
primary cancers of the brain in adults	• **glioblastoma multiforme:** * GBM, * grade IV astrocytoma, • *anaplastic astrocytoma:* grade III astrocytoma, • *astrocytoma:* grades I/II are benign, • *CNS lymphoma in AIDS patients* [~70% of adult primary CNS tumors are supratentorial, while ~70% of primary CNS tumors in children are infratentorial, the MC location being cerebellum (cystic astrocytoma, medulloblastoma).]
primary benign brain tumor in adults	• **meningioma,** • *acoustic neuroma*
tumors in cerebral cortex	• **metastasis,** • *GBM,* • *low-grade astrocytoma,* • *meningioma,* • *oligodendroglioma*
tumors in cerebellum	• **astrocytoma,** • *medulloblastoma,* • *cerebellar hemangioblastoma:* part of von Hippel-Lindau disease
intraspinal tumor in adults	*ependymoma*

Table continued on following page

Table 15–6. EPILEPSY, ALTERED INTRACRANIAL PRESSURE, CENTRAL NERVOUS SYSTEM TUMORS
Continued

Most Common...	Answer and Explanation
location for ependymomas in adults	*lumbosacral portion of spinal cord:* * involve filum terminale/conus medullaris, * aggressive tumors that invade nerve roots
primary CNS tumors seeding neuraxis	• **GBM,** • *medulloblastoma,* • *ependymoma*
risk factors of CNS tumors	• **AIDS,** • *neurofibromatosis,* • *Turcot's polyposis syndrome*
CNS tumors that calcify	• **meningioma,** • *oligodendroglioma:* * benign tumor, * frontal lobe, * often mixed in with astrocytoma
clinical findings associated with meningiomas	• *women > men,* • *neurofibromatosis association,* • *parasagittal area MC location,* • *push surface of brain,* • *may invade overlying skull:* increased bone density, • *enlarge during pregnancy:* contain progesterone receptors, • *intraspinal location:* 25%, • *MC tumor associated with new onset focal epileptic seizures in adults,* • *contain psammoma bodies*
clinical findings in GBM	• *may evolve from low-grade astrocytoma or arise de novo,* • *peak in 40–70-y-old age bracket,* • *target frontal lobes:* often cross the corpus callosum, • *necrotic/hemorrhagic tumors,* • *rarely metastasize out of neuraxis,* • *25–40% 5-y survival*
S/S of brain tumors	• **morning headache:** * presenting symptom in 50%, * may awaken patient at night, • *papilledema:* 10%, • *vomiting:* * more common in children than adults, * projectile and often not associated with nausea, * usually in AM before breakfast, • *altered mental status:* • *visual loss/weakness/altered consciousness:* due to plateaus of increased intracranial pressure that come and go, • *nuchal rigidity:* * leptomeningeal spread, * CSF glucose may be decreased, • *cranial nerve palsies,* • *sensorimotor deficits depending on site*
diagnostic tests used in working-up brain tumors	• **MRI,** • *lumbar puncture:* cytology to look for tumor cells
Rx of malignant brain tumors	• *chemotherapy,* • *radiation,* • *surgery:* * meningiomas, * acoustic neuromas

Table 15–6. EPILEPSY, ALTERED INTRACRANIAL PRESSURE, CENTRAL NERVOUS SYSTEM TUMORS
Continued

Most Common...	Answer and Explanation
cause of increased incidence of primary CNS lymphomas	*AIDS* [Most malignant CNS lymphomas are metastatic and involve leptomeninges. Complication of advanced AIDS (CD_4 T helper count <50 cells/μL). HIV/EBV viruses (100% of cases) are implicated. High-grade lymphomas. Multifocal and involve CNS parenchyma (space-occupying lesion).]
CNS causes of calcification	• **old age:** calcified pineal gland, • *meningioma,* • *low-grade astrocytoma,* • *oligodendroglioma,* • *hypoparathyroidism:* basal ganglia, • *tuberous sclerosis,* • *AVM:* tram track appearance of vessels, • *cysticercosis,* • *old subdural hematoma,* • *primary HPTH,* • *calcified atherosclerotic fusiform aneurysm*

Question: Which of the following CNS disorders are associated with noncommunicating hydrocephalus? **SELECT 3**
- (A) Aqueductal stenosis
- (B) Subarachnoid hemorrhage
- (C) Lead encephalopathy
- (D) Vitamin A toxicity
- (E) Pseudotumor cerebri
- (F) Choroid plexus papilloma
- (G) Ependymoma of fourth ventricle
- (H) Alzheimer's disease
- (I) Medulloblastoma

Answers: (A), (G), (I): Aqueductal stenosis **(choice A)** is the most common cause of hydrocephalus in adults and type of noncommunicating hydrocephalus. A subarachnoid hemorrhage is the most common cause of a communicating type of hydrocephalus owing to blood blocking the arachnoid granulations along the convexity of the brain **(choice B is incorrect)**. Lead poisoning **(choice C is incorrect)**, vitamin A toxicity **(choice D is incorrect)**, and pseudotumor cerebri **(choice E is incorrect)** are associated with increased intracranial pressure but no evidence of hydrocephalus. A choroid plexus papilloma is a common cause of a communicating hydrocephalus due to an increase in production of CSF **(choice F is incorrect)**. Ependymomas of the fourth ventricle **(choice G)** and medulloblastomas, which are located in the cerebellum **(choice I)** produce a noncommunicating hydrocephalus by blocking the exit of CSF through the foramina. Alzheimer's disease leads to cerebral atrophy, which causes hydrocephalus ex vacuo owing to loss of brain substance rather than an increase in intracranial pressure **(choice H is incorrect)**.

AIDS = acquired immunodeficiency syndrome, ALL = acute lympho-blastic leukemia, AVM = arteriovenous malformation, Cl⁻ = chloride ion, CNS = central nervous system, CPR = cardiopulmonary resuscita-tion, CSF = cerebrospinal fluid, CT = computed tomography, EBV = Epstein-Barr virus, EEG = electroencephalogram, GABA = γ-aminobu-tyric acid, GBM = glioblastoma multiforme, HIV = human immunodefi-ciency virus, HPTH = hyperparathyroidism, HTN = hypertension, MC = most common, MCC = most common cause, MRI = magnetic resonance imaging, RHF = right heart failure, R/O = rule out, Rx = treatment, SIADH = syndrome of inappropriate antidiuretic hormone, S/S = signs and symptoms, SVC = superior vena cava, TIA = transient ischemic attack, UMN = upper motor neuron.

Table 15–7. CENTRAL NERVOUS SYSTEM INFECTIONS, NEUROLOGIC DISORDERS IN ACQUIRED IMMUNODEFICIENCY SYNDROME, DEMYELINATING DISORDERS

Most Common...	Answer and Explanation
types of CNS infections	• **leptomeningitis:** pia mater inflammation, • *encephalitis:* brain inflammation, • *meningo-encephalitis:* combination of above, • *cerebral abscess,* • *pachymeningitis:* epidural in-flammation, • *subdural abscess*
methods of transmission of CNS infection	• **hematogenous,** • *traumatic,* • *ascending:* e.g., rabies, • *local extension:* e.g., * mastoid-itis, * sinusitis
method of transmission of leptomeningitis	*hematogenous*
S/S of leptomeningitis	• **fever,** • *headache,* • *nuchal rigidity,* • *al-tered sensorium* [Triad of fever, nuchal rigid-ity, and altered sensorium is present in ~65% of patients.]
S/S of encephalitis	• **mental status alterations,** • *drowsiness,* • *headache*
CSF differences between viral and bacterial meningitis	• *viral:* * normal glucose, * lymphocyte-domi-nant smear (neutrophil dominant in first 48 h), • *bacterial:* * low glucose, * neutrophil dominant smear, * positive Gram stain
cause of aseptic meningitis	*virus:* * aseptic meningitis refers to a patient with S/S of meningitis and CSF findings of meningitis but Gram stain/bacterial cultures are negative, * most are viral
causes of viral meningitis in summer	• **enteroviruses:** * 85%, * coxsackievirus MC, • *HIV,* • *CMV,* • *HSV 1,2,* • *human herpes viruses 6, 7,* • *EBV,* • *Colorado tick fever virus*

Table 15–7. CENTRAL NERVOUS SYSTEM INFECTIONS, NEUROLOGIC DISORDERS IN ACQUIRED IMMUNODEFICIENCY SYNDROME, DEMYELINATING DISORDERS *Continued*

Most Common...	Answer and Explanation
cause of viral meningitis in winter and spring	*mumps*
childhood disease causing self-limited viral meningitis	*mumps:* * 15%, * low CSF glucose, * deafness may occur
viral cause of hemorrhagic necrosis of the temporal lobes	*HSV-1*
clinical findings of HSV-1 encephalitis	• *fever,* • *headache,* • *simultaneous herpes labialis in 10–15%,* • *seizures,* • *CSF findings:* * elevated pressure, * high WBC count, * increased RBCs, * normal/low glucose, • *MRI better than CT for Dx,* • *CSF PCR to detect HSV DNA:* brain Bx no longer recommended, • *EEG* shows periodic lateralized epileptiform discharges
Rx of HSV encephalitis	*acyclovir*
vector of encephalitis due to arborviruses	*mosquito:* * infection occurs in summer months, * most cases are subclinical
arbovirus infection in the United States	*St. Louis encephalitis:* English sparrows are the natural host
arbovirus infection with greatest mortality	*Eastern equine encephalitis:* * 50% mortality, * wild birds natural host, * low CSF glucose
childhood meningitis transmitted by rodent urine	*lymphocytic choriomeningitis:* * due to an RNA virus that infects mice, * CSF has profound lymphocytosis, * >25% have permanent neurologic damage
childhood disease associated with a self-limited cerebellitis	*varicella*

Table continued on following page

Table 15–7. CENTRAL NERVOUS SYSTEM INFECTIONS, NEUROLOGIC DISORDERS IN ACQUIRED IMMUNODEFICIENCY SYNDROME, DEMYELINATING DISORDERS *Continued*

Most Common...	Answer and Explanation
cause of rabies in the United States	• **skunk bite,** • *raccoon:* Northeast, • *bats,* • *fox,* • *coyotes,* • *dogs:* rare [See Table 2–2 for full discussion.]
clinical findings of poliovirus infection	• **flaccid paralysis:** * paraplegia, * quadriplegia, * paralysis less severe in children, • *CN palsies:* bulbar involvement, • *post-polio syndrome:* 25–35 years later [Virus first infects tonsils → Peyer's patches → regional lymph nodes → hematogenous spread. Paralysis due to viral destruction of anterior horn cells in spinal cord/medulla. Outbreaks occur in summer. See Table 2–2.]
types of slow virus disease	• **PML,** • *SSPE,* • *CJ* [See Table 15–2]
cause of PML	*papovavirus* (JC virus, SV 40 virus): * produces subacute demyelination of CNS white matter, * infects/destroys oligodendrocytes
clinical associations in PML	• **AIDS,** • *lymphoproliferative disease,* • *immunosuppression from organ transplant*
clinical findings in PML	• *solitary brain lesions,* • *progressive dementia:* * invariably fatal, • *Dx:* * brain Bx, * PCR detecting viral DNA, • *no Rx*
cause of SSPE	*rubeola virus:* * part of primary infection or complication of live virus vaccine, * virus invades oligodendrocytes and produces extensive demyelination
clinical findings in SSPE	• *MC in children <11 years old,* • *progressive mental deterioration,* • *death in 1–2 y,* • *brain Bx necessary for Dx,* • *no Rx*
risk factors for bacterial meningitis	• *acute otitis media,* • *alcoholism,* • *altered immune states:* e.g., * splenectomy, * hypogammaglobulinemia, • *pneumonia,* • *DM,* • *sinusitis,* • *CSF leak*
causes of bacterial meningitis in children between 1 mth and 18 y old	• ***Neisseria meningitidis:*** gram-negative diplococcus, • *Streptococcus pneumoniae:* gram-positive diplococcus, • *Haemophilus influenzae:* * gram-negative coccobacillus, * immunization has dramatically reduced its incidence

Table 15-7. CENTRAL NERVOUS SYSTEM INFECTIONS, NEUROLOGIC DISORDERS IN ACQUIRED IMMUNODEFICIENCY SYNDROME, DEMYELINATING DISORDERS *Continued*

Most Common...	Answer and Explanation
cause of bacterial meningitis in adults	*Streptococcus pneumoniae*
cause of bacterial meningitis post-neurosurgery or head trauma	*Streptococcus pneumoniae*
cause of ventriculitis/meningitis in ventriculoperitoneal shunt	• **Staphylococcus epidermidis:** gram-positive coccus, • *Staphylococcus aureus:* gram-positive coccus, • *Escherichia coli:* gram-negative rod
bacterial meningitis associated with sterile subdural effusions	*Haemophilus influenzae:* * subdural effusions are sterile, * may produce focal neurologic signs
bacterial causes of meningitis in immunosuppressed adults and elderly	• **Streptococcus pneumoniae,** • *Listeria monocytogenes:* gram-positive rod
complications of meningitis	• **temporary paralysis,** • *permanent deafness,* • *mental retardation,* • *hydrocephalus,* • *epilepsy,* • *CN VI palsy,* • *Waterhouse Friderichsen syndrome:* see Table 11-4
empiric Rx of suspected bacterial meningitis	*ceftriaxone*
Rx of *Streptococcus pneumoniae* meningitis	*IV penicillin G:* * skin test penicillin allergic patients, * desensitize if necessary
Rx of *Neisseria meningitidis* meningitis	*IV penicillin G:* all family members in contact with patient should be Rx with rifampin to eradicate carrier state (nasopharynx)
Rx of *Haemophilus influenzae* meningitis	*IV ceftazidime + gentamicin*
Rx of *Staphylococcus epidermidis* meningitis	*IV vancomycin:* shunt may have to be removed

Table continued on following page

Table 15–7. CENTRAL NERVOUS SYSTEM INFECTIONS, NEUROLOGIC DISORDERS IN ACQUIRED IMMUNODEFICIENCY SYNDROME, DEMYELINATING DISORDERS *Continued*

Most Common...	Answer and Explanation
Rx of *Listeria monocytogenes* meningitis	*IV ampicillin + aminoglycoside*
recommendation for dexamethasone in Rx of bacterial meningitis	*controversial:* most recommend its use to prevent neurologic complications
complications associated with TB meningitis	• **noncommunicating hydrocephalus,** • *stroke:* vasculitis, • *SIADH* [Complication of primary TB in children. Involves base of brain and produces a vasculitis (stroke potential) and scarring (hydrocephalus potential).]
CSF findings in TB meningitis	• *high protein,* • *low glucose,* • *<500 cells/µL:* lymphocytes/monocytes, • *low chloride*
Rx of TB meningitis	*INH + RIF + ETB + PZA + dexamethasone*
types of neurosyphilis	• **meningovascular,** • *paretic form,* • *tabes dorsalis,* • *gumma:* presents as a mass lesion
clinical findings in meningovascular syphilis	• **acute/subacute meningitis,** • *vasculitis:* * endarteritis obliterans, * stroke potential, * focal neurologic signs, • *may progress to paresis or tabes*
clinical findings in paretic type of neurosyphilis	• **chronic meningoencephalitis,** • *progressive dementia,* • *frontal lobe atrophy,* • *generalized limb weakness,* • *organisms present in brain*
clinical findings in tabes dorsalis	• *attacks posterior root ganglia and cord,* • *lancinating pain,* • *wide-based gait,* • *absent DTRs,* • *sphincter dysfunction,* • *Argyll Robertson pupil:* ~95%, • *loss of proprioception,* • *Charcot joint:* see Table 12–1
CSF findings in neurosyphilis	• **positive VDRL:** * 25–55%, * best initial test, • *positive CSF FTA-ABS:* * 80–95%, * CDC does not recommend this study (? its meaning), • *oligoclonal bands on CSF high resolution electrophoresis:* * 75%, * indicates demyelination, • *high CSF protein,* • *CSF lymphocytosis:* 200–300 cells/µL, • *normal CSF glucose*

Table 15–7. CENTRAL NERVOUS SYSTEM INFECTIONS, NEUROLOGIC DISORDERS IN ACQUIRED IMMUNODEFICIENCY SYNDROME, DEMYELINATING DISORDERS *Continued*

Most Common...	Answer and Explanation
Rx of neurosyphilis	*IV aqueous penicillin* (12–24 million units) or *IM procaine penicillin* (2.4 million units)
CNS clinical/lab findings in the disseminated phase of early Lyme disease	• **fluctuating symptoms of meningitis plus bilateral CN VII Bell's palsy and peripheral radiculoneuropathy,** • *CSF findings:* * cell count <100 cells/µL, * pleocytosis, * normal to low glucose, * increased protein [See Table 12–1.]
CNS clinical findings in late stage Lyme disease	• **encephalopathy with mental status abnormalities,** • *axonal peripheral neuropathy*
Rx of CNS Lyme disease	*ceftriaxone*
systemic fungal cause of meningitis	*Cryptococcus neoformans:* particularly in immunocompromised hosts
types of CNS abscesses	• **brain,** • *epidural,* • *subdural*
cause of solitary cerebral abscess	*extension of infection from adjacent focus of infection:* e.g., * sinusitis, * mastoiditis
cause of multiple cerebral abscesses	*hematogenous spread:* e.g., * cyanotic CHD, * bronchiectasis
sign of cerebral abscess	*hemiplegia*
CSF findings in cerebral abscess	• *normal glucose,* • *increased protein,* • *increased leukocytes*
cause of epidural abscess	*direct extension:* e.g., * adjacent osteomyelitis, * mastoiditis, * paranasal sinus infection
clinical findings of an epidural abscess	• **fever with neutrophilic leukocytosis,** • *local findings of pain, swelling overlying abscess,* • *venous sinus thrombophlebitis,* • *extension through dura to produce subdural abscess, meningitis,* • *Rx with antibiotics,* • *surgical drainage may be necessary*
cause of subdural abscess	*infection of paranasal sinuses or middle ear*

Table continued on following page

Table 15–7. CENTRAL NERVOUS SYSTEM INFECTIONS, NEUROLOGIC DISORDERS IN ACQUIRED IMMUNODEFICIENCY SYNDROME, DEMYELINATING DISORDERS *Continued*

Most Common...	Answer and Explanation
clinical findings of a subdural abscess	• **fever with neutrophilic leukocytosis,** • *seizures,* • *hemiparesis,* • *localized with CT/ MRI,* • *must surgically drain and Rx with antibiotics,* • *mortality 25%,* • *COD:* venous sinus thrombosis with infarction
cause of frontal lobe abscess in DKA	*Mucor:* * invades brain through cribriform plate, * hyperglycemia increases proliferation
Rx of rhinocerebral mucormycosis	*amphotericin B*
fungal cause of meningitis in immunocompromised patients	*Cryptococcus neoformans:* * India ink test has 50–60% sensitivity, * perform latex agglutination if India ink test is negative
Rx of *Cryptococcus neoformans* in CNS	*amphotericin B + flucytosine*
type of malaria involving the CNS	*Plasmodium falciparum*
Rx of cerebral malaria	*IV quinidine or quinine:* exchange transfusion may be necessary in severe parasitemia
protozoa producing meningoencephalitis after swimming in fresh water	*Naegleria fowleri*
Rx of amebic meningoencephalitis	*amphotericin B*
parasitic cause of focal epileptic seizures worldwide	*cysticercosis due to Taenia solium:* eggs ingested by humans from an infected human host (definitive host) become larvae (intermediate host), which invade CNS (50–70%), eyes, skin, and other sites
clinical findings in CNS cysticercosis	• **focal epileptic seizures,** • *hemiparesis,* • *ataxia,* • *ring-enhancing lesion(s) on CT*
Rx of CNS cysticercosis	*praziquantel + corticosteroids*

**Table 15–7. CENTRAL NERVOUS SYSTEM INFECTIONS,
NEUROLOGIC DISORDERS IN ACQUIRED
IMMUNODEFICIENCY SYNDROME,
DEMYELINATING DISORDERS** Continued

Most Common...	Answer and Explanation
route of transmission of HIV into the CNS	• **monocytes/macrophages:** reservoir of HIV, • *astrocytes lining blood-brain barrier:* oligodendrocytes and microglial cells also infected by HIV
reservoir cell of HIV in CNS	*microglial cells:* form multinucleated giant cells to concentrate HIV
CNS neurologic disorder in AIDS	• **AIDS dementia complex** (ADC), • *toxoplasmosis,* • *primary CNS lymphoma:* see Table 15–6, • *CMV encephalitis,* • *cryptococcal meningitis,* • *PML,* • *vacuolar myelopathy,* • *aseptic meningitis,* • *peripheral neuropathy:* Guillain-Barré-like syndrome of ascending paralysis
clinical findings in ADC	• *motor impairment:* e.g., * tremors, * ataxia, * spasticity, • *cognitive deficits:* e.g., * memory loss, * concentration deficits, • *behavioral dysfunction:* e.g., * social withdrawal, * hallucinations, * delusions
MRI findings in ADC	*diffuse cerebral atrophy*
Rx of ADC	*high-dose zidovudine* (AZT)
cause of space-occupying lesion in CNS in AIDS	*Toxoplasma gondii:* * sporozoan, * produces multiple, ring-enhanced lesions
clinical findings in *Toxoplasma* encephalitis	• **focal neurologic deficits:** ~70%, • *confusion,* • *headache,* • *focal epileptic seizures*
indication/Rx for chemoprophylaxis against toxoplasmosis in AIDS	• *seropositive for Toxoplasma,* • *CD_4 T helper count <100 cells/μL,* • *Rx:* TMP/SMX [Test for IgG antibodies against *Toxoplasma* is part of initial work-up in HIV-positive patients.]
Rx of CNS toxoplasmosis	*pyrimethamine + clindamycin or sulfadiazine:* TMP/SMX prophylaxis against *Pneumocystis carinii* offers some protection against toxoplasmosis

Table continued on following page

Table 15–7. CENTRAL NERVOUS SYSTEM INFECTIONS, NEUROLOGIC DISORDERS IN ACQUIRED IMMUNODEFICIENCY SYNDROME, DEMYELINATING DISORDERS *Continued*

Most Common...	Answer and Explanation
clinical findings in vacuolar myelopathy	*subacute combined degeneration of spinal cord:* * posterior column + lateral corticospinal tract disease, * similar to B_{12} deficiency
CNS viral infection in AIDS	*CMV*
cause of lumbosacral polyradiculomyo-pathy in AIDS	*CMV*
Rx of CMV infections in AIDS	*ganciclovir:* foscarnet is used in cases resistant to ganciclovir
CNS fungal infection in AIDS	*Cryptococcus neoformans*
mechanisms of demyelination	• **autoimmune destruction of myelin sheath,** • *destruction of oligodendrocytes (Schwann cells in PNS)*
demyelinating diseases	• **multiple sclerosis** (MS), • *transverse myelitis,* • *optic neuritis,* • *Devic's syndrome,* • *nutritional disorders:* e.g., * B_{12} deficiency, * Marchiafava-Bignami (demyelination of corpus callosum in alcoholics with thiamine deficiency), • *acute disseminated encephalomyelitis:* post-infectious childhood disease like measles or post-vaccination, • *viral disease:* e.g., * SSPE, * PML
effect of demyelination on nerve impulses	*slows or blocks nerve impulses*
causative factors implicated in MS	• **autoimmune disease:** * antibodies directed against myelin sheath, * more common in women, • *HLA DW2 haplotype:* 65%, • *genetic relationship:* increased incidence in monozygotic twins, • *viral inciting agent:* e.g., * herpesvirus 6, * measles, * retrovirus, • *northern/southern latitudes* [Targets individuals between 20 and 40 y old.]
symptoms of MS	• **paresthesias,** • **unilateral visual impairment:** optic neuritis, • *unsteadiness,* • *diplopia,* • *vertigo,* • *muscle weakness/fatigue,* •

Table 15–7. CENTRAL NERVOUS SYSTEM INFECTIONS, NEUROLOGIC DISORDERS IN ACQUIRED IMMUNODEFICIENCY SYNDROME, DEMYELINATING DISORDERS *Continued*

Most Common...	Answer and Explanation
Continued	*scanning speech:* sound drunk, • *urinary disturbances* [Symptoms follow an episodic course of neurologic dysfunction punctuated by acute relapses/remissions. ~70% remain functional 10 y after first attack.]
signs of MS	• **optic neuritis:** see Table 15–2, • *intention tremor,* • *nystagmus:* see Table 15–2, • *preservation of intellect,* • *bilateral INO:* see Table 15–2, • *lower extremity spasticity,* • *labile mood,* • Lhermitte's sign: electric shock-like sensation radiating to extremities with neck flexion
highly predictive isolated findings suggesting MS	*involvement of optic nerve, brain stem, or spinal cord*
lab/radiologic findings in MS	• *imaging:* MRI most sensitive for detecting plaques, • *evoked potentials:* see Table 15–1, • *CSF findings:* see Table 15–1: * increased protein, * oligoclonal bands, * <50 cells/μL (usually T lymphocytes), * normal glucose, * increased MBP (♦ encephalitogenic protein, ♦ not useful)
clinically definite findings in MS	*evidence by history/neurologic exam or both of two distinct attacks separated in time with objective evidence of neurologic dysfunction in separate areas of the central white matter:* one objective sign can also be * oligoclonal bands in CSF, * positive evoked potential, or * MRI lesions
favorable signs in MS	• *onset <40 years of age,* • *female sex,* • *optic neuritis,* • *sensory finding:* paresthesias first manifestation, • *infrequent recurrences*
unfavorable signs in MS	• *onset >40 years of age,* • *cerebellar/pyramidal tract involvement as first manifestation,* • *frequent recurrences*
Rx for MS	• **interferon-β:** decreases number of relapses, • *ACTH injections,* • *methylprednisolone*

Table continued on following page

Table 15–7. CENTRAL NERVOUS SYSTEM INFECTIONS, NEUROLOGIC DISORDERS IN ACQUIRED IMMUNODEFICIENCY SYNDROME, DEMYELINATING DISORDERS *Continued*

Most Common...	Answer and Explanation
clinical findings in Devic's syndrome	*bilateral optic nerve neuritis + transverse myelitis*
clinical finding in acute transverse myelitis	• *previous URI* (e.g., enterovirus) *or vaccination often precedes the neurologic dysfunction*, • *other associations:* * SLE, * MS, * TB, * syphilis, * herpes zoster, * malignancy, • *rapid onset of ascending or transverse spinal cord dysfunction:* * midthoracic, * high thoracic–low cervical region, • *weakness/paresthesias in lower extremities*, • *Brown-Séquard syndrome* [Delayed-type of immune destruction of myelin. One-third recover spontaneously.]
diagnostic findings in acute transverse myelitis	• *MRI:* best imaging test to R/O other causes of spinal cord dysfunction, • *CSF:* * increased protein, * <100 cells (usually lymphocytes)/ μL
Rx of acute transverse myelitis	• *IV dexmethasone*, • *Rx infection, if present*, • *radiotherapy if due to malignancy*

Question: Which of the following conditions are associated with an increased CSF protein with low glucose? **SELECT 3**
  (A) Multiple sclerosis
  (B) Cryptococcosis in AIDS
  (C) Cerebral abscess
  (D) Guillain-Barré syndrome
  (E) Neurosyphilis
  (F) Leptomeningeal spread of cancer
  (G) Mumps meningoencephalitis
  (H) *Neisseria meningitidis* meningitis
  (I) Enterovirus meningitis

Answers: (F), (G), (H): Multiple sclerosis, cryptococcosis in AIDS, a cerebral abscess, Guillain-Barré syndrome, neurosyphilis, and an enterovirus cause of meningitis all have an increase in CSF protein with a normal CSF glucose (**choices A, B, C, D, E, I are incorrect**). Leptomeningeal spread of cancer (**choice F**), mumps meningoencephalitis (**choice G**), and *Neisseria meningitidis* meningitis (**choice H**) are all associated with a high CSF protein and a low CSF glucose.

ACTH = adrenocorticotropic hormone, ADC = AIDS dementia complex, AIDS = acquired immunodeficiency virus, AZT = zidovudine, Bx = biopsy, CDC = Center for Disease Control and Prevention, CHD = congenital heart disease, CJ = Creutzfeldt-Jakob syndrome, CMV = cytomegalovirus, CN = cranial nerve, CNS = central nervous system, COD = cause of death, CSF = cerebrospinal fluid, CT = computed tomography, DKA = diabetic ketoacidosis, DM = diabetes mellitus, DTRs = deep tendon reflexes, Dx = diagnosis, EBV = Epstein-Barr virus, EEG = electroencephalogram, ETB = ethambutol, FTA-ABS = fluorescent treponema antibody absorption test, HIV = human immunodeficiency virus, HLA = human leukocyte antigen, HSV = herpes simplex virus, Ig = immunoglobulin, IM = intramuscular, INH = isoniazid, INO = internuclear ophthalmoplegia, IV = intravenous, LA = latex agglutination, MBP = myelin basic protein, MC = most common, MRI = magnetic resonance imaging, MS = multiple sclerosis, PCR = polymerase chain reaction, PML = progressive multifocal leukoencephalopathy, PNS = peripheral nervous system, PZA = pyrazinamide, RBC = red blood cell, RIF = rifampin, R/O = rule out, Rx = treatment, SIADH = syndrome of inappropriate antidiuretic hormone, SLE = systemic lupus erythematosus, S/S = signs and symptoms, SSPE = subacute sclerosing panencephalitis, TB = tuberculosis, TMP/SMX = trimethoprim/sulfamethoxazole, URI = upper respiratory infection, VDRL = Veneral Disease Research Laboratory, WBC = white blood cell.

Table 15–8. SPINAL CORD DISORDERS, NEUROCUTANEOUS DISORDERS, CRANIOCERVICAL JUNCTION ABNORMALITIES, AND PERIPHERAL NERVE DISORDERS

Most Common...	Answer and Explanation
mechansism of spinal cord injury	• **dislocation with or without fracture at the atlas-axis junction**, • *fracture-dislocations with or without bony fragmentation at other spinal levels*, • *penetrating missile or stab wounds*
locations for dislocations of spine	• *C7–T1 junction*, • *T12–L1 junction*
hallmarks of spinal cord dysfunction	*interruption of motor, sensory, autonomic function below a level of injury*
spinal cord segments involved in bulbocavernous reflex	*S1 and S2:* * reflex dependent on intact S1/S2, * stimulus to glans penis/vaginal wall should cause anal sphincter contraction around examiner's finger, * absence of reflex with spinal cord injury indicates S1/S2 involved

Table continued on following page

Table 15–8. SPINAL CORD DISORDERS, NEUROCUTANEOUS DISORDERS, CRANIOCERVICAL JUNCTION ABNORMALITIES, AND PERIPHERAL NERVE DISORDERS *Continued*

Most Common...	Answer and Explanation
types of shock associated with spinal injures	• *spinal cord shock,* • *neurogenic shock*
clinical findings in spinal shock	• *occurs soon after either complete/partial spinal cord injuries,* • *absence of motor, sensory, autonomic function below level of injury,* • *spinal shock disappears in 1–3 d,* • *previously flaccid muscle becomes spastic,* • *DTRs exaggerated,* • *positive Babinski's*
clinical findings in neurogenic shock	• **dysfunction of descending sympathetic pathways,** • *heart/BV nonresponsive to sympathetic responses*: * no compensatory tachycardia, * bradycardia present, • *vasomotor tone decreased*: pooling of blood
differences of neurogenic vs hypovolemic shock and intracranial hypertension	• *neurogenic shock*: hypotension + sinus bradycardia, • *hypovolemic shock*: hypotension + sinus tachycardia, • *intracranial HTN*: diastolic HTN + sinus bradycardia
findings in complete spinal cord injury	• **sine qua non of complete injury is lack of anal sphincter tone/sensations in perianal area after 24 h**, • *flaccid motor paralysis below level of damage,* • *total anesthesia in same distribution as motor paralysis,* • *bladder dysfunction,* • *immediate onset of priapism*: delayed onset due to an incomplete spinal cord injury that has progressed to complete spinal cord injury, • *superficial reflexes and DTRs absent below level of lesion,* • *absent sweating/skin vasomotor tone*
findings in anterior cord syndrome	• *cause*: hyperflexion injury in cervical region: e.g., * trauma, * acute central intervertebral disk disease, * anterior spinal artery occlusion, • *anterior half of cord damaged*: includes central gray matter and fibers of spinothalamic tract that cross center, * no posterior column dysfunction, • *tetraparesis/-plegia,* • *bilateral pain/temperature impairment below lesion,* • *urinary retention*

Table 15–8. SPINAL CORD DISORDERS, NEUROCUTANEOUS DISORDERS, CRANIOCERVICAL JUNCTION ABNORMALITIES, AND PERIPHERAL NERVE DISORDERS *Continued*

Most Common...	Answer and Explanation
findings in central cord syndrome	• *cause*: hyperextension of cervical region, • *sites of damage*: * central gray matter, * fibers of lateral spinothalamic tracts that cross center, • *quadriplegia*, • *upper extremities more involved than lower*
findings in Brown-Séquard syndrome	• *causes*: * **penetrating injury**, * radiation myelopathy, • *hemisection of spinal cord*, • *ipsilateral*: * loss of position/vibration sense, * spastic hemiparesis, * vasomotor paralysis below level of lesion, • *contralateral*: * loss of pain/temperature below the T12 level, * loss of sensation in perineum/genitals
findings in posterolateral cord syndrome	• *cause*: * MS, * AIDS vacuolar myelopathy, * B$_{12}$ deficiency, • *loss of position/vibratory sensation*: posterior column, • *preservation of pain/temperature sensation*: intact crossed spinothalamic tracts, • *spastic paraparesis*: lateral corticospinal tract involved
findings in anterior commissure syndrome	• *cause*: syringomyelia, • *bilateral loss of pain/temperature sensation*, • *weakness of intrinsic muscles of hand*, • *bladder/bowel incontinence*
Rx of spinal cord injury	• **immobilization:** e.g., rigid cervical collar, • *correct hypotension with crystalloids or pneumatic antishock garment*, • *corticosteroids*: reduce cord edema, • *prophylactic antibiotics for penetrating injuries*, • *NG tube*: if paralytic ileus occurs, • *neurosurgical consult*, • *avoid lumbar puncture*, • *prevent complications*: e.g., * pressure ulcers, * pneumonia, etc.
cause of spinal cord concussion	*high-velocity missile wounds passing close to spinal canal*: S/S resolve rapidly
causes of spinal cord compression	• **trauma**, • *epidural tumor*, • *herniated intervertebral disk*, • *epidural/subdural abscess/hematoma*, • *AVM*
causes of extradural hematomas	• **trauma**, • *anticoagulants*, • *AVM*, • *hemophilia*

Table continued on following page

**Table 15–8. SPINAL CORD DISORDERS,
NEUROCUTANEOUS DISORDERS, CRANIOCERVICAL
JUNCTION ABNORMALITIES, AND PERIPHERAL NERVE
DISORDERS** *Continued*

Most Common...	Answer and Explanation
extradural spinal tumors leading to cord compression	*metastatic breast, prostate, lung* [85% have evidence of vertebral metastasis.]
site for extradural compression of cord due to cancer	• **thoracic**: 70%, • *lumbar*: 20%, • *multiple noncontiguous sites*: 10–40%, • *cervical*: 10%
clinical findings in extradural compression on the cord	• **pain comes first**, • *second*: corticospinal tract dysfunction: * weakness, * spasticity, * hyperreflexia, • *third*: posterior column disease: * paresthesias, * loss of vibration/position sense, • *bladder/bowel dysfunction if conus medullaris or cauda equina compressed* [Distal signs occur before proximal signs.]
Rx of spinal cord compression	• *MRI entire spine to identify all lesions,* • *dexamethasone,* • *radiation for metastatic lesions*: >80% ambulatory after radiation, • *neurosurgical consultation*
clinical findings of spinal cord compression	• *back pain at level of compression,* • *difficulty with walking,* • *sensory impairment,* • *urinary retention with overflow incontinence*
noncompressive spinal cord lesion associated with weakness	*acute transverse myelitis*: see Table 15–7
cause of paraplegia following hypotension in surgery	*ischemic infarction of cord*: in watershed area between descending anterior spinal artery and aberrant ascending spinal artery of Adamkiewicz
intradural spinal tumors	• **meningioma**: * **thoracic region**/foramen magnum, * increased CSF protein, • *neurofibroma*: * arise from dorsal root, * radicular pain, * association with NF, * increased CSF protein
intramedullary spinal tumors	• **ependymoma**: see Table 15–6, • *astrocytoma*

Table 15–8. SPINAL CORD DISORDERS, NEUROCUTANEOUS DISORDERS, CRANIOCERVICAL JUNCTION ABNORMALITIES, AND PERIPHERAL NERVE DISORDERS *Continued*

Most Common...	Answer and Explanation
phakomatoses	• **neurofibromatosis**: see Table 3–2, • *Sturge-Weber syndrome:* see Table 5–3, • *tuberous sclerosis* [Phakomatoses are ectodermal/CNS abnormalities.]
CNS findings in neurofibromatosis	• *meningioma,* • *acoustic neuromas*: often bilateral, • *optic gliomas*
S/S of Sturge-Weber syndrome	• *port-wine stain in the trigeminal nerve distribution,* • *ipsilateral AV malformation,* • *mental retardation*
S/S of tuberous sclerosis	• *AD disease*: * 25%, * remainder are new mutations, • *epileptic seizures*: 80%, • *mental retardation*: 60%, • *hamartomas*: * subependymal astrocytic proliferations on ventricle walls, * bilateral angiomyolipomas of the kidneys (80%), • *adenoma sebaceum of skin,* • *subungual fibromas,* • *shagreen patches*: connective tissue nevus, • *hypopigmented macules,* • *rhabdomyoma of heart*: MC primary heart tumor in children
open neural tube defect	*spina bifida occulta*: * dimple/tuck of hair over L5–S1, * failure of closure of vertebral arch
craniocervical junction abnormalities	• **syringomyelia**, • *Arnold-Chiari syndrome*
site for syringomyelia	*fluid-filled cavity* (syrinx) *in central portion of cervical spinal cord*: * MRI demonstrates cord enlargement, * proceeds distally
clinical findings in syringomeylia	• *destruction of crossed lateral spinothalamic tracts*: * loss of pain/temperature in cape-like distribution, * patients burn hands and cannot feel it, • *atrophy of intrinsic hand muscle*: anterior horn destruction confused with ALS, • *areflexia in upper extremities*: destruction of LMNs, • *hyperreflexia in lower extremities*: lateral corticospinal tract, • *Horner's syndrome*: * miosis, * lid lag, * anhidrosis, • *associations*: * intraspinal tumors, * Arnold-Chiari syndrome, • *independent cavities may occur in medulla*: syringobulbia

Table continued on following page

Table 15–8. SPINAL CORD DISORDERS, NEUROCUTANEOUS DISORDERS, CRANIOCERVICAL JUNCTION ABNORMALITIES, AND PERIPHERAL NERVE DISORDERS *Continued*

Most Common...	Answer and Explanation
clinical findings in Arnold-Chiari syndrome	• *elongation of medulla oblongata/cerebellar tonsils through foramen magnum*, • *platybasia*: flat base of skull, • *meningomyelocele*, • *hydrocephalus*: ~50%, • *syringomyelia*
types of peripheral neuropathy	• *mononeuropathy*: dysfunction of one nerve, • *polyneuropathy*: dysfunction of more than one nerve, • *motor neuropathy*, • *sensory neuropathy*, • *mixed*
sites of median nerve entrapment	• **wrist**: * carpal tunnel syndrome, * see Table 12–1, • *pronator muscle in forearm*
sites of ulnar nerve entrapment	• **elbow**, • *wrist* [Loss of dorsal interosseous muscles produces claw hand. Numbness of 5th digit and contiguous half of ring finger.]
site of radial nerve entrapment	*humeral groove*: radial nerve palsy with wrist drop
site of brachial plexus entrapment	*thoracic outlet*: thoracic outlet syndrome
clinical findings in thoracic outlet syndrome	• **neurovascular compression syndrome**: * cervical rib, * tight scalenus anticus muscles, * common in weight lifters, • *arm falls asleep at night*, • *pain, paresthesias, numbness in one or more brachial plexus nerve trunks*, • *radial pulse weakens when head is turned to side of the lesion*: Adson's test, • *subclavian artery bruit*, • *arteriography confirmatory test*
site of sciatic nerve entrapment	*sciatic notch in buttocks*
site of peroneal nerve entrapment	*behind knee*: * common in people who cross their legs, * slapping gait
site of lateral femoral nerve entrapment	*inguinal ligament*: * produces meralgia paresthetica, * numbness/burning sensation over lateral thigh when walking/prolonged standing
cause of intervertebral disk disease	*degeneration of fibrocartilage/nucleus pulposus*: * ruptured disk may herniate posteriorly and compress nerve root and/or spinal cord, * pain radiates from low back, to buttocks, down leg, below knee: sciatica

Table 15–8. SPINAL CORD DISORDERS, NEUROCUTANEOUS DISORDERS, CRANIOCERVICAL JUNCTION ABNORMALITIES, AND PERIPHERAL NERVE DISORDERS *Continued*

Most Common...	Answer and Explanation
disk herniation	*L5–S1*
S/S of herniation of L5–S1 disk	• *pain*: S1 distribution: * back of thigh, * back of calf, * lateral foot, • *sensory loss*: * lateral/posterior calf, * plantar aspect of foot, • *reflex loss*: Achilles' reflex, • *motor deficit*: * plantar flexion, * eversion of foot
S/S of herniation of L3–L4 disk	• *pain*: L4 distribution: down to medial malleolus, • *sensory loss*: medial leg to malleolus, • *reflex loss*: knee jerk, • *motor deficit*: * inversion of foot, * quadriceps
S/S of herniation of L4–L5 disk	• *pain*: L5 distribution: * back of thigh, * lateral calf, * dorsum of foot, • *sensory loss*: * dorsum of foot, * webbed space between great toe, • *reflex loss*: none, • *motor deficit*: * dorsiflexion of toes/foot
S/S of herniation of C4–C5 disk	• *pain*: C5 distribution: * medial scapula, * lateral border arm, • *sensory loss*: lateral border upper arm, • *reflex loss*: biceps, • *motor deficit*: * deltoid, * supraspinatus, * infraspinatus, * rhomboids
S/S of herniation of C5–C6 disk	• *pain*: C6 distribution: * lateral forearm, * thumb, * index finger, • *sensory loss*: * lateral forearm, * index finger, • *reflex loss*: supinator, • *motor deficit*: * biceps, brachioradialis, * pronators/supinators of forearm
S/S of herniation of C6–C7 disk	• *pain*: C7 distribution: * posterior arm, * lateral hand, * mid-forearm, * medial scapula, • *sensory loss*: * mid-forearm, * middle finger, • *reflex loss*: triceps, • *motor deficit*: * latissimus dorsi, * triceps, * pectoralis major, * wrist flexors
S/S of lateral recess syndrome in lumbar spine (facet syndrome)	• *osteophyte on superior articular facet*, • *radicular pain*, • *unilateral/bilateral pain/paresthesias in L5 or S1*, • *pain brought on by walking/standing and relieved by sitting*, • *negative straight leg test*: positive straight leg test indicates a ruptured intervertebral disk

Table continued on following page

Table 15–8. SPINAL CORD DISORDERS, NEUROCUTANEOUS DISORDERS, CRANIOCERVICAL JUNCTION ABNORMALITIES, AND PERIPHERAL NERVE DISORDERS *Continued*

Most Common...	Answer and Explanation
S/S of lumbar stenosis	• *patients >50 y old,* • *symptoms usually bilateral,* • *pain dull/aching,* • *whole extremity involved,* • *pain provoked by walking/standing and relieved by sitting or leaning forward,* • *feeling of deadness in leg*
mechanisms of peripheral neuropathy	• *demyelination*: often segmental, • *axonal degeneration,* • *combination of the two*
S/S of segmental demyelination	• *distal symmetric "glove and stocking" distribution,* • *burning feet,* • *formication*: "feels like insects are biting my legs"
S/S of axonal degeneration	• *denervation,* • *muscle fasciculations/atrophy,* • *muscle weakness,* • *absent DTRs*
cause of distal sensorimotor peripheral neuropathy	• **DM,** • *alcohol,* • *nutritional*: * thiamine deficiency, * pyridoxine deficiency, • *Pb poisoning,* • *drugs*: * vincristine, * isoniazid, • *autoimmune*: Guillain-Barré, • *paraneoplastic syndrome,* • *amyloidosis,* • *toxins*: diptheria
clinical findings in DM neuropathy	• *pathogenesis*: * osmotic damage to Schwann cells, * vascular (focal involvement of two or more nerves), • *sensory changes*: see above, • *motor changes*: see above, • *MCC diabetic ulcers*: cannot feel pain, • *Rx*: * glycemic control, * amitriptyline
cause of acute inflammatory polyradiculo-neuropathy	*Guillain-Barré syndrome* (GBS): * autoimmune demyelinating disease, * destruction myelin sheath of spinal/cranial nerves
clinical findings in GBS	• *precipitating conditions*: * **viral illness** (♦ 50%, ♦ respiratory or GI), * autoimmune disease, * lymphoreticular malignancy, • *afebrile,* • *LMN weakness/paresthesia/pain begins in lower extremities and ascends to involve upper extremities/muscles of respiration*: intubation/respiratory support, • *CN involvement >50%,* • *cardiovascular*: * HTN, * cardiac arrhythmias, • *autonomic neuropathy,* • *bowel/bladder dysfunction rare,* • *recovery over several weeks to months*

Table 15–8. SPINAL CORD DISORDERS, NEUROCUTANEOUS DISORDERS, CRANIOCERVICAL JUNCTION ABNORMALITIES, AND PERIPHERAL NERVE DISORDERS *Continued*

Most Common...	Answer and Explanation
CSF findings in GBS	• *increased protein*: often >100 mg/dL, • *≤20 cells* (lymphocytes)/μL, • *normal glucose*, • *oligoclonal bands present*
Rx of GBS	• **plasmapheresis/IV gamma-globulin**, • *respiratory support if necessary*, • *steroids may exacerbate condition*
COD in GBS	*cardiac arrhythmias*
clinical findings in uremic neuropathy	• *mixed sensory/motor neuropathy*, • *restless legs*, • *calf cramps*, • *improves with dialysis*
clinical findings in tick paralysis	• *ascending motor paralysis similar to GBS*, • *decreased DTRs*, • *reverses with tick removal*
clinical findings in neuropathy secondary to leprosy	• *tuberculoid*: mononeuritis due to nerve injury, • *lepromatous*: * direct nerve invasion, * diminished pain/temperature sensation
neuropathies associated with sarcoidosis	• *symmetric polyneuropathy*, • *single/multiple CN neuropathies*: CN VII MC
cancer associated with paraneoplastic neuropathy	*lung cancer*: * autoantibodies, * primarily sensory
type of neuropathy noted in amyloidosis	*autonomic neuropathy*: primarily sensory
causes of nutritional polyneuropathy	• **thiamine deficiency**: alcoholic, • *pyridoxine deficiency*: post-INH Rx, • *vitamin E deficiency*, • B_{12} *deficiency* [Distal, symmetric sensorimotor neuropathy is MC type.]
heavy metals associated with neuropathy	• **Pb**: * motor neuropathy, * chelation Rx, • *arsenic*: chelation Rx, • *mercury*: Rx with vitamin E/selenium [See Table 7–4.]
drugs associated with toxic neuropathies	• *vincristine*: sensorimotor, • *cisplatin*: sensory, • *nitrofurantoin*: sensorimotor, • *high doses of pyridoxine*: sensory, • *phenytoin*, • *dapsone*
genetic cause of peripheral neuropathy	*Charcot-Marie-Tooth* (CMT) *disease*

Table continued on following page

Table 15–8. SPINAL CORD DISORDERS, NEUROCUTANEOUS DISORDERS, CRANIOCERVICAL JUNCTION ABNORMALITIES, AND PERIPHERAL NERVE DISORDERS *Continued*

Most Common...	Answer and Explanation
clinical findings in CMT disease	• *involves peroneal nerve,* • *muscle atrophy lower legs:* "inverted bottle" or "stork leg" *appearance,* • *pes cavus,* • *stocking/glove sensory loss,* • *decreased ankle DTR*
causes of autonomic neuropathy	• **DM**: *see Table 11–5,* • *amyloidosis,* • *GBS,* • *AIP: see Table 14–1,* • *MS*
clinical findings in autonomic neuropathy	• *orthostatic hypotension,* • *bowel/bladder dysfunction,* • *impotency,* • *peristalsis dysfunction*
disorders with primarily motor neuropathy	• **GBS,** • *chronic inflammatory demyelinating polyneuropathy,* • *AIP,* • *Pb poisoning,* • *organophosphate poisoning,* • *hypoglycemia,* • *diabetic proximal motor neuropathy* [Steroids contraindicated in GBS, but indicated in chronic inflammatory demyelinating polyneuropathy.]

Question: Multiple cranial nerve palsies, peripheral neuropathy, and autonomic neuropathy are most often associated with which of the following disorders? **SELECT 2**

(A) Multiple sclerosis
(B) Guillain-Barré syndrome
(C) B$_{12}$ deficiency
(D) Syringomyelia
(E) Diabetes mellitus
(F) Pb poisoning

Answers: (B), (E): Multiple sclerosis produces multiple CN palsies leading to diplopia, autonomic neuropathy, but is not associated with peripheral neuropathies **(choice A is incorrect).** GBS **(choice B)** is an acute inflammatory demyelinating polyneuropathy that involves cranial nerves, peripheral nerves, and the autonomic nervous system. B$_{12}$ deficiency is associated with subacute combined degeneration of the spinal cord and peripheral neuropathy, but is not associated with CN palsies **(choice C is incorrect).** Syringomyelia involves CNs in the lower brain stem (syringobulbia) and the autonomic nervous system, however, it is not associated with peripheral neuropathy **(choice D is incorrect).** Diabetes mellitus **(choice E)** is the most common overall cause of multiple CN palsies, autonomic neuropathy, and peripheral neuropathy. Pb poisoning primarily produces peripheral neuropathy **(choice F is incorrect).**

AD = autosomal dominant, AIDS = acquired immunodeficiency syndrome, AIP = acute intermittent porphyria, ALS = amyotrophic lateral sclerosis, AV = arteriovenous, AVM = arteriovenous malformation, BV = blood vessel, C = cervical, CMT = Charcot-Marie-Tooth, CN = cranial nerve, CNS = central nervous system, COD = cause of death, CSF = cerebrospinal fluid, DM = diabetes mellitus, DTRs = deep tendon reflexes, GBS = Guillain-Barré syndrome, GI = gastrointestinal, HTN = hypertension, INH = isoniazid, IV = intravenous, L = lumbar, LMN = lower motor neuron, MC = most common, MCC = most common cause, MRI = magnetic resonance imaging, MS = multiple sclerosis, NF = neurofibromatosis, NG = nasogastric, PA = pernicious anemia, Pb = lead, Rx = treatment, S = sacral, S/S = signs and symptoms, T = thoracic.

■ INDEX

A
a wave, 107
  giant, 108
Abdomen, abscess in, 427
Abetalipoproteinemia, 116
Acanthosis nigricans, 670, 692
Acceleration-deceleration injury, 747
Acetaldehyde-protein complex, in
  alcohol-related liver fibrosis, 435
Acetaminophen, interstitial nephritis
  from, 513
  poisoning from, 255
Acetazolamide, 482
Acetylcholine, drug blockage of, 637
Acetylcholine esterase, blockage of, in
  organophosphate poisoning, 260
Achalasia, 372–373
Achlorhydria, 378
  vitamin deficiency and, 460
Acid(s), ingestion of, esophageal effect
  of, 255
Acid-base balance, disorders of, 193
  in bulimia nervosa, 449
  in cirrhosis, 438
Acidosis, metabolic. See *Metabolic
  acidosis.*
  respiratory. See *Respiratory acidosis.*
Acne rosacea, 668
Acne vulgaris, 667
Acoustic neuroma, 737
  autosomal dominant syndrome with,
  80
Acquired immunodeficiency syndrome
  (AIDS), 645–653
  anemia in, 300, 650
  aphthous ulcer in, 369
  bacterial infections in, 649
  blindness in, 651, 732
  bone marrow in, 307, 650
  CD4+ helper T cell count in, 648,
  652
  central nervous system in, 773
  cutaneous lesions in, 650
  cytomegalovirus infection in, 651,
  774
  death in, 653
  diarrhea in, 397, 650
  drug treatment of, 651–652
  epileptic seizures in, 651
  esophagitis in, 374
  fungal infections in, 649, 774
  glomerulonephritis in, 500
  hepatitis in, 650
  Histoplasma capsulatum infection
  in, 397
  hyponatremia in, 491

Acquired immunodeficiency syndrome
  (AIDS) *(Continued)*
  immunologic abnormalities in, 647
  lumbosacral polyradiculomyopathy
  in, 774
  lymphoma in, 650
  malignancy in, 648
  Mycobacterium avium-intracellulare
  infection in, 397
  neutropenia in, 650
  opportunistic infections in, 649
  prophylaxis against, 652–653
  oral manifestations of, 368
  prevention of, 653
  racial distribution of, 645
  squamous cell cancer in, anal, 650
  toxoplasmosis in, 773
  viral infections in, 649
  central nervous system, 774
  wasting syndrome in, 651
  Whipple's-like syndrome in, 650
Acrochordon, 692
Acromegaly, 556
Actinic keratosis, 82, 664
Actinomyces israelii infection, 215,
  369
Actinomycetes, thermophilic,
  inhalation of, 223
Activated charcoal, for poisoning, 254
Addison's disease, 370, 585–586, 587
Adenovirus, in hemorrhagic cystitis,
  524
Adrenal gland, cortex of,
  steroidogenesis in, 550
α-Adrenergic blockers, 131
β-Adrenergic blockers, diuretics with,
  130, 131, 133
  for acute myocardial infarction, 164,
  167
  for atrial fibrillation, 151
  for mitral valve prolapse, 174
  for torsade de pointes, 153
  for ventricular premature beats, 152
  in angina prevention, 162
  in hypertrophic cardiomyopathy,
  179
  poisoning from, 256
Adrenergic drugs, mechanism of, 131
Adrenocorticotropic hormone,
  deficiency of, 551–553
  function of, 550
Adult respiratory distress syndrome
  (ARDS), 207
Afibrinogenemia, cryoprecipitate for,
  352
Aflatoxin, in hepatocellular carcinoma,
  73, 464

789

Collagen vascular disease *(Continued)*
interstitial lung disease from, 225
myocarditis from, 178
pleural fluid glucose levels in, 237
small intestinal diverticula in, 400
with pericarditis, 181
Colles' fracture, 634
Colon, cancer of, 410–411. See also
Colorectal cancer.
diseases of, 399–413
signs/symptoms of, 358
diverticulitis of, 400
diverticulosis of, 399–400
function of, 384
motility of, constipation and, 366
obstruction of, 403
vascular supply of, 401
Colonoscopy, colorectal cancer
confirmation with, 7
Colorectal cancer, 409–410. See also
Colon, cancer of.
genetic precursor for, 83
inflammatory bowel disease with, 83
marker for, 78
metastatic, 71, 411
precursor for, 82
premalignant dysplastic polyp of,
409
risk factors for, 21, 30, 83
screening/confirmatory tests for, 7
secondary prevention of, 21
staging of, 410
Colposcopy, cervical cancer
confirmation with, 7, 19
Coma, 711
death in, 255
Glasgow Coma Scale in, 713
management of, 255, 714
myxedema, 564
psychogenic, 713
Complement, activation of, 656
deficiency of, 643
in disseminated gonococcemia,
620, 644
in classical/alternative pathway dysfunction, 643
tests of, 641–644
Complete blood count (CBC),
pseudoanemia in, 9
parameters reported in, 269
Complete heart block, 154
Computed tomography, in renal
disease, 468
in respiratory disease, 192
magnetic resonance imaging vs., in
diagnosis of central nervous system disorders, 707–708
Concussion, cerebral, 747
Condyloma acuminatum, 540, 676

Congenital heart disease, 156–158
adult vs. childhood, 156
cyanotic, 156
complications of, 157
death from, 158
infectious endocarditis in, prophylaxis for, 158
occlusive, treatment of, 162
Congenital rubella syndrome, 25
Conjunctivitis, allergic, 654
Connective tissue, malignant tumors
of, 67
mixed connective tissue disease of,
627
Consciousness, disorders of, 709–720
Constipation, 366
Continine, plasma/urine levels of, 30
Continuous positive airway pressure
(CPAP), 243
Coombs' test, 656
direct, 272
indirect, 273, 278
Copper, deficiency of, 462
excretion of, defect in, 434
Cor pulmonale, 211
Coronary artery, atherosclerosis of, 120
blood flow in, in myocardial oxygen
supply, 159
congenital malformation of, 158
left anterior descending, distribution
of, 158
thrombosis in, 159
left circumflex, distribution of, 159
right, distribution of, 159
thrombosis in, 159
vasodilatation of, 160
Coronary heart disease, diabetic
treatment in, 597
lipid ratio in, 111
prevention of, 111
risk factor for, 113
screening for, 111
Corticospinal tract, in muscular
weakness, 741
injury to, 712
Corticosteroids, anabolic, liver tumor
with, 438
for autoimmune hemolytic anemia,
299
for immune thrombocytopenia, 330
for sarcoidosis, 225
lipid effect of, 113
neutrophilic leukocytosis with, 281
peripheral blood findings with, 306
psoriasis exacerbation by, 665
synthesis of, 582
Cortisol, caffeine effect on, 10
in bone metabolism, 551
in collagen synthesis, 550